Core Curriculum for

VASCULAR NURSING

Core Curriculum for

VASCULAR NURSING

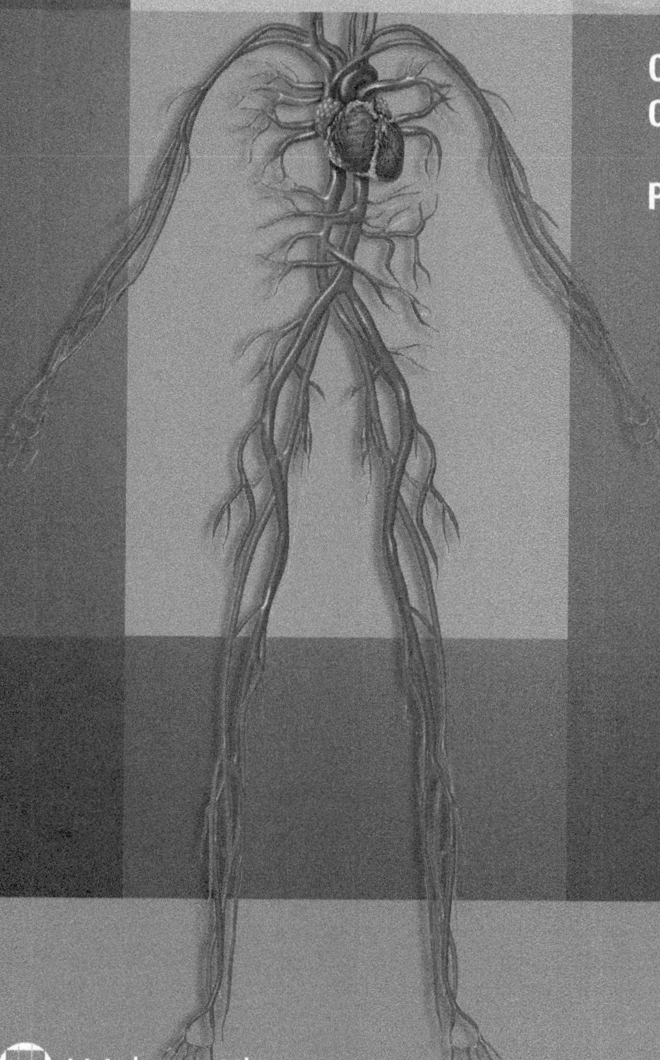

Cynthia Rebik Christensen, MSN, CVN, ARNP-BC

Patricia A. Lewis, MSN, APRN

Wolters Kluwer

Philadelphia • Baltimore • New York • London
Buenos Aires • Hong Kong • Sydney • Tokyo

SVN Society for Vascular Nursing

Acquisitions Editor: Shannon W. Magee
Product Development Editor: Maria M. McAvey
Senior Marketing Manager: Mark Wiragh
Editorial Assistant: Zachary Shapiro
Production Project Manager: Priscilla Crater
Creative Director: Doug Smock
Manufacturing Coordinator: Kathleen Brown
Prepress Vendor: Aptara, Inc.

Two Commerce Square
2001 Market Street
Philadelphia, PA 19103 USA
LWW.com

9 8 7 6 5 4 3 2

Printed in the United States of America

Library of Congress Cataloging-in-Publication Data

Core curriculum for vascular nursing / [edited by] Cynthia Rebik Christensen, Patricia A. Lewis. – Second edition.
p. ; cm.
Preceded by: Core curriculum for vascular nursing / Patricia A. Lewis, editor. c2007.
Includes bibliographical references and index.
ISBN 978-1-4511-9232-2 (alk. paper)
I. Christensen, Cynthia Rebik, editor. II. Lewis, Patricia A., editor. III. Society for Vascular Nursing, publisher.
[DNLM: 1. Cardiovascular Nursing–methods–Outlines. 2. Vascular Diseases–nursing–Outlines. WY 18.2]
RC674
616.1'02310711–dc23

2014019996

Care has been taken to confirm the accuracy of the information presented and to describe generally accepted practices. However, the author(s), editors, and publisher are not responsible for errors or omissions or for any consequences from application of the information in this book and make no warranty, expressed or implied, with respect to the currency, completeness, or accuracy of the contents of the publication. Application of this information in a particular situation remains the professional responsibility of the practitioner; the clinical treatments described and recommended may not be considered absolute and universal recommendations.

The author(s), editors, and publisher have exerted every effort to ensure that drug selection and dosage set forth in this text are in accordance with the current recommendations and practice at the time of publication. However, in view of ongoing research, changes in government regulations, and the constant flow of information relating to drug therapy and drug reactions, the reader is urged to check the package insert for each drug for any change in indications and dosage and for added warnings and precautions. This is particularly important when the recommended agent is a new or infrequently employed drug.

Some drugs and medical devices presented in this publication have Food and Drug Administration (FDA) clearance for limited use in restricted research settings. It is the responsibility of the health care provider to ascertain the FDA status of each drug or device planned for use in his or her clinical practice.

Contributors

Anne M. Aquila, MSN, RN, ACNS-BC
Virginia Capasso, PhD, ANP-BC, CWS
Cynthia Rebik Christensen, MSN, CVN, ARNP-BC
Rita C. Clark, MS, BSN, RN, CVN
Jeanne E. Doyle, BS, RN-BC
Karen R. Fitzgerald, MSN, RN, NP, CVN
Phyllis Gordon, MSN, APRN, ACNS-BC
Melody S. Heffline, MSN, RN, ACNS-BC, ACNP-BC
Debra Kohlman-Trigoboff, RN, MS, ACNP-BC, CVN
Cynthia Lewis, MSN, RN, ACNS-BC
Patricia A. Lewis, APRN, MSN
Victoria Latessa, MSN, ANP, ACNP, BC
Marge Lovell, RN, CCRC, Bed, Med
Ellen Malone, ACNP-BC
Patricia Matula, RN, MSN
Monica Melo, MSN, RN, ACNS-BC, CWOCN, CFCN
Renee Mosier, PharmD
Christine M. Pontuso, BSN, RN
Kathleen Rich, PhD, RN, CCNS, CCRN-CSC, CNN
Carolyn Robinson, RN, MSN, ANP-BC
Marie Rossi, BS, RN, CVN
Lori L. Schirmer, PharmD, BCPS, BCNSP
Katie Schmidt, FNP
Nancy D. Shebel, MSN. NP-c, MHA, BSNS, RN, RVT
Mary Sieggreen, MSN, RN, CVN, CNS-BC, NP
Leslie Beth Sossoman, ACNP, CPHQ, CVN
Robyn Strauss, ACNS-BC, RN, MSN, WCC
Tiffany K. Street, RN, MSN, ACNP
Michelle Tinkham, RN, BSN, CNOR, RNFA
Diane Treat-Jacobson, PhD, RN, FAAN
M. Eileen Walsh, PhD, APN, RN-BC, FAHA

Foreword

"Variability is the law of life, and as no two faces are the same, so no two bodies are alike, and no two individuals react alike and behave alike under the abnormal conditions which we know as disease."

—Sir William Osler, a Canadian physician known as the "Father of Modern Medicine."

Vascular disease presents in many clinical forms, several of which are asymptomatic and coexistent with other cardiovascular diseases. Disorders of the circulatory system (arteries, veins, and lymphatics), exclusive of the heart, comprise vascular disease. Peripheral arterial disease (PAD), one of the major vascular disorders, affects approximately 8.5 million adults age 40 or older in the United States (Go et al., 2013). PAD is a common manifestation of systemic atherosclerosis and is associated with a high risk of stroke, myocardial infarction, and cardiovascular death. Earlier recognition of the clinical manifestations of vascular disease and utilization of the guideline-directed medical therapy will lead to earlier identification of patients with vascular disorders, improved quality of life, and continuity of care for patients with cardiovascular disease.

Through excellence in clinical practice, education, research, and professional networking, the vascular nurse can provide optimal care for patients with vascular disease. The purpose of this book is to provide the core knowledge needed by the novice entering the specialty of vascular nursing. It can also serve as a manual for the nursing instructor, as a study guide for cardiovascular certification, and as a reference for the experienced vascular clinician caring for the challenging vascular patient.

The Core Curriculum for Vascular Nursing has been written by vascular nursing experts bringing into one book their breadth of knowledge. Topics include the evolution of vascular nursing, vascular assessment and diagnosis, vascular nursing research, and guideline-directed medical, endovascular, and surgical therapy for the treatment of carotid artery stenosis, aortic aneurysm, renal artery stenosis, vascular access, venous disease, vascular trauma, amputations, and lymphedema. SVN hopes this text becomes a useful tool in appreciating and addressing what Dr. Osler identifies as the *"variability as the law of life"* as it relates to vascular disease.

CITATION

Go, A.S., Mozaffarian, D., Roger, V. L., Benjamin, E.J., Berry, J.D., Borden, W.B.,...Turner, M.B. (2013). Heart disease and stroke statistics – 2013 report: A report from the American Heart Association. *Circulation, 127*(1): e6–e245.

Debra Kohlman-Trigoboff, RN, MS, ACNP-BC, CVN
Society for Vascular Nursing President 2013-2014

Contents

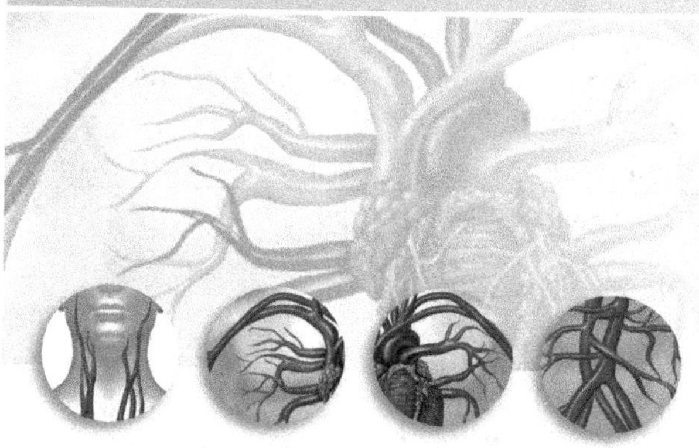

CHAPTER 1

The Evolution of Vascular Nursing

Jeanne Doyle

Introduction

As the specialties of peripheral vascular surgery, and more recently, vascular medicine, have emerged in the last half-century, so has the specialized body of knowledge that defines vascular nursing practice. With rapid advancements in the diagnosis and management of a wide array of vascular diseases, nurses in nearly all health care settings are now caring for patients with unique needs, in an ever-expanding practice environment.

In the early 1980s, in concert with these advancements, and under the leadership of a core group of self-proclaimed "vascular nurses," a new nursing specialty began to emerge. The founding officers and Board of Trustees members (see Table 1-1) recognized the need for ***nursing*** to define the scope and standards of our specialty practice. Originally incorporated as the Society for Peripheral Vascular Nursing (SPVN, 1982), and re-named the Society for Vascular Nursing (SVN, 1990), the formal establishment of this organization served to solidly validate vascular nursing as a unique specialty.

The charter members, and the many leaders that followed, have fostered the Society's vision to be the premier vascular nursing organization whose members are improving outcomes for persons living with vascular disease. Our mission is to provide a professional community for vascular nurses focused on advancing the care of persons living with vascular disease through excellence in clinical practice, education, and research. With its focus on the Core Values of Excellence, Respect and Advocacy, SVN has continued to positively influence the quality of care delivery for vascular patients for the past three decades. In addition, and importantly, the Society continues to play a vital role in the multidisciplinary vascular specialty arena. An example of this collaborative work is evidenced in SVN's endorsement of the *ACC/AHA 2005 Practice Guidelines for the Management of Patients with Peripheral Artery Disease* (Hirsch et al., 2006) and *the 2012 ACCF/AHA/ACR/SCAI/SIR/STS/SVM/SVN/SVS Key Data Elements and Definitions for Peripheral Atherosclerotic Vascular Disease: A Report of the American College of Cardiology Foundation/American Heart Association Task Force on Clinical Data Standards (Writing Committee to Develop Clinical Data Standards for Peripheral Atherosclerotic Vascular Disease)* (Creager et al., 2012).

As a key component of its first 5-year strategic plan in 1983, the Society recognized the significance of and need for a specialty certification process, to help ensure the competency of nurses caring for vascular patients. This commitment evolved into the establishment of *Certified Vascular Nurse* (CVN) credentialing for nurses successfully completing a certification examination developed by the Vascular Nursing Certification Board, a self-governed entity within the Society as a whole. More recently, the administration of the credentialing process was adopted by the American Nurses Credentialing Center via the Cardiac/Vascular Nurse examination, in collaboration

TABLE 1-1 The Following Vascular Nurses Served as Charter Members of the Society for Peripheral Vascular Nursing, Incorporated in 1982

Officers	Trustees
President **Jeanne Doyle, BS, RN** Boston, MA **Vice President** **Patricia Baum, BSN, RN** Worcester, MA **Secretary/Treasurer** **Patricia McGlone, MSN, RN** Columbus, OH	**Mitzi Andrews-Ekers, BSN, RN** Columbus, OH **Victora Fahey, BSN, RN** Chicago, IL **Jacqueline Helt, BSN, RN** New York, NY **Nancy Jasinkowski, RN** Toledo, OH **Sheila White-Flores, MSN, RN** New York, NY

with SVN. The certification process provided the driving force behind the publication of this Core Curriculum.

Vascular Nursing Practice

Nurses caring for patients and families with vascular disease practice in a wide variety of settings, from acute care to the community. SVN offers all nurses a network for sharing best practices, with an emphasis on evidence-based practice. The Scope and Standards of Vascular Nursing Practice (2004, update anticipated in 2014), written by nurse expert members of SVN in collaboration with the American Nurses Association, provides the framework for defining our patient population, and outlining the behavior, responsibilities, functions, and skills of both the vascular nurse generalist and the advanced practice vascular nurse. The practice of every vascular nurse should be guided by this document.

In its effort to continually improve clinical outcomes and enhance continuity of care in specified patient populations as we go forward, the Society's Practice and Research Committee has been charged with developing guidance documents to meet this goal. The first such guideline, entitled the Clinical Practice Guideline for Patients Undergoing Endovascular Repair of Abdominal Aortic Aneurysms (AAA), was published in the June 2009 issue of the Journal of Vascular Nursing. Practice Guidelines for care of patients undergoing carotid endarterectomy and carotid artery stenting have been published subsequently, and are available to the membership of the Society's website.

Vascular Nursing Education

Vascular nursing is ever-evolving. Advances in diagnostic and interventional technology will continue to influence the care we provide to vascular patients. It is incumbent upon each vascular nurse to actively participate in continuing education activities to assure that his/her knowledge remains current. One vital way that SVN helps to educate vascular nurses is through its national convention. What began as a half-day program of didactic content (San Francisco, 1983) has evolved into an annual 2- to 3-day comprehensive educational program covering state-of-the-art topics pertinent to the specialty, presented by internationally recognized vascular experts from all disciplines. The convention also provides an important forum for networking with vascular nurses from around the country, and indeed, around the globe.

In addition, the Society's early publication of a newsletter, which served primarily as a communication tool for the membership, gradually evolved into the peer-reviewed *Journal of Vascular*

Nursing, a prestigious quarterly periodical with an Editorial Board of expert vascular nurses. The *Journal* is recognized as a key resource for nurses in all practice areas. Also, the use of varied electronic media, along with continued enhancements of the Society's website, www.svnnet.org, help to maintain effective communication with the membership.

And as previously mentioned, SVN strongly supports and promotes specialty certification in cardiac/vascular nursing as a tool to promote excellence in practice. It is with this latter focus in mind that this Vascular Nursing Core Curriculum was developed.

Patient/Community Education

As we better understand underlying disease processes and their associated risk factors, vascular nurses will play an even greater role in promoting arterial, venous, and lymphatic disease awareness and prevention. One notable example of the Society's commitment in this regard was the launch of the "A Step Ahead" program at the national convention in Washington, DC, in 1993, as well as at a press conference on Capitol Hill that same year. This nurse-managed peripheral artery disease (PAD) public screening and education program served as the framework for a large scale community-based research study designed to measure PAD awareness, physician recognition, and treatment intensity (Hirsch et al., 2001). The results of this study pointed to the under-diagnosis of PAD in primary care, and led to the convening of a 2-day PAD Public Education Strategy meeting at the National Heart Lung and Blood Institute (NHLBI)/National Institutes of Health (NIH) in 2003 (Hirsch, Gloviczki, Drooz, Lovell, & Creager, 2004). SVN was one of 17 professional societies and public health associations participating in this forum.

Vascular Nursing Research

Nursing research, the foundation for evidence-based practice, is critical to the advancement of nursing, and the key to professional accountability (Kraus, 2000). In its Position Statement on Vascular Nursing Research, SVN submits that "all registered professional nurses need to clarify problems relevant to their vascular nursing practice setting, ask critical questions about the applicability of research findings to the vascular patient population, participate in data collection, and understand the value and relevance of vascular nursing research (2002)."

The Society conducted its own Vascular Nursing Research Priorities Delphi Study in the early 1990s (Hatton & Nunnelee, 1995) and replicated it in 2001 (Wipke-Tevis, 2001). This effort was designed to gain consensus and stimulate vascular nursing research by clinicians and expert researchers. In addition, the Society's commitment to research is evidenced by its grant support of proposals reviewed and approved for grant funding by the SVN Research Committee.

Summary

In its 32-year history, the Society for Vascular Nursing has continued to outline the scope and define the standards of vascular nursing practice. Working collaboratively, SVN's members have contributed immeasurably to promoting excellence in quality care for persons with vascular disease. As *the* recognized experts in vascular nursing, we must continue to chart the course. Efforts aimed at fostering collaborative educational and research initiatives with other vascular specialty societies will be key to optimizing clinical outcomes for our patients, and should be a focus of the Society in the years to come.

The Society's core purpose and values continue to serve us well as we approach the future. Through 2015, our Society remains focused on three strategic priorities:

- SVN will be the premier resource for vascular nursing, encouraging innovation in vascular nursing practice, education, and research.

- SVN will advance the science of vascular nursing, translate evidence into practice, and improve outcomes for persons living with vascular disease.
- SVN will position its members as advocates for nurses and persons living with vascular disease.

Goals and objectives designed to meet the specific outcomes outlined in this plan are clearly articulated and measurable. Ongoing assessment will help to guide our continued evolution.

Despite our many notable achievements, we will (hopefully) always remain a work in progress, constantly striving to enhance our professional development while remaining focused on the ever-changing needs of our patients.

The evolution of our specialty and our Society is a dynamic journey, and future challenges are both daunting and exciting. I urge you to keep pace with current clinical practice as a means of optimizing quality patient care. This comprehensive Core Curriculum provides a springboard for attaining *your* certification as a cardiac/vascular nurse, a tangible indicator of *your* expertise in our specialty, and an important component of *your* professional development. Our patients deserve to be cared for by the most competent vascular nurses... wouldn't you agree?

Jeanne Doyle, BS, RN-BC
Founding President, Society for Vascular Nursing

REFERENCES

Creager, M. A., Belkin, M., Bluth, E. I., Casey, D. E., Jr., Chaturvedi, S., Dake, M. D.,... Ziffer, J. A. (2012) 2012 ACCF/AHA/ACR/SCAI/SIR/STS/SVM/SVN/SVS key data elements and definitions for peripheral atherosclerotic vascular disease: A report of the American College of Cardiology Foundation/American Heart Association Task Force on Clinical Data Standards (Writing Committee to develop clinical data standards for peripheral atherosclerotic vascular disease). *Circulation, 125,* 395–467.

Hatton, J. M., & Nunnelee, J. D. (1995). Research priorities in vascular nursing. *Journal of Vascular Nursing, 13*(1), 1–7.

Hirsch, A. T., Criqui, M. H., Treat-Jacobson, D., Regensteiner, J. G., Creager, M., Olin, J. W.,... Hiatt, W. R. (2001). Peripheral arterial disease detection, awareness, and treatment in primary care. *Journal of the American Medical Association, 286*(11), 1317–1324.

Hirsch, A. T., Gloviczki, P., Drooz, A., Lovell, M., & Creager, M. A. (2004). Mandate for creation of a national peripheral arterial disease public awareness program: An opportunity to improve cardiovascular health. *Journal of Vascular Nursing, 22*(1), 24–31.

Hirsch, A. T., Haskal, Z. J., Hertzer, N. R., Bakal, C. W., Creager, M. A., Halperin, J. L.,... White, R. A. (2006). ACC/AHA 2005 Practice guidelines for the management of patients with peripheral arterial disease (lower extremity, renal, mesenteric, and abdominal aortic): A collaborative report from the American Association for Vascular Surgery/Society for Vascular Surgery, Society for Cardiovascular Angiography and Interventions, Society for Vascular Medicine and Biology, Society of Interventional Radiology, and the ACC/AHA Task Force on Practice Guidelines. *Circulation, 113,* e463–e465.

Kraus, V. L. (2000). The research basis for practice: The foundation if evidence-based practice. In J. V. Hickey, R. M. Oiumette, & S. L. Venegoni (Eds.), *Advanced practice nursing: Changing roles and clinical applications* (2nd ed., pp. 317–329). Philadelphia, PA: Lippincott.

Society for Vascular Nursing. (2009). 2009 clinical practice guideline for patients undergoing endovascular repair of abdominal aortic aneurysms (AAA). *Journal of Vascular Nursing, 27,* 48–63.

Society for Vascular Nursing, & American Nurses Association. (2004). *Scope and standards of vascular nursing practice.* Washington, DC: Nursesbooks.org

Wipke-Tevis, D. D. (2001). The vascular research priorities survey: An update. *Journal of Vascular Nursing, 19*(3), 101–102.

SUGGESTED READING

Society for Vascular Nursing. (2000). *Position statement on vascular nursing research.* Pensacola, FL.

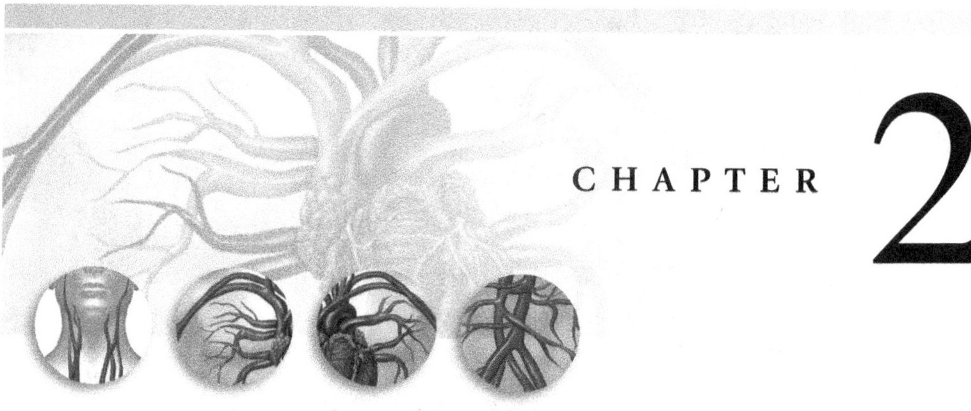

CHAPTER 2

Vascular Nursing Research and Evidence-Based Practice

Patricia Matula
Kathleen Rich
First Edition Author: *Patricia Matula*

OBJECTIVES

1. Define the research process.
2. Identify key areas of nursing research related to vascular nursing.
3. Differentiate between quantitative and qualitative designs.
4. Discuss the relationship between research and evidence-based practice.
5. Describe the process for evidence-based practice.

Introduction

The spirit of inquiry and dedication to life-long learning is critical to overcoming the barriers to research and disseminating evidence into vascular nursing practice. The statistic that "it takes an average of 17 years to move research into practice" persists in many healthcare institutions. Point-of-care clinicians need to have the tools to use research evidence in their practices to improve patient outcomes (Institute of Medicine of the National Academies, 2010).

I. Vascular Research

A. **Definition:** A scientific process that uses a systematic inquiry to answer questions or solve problems related to vascular nursing. In addition, it validates and refines existing knowledge that directly and indirectly influences clinical vascular nursing practice.

B. Purpose of Vascular Research

1. Generate new scientific knowledge and expand previously generated knowledge for the practice of vascular nursing.
2. Create research-based and evidence-based nursing care that ensures quality and cost-effective outcomes (Sigma Theta Tau Nursing Practice and Education Consortium, 2005).

3. Identify the experience of the patient and family in all types and stages of vascular disease.
4. Identify the impact of vascular disease on patients, family, and the healthcare economy.
5. Identify attitudes and characteristics of nurses caring for the vascular patient.
6. Demonstrate the efficacy of nursing in the changing healthcare arena.
7. Define the specialty of vascular nursing.
8. Identify research priorities in vascular nursing.

C. Importance of Vascular Research to Practice

1. Nurse related
    a. Defining the specialty and the specific body of knowledge for nursing is essential.
    b. Knowledge related to patient response allows congruence between nurse and patient information.
    c. The use and practice of research is one of the expectations of nursing, by both the Society for Vascular Nursing and the American Nurses Association (SVN and ANA standards of practice).
    d. The use of research provides a current and legally defensible practice of the specialty.
    e. Knowledge of current professional research is essential for professional pride and growth.
    f. Dissemination of research is a professional responsibility.
2. Patient/practice related
    a. Create a research-supported, evidence-based infrastructure that ensures current nursing practice is consistent with best available knowledge.
    b. Quantifying outcomes in relation to interventions is necessary for appropriate utilization of research.
    c. Research provides a patient worldview for nurses (Institute of Medicine of the National Academies, 2011).
3. Cost related
    a. Research-supported, evidenced-based vascular nursing practice may improve nursing efficiency resulting in institutional cost savings.
    b. Delivering research-supported vascular nursing practice may lessen avoidable hospital admissions and readmissions, thus reducing payer and provider costs.

D. Outline of a Study (see Table 2-1)

E. Study Designs: Methods used to examine the relationships between and among variables measured.

1. Quantitative (deductive) studies: used to explain and predict phenomena, evaluate the effectiveness of interventions, create evidence for cause and effect, test theory or instruments, and evaluate the effectiveness of interventions.
    a. An independent variable is the stimulus or activity manipulated to create an effect on the dependent variable. Control is critical to quantitative designs to ensure consistency of methods and minimize the role of chance.

TABLE 2-1 Outline of a Study

Study Component	Definition
Research problem	States the area of concern or gap in knowledge that generated the study.
Research question	A very concise query that identifies precisely what the researcher is trying to answer through the study. The research question guides the study. In more advanced research, the investigator may make a predictive statement regarding answers to a research question. This is known as a hypothesis.
Literature review	A summary of published and, if appropriate, unpublished research and other supporting literature regarding the research problem.
Design	The study structure and overall plan in quantitative research.
Methods	How the study is specifically being conducted. This includes who is conducting the study, study location, sample selection and sample size, variables being measured and controlled for and excluded, type of equipment or instruments being used, what measurements are being obtained.
Data analysis	Describes the statistics being used to organize and assess the data findings.
Results and conclusions	Results are the specific data measurements obtained from the analysis. Conclusions are the interpretation of those results by the researcher. Conclusions often include recommendations for nursing practice and further research.

b. A dependent variable is the behavior, response, or outcome the researcher wants to explain.
c. Sampling is the process of selecting a portion of the population to participate in the study. Researchers conduct a power analysis to determine what the sample size needs to be to minimize finding based on chance.
d. Validity is the extent to which the variable or intervention measures what it is supposed to measure. Internal validity refers to integrity of the design. External validity refers to the appropriateness by which results can be applied to nonstudy patients or populations. Note: Type I error: The researcher concludes that a relationship exists when there is none (reject the null hypothesis). Type II error: The researcher concludes that no relationship exists when in fact it does (accept the null hypothesis).
e. Common examples of designs used in quantitative research studies are described in Table 2-2.

TABLE 2-2 Study Designs

Study Design Key Feature
Observational Studies
1. Cohort study (longitudinal): a group followed over time
2. Cross-sectional study (prevalence): a group examined at one point in time
3. Case-control study: two groups, based on the outcome
Experimental Studies
1. Randomized controlled trial: two groups created by a random process and a blinded intervention
2. Quasiexperimental: absence of random assignment or control group

Adapted with permission from Hulley, S. B., Cummings, S. R., Browner, W. S., Grady, D., Hearst, N., & Newman, T. B. (2001). The anatomy and physiology of clinical research. In *Designing clinical research* (2nd ed.). Philadelphia, PA: Lippincott Williams & Wilkins.

2. Qualitative inductive studies: use an interactive, systematic, subjective approach to describe life experiences and give them meaning (Burns & Grove, 2011).
   a. Methods allow the researcher to gain insight by discovering meaning through a purposeful sample (participants are selected because they have common characteristics).
   b. Data are collected in words as opposed to numbers.
   c. Methods explore the richness and complexity of the phenomena. If the research study is not a pilot, then conducting a power analysis is appropriate. A power analysis allows the researcher to find a statistically significant difference when the null hypothesis is in fact false. A null hypothesis is a hypothesis which the researcher tries to disprove, reject, or invalidate. The power of a study is determined by three factors: the sample size, the alpha level, and the effect size.
   d. Trustworthiness: a method of appraising qualitative research according to Lincoln and Guba (1985).
      1) Credibility (parallels internal validity): documentation of processes, period of engagement, data appropriateness (purposeful sample), adequacy of database (saturation), use of multiple data sources (saturation), validation of data and findings with participants.
      2) Transferability (external validity): extent to which research findings can be applied to experiences of those in similar situations.
      3) Dependability (reliability): requires meticulous documentation of the research process.
      4) Confirmability (objectivity): extent to which the findings and interpretation are grounded in data.
   e. Common approaches to qualitative research include the following:
      1) *Phenomenological research* describes the experience as lived by the participant. Data are generated through observation, interview, videotape, and/or writings of the participants.
      2) *Grounded theory* is rooted in sociology and approaches data to develop theories about phenomena being studied. The theory then explains the social process.
      3) *Ethnography* is rooted in anthropology and studies the culture of people. The outcome is a detailed description of phenomena as observed through immersion in the culture.
      4) *Historical research or historiography* studies past events in a systematic method. The result is a retelling of the events and their meaning.
      5) *Content analysis* uses numbers to represent frequency, order, or intensity of words or phrases. Theoretical categories are then identified.

F. **Epidemiology** studies the distribution and determinants of disease frequency in populations. It scrutinizes illness patterns within a population and then attempts to ascertain why some individuals develop a disease whereas others do not (Greenberg, Daniels, Flanders, Eley, & Boring, 2005).

1. Determine what factors might be associated with disease (risk factors).
2. The higher the correlation, the more certain the association.
3. Two basic types of studies retrospective, whether the events have already happened or prospective, whether the events may happen in the future.

4. The Framingham Heart Study is the largest database on risk factors for cardiovascular disease.

G. **Measurement** is the process of assigning numbers to objects, events, or situations according to a rule. Levels of measurement:

1. Nominal: lowest level of measurement. Data can be organized into categories but cannot be manipulated.
2. Ordinal scale: data can be ranked but the intervals are not necessarily equal. The number is significant in terms of position.
3. Interval scale: order and equal distance between intervals. Mutually exclusive categories, such as temperature.
4. Ratio scale: highest level of measurement.

H. Protection of Human Subjects

1. All nursing research must be approved by an Institutional Review Board (IRB). An Investigational Review Board is a multidisciplinary group (physicians, nurses, chaplains, administration, legal, community persons) that is responsible for assuring that all research projects conducted within the facility that require human or animal subjects are in accordance with the appropriate federal regulations.
2. Informed consent: The knowing consent of an individual or legally authorized representative to decide whether or not to participate in a research study without undue inducement or any elements of fraud, force, deceit, duress, constraint, or coercion.
3. Elements of informed consent
   a. Decisional capacity: The participant has the ability to understand and make decisions.
   b. Disclosure: The relevant risks, benefits, alternative treatments, and uncertainties have been discussed with the participant.
   c. Understanding: The participants understand at least what the researcher believes they need to understand to authorize the study.
   d. Voluntary: The participant agrees to the interventions without undue duress.
   e. Consent: A written form documenting the acceptance of the intervention has been completed. The participant understands consent can be withdrawn at any time.

II. Evidence-Based Practice (Melnyk & Fineout-Overholt, 2011)

A. **Definition:** Evidence-based practice (EBP) is a problem-solving approach to clinical practice that integrates the following—a systematic search for and critical appraisal of the most relevant evidence to answer a burning clinical question; one's own expertise; and patient preferences and values.

B. Steps to Evidence-Based Practice

1. Ask the burning clinical question.
2. Collect the most relevant and best evidence and rank using a hierarchal approach (Long, 2009).
   a. Systematic reviews, meta-analyses (strongest).

   b. Randomized controlled trials.
   c. Controlled trials without randomization.
   d. Cohort or case-controlled studies.
   e. Descriptive or qualitative studies.
   f. Expert opinions or case reports (least strong).
3. Critically appraise and grade the evidence using an accepted grading scale.
4. Integrate all evidence with one's clinical expertise, patient preferences, and values in making a practice decision or change.
5. Evaluate the practice decision or change.

C. Ask the Burning Question using a PICO Format, then Modify the Below Subletters as Follows:

1. Patient population or Problem (describes the group of patients or problem identified).
2. Intervention of interest (cause, prevention, treatment strategy).
3. Comparison of interest (if appropriate, what is the main alternative).
4. Outcome (what could this intervention really affect).

D. Collect the Most Relevant and Best Evidence.

1. Systematic reviews or meta-analyses (COCHRANE, Joanna Briggs Institute).
2. Clinical practice guidelines (National Guideline Clearinghouse).
3. Randomized controlled trials (MEDLINE or Cumulative Index of Nursing and Allied Health Literature [CINAHL]).
4. All other types of studies: single descriptive or qualitative studies.
5. Expert opinion or reports of expert committees.

E. Critically Appraise the Evidence.

1. What was the sample size?
2. What were the results of the study?
3. Are the results valid?
4. Will the results help me in caring for my patients?

F. Integrate the Evidence from the Literature with the Following:

1. Healthcare provider's expertise.
2. Clinical assessment of the patient and available healthcare resources.

G. Evaluate Effectiveness.

1. How did the treatment work?
2. How effective was the clinical decision with a particular patient or practice pattern?

III. Use of Evidence-Based Practice Nursing Models

A. EBP Nursing Models Assist the Nurse into Moving Evidence into Practice.

B. EBP Nursing Models can Organize the Method Strategies, Improve use of Resources, Maximize Nursing Time, and allow for a More Complete Implementation (Gawlinski & Rutledge, 2008).

C. Each Model Follows a Specific Algorithm or Series of Steps in this Process.

D. There are Several Different Models Available: Selection is Dependent on the One that Best Meets the Needs of the Individual Institution.

E. Examples of Commonly Utilized EBP Nursing Models include Iowa Model of Evidence-Based Practice to Promote Quality of Care, Stetler's Model, and John Hopkins Nursing Model.

Research Terms

Absolute risk: The observed or calculated probability of an event in the population under study.

Absolute risk difference: The difference in the risk for disease or death between an exposed population and an unexposed population.

Absolute risk reduction (ARR): The difference in the absolute risk (rates of adverse events) between study and control populations.

Bias (Syn: systematic error): Deviation of results or inferences from the truth, or processes leading to such deviation.

Blind(ed) study (Syn: masked study): A study in which observer(s) and/or subjects are kept ignorant of the group to which the subjects are assigned, as in an experimental study, or of the population from which the subjects come, as in a nonexperimental or observational study. When both observer and subjects are kept ignorant, the study is termed a **double-blind** study. When the statistical analysis is also done in ignorance of the group to which subjects belong, the study is sometimes described as **triple blind.** The purpose of "blinding" is to eliminate sources of bias.

Case series: Report of a number of cases of a particular disease.

Case-control study: Retrospective comparison of exposures of persons with disease (cases) with those of persons without the disease (controls) (see **Retrospective study**).

Causality: The effect of a treatment or intervention on an outcome. Three conditions necessary to establish causality are (a) a strong correlation between proposed cause and effect; (b) the proposed cause must precede the effect in time; and (c) the proposed cause must be present every time the effect occurs.

Cohort study: Follow-up of exposed and nonexposed defined groups, with a comparison of disease rates during the time covered.

Comparison group: Any group to which the index group is compared; usually, synonymous with **control group.**

Comorbidity: Coexistence of a disease or diseases in a study participant in addition to the index condition that is the subject of study.

Confidence interval (CI): The range of numerical values in which we can be confident (to a computed probability, such as 90% or 95%) that the population value being estimated will be found.

Confidence intervals indicate the strength of evidence; when confidence intervals are wide, they indicate less precise estimates of effect. The larger the trial's sample size, the larger the number of outcome events and the greater the confidence that the true relative risk reduction is close to the value stated. Thus, the confidence intervals narrow, and "precision" is increased. In a "positive finding" study, the lower boundary of the confidence interval, or lower confidence limit, should still remain important or clinically significant if the results are to be accepted. In a "negative finding" study, the upper boundary of the confidence interval should not be clinically significant if you are to confidently accept this result.

Effectiveness: A measure of the benefit resulting from an intervention for a given health problem under usual conditions of clinical care for a particular group; this form of evaluation considers the **efficacy** of an intervention and its acceptance by those to whom it is offered, answering the question, "Does the practice do more good than harm to people to whom it is offered?" (see **Intention-to-treat analysis**).

Efficacy: A measure of the benefit resulting from an intervention for a given health problem under the ideal conditions of an investigation; it answers the question, "Does the practice do more good than harm to people who fully comply with the recommendations?"

Exclusion criteria: Conditions that preclude entrance of candidates into an investigation, even if they meet the inclusion criteria.

Experimental event rate (EER): The percentage of intervention/exposed group who experienced the outcome in question.

Follow-up: Observation over a period of time of an individual, group, or initially defined population whose relevant characteristics have been assessed to observe changes in health status or health-related variables.

Gold standard: A method, procedure, or measurement that is widely accepted as being the best available.

Hypothesis: A statement of predicted relationships between variables in a study.

Incidence: The number of new cases of illness commencing or of persons falling ill during a specified time period in a given population (see also **Prevalence**).

Intention-to-treat analysis: A method for data analysis in a randomized clinical trial in which individual outcomes are analyzed according to the group to which they have been randomized, even if they never received the treatment they were assigned. By simulating practical experience, it provides a better measure of **effectiveness** (versus **efficacy**).

Interviewer bias: Systematic error caused by the interviewer's subconscious or conscious gathering of selective data.

Lead-time bias: If prognosis study patients are not all enrolled at similar, well-defined points in the course of their disease, differences in outcome over time may merely reflect differences in duration of illness.

Likelihood ratio: Ratio of the probability that a given diagnostic test result will be expected for a patient with the target disorder rather than for a patient without the disorder.

Number needed to treat (NNT): The number of patients who must be exposed to an intervention before the clinical outcome of interest occurs, for example, the number of patients needed to treat to prevent one adverse outcome.

***p* value:** The statistical test of the assumption that there is no difference between an experimental intervention and a control p value. When a test of difference is significant at the 0.05 levels (p is usually 0.05) the researcher may conclude that there is a 95% probability that the two groups are different and the difference is not caused by chance.

Predictive value: In screening and diagnostic tests, the probability that a person with a positive test is a true positive (i.e., has the disease), or that a person with a negative test truly does not have the disease. The predictive value of a screening test is determined by the **sensitivity** and **specificity** of the test and by the prevalence of the condition for which the test is used.

Prevalence: The proportion of persons with a particular disease within a given population at a given time.

Prospective study: Study design in which one or more groups (**cohorts**) of individuals who have not yet had the outcome event in question are monitored for the number of such events that occur over time.

Randomized controlled trial: Study design in which treatments, interventions, or enrollment into different study groups are assigned by random allocation rather than by conscious decisions of clinicians or patients. When the sample size is large enough, this study design avoids problems of bias and confounding variables by ensuring that known and unknown determinants of outcome are evenly distributed between treatment and control groups.

Relative risk (RR): The ratio of the probability of developing, in a specified period of time, an outcome among those receiving the treatment of interest or exposed to a risk factor compared with the probability of developing the outcome if the risk factor or intervention is not present.

Relative risk reduction (RRR): The extent to which a treatment reduces a risk in comparison with patients not receiving the treatment of interest.

Reproducibility (repeatability, reliability): The results of a test or measure are identical or closely similar each time it is conducted.

Retrospective study: Study design in which data for individuals who had an outcome event in question are collected and analyzed after the outcomes have occurred (see also **Case–control study**).

Risk factor: Patient characteristics or factors associated with an increased probability of developing a condition or disease in the first place. Compare with **prognostic factors.** Risk or prognostic factors do not necessarily imply a cause-and-effect relationship.

Selection bias: A bias in assignment or a **confounding variable** that arises from study design rather than by chance. These can occur when the study and control groups are chosen so that they differ from each other by one or more factors that may affect the outcome of the study.

Sensitivity (of a diagnostic test): The proportion of truly diseased persons, as measured by the gold standard.

Specificity (of a diagnostic test): The proportion of truly nondiseased persons, as measured by the gold standard, who are so identified by the diagnostic test under study.

Strength of inference: The likelihood that an observed difference between groups within a study represents a real difference rather than mere chance or the influence of confounding factors, based on p values and confidence intervals. Strength of inference is weakened by various forms of bias and by small sample sizes.

Variable: Anything that varies; any property that takes on different values.

REFERENCES

Burns, N., & Grove, S. (2011). *Understanding nursing research: Building an evidence-based practice* (5th ed.). Philadelphia, PA: Elsevier.

Gawlinski, A., & Rutledge, D. (2008). Selecting a model for evidence-based practice changes. *Advanced Critical Care, 19*(3), 291–300.

Greenberg, R. S., Daniels, S. R., Flanders, W. D., Eley, J. W., & Boring III, J. R. (2005). Chapter 1. Introduction to epidemiology. In R. S. Greenberg, S. R. Daniels, W. D. Flanders, J. W. Eley, & J. R. Boring III (Eds.), *Medical epidemiology* (4th ed.). New York, NY: McGraw-Hill. Retrieved from http://www.accessmedicine.com/content.aspx?aID=545000, accessed December 8, 2011.

Hulley, S. B., Cummings, S. R., Browner, W. S., Grady, D., Hearst, N., & Newman, T. B. (2001). *Designing clinical research* (2nd ed.). Philadelphia, PA: Lippincott Williams & Wilkins.

Institute of Medicine of the National Academies. (2010). *Redesigning the clinical effectiveness research paradigm: Innovation and practice based approaches workshop summary.* Washington, DC: National Academy Press.

Institute of Medicine of the National Academies. (2011). *The future of nursing: Leading change, advancing health.* Washington, DC: National Academy Press.

Lincoln, Y. S., & Guba, E. G. (1985). *Naturalistic inquiry.* Beverly Hills, CA: Sage.

Long, C. (2009). Weighing in on the evidence. In N. Schmidt & J. Brown (Eds.), *Evidence-based practice for nurses* (pp. 315–331). Boston, MA: Jones and Bartlett.

Melnyk, B. M., & Fineout-Overholt, E. (2011). *Evidence-based practice in nursing & healthcare: A guide to best practice* (2nd ed.). Philadelphia, PA: Lippincott Williams & Wilkins.

Sigma Theta Tau International Honor Society of Nursing. (2005). *Position statement on evidence-based nursing.* Indianapolis, IN: Sigma Theta Tau International. Retrieved from http://www.nursingsociety.org/aboutus/PositionPapers/Pages/EBN_positionpaper.aspx, accessed September 1, 2013.

SUGGESTED READINGS

Baas, L. (2010). *Nursing review and resource manual: Cardiac vascular nursing* (3rd ed.). Silver Spring, MD: ANCC's Institute for Credentialing Innovation.

Buckingham, J., Fisher, B., & Saunders, D. (rev. 2008). *Evidence-based medicine tool kit.* Evidence-Based Medicine Working Group, originally published in *JAMA*. Retrieved from http://www.med.ualberta.ca/#

Polit, D., & Beck, C. (2010). *Essentials of nursing research* (7th ed.). Philadelphia, PA: Wolters Kluwer-Lippincott, Williams & Wilkins.

Titler, M. G., Kleiber, C., Rakel, B., Budreau, G., Everett, L., Steelman, V., ... Goode, C. (2001). The Iowa model of evidence-based practice to promote quality care. *Critical Care Nursing Clinics of North America, 13*(4), 497–509.

Anatomy and Physiology of the Vascular System

Diane Treat-Jacobson

OBJECTIVES

1. Describe the anatomy and physiology of the arterial, venous, and lymphatic systems.
2. Describe the changes that occur in the vascular system with aging.

Introduction/Overview

This chapter reviews the structure and function of the three major components of the vascular system: the arterial, venous, and lymphatic systems. The purpose of the vascular system is to transport blood from the heart to all parts of the body, to allow for the exchange of substances between the blood and the tissues, and to return blood to the heart. The vessel size, wall thickness, and internal pressure within vessels vary depending on vessel type and function.

I. Arterial Circulation (Graham & Ford, 1999; Guyton & Hall, 2000; Spence, 1982; Tottora & Grabowski, 2003)

A. General Arterial Anatomy and Physiology: Conductive versus Distributive Vessels

1. Conductive vessels are relatively straight with few branches
2. Distributive vessels arise from conductive arteries and have multiple branches
3. Arteries, arterioles, capillaries
   a. Arteries transport blood to the tissues under high pressure (mean pressure 100 mm Hg)
   b. Arterioles: the last small branch of the arterial system; controls flow into the capillary. Proximal pressure approximately 85 mm Hg and distal pressure approximately 30 mm Hg
   c. Capillary: fluid, nutrients, electrolytes, and hormones are exchanged between the blood and the interstitial fluid. Arterial end capillary pressure approximately 30 mm Hg; venous end capillary pressure approximately 10 mm Hg

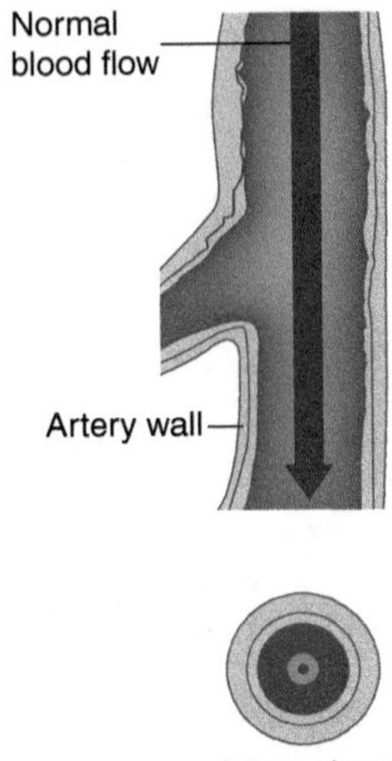

FIGURE 3-1. Cross-section of arterial wall.

B. Arterial Structure (see Fig. 3-1)

1. Intima
   a. The innermost layer, lining the lumen of the arterial wall
   b. Consists of a single layer of endothelial cells
   c. Separated from the media by the internal elastic membrane
   d. Nutrients obtained by diffusion from the arterial lumen
2. Media
   a. Thick layer of smooth muscle cells, collagen, and elastic fibers
   b. Separated from the adventitia by the external elastic membrane
   c. Inner portion receives nutrients by diffusion from the arterial lumen; outer portion receives nutrients from small blood vessels that penetrate the arterial wall
3. Adventitia
   a. Outer layer of the artery
   b. Composed of connective tissue, collagen, and elastic fibers
   c. Provides majority of strength of the arterial wall
   d. Nutrients obtained from small blood vessels that penetrate the arterial wall

C. Arteries of the Head and Neck (see Fig. 3-2)

1. After arising from the aortic arch, the brachiocephalic artery divides into the right subclavian artery and the right common carotid artery
2. Right and left common carotid arteries supply most of the blood to the head and neck
3. Common carotid arteries bifurcate as follows:
   a. Carotid sinus: formed at the point of bifurcation
   b. Right and left external carotid arteries
      1) Supply most of head and neck except for the brain
      2) Lie more superficially than the internal carotid arteries
      3) Terminate as the maxillary and superficial temporal arteries supplying muscles of mastication, the nose, pharynx, palate, teeth, and some neck muscles
      4) Give off the occipital artery to the posterior region of the scalp

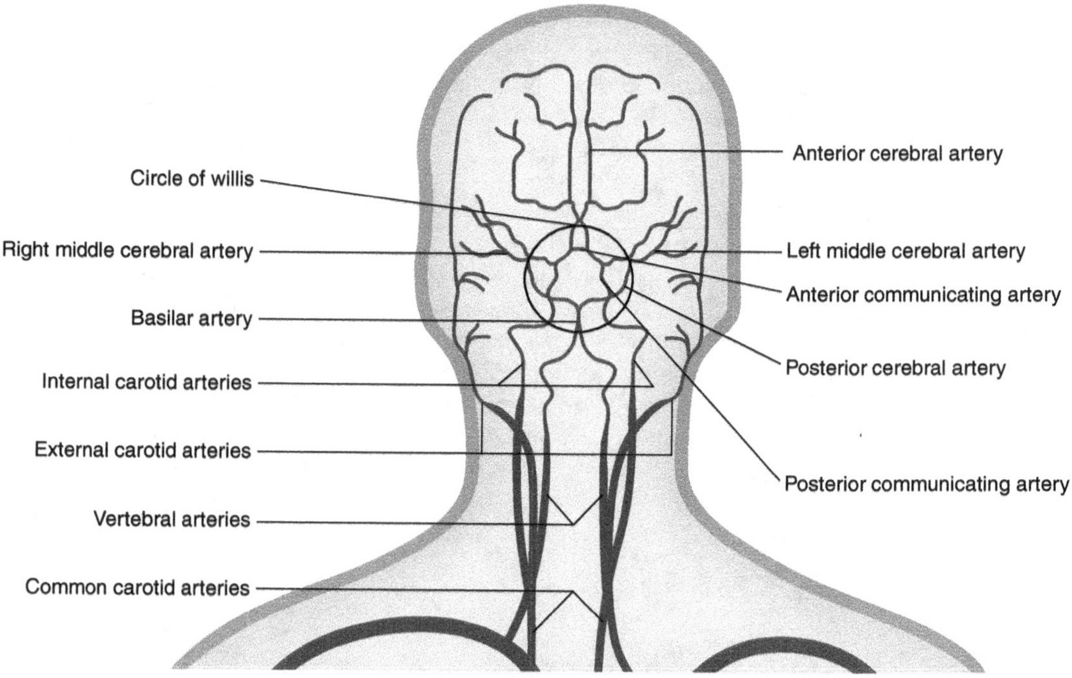

FIGURE 3-2. Arteries of the head and neck.

5) Send branches to supply the thyroid gland, tongue, skin, and muscles of the face

c. Right and left internal carotid arteries
   1) Enter the cranial cavity through the carotid canal of the temporal bone
   2) Supply the brain through the terminal branches: the anterior cerebral artery, the middle cerebral artery
   3) Right and left internal carotid arteries are connected by the anterior communicating artery

d. Vertebral artery
   1) First branch of the subclavian artery
   2) Reaches the cranial cavity by passing through the transverse foramen of the cervical vertebrae and the foramen magnum
   3) Right and left vertebral arteries join to form the basilar artery
   4) Basilar artery supplies pons and cerebellum
   5) Basilar artery terminates as the right and left posterior cerebral arteries

e. Circle of Willis
   1) Anterior communicating artery, anterior cerebral artery, posterior communicating artery, and posterior cerebral artery join to form the Circle of Willis
   2) Provides the potential for collateral flow to compensate for the loss of a carotid or vertebral artery

D. Arteries of the Upper Extremities

1. Supplied by the subclavian arteries
2. First branches off the subclavian artery do not supply the upper limbs
   a. Thyrocervical trunk sends branches to lower neck and dorsal scapular regions
   b. Costocervical trunk sends branches to the intercostal region

c. Internal thoracic (internal mammary artery) supplies branches to the thoracic and intercostal muscles
3. Subclavian artery becomes the axillary artery after passing through the clavicle
   a. Branches to the lateral wall of the thorax
      1) Thoracocranial trunk
      2) Lateral thoracic artery
      3) Subscapular artery
      4) Thoracodorsal artery
   b. Branches to region around proximal end of the humerus (circumflex arteries)
   c. Becomes brachial artery, traveling down medial side of humerus and supplying muscles of the arm
   d. Brachial artery branches as follows:
      1) Ulnar artery down anterior surface of forearm along ulna
      2) Radial artery down anterior surface of forearm along radius
      3) Ulnar and radial arteries join in the hand through interconnecting branches of the superficial and deep palmar arteries
      4) Digital arteries arise from the palmar arches and supply the fingers

E. Aorta (see Fig. 3-3)

1. Ascending aorta
   a. Passes in front of the pulmonary artery
   b. Branches include right and left coronary arteries

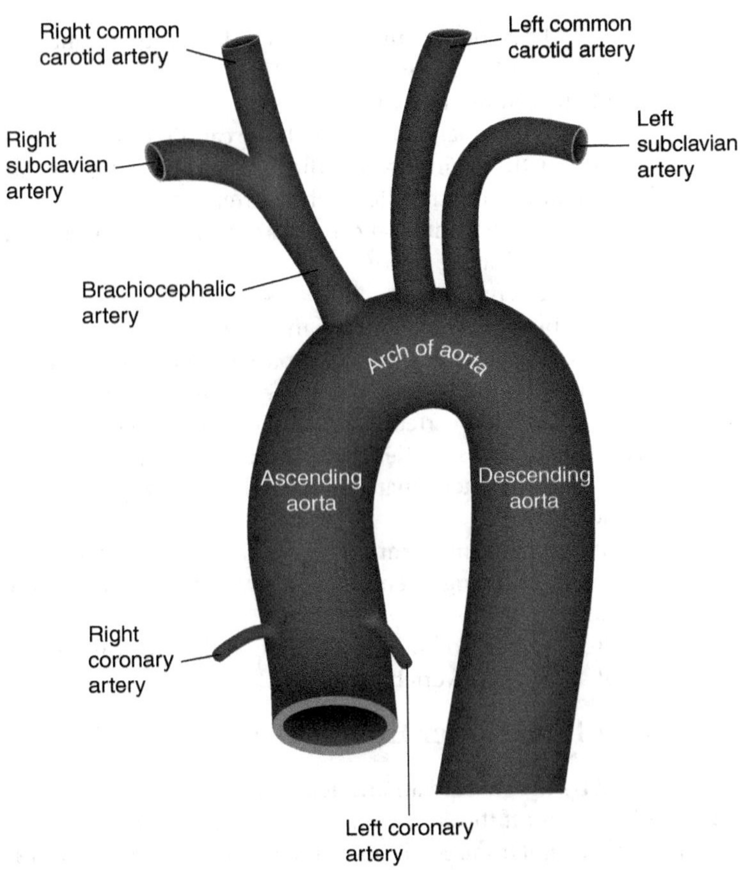

FIGURE 3-3. Aortic arch.

2. Aortic arch
   a. Aorta arches dorsally as it leaves the pericardial sac
   b. Branches include brachiocephalic artery, left common carotid artery, and left subclavian artery
   c. Furnishes all blood to head, neck, and upper limbs
3. Thoracic aorta gives rise to the following:
   a. Posterior intercostal arteries
   b. Bronchial artery
   c. Esophageal artery
   d. Superior phrenic artery

F. Abdominal Aorta/Mesenteric Arteries

1. Lumbar arteries supply posterior abdominal walls
2. Inferior phrenic arteries supply underside of diaphragm
3. Celiac artery
   a. Arises just below inferior phrenic arteries
   b. Divides as follows:
      1) Left gastric artery supplies lower part of esophagus and part of the stomach
      2) Splenic artery
         a) Supplies the spleen
         b) Gives branches to the pancreas and stomach
         c) Branches to the left gastroepiploic artery supplies greater curvature of the stomach
      3) Hepatic artery
         a) Supplies liver
         b) Sends branches to the stomach, duodenum, pancreas, and gallbladder
4. Superior mesenteric artery
   a. Arises below celiac artery
   b. Supplies all of small intestine, cecum, and the ascending and transverse colon of the large intestine
5. Suprarenal arteries
   a. Branch from the aorta at the level of the superior mesenteric artery
   b. Supply adrenal glands
6. Renal arteries
   a. Arise from aorta inferior to superior mesenteric artery
   b. Supply the kidneys
7. Ovarian arteries (women)
   a. Arise from aorta below renal arteries
   b. Supply ovaries
   c. Send branches to the ureters and uterine tubes
8. Testicular (internal spermatic) arteries (men)
   a. Arise from aorta below renal arteries
   b. Pass through inguinal canal to the scrotum; supply the testes
9. Inferior mesenteric artery
   a. Final branch of abdominal aorta
   b. Supplies part of transverse colon, descending colon, sigmoid colon, and rectum

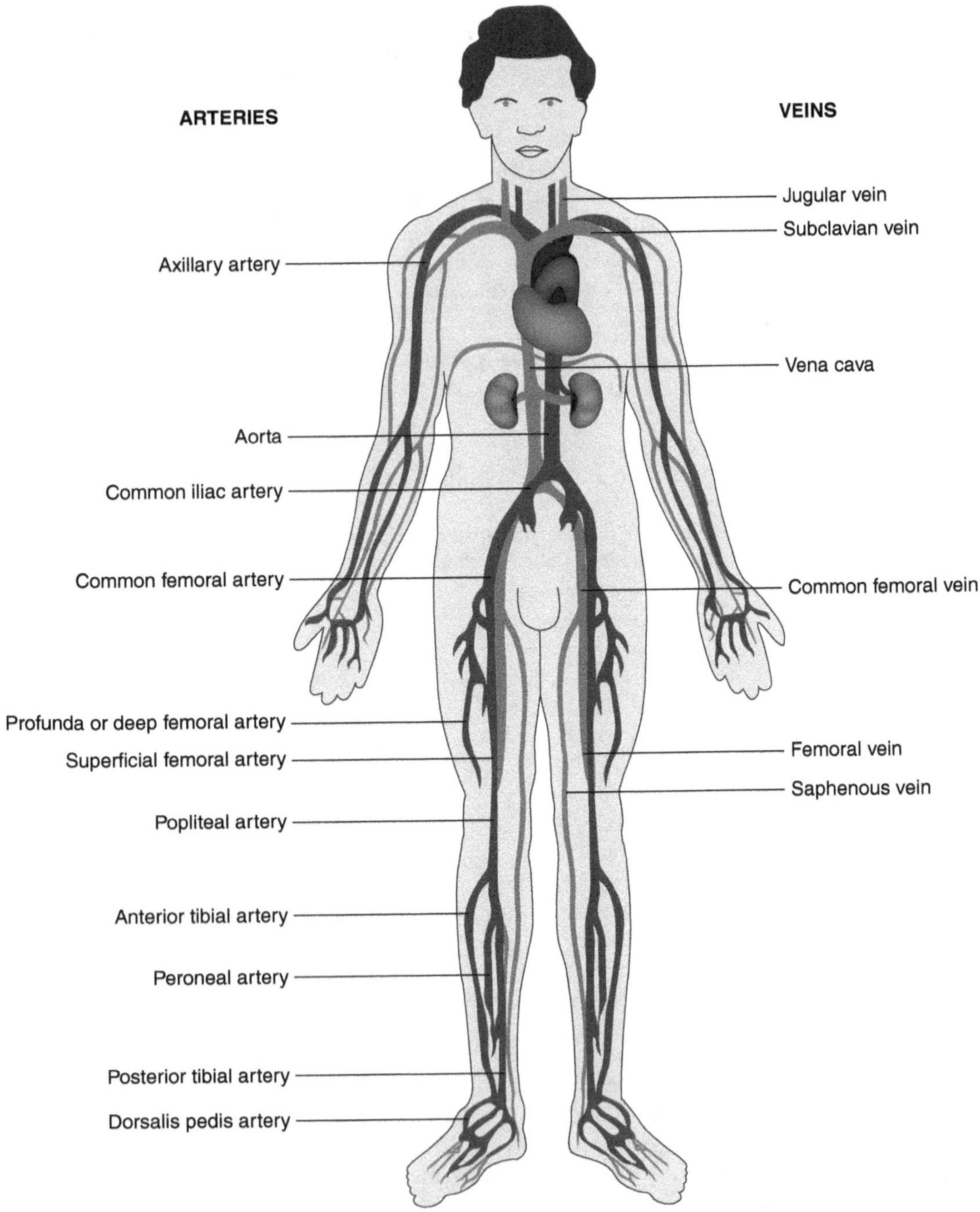

FIGURE 3-4. Arterial and venous anatomy.

G. Arteries of the Lower Extremities.

The distal aorta branches into common iliac arteries, which divide as follows (see Fig. 3-4):

1. Internal iliac (hypogastric) arteries
   a. Enter pelvic cavity
   b. Divide into branches that supply the pelvic viscera (urinary bladder, uterus, vagina, and rectum), muscles of gluteal and lumbar regions, walls of pelvis, external genitalia, and medial region of thigh

2. External iliac arteries
   a. Continuation of common iliac artery
   b. Supplies branches to the muscles and skin of the lower abdominal wall
3. Common femoral artery begins on entry to thigh; divides into the following:
   a. Superficial femoral artery supplies muscles of the anterior thigh
   b. Profunda femoral artery supplies muscles of posterior compartment of the thigh
4. Popliteal artery arises from the superficial femoral artery at the level of the knee
   a. Passes behind the knee, through the popliteal fossa
   b. Supplies muscles and skin of the area
5. Anterior tibial artery
   a. Supplies muscles of the anterior compartment of the leg
   b. Passes in front of the ankle, becomes dorsalis pedis artery, which supplies the dorsum of the foot and connects with plantar arch on dorsum of foot
6. Posterior tibial artery continues downward behind tibia and supplies muscles of posterior compartment of leg
   a. Divides into medial and lateral plantar arteries, which supply the sole of the foot and form the plantar arch
   b. Gives rise to peroneal artery, which supplies the peroneal muscles in the lateral compartment of leg

II. Venous Circulation (Guyton & Hall, 2000; Rohrer, 1999; Spence, 1982; Tottora & Grabowski, 2003)

A. General Venous Anatomy and Physiology. Acts as a conduit for transport of blood from the tissues back to the heart

1. Characterized as follows:
   a. Intermittent flow
   b. Collapsible tubes
   c. A low-pressure system
   d. Flow against the force of gravity
   e. Being able to accommodate large shifts in volume with limited changes in pressure (compliance)
   f. Serves as a reservoir for intervascular volume
2. Veins (see Fig. 3-5)
   a. Have a larger lumen and thinner walls and are more numerous than arteries
   b. Composed of three layers, similar to arteries: intima, media, adventitia
   c. Media is thinner than in arteries and has few muscle fibers
   d. Adventitia is thicker than media with little elastic material
   e. Walls of veins receive nourishment through vasa vasorum
   f. Venous return in lower extremities is aided by the calf muscle pump; leg muscles contract around veins; blood is squeezed from veins toward heart
   g. One-way valves prevent retrograde flow
3. Venules
   a. Collect blood from capillaries and become progressively larger veins
   b. Composed of an inner lining of epithelium (intima), surrounded by fibrous tissue

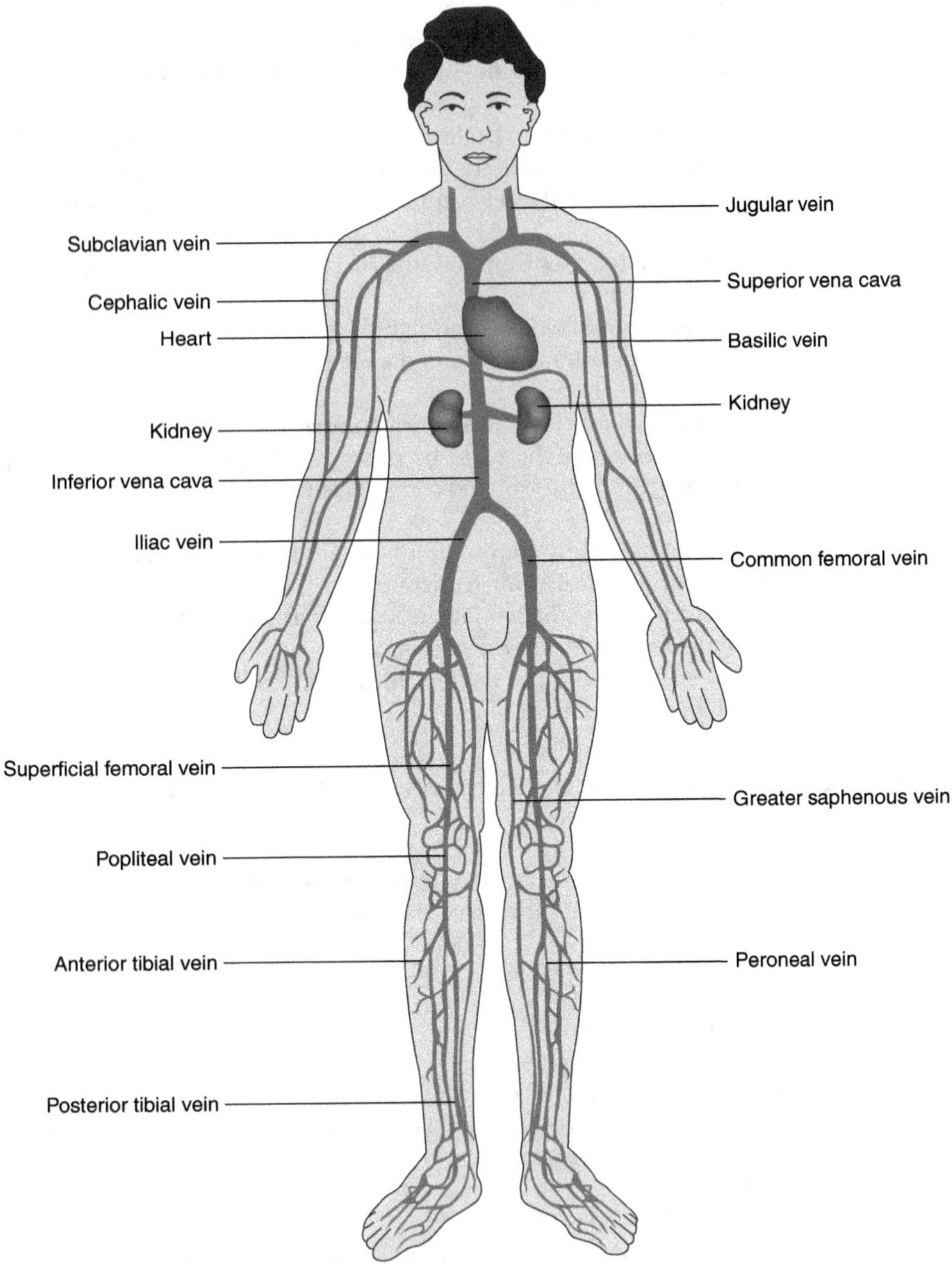

FIGURE 3-5. Venous anatomy.

4. Capacity of the venous system is larger than that of the arterial system
5. Classification of veins
   a. Deep veins travel alongside an artery and have the same name as the artery
   b. Superficial veins lie just beneath skin, return blood from skin and subcutaneous regions to the deep veins; names do not correspond to an artery
   c. Communicating or perforator veins channel flow from the superficial to the deep veins

B. Veins of the Head and Neck

1. Internal jugular vein
   a. Major venous drainage from the brain
   b. Leaves brain through the jugular foramen
   c. Travels alongside carotid artery and vagus nerve
   d. Joins with subclavian vein to form an innominate vein
2. Vertebral vein
   a. Drains posterior regions of the head
   b. Passes through transverse foramina of the cervical vertebrae
   c. Joins an innominate vein
3. External jugular vein
   a. Drains superficial regions of the head and neck
   b. Passes superficially down the neck
   c. Empties into subclavian vein
   d. Subclavian and internal jugular veins join to form the innominate vein
   e. Innominate veins join to form the superior vena cava
   f. Superior vena cava empties into the right atrium of the heart

C. Upper Extremities

1. Deep veins of upper extremities follow the paths of the arteries and have the same names
   a. Deep veins of forearm
      1) Paired veins consisting of the following:
         a) Ulnar vein
         b) Radial vein
         c) Interosseous vein
      2) Converge to form the paired brachial veins
   b. Brachial veins (paired)
      1) Travel through the elbow and upper arm
      2) Provide drainage to the upper arm
      3) Join to form axillary vein in upper arm
   c. Axillary vein
      1) Travels through the area of the shoulder
      2) Becomes the subclavian vein at the lateral border of the first rib
2. Superficial veins
   a. Cephalic vein
      1) Arises from lateral side of dorsal veins of hand and continues up lateral side of the arm
      2) At the level of shoulder, it goes deep and empties into the axillary vein
   b. Basilic vein
      1) Arises from the medial side of the dorsal veins of the hand
      2) Ascends along the medial-posterior side of the forearm
      3) Joins with the brachial vein at the level of the elbow
      4) Median cubital vein is one of seven branches between cephalic and basilic veins
3. All blood from the upper extremities is returned to the heart through the superior vena cava

D. Veins of the Thorax

1. Venous blood from the thorax empties into superior vena cava via the azygos system of veins
2. Azygos vein
   a. Begins in upper right lumbar region and enters thorax through the diaphragm
   b. Continues up posterior wall of thorax to the right vertebral column, empties into superior vena cava
3. Hemiazygos vein
   a. Follows similar path on left side of thorax
   b. Empties into azygos vein in the middle thorax
4. Azygos system also receives the accessory hemiazygos, intercostals, bronchial, esophageal, and pericardial veins

E. Veins of the Abdomen and Pelvis

1. Inferior vena cava
   a. Returns blood from the lower body
   b. Formed by the right and left common iliac veins at the level of fifth vertebra
   c. Receives tributaries from the lumbar, renal, suprarenal, hepatic, and right testicular or ovarian veins (left testicular or ovarian veins drain into left renal vein)
2. Hepatic portal system
   a. Consists of three large veins that drain the venous blood from the stomach, intestines, spleen, and pancreas
   b. Inferior mesenteric vein from the large intestine
   c. Superior mesenteric vein from the small intestine, pancreas
   d. Splenic vein
   e. Join to form the hepatic vein, which enters the liver and then drains into the inferior vena cava
   f. Hepatic portal system provides opportunity to remove nutrients and other substances from the blood as it passes through the liver

F. Veins of the Lower Extremities

1. Deep veins usually travel along with the arteries and are often given the same names
   a. Peroneal veins (paired) drain muscles of the calf
   b. Posterior tibial veins (paired) drain muscles of the calf
   c. Anterior tibial veins (paired) drain muscles of the calf
   d. Popliteal vein
      1) Formed by the convergence of the tibial and peroneal veins at the level of the knee
      2) Becomes superficial femoral vein as it reaches the lower thigh
   e. Superficial femoral vein
      1) Ascends through the thigh
      2) Joins with the profunda femoris vein to form the common femoral vein
   f. Profunda femoris vein
      1) Begins at the level of the mid-thigh
      2) Drains the muscles of the thigh

g. Common femoral vein
   1) Formed by the convergence of the superficial femoral and the profunda femoris veins at the level of the groin
   2) Renamed the external iliac vein as it crosses the inguinal ligament
h. External iliac vein provides drainage to the pelvis
i. Internal iliac (hypogastric) vein
   1) Provides venous drainage to the pelvis
   2) Combines with the external iliac vein to form the common iliac vein in the pelvis
j. Common iliac veins join to form the inferior vena cava

2. Superficial veins
   a. Dorsal venous arch on top of foot
   b. Greater saphenous vein
      1) Longest vein in the body
      2) Travels along the medial side of the foot, leg, and thigh
      3) Joins with the femoral vein just below the inguinal ligament
   c. Lesser saphenous vein
      1) Travels along the lateral side of the foot
      2) Crosses posterior surface of the leg
      3) Joins the popliteal vein behind the knee
3. Perforators
   a. 4 to 6 major perforating veins in each leg
   b. Located near the medial malleolus, medial calf, and distal medial thigh
   c. Valves allow flow of blood only from superficial to deep and prevent reflux in the opposite direction

III. Lymphatic Circulation (Bergan, 1999; Guyton & Hall, 2000; Spence, 1982; Tottora & Grabowski, 2003)

A. General Structure and Function

1. Interstitial fluid bathes all cells
2. Normally, slightly more fluid leaves the capillaries than enters
3. The lymphatic system is an extensive capillary network that collects excess interstitial fluid from organs and tissues into lymphatic vessels, where it is called lymph
4. The capillary network connects to an elaborate system of collecting vessels
5. Transports lymph to blood stream
6. Provides the only route for proteins and other large particles that cannot be absorbed into the capillary to travel back to the blood
7. Larger lymphatic vessels generally travel alongside veins and pass through one or more lymph nodes
8. Lymphatic vessels empty as follows:
   a. Cisterna chyli lies in front of the upper lumbar portion of the vertebral column, close to the celiac artery, and receives lymphatic vessels that drain the lower limbs and the viscera of the abdominal and pelvic cavity
   b. Thoracic duct arises from the cisterna chyli and returns lymph to the bloodstream from the left side of the thorax, upper arms, and left side of the head and neck
   c. Right lymphatic duct returns lymph to the bloodstream from the right upper arm and the right side of the thorax, neck, and head

9. Lymphatic system also functions to remove or destroy bacteria and other foreign particles and plays a role in other immune responses, such as manufacture of antibodies and other cell-mediated immunity processes

B. Mechanisms of Lymphatic Flow

1. Lymph is returned back to circulatory system at a rate of approximately 2 to 4 L every 24 hours
2. Interstitial fluid pressure is a determinant of the rate of flow. Factors influencing interstitial fluid pressure include the following:
   a. Elevated capillary pressure
   b. Decreased plasma colloid osmotic pressure
   c. Increased interstitial fluid protein
   d. Increased capillary permeability
3. Lymph flow is aided by the "milking" action of the muscles on lymph vessels
4. One-way valves in the lymphatic vessels prevent backflow of lymph in the vessels
5. Negative pressure in the thoracic cavity on inspiration promotes lymphatic flow

IV. Age-Related Changes in the Vascular System

A. Changes with Aging Occur in the Intima and Media

B. Age-Related Changes Usually Affect Large and Medium-Sized Vessels

C. Specific Age-Related Changes

1. Increased intimal thickness
2. Increased intimal collagen content
3. Decreased intimal elasticity
4. Degeneration of internal elastic membrane
5. Calcification of elastic tissue
6. Degeneration of smooth muscle in media secondary to inhibition of diffusion of nutrients following intimal thickening

REFERENCES

Bergan, J. J. (1999). Lymphedema. In V. Fahey (Ed.), *Vascular nursing* (3rd ed., pp. 33–48). Philadelphia, PA: WB Saunders.

Graham, L., & Ford, M. B. (1999). Arterial disease. In V. Fahey (Ed.), *Vascular nursing* (3rd ed., pp. 2–20). Philadelphia, PA: WB Saunders.

Guyton, A. C., & Hall, J. E. (Eds.). (2000). *Textbook of medical physiology* (10th ed.). Philadelphia, PA: WB Saunders.

Rohrer, M. J. (1999). The systemic venous system: Basic considerations. In V. Fahey (Ed.), *Vascular nursing* (3rd ed., pp. 21–32). Philadelphia, PA: WB Saunders.

Spence, A. P. (1982). *Basic human anatomy.* Menlo Park, CA: Benjamin/Cummings.

Tottora, G. J., & Grabowski, S. R. (Eds.). (2003). *Principles of anatomy and physiology* (10th ed.). New York, NY: John Wiley & Sons.

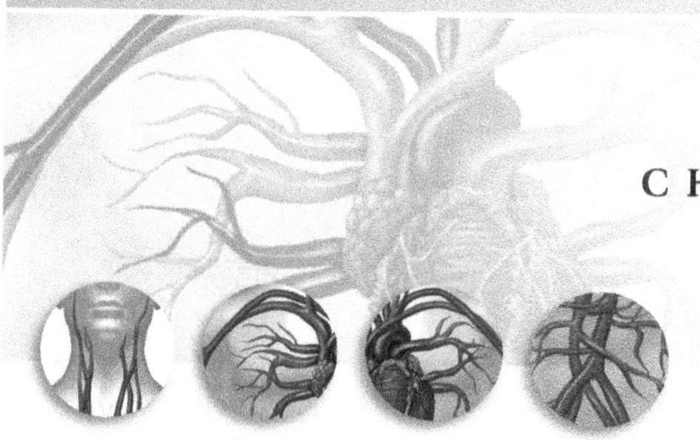

CHAPTER 4

Peripheral Vascular Assessment

Cindy Lewis

OBJECTIVES

1. Develop a systematic approach for assessing the peripheral vascular system.
2. Determine the components of a comprehensive health history.
3. Identify the skills and techniques required in performing a physical examination of the peripheral vascular system.

Overview/Introduction

The physical examination serves as the foundation on which therapeutic interventions, diagnostic tests, and nursing diagnoses can be determined. This chapter reviews the systematic order of assessment including a complete history followed by physical assessment involving inspection, palpation, and auscultation. Visual, tactile, auditory, and olfactory senses as well as nonverbal behaviors should be evaluated. The assessment should be performed bilaterally, comparing one extremity or side to the other.

I. Preparation for the History and Physical Examination

A. Preparing the Patient

1. Provide privacy
2. Eliminate drafts, control room temperature, and provide blankets as needed
3. Help the patient assume proper positions during the examination so that the body parts are accessible and comfort maintained
4. Minimize patient anxiety and fear by conveying an open, receptive, and professional approach. Explain thoroughly what will be done, what they can expect to feel, and how they can cooperate
5. An explanation of the history and physical examination should occur prior to its initiation to enhance patient compliance and contribution to the examination. Use simple terms when describing the steps of the examination
6. Use a relaxed voice tone and facial expressions to put the patient at ease
7. Encourage the patient to ask questions and mention any discomforts during the examination

B. Preparing the Environment

1. Provide good lighting, a warm comfortable room, and full exposure to all extremities
2. Ensure privacy
3. Control outside noises and prevent interruptions

C. Preparing the Equipment

1. A Doppler, stethoscope, and sphygmomanometer may be utilized to enhance the examination
2. Gloves should be worn during the physical examination

II. Patient History

A. Careful Questioning is important in obtaining a comprehensive history and is the key to an accurate assessment, nursing diagnosis, and treatment plan

1. Chief complaint/history of present illness: the chief complaint is the reason the patient is seeking medical attention. The disease may often be localized by history alone. It is important to listen and to ask specific questions about the patient's complaints
   a. Symptoms
      1) Location
      2) Character (severity of symptoms)
      3) Date of onset
      4) Precipitating factors (stress, activity, medication)
      5) Relief methods/alleviating factors
      6) Frequency
      7) Duration
      8) Progression
   b. Comprehensive pain assessment
      1) Intermittent claudication
      2) Ischemic rest pain
2. Significant medical surgical history
   a. Allergic reactions
   b. African American ethnicity
   c. Atherosclerosis
   d. Advanced age (>60)
   e. Cardiac history (history of angina, arrhythmias, myocardial infarction)
   f. Cellulitis, gangrene, wounds
   g. Clotting abnormalities (polycythemia vera, antithrombin III deficiency)
   h. Collagen vascular disease
   i. Diabetes mellitus
   j. Gout
   k. Hypercholesterolemia, reduced high-density lipoprotein (HDL-C), elevated triglycerides, hyperhomocysteinemia
   l. Hypertension (age of onset, severity, medications)
   m. Infections
   n. Malignancy
   o. Male gender

   p. Neurologic events or disorders: cerebrovascular or peripheral, strokes, seizures, loss of motor, sensory function, speech deficits, visual disturbances, dizziness, syncope, epilepsy, Parkinson disease, multiple sclerosis, migraine headaches, dementia
   q. Osteomyelitis
   r. Past injuries/spinal cord injuries
   s. Past surgical procedures
   t. Pregnancies
   u. Renal disease
   v. Use of oral contraceptives
   w. Venous thromboembolism
3. Medications that could alleviate and/or cause symptoms (include herbal medications)
4. Family history
   a. Arterial disease (cerebral, coronary, peripheral, or aneurysmal disease)
   b. Venous disease
   c. Cholesterolemia
   d. Clotting abnormalities
   e. Diabetes mellitus
5. Psychosocial history
   a. Occupational history—(current and past) type of work (i.e., standing all day, athlete)
   b. Tobacco use
   c. Drug abuse (i.e., amphetamines, opioids, illicit drugs)
   d. Current activity level, standing patterns
   e. Stress level/emotional state
   f. Dietary intake/obesity
   g. Alcohol intake
   h. Activities of daily living
   i. Walking or exercise regime
   j. Hygiene habits/foot and leg care
   k. Changes in lifestyle precipitated by signs and symptoms

III. Peripheral Vascular Assessment (see also Tables 4-1 and 4-2)

A. Head

1. Inspection
   a. Determine orientation to person, place, and time
   b. Assess for
      1) Pupil reactions, size, reaction to light
      2) Visual changes/blurred vision
      3) Facial symmetry
      4) Tongue deviation
      5) Speech
      6) Swallowing difficulties
   c. Check for large, bounding, or pulsatile carotid pulse. May be visible at the base of right side of neck if long-standing hypertension, tortuous carotid artery aneurysm, or carotid body tumor
   d. Inspect for jugular vein distention (JVD) (pressure)—note character of pulse
   e. Assess for weakness/numbness and motor movement in face

TABLE 4-1 Peripheral Vascular Assessment Parameters

Characteristics	Inadequate Arterial Supply	Inadequate Venous Supply
Skin color	Elevational pallor, dependent rubor	Brawny, brown, cyanotic when down
Skin texture	Thin, shiny, dry	Flaking, stasis, dermatitis, mottled
Paresthesias	Possible	Absent
Pulses	Weak or absent	Normal, strong and symmetrical
Temperature	Cool	Warm
Pain	Acute, sharp, gnawing lessens with rest, and limb dependent	Aching, cramping, lessens with limb elevated
Hair loss	Present, especially lower legs, feet, toes	Absent
Nails	Thick, brittle	Normal
Capillary refill	>3 s	<3 s
Edema	None or mild, usually unilateral	Usually present foot to calf, unilateral or bilateral
Skeletal muscle	Atrophy possible	Normal
Impotence	May be present with aortoiliac disease	Absent
Varicose veins	Absent	Possible
Ulceration	At pressure points, painful, pale dry, little drainage, well demarcated with eschar or dried; surrounded by fibrous tissue; granulation tissue scant and pale	Often at the ankle, painless, pinkish moist, large drainage, irregular, dry, and scaly, surrounded by dermatitis; granulation tissue healthy

2. Palpation
   a. Carotid pulse
      1) Palpate one side at a time
      2) Technique: place index and third fingers in groove at the medial edge of sternocleidomastoid muscle, just below the angle of jaw
      3) Assess in relation to other data collected
      4) Evaluate rate, rhythm, equality, amplitude
      5) Decreased or absent carotid or brachial equals diffuse process involving aortic arch and its major branches
      6) Palpate facial and superficial temporal pulses. These are continuation of carotid artery (external)—they do not supply brain directly but a strong pulse indicates an open, common carotid
   b. Jugular vein—principle vein from head
      1) Frequently seen in CHF, mechanical obstruction, neoplastic, inflammatory, or vascular masses
      2) Inspect JVD (pressure)—note character of pulse
      3) Elevate HOB to 45 degrees—check effect. Frequently distended when patient supine
      4) Check variation with respiration; tends to collapse on inspiration and refill during expiration
      5) Evaluate bilaterally—difficult to check in obese or full-necked individuals
3. Auscultation
   a. Important to make sure document preoperative. Bruits—abnormal low-pitched crackling, whooshing, or windy sound, produced as blood flows through irregular and stenotic lumen. Indicates turbulence, local obstruction, or transmission of murmurs because of increased resistance to flow
   b. Auscultate with bell of stethoscope while patient holds his breath and head turned to side

TABLE 4-2 Skin Color Variations

Color	Condition	Cause	Assessment Location
Blue (cyanosis)	Increased amount of deoxygenated hemoglobin, associated with hypoxia	Heart or lung disease, cold environment	Nail beds, lips, mouth, skin (severe cases)
Pallor (decrease in color)	Reduced amount of oxyhemoglobin	Anemia, shock	Face, skin, nail beds, conjunctivae, lips
	Reduced blood flow		Skin, nail beds, conjunctivae, lips
	Congenital or autoimmune condition causing lack of pigment	Vitiligo	Patchy areas on skin
Yellow-orange (jaundice)	Increased deposition of bilirubin in tissues	Liver disease, destruction of red blood cells	Sclerae, mucous membranes, skin
Red (erythema)	Dilation of blood vessels or increased blood flow	Fever, direct trauma, blushing, alcohol intake	Face, area of trauma
Tan-brown	Increased amount of melanin	Suntan, pregnancy, endocrine disorder	Areas exposed to sun, face, areolas, nipples

B. Arms (can have claudication or venous pain symptoms as in legs)

1. Chief complaint
   a. Arterial insufficiency associated with acute onset of pain, chronic exertional muscle fatigue of upper arm, Raynaud phenomenon (cold sensitivity)
   b. Acute arterial insufficiency associated with severe pain, pallor, pulselessness, poikilothermia, late paresthesias, and paralysis usually due to embolism, proximal thrombosis, subclavian artery aneurysm, or arterial injury
   c. Muscle fatigue and discomfort after prolonged use of arm is similar to intermittent claudication of lower extremity
   d. Thoracic outlet syndrome associated with fatigue, paresthesias, numbness in arm with activity
   e. Symptoms initiated by elevation or hyperabduction of arm may indicate neurovascular compression
2. Inspection
   a. Size, symmetry, and muscle tone/atrophy
   b. Color and texture of skin and nail beds—nails grow slow or not at all—dry, brittle, thick. Inspect for erythema (rubor) if suspect thrombophlebitis
   c. Assess temperature of limb
   d. Inspect for any breaks in the skin; fingertip lesions along nail edge, skin ulcerations, or gangrene
   e. Edema—chronic arm swelling may be due to chronic venous or lymphatic occlusion. Unilateral swelling and the presence of dilated superficial veins around the shoulder suggest subclavian vein thrombosis
   f. Venous pattern
      1) Storage function of venous system renders it susceptible to venous insufficiency, stasis, and thrombus formation
      2) Inspect for dilated, tortuous veins, pain, swelling, muscle tenderness (venous thrombophlebitis), and thin, shiny, bluish/brown, irregularly pigmented skin (venous stasis)

g. Arterial pattern
    1) Upper arterial insufficiency associated with itching-type pain, chronic exertional muscle fatigue, weakness, or cold sensitivity
    2) Assess for paresthesias, pallor, paralysis/numbness, cold sensitivity
h. Assess for weakness, numbness, and motor movement in arms (compare bilaterally)
i. Have patient flex and extend fingers
j. Test sensory function
k. If suspect Raynaud's, inspect fingers for tapering (waxy appearance), joint mobility, skin tautness, or signs of scleroderma including shiny atrophic skin

3. Palpation
    a. Subclavian: large artery at the base of neck supplies blood to arm
    b. Axillary: main artery to arm; branches off subclavian—palpable in axillary space
    c. Brachial: groove between biceps and triceps muscles above the elbow; feeds upper arm to elbow
    d. Radial: most common pulse palpated; compare volume on both arms—located on the thumb side of wrist
    e. Ulnar: flexor surface of wrist medially; easily felt
        1) Two vascular branches of hand and fingers interconnected (palmar arch) so circulation to hands and fingers doubly protected against possible arterial occlusion—flow in either direction possible since no valves
        2) If suspect arterial insufficiency, palpate these. Arterial occlusion in arms less common than legs. If pulses decreased markedly, question thromboangiitis obliterans, Buerger disease, or emboli—always compare to opposite arm
    f. Allen test (tests patency of ulnar and radial arteries)
        1) Have patient place his hands in his lap, palm up. Compress radial and ulnar arteries. Have patient open and close his fist tightly. Have patient open his hand to relaxed position. Release radial and observe the color of his palm—should turn pink promptly. Repeat—releasing ulnar artery. Persistence of pallor when one artery released indicates occlusion of the other (Pagana & Pagana, 1999)
    g. Palpate epitrochlear node
        1) Flex arm 90 degrees; reach under arm and feel in groove between biceps/triceps. Check for presence of node; size, consistency, tenderness. May be enlarged secondary to lesion in its drainage area or with generalized lymphadenopathy

4. Pulse grading
    a. 0 = absent, not palpable
       +1/4 = pulse is diminished, barely palpable, easily obliterated by pressure
       +2/4 = difficult to palpable, obliterated with pressure
       +3/4 = easy to palpate, not easily obliterated with pressure (normal)
       +4/4 = pulse is strong, bounding, or hyperactive, not obliterated with pressure (Seidel, Ball, Dains, & Benedict, 2006)
    b. Document presence or absence of pulses by palpation and Doppler signals

5. Auscultation
    a. Blood pressure: Assess bilaterally initially. If equal, can assess unilaterally for subsequent checks

6. Capillary refill time
   a. Evaluates the arterial supply to the small peripheral vessels since the capillary bed is the farthest portion of the vascular system from the heart
   b. Determines peripheral perfusion and cardiac output
   c. Blanch fingernail beds. Color should return in ≤3 seconds
7. Pulse oximetry
   a. Measures arterial oxygen saturation noninvasively
   b. Hypotension, hypothermia, and vasoconstriction reduce arterial blood flow
   c. Finger movement may interfere with accurate interpretations

C. Abdomen

1. Chief complaint—large aneurysm; may cause duodenal compression with weight loss and indigestion
2. Lower extremity edema secondary to iliac vein compression may occur
3. Turbulent blood flow within the aneurysm may cause distal embolization in which the patient may present with a blue toe or a painful toe
4. Symptomatic aneurysm (leaking or ruptured) may be accompanied by
   a. Abdominal pain
   b. Pain radiating toward the back or groin
   c. Syncope
   d. Shock
   e. Hypotension
   f. Tenderness may occur in the presence of inflammatory aneurysms
   g. Discoloration of the abdomen, flank, or scrotum due to extravasation of blood
   h. Sudden, acute foot or leg pain
   i. Bloody stools
5. Intestinal angina may occur with mesenteric ischemia. Pain occurs 15 to 30 minutes after eating (postprandial pain). May result from narrowing of superior mesenteric artery. Lower limb symptoms related to narrowing of iliac or femoral arteries or calf vessels
6. Acute intestinal ischemia may present with severe abdominal pain followed by vomiting and/or diarrhea
7. Uncontrollable hypertension and new onset of renal failure may be indicative of narrowing of the renal arteries causing renovascular hypertension
8. Sexual impotence, characterized by inability to maintain an erection, is a common complaint associated with aortoiliac occlusive disease. Medications, psychological factors, or diabetes may also cause impotence
9. Inspection
   a. Patient in supine position—note
      1) Contour of abdomen
      2) Obesity
      3) Ascites
      4) Pulsations
      5) Distention
      6) Discoloration
      7) Incisions from previous surgery
      8) Blue toe syndrome may be present secondary to an embolic source in the aorta

10. Palpation
    a. Aorta bifurcates at the level of the umbilicus; aortic pulse may be felt above this level in nonobese patients
    b. Normal size of aorta approximates the width of the thumb
    c. Press fingers firmly, deep into the abdomen to identify aortic pulsation
    d. If the pulse is prominent or feels wide, place thumb along one side of the aorta and the fingers along the other side
    e. Abdominal aortic aneurysm should be suspected if the width is larger than 4 to 5 cm (Fink et al., 2000)
    f. If mass extends to xiphoid and costal margins, suspect suprarenal or thoracoabdominal aneurysm
    g. Iliac artery aneurysms of significant size may be palpable on a rectal examination
    h. Assess for abdominal tenderness or referred pain; may indicate rupture, leak, or inflammation
11. Auscultation
    a. Check presence of bruits
    b. Aortoiliac disease may cause bruits in the middle and lower areas of the abdomen
    c. Renal artery bruits may be faint and localized in the upper abdominal quarter, just lateral to the midline
    d. Mesenteric artery bruits are associated with epigastric bruits

D. Legs

1. Chief complaint. May be asymptomatic, a pulse deficit, bruit, or abnormal pulsation or aneurysm
2. History
    a. Pain—usually most frequent symptom. Pain on exercise, relieved by rest. Sharp pain distal to the obstruction due to shunting of cutaneous blood to muscles ischemic from activity. Site of pain always distal to site of occlusion. Most common site of occlusion is femoral/popliteal artery. May occur on both sides—unilateral most frequent, but over time, may be bilateral
    b. Degree of pain depends on whether acute or chronic onset, severity of disease (extent of blood flow reduction), and adequacy of collateral blood supply
    c. Assess temperature and color. Numbness/tingling of toes/coldness indicates arterial insufficiency or diabetic neuropathy. More common with arterial than venous disease; feet have pale color. If due to diabetic neuropathy, usually bilateral
    d. Chronic arterial insufficiency causes two types of pain: intermittent claudication and ischemic rest pain
    e. Intermittent claudication: Described as ache, cramp, tiredness in muscle. Symptoms consistent each time the person walks. Results from inadequate oxygenation of muscle during exercise; since have sufficient blood flow in resting state. Level of arterial involvement usually a level above the area of pain (e.g., buttock/hip pain with aortoiliac artery disease, thigh pain with iliofemoral artery disease, pain in upper two-thirds of calf with superficial femoral artery disease, pain in lower third of calf with popliteal artery disease, and foot claudication with tibial or peroneal artery disease)

1) Pain during exercise, relieved with rest basically caused by ischemia from inadequate flow to muscle during period of increased demand (angina of leg)
2) Two theories for pain caused by
    a) Lactic acid which accumulates during ischemia occlusion/stenosis or
    b) Stimulated by chemical agents—bradykinin and histamine that are formed during muscle cell damage. Protective symptom designed to limit walking and weight bearing of ischemic muscle—warns of impending tissue damage
3) Should exercise limb to point of claudication or just prior, to stimulate collateral development of increased blood flow
4) Venous claudication is pain associated with post-phlebotic venous insufficiency. Mimics arterial claudication except "bursting" in nature rather than aching. May involve entire leg and often associated with swelling. Deep vein thrombosis is associated with little or no pain. Thrombophlebitis associated with tenderness or pain along vein course, varicose veins associated with heaviness and cramping in the calf

f. Nocturnal leg muscle cramps—occur at rest, relieved with activity or massage, not related to arterial disease

g. Ischemic rest pain—constant, hot, burning pain in foot, usually across the metatarsal head—unrelated to walking. Worse with elevation, somewhat decreased by dependency. Atrophy of skin, thick nails, loss of hair—trophic changes caused by tissue malnutrition from poor perfusion usually present. Affects toes first. Pain can become more proximal to forefoot later
    1) Occurs when tissue perfusion increasingly impaired affecting nutrition of resting tissues due to severe/advanced arterial occlusion. Inability to clear tissue metabolites from distal network
    2) Unremitting, constant pain indicates failure of collateral circulation to prevent ischemia
    3) May progress until gangrene ensues. Ischemic gangrene is dry and has no odor
    4) Dependency may bring relief (elevation or cold increases pain)

h. Impotence—found with aortoiliac obstruction (Leriche syndrome)

3. Inspection
    a. Provide privacy; remove stockings or socks; both feet
    b. Size, symmetry, and edema. Check for unilateral and/or bilateral edema and muscle atrophy
    c. Check for foot drop
    d. Check color; pink is normal. Pale, dusky color indicates arterial insufficiency. Cyanosis may be due to venous problem. Dusky, blue, cyanotic, or mottled discoloration usually means inadequate venous return
    e. Assess texture; hair distribution on lower legs, feet, and toes
    f. Assess for smooth, shiny skin, thick brittle nails with or without fungal infection and tapering of toes
    g. Assess temperature; reliable indicator of blood flow in dermal vessels—compare sides, using back of hand. Coldness indicates arterial insufficiency especially when one sided; if bilateral, question environment, anxiety. Hot temperature is suggestive of venous congestion. Symmetrical coolness usually indicates peripheral constriction. Asymmetrical coolness may represent arterial insufficiency

h. Check for pigmentation, rashes, scars, tissue loss, and venous pattern
i. Check for ulcers; assess site, size, surface, edge, duration, infection, and pain. Pressure sores due to decreased arteriole and capillary blood flow. Check for gangrene
j. Check veins when standing. Inspect for dilated tortuous veins
   1) If suspect chronic arterial insufficiency, elevate legs 12 inches off bed—move feet and ankles up and down for 30 to 60 seconds (drains feet of venous blood, permits evaluation of tissue color produced by arterial blood. Inspect for pallor—mild is normal). Red/purple with dependence (rubor) is chronic vasodilation in response to ischemia. Cyanosis is associated with obstructions. Degree of pallor indicates degree of arterial impairment
   2) Then have patient sit on edge of bed—dangle feet—check the amount of time required for color to return. Normal is ≤10 seconds. Dependent rubor due to oxyhemoglobin in corpuscles. Skin tissues are cold, so cannot readily take up oxygen nor can hemoglobin give up oxygen. Occurs with loss of 90% capacity (Fahey & White, 2004)
k. Check filling of veins of feet and ankles. Check capillary refill—press on toenails—check time for color to return—normal is ≤3 seconds. Delayed filling signifies arterial obstruction. Check for gangrene. Check location, color, drainage, and size. Usually occurs on bony prominences of toes, heels, and bunions
l. Assess for weakness, numbness, and motor movement in legs

4. Palpation
   a. Arteries—check for symmetry and regularity of beat. Listen for bruits. Listen with Doppler. Doppler pulse and palpable pulse do not indicate equal flow
   b. After completing pulse evaluation use back of hand to assess skin temperature. Symmetrical coolness may represent arterial insufficiency
      1) Abdominal aorta—check for palpable pulsatile masses, especially if elderly
      2) Common iliac—main artery to legs, comes off abdominal aorta and branches into external and internal iliac
      3) Femoral—groin to knee—midway between anterior superior iliac spine and symphysis pubis. Check for tenderness in area. Two hands helpful for palpation
      4) Popliteal—knee to mid-calf—posterior knees—deeper, diffuse, usually difficult to find. Use two hands, flex knee, or have patient prone. Popliteal aneurysm is the second most common site for aneurysm after abdominal. Feel above the posterior knee if cannot locate pulse
      5) Posterior tibial—medial and posterior from mid-calf to foot—behind and slightly below medial malleolus. Critical in diagnosis. If cannot find in nonedematous foot, suspect arterial occlusion
      6) Dorsalis pedis (pedal)—supplies foot—most common pulse evaluated—can be congenitally absent (5%). Like hand, foot is doubly protected by interconnecting arch between two chief arterial branches (pedal arch)
   c. Veins
      1) Deep leg veins: deep veins are supported by surrounding muscle and fascia. Veins from legs and lower trunk drain into inferior vena cava. Deep veins carry 90% of venous return from lower extremities (Porth & Matfin, 2009)

a) Femoral
b) Popliteal
c) Anterior–posterior tibial
d) Peroneal plantar arch

2) Superficial leg veins: in contrast to deep veins, superficial veins are located subcutaneously and supported poorly by fat and skin
a) Great saphenous—dorsum of foot to medial malleolus to medial aspect of leg
b) Small saphenous vein
c) Communicating or perforating veins—connects saphenous system with veins of deep system
d) Deep, superficial, and communicating veins all have thin valves 10 to 12 cm apart, arranged so venous blood can flow from superficial to deep toward heart not in opposite direction

d. Lymphatics: Check size, consistency, and tenderness. Should be small, mobile, nontender. Tenderness indicates lymphadenitis. Two groups of superficial inguinal nodes
1) Vertical group—lies close to upper portion of great saphenous vein (drains corresponding area of leg)
2) Horizontal group—lies below inguinal ligament—drains skin of lower abdomen, external genitalia, anal canal, lower vagina, gluteal area

e. Allen maneuver—compress pedal and posttibial while foot elevated then let foot down to observe color

f. Edema grading scale
1) 0 = absent
+1 = slight indentation, disappears rapidly
+2 = indentation rapidly noticeable, disappears within 10 to 15 seconds
+3 = deep indentation, lasts more than a minute; extremity looks fuller and swollen
+4 = marked, deep indentation; may be visible after 2 to 5 minutes; extremity is grossly distorted (Porth & Matfin, 2009)
2) Cardiac edema is usually dependent: feet, ankles, back, flanks (common sign of CHF)
3) Unilateral edema indicates occlusion of a major vein
4) Chronic arterial occlusion presents as mild, nonpitting edema

g. Homans' sign (not considered reliable indicator; trauma to vein or muscle, reduced mobility, and increased blood clotting are considered reliable risk factors) (Bonham et al., 2009; Wound, Ostomy, and Continence Nurses Society [WOCN], 2012)

Palpate calves for tenderness, on dorsiflexion of elevated leg—check firmness or warmth. Measure leg circumference and capillary refill. Positive Homans' sign may indicate a leg problem although a deep venous thrombosis is found only 50% of the time

h. Arterial/brachial index (ABI)—check with Doppler-pedal and brachial systolic pressures; detects decrease in blood flow before clinical signs apparent. Arterial occlusion and claudication can be present even though pulses persist
1) With patient lying flat, measure blood pressure of left and right arms. If the blood pressures differ from arm to arm, use the higher of the two blood pressures and record. Next, apply blood pressure cuff over the ankles. Take blood pressure reading over dorsalis pedis

and posterior tibial artery on right leg and left leg. Calculate the ankle/brachial index by dividing the systolic reading at the dorsalis pedis/posterior tibial level by the systolic reading at the arm (brachial artery)

2) If ankle ≥ brachial (≥0.90) peripheral pressure normal
3) If ankle < brachial, suspect partial arterial obstruction proximal to vessel measures
4) If ankle < 20% of brachial, pressure indicates severe ischemia, rest pain, gangrene
   a. Ankle/brachial index interpretation
      1.30: abnormally high range, suggests poorly compressible calcified arteries
      1.0: to 1.3: "normal" range
      ≤0.9: lower extremity arterial disease (LEAD)
      ≤0.6 to 0.8: borderline perfusion
      ≤0.5: severe ischemia (Bonham et al., 2008; Hirsch et al., 2006; WOCN, 2012)
5) The lower the ankle pressure, the higher the risk of ischemic injury. Monitors significant changes in patient's norm. Useful to monitor before and after surgery, and for bypass graft surveillance

IV. Key Points

A. History Review, Including Risk Factors

1. Chief complaints
2. Pain history
3. Significant medical/surgical history
4. Medications
5. Family history
6. Psychosocial history

B. Physical Examination

1. Arterial problems are suspected in the presence of dependent rubor or atrophy. Dependent rubor occurs when the legs are dangled; lower legs become red
2. Venous insufficiency is suspected in the presence of edema, flaking skin, and brown pigmentation
   a. Inspection
      1) Skin color—look for dependent rubor, flaking skin, brown pigmentation
      2) Temperature—look for signs of heat, redness, calf tenderness, thrombophlebitis
      3) Hair pattern
      4) Presence of edema or atrophy of lower extremities, ulcers
      5) Weakness, movement
   b. Palpation
      1) Vascular tone, turgor
      2) Skin temperature
      3) Pulses; note amplitude and symmetry
      4) Capillary refill time

c. Auscultation
   1) Listen closely over the carotid, abdominal, renal, and iliac arteries for bruits
   2) Blood pressure

REVIEW QUESTIONS

1. A 5-minute peripheral vascular assessment should include
   a. Inspection
   b. Palpation
   c. Auscultation
   d. All of the above

2. Pain, pallor, and absent pulses in an extremity are signs of
   a. Chronic venous insufficiency
   b. Acute venous insufficiency
   c. Chronic arterial insufficiency
   d. Acute arterial insufficiency

3. Leg pain precipitated by exercise and relieved by rest is known as
   a. Embolization
   b. Intermittent claudication
   c. The Somogyi phenomenon
   d. Traumatic pain

4. What color change occurs when the legs of a patient with arterial insufficiency are placed in a dependent position?
   a. Cyanosis
   b. Pallor
   c. Rubor
   d. Brown hyperpigmentation

5. Normal capillary refill time is less than
   a. 1 second
   b. 3 seconds
   c. 5 seconds
   d. 10 seconds

6. Blood pressure readings in the arms and legs
   a. Are equal
   b. Vary greatly
   c. Differ by 10 mm Hg; arm readings are higher
   d. Differ by 10 mm Hg; leg readings are higher

7. Which maneuver evaluates the presence of an occlusion in the ulnar artery?
   a. The Allen test
   b. The Trendelenburg test
   c. Eliciting Homans' sign
   d. Eliciting Chvostek sign

8. Which sign is NOT associated with arterial insufficiency?
   a. Pain at rest
   b. Decreased pulses

c. Thickened nails
d. Brown pigmentation of the ankles

9. What increases your risk for atherosclerosis?
   a. High carbohydrate diet
   b. Blood pressure 120/80
   c. Smoking
   d. Chronic pain

10. What is the most common symptom associated with arterial disease?
    a. Swelling
    b. Pain
    c. Skin changes
    d. Unsightly veins

ANSWERS/RATIONALE

1. **d.** A 5-minute peripheral vascular assessment includes inspection, palpation, and auscultation techniques.
2. **d.** Arterial disease is characterized by pain, pallor, and absent pulses. Venous disease is characterized by dilated veins, pain, swelling, and hyperpigmentation.
3. **b.** Intermittent claudication is pain during exercise, relieved with rest. Caused by ischemia from inadequate blood flow to muscle during period of increased demand.
4. **c.** With arterial disease, if the extremity is elevated, pallor will occur since venous blood drained from the extremity evaluates tissue color produced by arterial blood. If the extremity is dependent, rubor occurs due to chronic vasodilatation in response to the underlying ischemia.
5. **b.** Normal capillary refill time is less than 3 seconds. Capillary refill time evaluates peripheral perfusion and cardiac output.
6. **a.** Normal arterial/brachial index (ABI) is 1.0 to 1.3. Ankle and brachial blood pressure readings should be equal in the absence of any disease.
7. **a.** The Allen test evaluates the patency of the ulnar and radial arteries. Persistence of pallor when one artery is released indicates occlusion of the other.
8. **d.** Brown hyperpigmentation of the skin is associated with venous disease (due to breakdown of red blood cells into deposits of hemosiderin that stain the tissue a characteristic brownish color).
9. **c.** Smoking is a significant risk factor for peripheral vascular disease. Hypertension, high cholesterol, high-fat diet, heart disease, diabetes, obesity, and family history are other significant risk factors.
10. **b.** The most common presenting symptom in lower extremity arterial disease is pain. The degree of pain depends on whether the problem has an acute or chronic onset, the severity of the disease (the extent of flow reduction), and the adequacy of collateral vessels.

REFERENCES

Bonham, P. A., Flemister, B. G., Goldberg, M., Crawford, P., Johnson, J. J., & Varnado, M. F. (2009). What's new in lower-extremity arterial disease? WOCN's 2008 Clinical Practice Guideline. *Journal of Wound, Ostomy and Continence Nursing, 36*(1), 37–44.

Fahey, V. A., & White, S. A. (2004). Physical assessment of the vascular system. In V. A. Fahey (Ed.), *Vascular nursing* (4th ed., pp. 53–72). Philadelphia, PA: W.B. Saunders.

Fink, H. A., Lederle, F. A., Roth, C. S., Bowles, C. A., Nelson, D. B., & Haas, M. A. (2000). The accuracy of physical examination to detect abdominal aortic aneurysm. *Archives of Internal Medicine, 160*(6), 833–836.

Hirsch, A. T., Haskal, Z. J., Hertzer, N. R., Bakal, C. W., Creager, M. A., Halperin, J. L., ... White, R. A. (2006). ACC/AHA 2005 practice guidelines for the management of patients with peripheral arterial disease (lower extremity, renal, mesenteric, and abdominal aortic): Executive summary. *Circulation, 113*, 1474–1547. doi:10.1161/CIRCULATIONAHA.106.173994 Retrieved from http://circ.ahajournals.org/content/113/11/1474

Pagana, K., & Pagana, T. (1999). *Diagnostic testing and a nursing implications: A case study approach* (5th ed.). St. Louis, MO: Mosby.

Porth, C. M., & Matfin, G. (2009). *Pathophysiology: Concepts of altered health states* (8th ed.). Philadelphia, PA: Wolters Kluwer Health/Lippincott, Williams and Wilkins.

Seidel, H. M., Ball, J. W., Dains, J. E., & Benedict, G. W. (2006). *Mosby's guide to physical examination* (6th ed.). St. Louis, MO: Mosby.

Wound, Ostomy, and Continence Nurses Society (WOCN). (2012). *Guideline for management of wounds in patients with lower-extremity neuropathic disease* (WOCN clinical practice guideline series; no. 3) (100 pp.). Mount Laurel, NJ: Wound, Ostomy, and Continence Nurses Society (WOCN).

SUGGESTED READINGS

Arain, F. A., & Cooper, L. T. (2008). Peripheral arterial disease: Diagnosis and management. *Mayo Clinic Proceedings, 83*(8), 944–950.

Hiatt, W. R., Hirsch, A. T., & Regensteiner, J. (2001). *Peripheral arterial disease handbook.* Boca Raton, FL: CRC Press.

Mourad, J.-J., Cacoub, P., Coller, J.-P., Becker, F., Pinel, J.-F., Huet, D., ... Priollet, P. (2009). Screening of unrecognized peripheral arterial disease (PAD) using ankle-brachial index in high cardiovascular risk patients free from symptomatic PAD. *Journal of Vascular Surgery, 50*(3), 572–580.

Treat-Jacobson, D., & Walsh, M. E. (2003). Treating patients with peripheral arterial disease and claudication. *Journal of Vascular Nursing, 21*(1), 5–14.

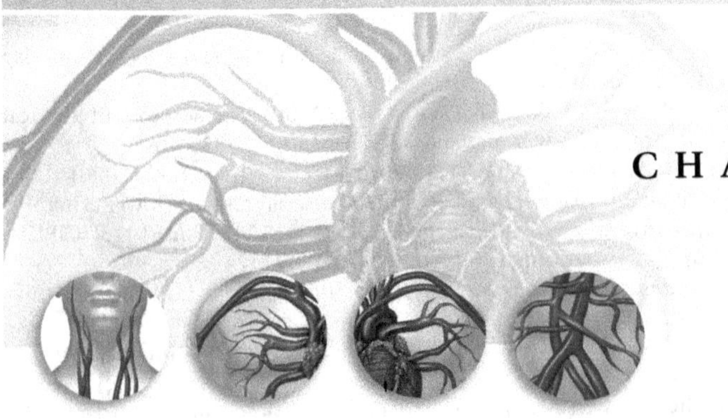

CHAPTER 5

Vascular Diagnostic Studies

Patricia A. Lewis
Marie Rossi
First Edition Author: *Patricia A. Lewis*

OBJECTIVES

1. Identify the purpose and clinical indications for invasive and noninvasive vascular diagnostic examinations.
2. List the elements of normal and abnormal results for vascular diagnostic examinations.
3. Correlate the findings from vascular examinations with appropriate nursing interventions.

Introduction

Vascular diagnostic studies are used as an adjunct to a thorough history and physical examination to detect disease in the arterial and venous systems, plan appropriate management or intervention, and follow disease progression. Invasive studies use various radiologic techniques combined with arterial or venous cannulation for instillation of radio-opaque contrast medium. Noninvasive testing uses ultrasound technology and Doppler principles to visualize vessels and analyze flow within the vascular bed under investigation. In addition to a discussion of the advantages and disadvantages of these general techniques, each test description provides information regarding test purpose, clinical indication, patient preparation, instrumentation, procedure, interpretation, limitations, complications and precautions, and nursing implications.

I. Overview

A. Objective Evaluation of the Circulatory System

1. History and physical examination
2. Methods of documenting site(s) of involvement
3. Functional impact of disease on patient's life

B. Invasive Vascular Examinations

1. Outline site(s) of disease
   a. Catheter cannulation of vessel with instillation of radio-opaque contrast medium provides outline of arterial or venous vascular system
   b. Highly accurate; considered "gold standard" for diagnosis of many disease conditions
2. Clinical benefits need to be weighed against risks and cost-effectiveness of procedure.
   a. Potential iatrogenic injury to vascular system and organ beds; exposure to x-rays, and complications of contrast
   b. Time consuming and expensive
3. Reserved for use when intervention is being considered
   a. Not useful for screening
   b. Limited use for following progression of disease or outcome of intervention because of cost and risks of procedure

C. Noninvasive Vascular Examinations

1. Based on Doppler ultrasound principles (Christian Doppler, circa 1840).
   a. Audible sound waves: 20 to 20,000 Hz. 1 Hz = 1 sound wave cycle/second
   b. Ultrasound: 1 to 30 MHz. Vascular ultrasound equipment uses 2 to 10 MHz
   c. Doppler effect: high-frequency sound beam generated from vibrating piezoelectric crystal in transducer meets moving structure (blood cell), reflected sound returns at different frequency (frequency shift) (see Fig. 5-1)

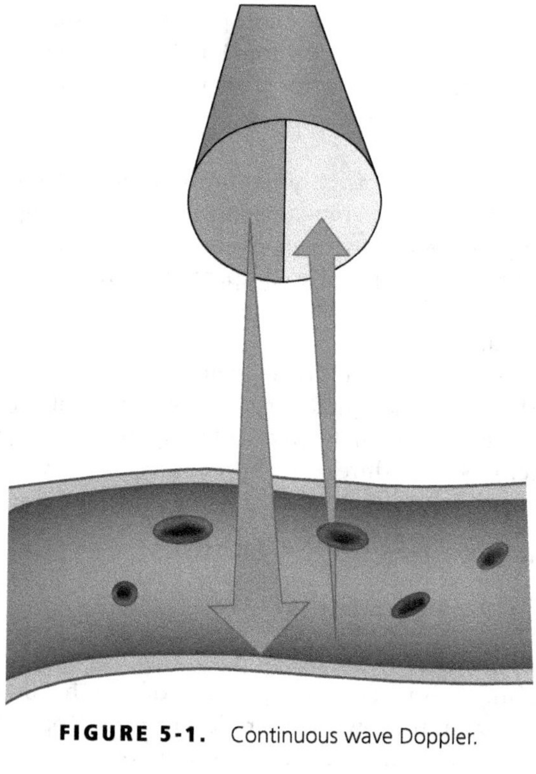

FIGURE 5-1. Continuous wave Doppler.

1) Speed of moving structure can be calculated from this frequency shift
2) Returning frequency increases if flow is toward the sound source (transducer); decreases if flow is away from sound source
3) Doppler equation: flow = returning frequency – sending frequency; dependent on angle of ultrasound beam directed at vessel (ideally, 60 degrees for most accurate signal processing) (Sanders, 1998)
4) Frequency of returning wave is converted into audible signal and visible waveform or sound spectrum on a screen that can be recorded as analog waveforms and analyzed by computer (spectral analysis)
5) Poiseuille law: speed of blood flow increases across an area of narrowing in a blood vessel, which results in higher frequency shifts on Doppler evaluation. At the same time, blood pressure in the vessel decreases beyond the area of narrowing because of loss of energy across the stenotic lesion. This is the basis for categorization of vascular stenosis

d. B-mode (brightness mode) ultrasound: reflected ultrasound produces two-dimensional (2D) image of anatomic structures (Ridgway, 1992; Rumwell & McPharlin, 1998)
   1) Reflected ultrasound displayed in shades of gray; the denser the tissue, the brighter the image. Example: calcified plaque is bright white; blood or fluid-filled lumen is black
   2) Real time: constantly rotating transducer produces moving images (pulsating vessel; moving organs)
e. Duplex ultrasound: combination of B-mode imaging with Doppler spectral analysis
   1) Anatomic and hemodynamic/physiologic information
   2) Color duplex imaging: frequency shift from moving red cells displayed with colors corresponding to direction of flow; blue, away from transducer (venous); red, toward transducer (arterial); mixed color, turbulent flow from mixed velocities across stenotic lesion (Wolf & Fobbe, 1995)

2. Advantages
   a. Provide noninvasive quantitative determination of severity of disease
   b. Suitable for screening, diagnosis, and follow-up evaluation
   c. Highly accurate with experienced technologist
   d. Relatively inexpensive compared with invasive testing without risks or complications
3. Disadvantages
   a. Results are operator dependent
   b. May not be adequate for operative intervention, although some surgeons rely solely on carotid duplex scanning results before endarterectomy procedures

II. Noninvasive Diagnostic Studies

A. Arterial Examinations

1. Ankle–brachial index (ABI)
   a. Purpose is to assess the presence of peripheral artery occlusive disease (PAD) in the lower extremities by using Doppler techniques combined with blood pressure evaluation of flow

b. Clinical indications
   1) Assess the patient who has complaints of claudication
   2) Evaluate patients who have suspected PAD by grading the severity of blood flow reduction
   3) Aid in determination of intervention methods for treating PAD
   4) Surveillance of disease progression before and after intervention
   5) Screening general population for presence of PAD

c. Patient preparation
   1) Explain procedure and complete history
   2) Remove appropriate clothing: shoes, socks, and long-sleeved shirts to expose feet, ankles, and arms
   3) Have patient lie supine with head slightly elevated in warm room for ≥10 minutes. Position for comfort and relaxation to minimize tremor, restlessness. Must be able to access all extremities easily

d. Instrumentation
   1) 5- to 10-MHz continuous wave Doppler and coupling gel
   2) Analog waveform equipment (desired but not absolute)
   3) Appropriate blood pressure cuffs for arms and ankles and sphygmomanometer

e. Procedure (see Figs. 5-2 and 5-3)
   1) Inflate blood pressure cuff to 20 mm Hg above systolic pressure, record systolic pressure as cuff is deflated using Doppler in right and left brachial, dorsalis pedis, and posterior tibial arteries
   2) If analog waveform is to be recorded, obtain tracings in all vessels before blood pressure recordings
   3) Calculate ratio of distal pressure/proximal pressure by dividing highest distal pressures on each limb by the highest brachial pressure. Example: ankle pressure of 60 mm Hg divided by brachial pressure of 120 mm Hg = 0.50

f. Findings/interpretation
   1) In absence of disease, no difference between proximal (brachial) and distal (ankle) pressures. Distal pressures may be slightly higher because of normal vascular resistance. Therefore, normal index = 1.00 to 1.20.

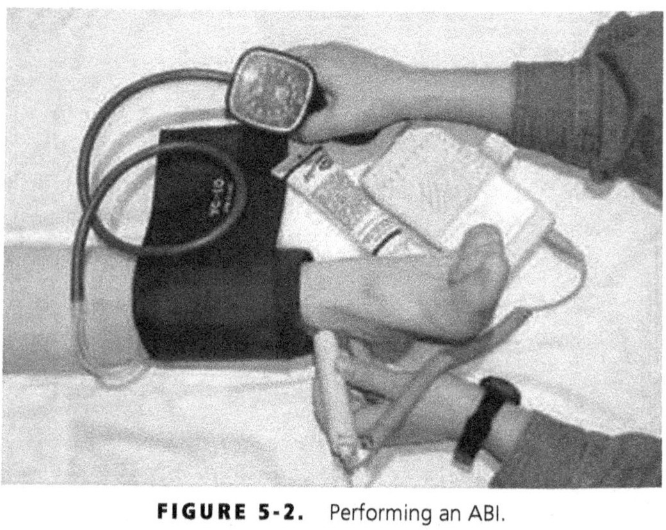

FIGURE 5-2. Performing an ABI.

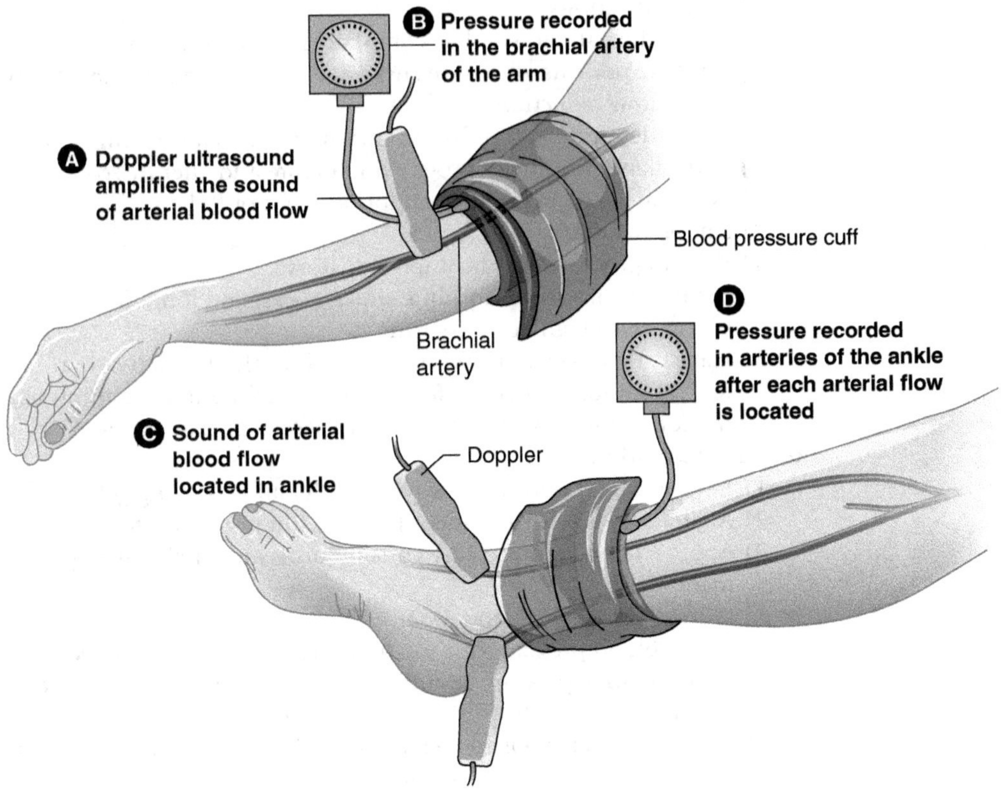

FIGURE 5-3. Cuff and Doppler placement for ABI.

2) As disease progresses, index drops, indicating reduced flow across stenotic lesion in arterial system; below diaphragm
3) Ratio is proportionate to degree of ischemia and is classified as follows

Normal	1.0 to 0.95
Mild	0.94 to 0.80
Moderate	0.75 to 0.40 (claudication level)
Ischemic	<0.40 (threatened tissue/limb loss)

Blackburn, D. R., & Peterson-Kennedy, L. (2004). Noninvasive vascular testing. In V. Fahey (Ed.), *Vascular nursing* (4th ed., pp. 73–96). St. Louis, MO: Saunders.

4) Ratio is useful for comparison studies/serial follow-up. Change of >0.15 (±) is indicative of deterioration or improvement
5) Analog waveform analysis (see Fig. 5-4)
   a) Normal: sharp systolic upstroke, narrow waveform, one or more diastolic (reversed) wave components

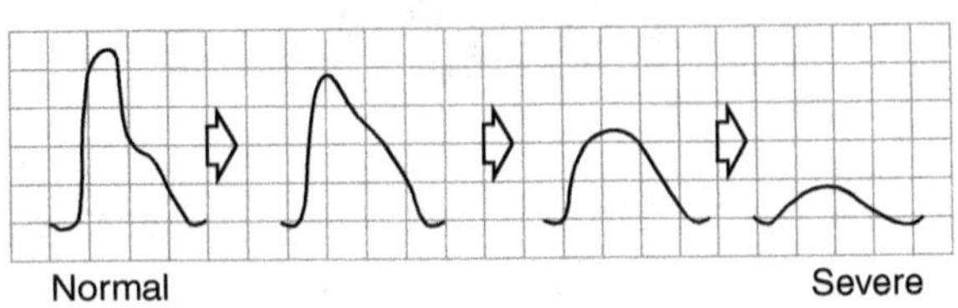

FIGURE 5-4. Analog readings.

b) Stenotic: absent diastolic component, widened systolic wave with blunting
c) Occluded or near occluded: marked flattening or widening; no diastolic component
d) Abnormal signal indicates stenosis proximal to or above site of recording

g. Limitations
1) Noncompressible vessels secondary to calcification of diabetes (Salles-Cunha et al., 2012), endstage renal disease—cause artificial elevation of pressures with index of ≥1.30. Must base examination on waveform analysis only.
2) Obesity: too large for appropriate cuff sizing
3) Acute deep vein thrombosis
4) Acute trauma, ulcerations, or indwelling intravenous (IV) line placement in areas needed for testing
5) Extensive dressings or casts at sites to be tested
6) Restlessness, tremor, inability to cooperate

h. Complications/precautions
1) Obtaining pressure readings immediately postoperatively following distal bypass revascularization may be contraindicated—check with surgeon. Waveform analysis acceptable
2) Appropriate precautions for wound infections. Avoid coupling gel in open wound
3) Avoid prolonged cuff inflation on any extremity

i. Nursing implications
1) Safe, accurate, reproducible, portable bedside test to assess vascular status on most patients, regardless of comorbidities
2) Implement appropriate vascular precautions and wound care as indicated

2. Segmental pressures and analog waveforms (see Fig. 5-5)
a. Purpose: to evaluate four segments of the arterial system in the lower extremity to identify the level of stenosis in the patient who is suspected of having PAD—aortoiliac, ileofemoral, femoral-popliteal, and distal circulation
b. Clinical indication: as above for ABI except not used for routine screening of general population
c. Patient preparation: as above for ABI
d. Instrumentation: as above for ABI with addition of blood pressure cuffs for upper thigh, lower thigh, below knee, and ankle
e. Procedure: After obtaining both brachial blood pressures as above, sequentially obtain analog waveforms and blood pressure on each segment of the lower extremities
1) All distal pressures are heard with the Doppler placed over the posterior tibial or dorsalis pedis artery, whichever is most audible
2) Calculate ABI as above for each extremity
f. Findings/interpretation: systolic pressure decreases and waveform changes below level of stenosis. Example: If pressures are diminished at high thigh, suspect aortoiliac disease. If not diminished until calf, suspect popliteal disease
1) If multiple levels of stenosis, systolic pressure measured distal to last area reflects additive changes, likely with ABI <0.5
2) Difference of >30 mm Hg between segments indicates disease

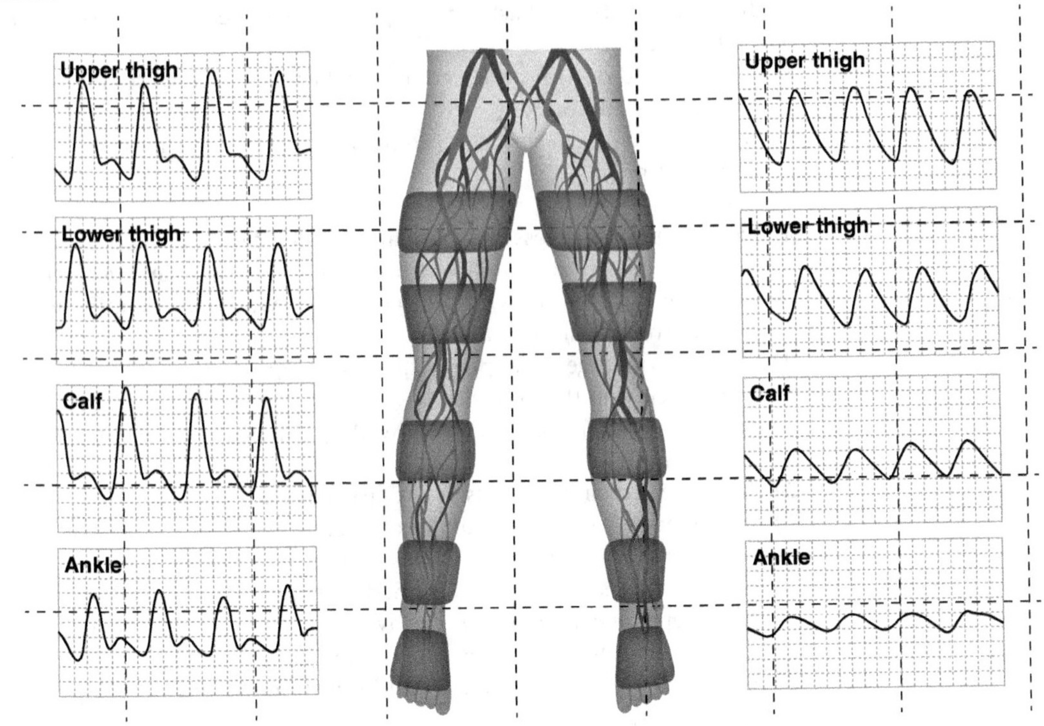

FIGURE 5-5. Segmental pressures and analog waveforms, Right leg = normal; Left leg = abnormal.

g. Limitations: as above for ABI
h. Complications/precautions: as above for ABI. Thigh cuff inflation may be painful; deflate as rapidly as possible while maintaining test accuracy
   1) Nursing implications: as above for ABI. Useful test to predict healing potential for amputation level. If thigh pressure exceeds 60 mm Hg, below knee amputation should heal

3. Toe pressures (Strandness, 1996)
   a. Purpose: assess distal arterial flow
   b. Clinical indications: patients who have diabetes or calcification of larger vessels of lower extremity, which make ABI calculation falsely elevated. Also useful for prediction of healing toe, forefoot, or digit amputation wounds
   c. Patient preparation: as for ABI
   d. Instrumentation: as for ABI with addition of 2.5 × 9 cm toe cuff
   e. Procedure: Obtain brachial systolic Doppler pressures as above. Place toe cuff around great toe of each foot, auscultate for arterial signal, obtain waveform tracing and pressure. Calculate toe/brachial index
   f. Findings/interpretation: normal toe pressure = 60 mm Hg
      1) Normal toe/brachial index (toe systolic pressure index) ≥0.60
      2) Variability of measurement is ± 0.17
      3) Hemodynamically significant lesion ≥0.60 or toe pressure between 30 and 60 mm Hg
      4) Rest pain/ischemia ≥0.15 or toe pressure less than 30 mm Hg
   g. Limitations: often difficult to auscultate toe arterial signal, especially when abnormal or if patient cannot maintain immobility during test. Pencil probe–style of Doppler is helpful

h. Complications/precautions: as above for ABI
i. Nursing implications: helpful in predicting healing of open lesions. If toe systolic pressure is less than 30 mm Hg, healing is unlikely without revascularization

4. Exercise testing
   a. Purpose: to differentiate between circulatory and neurologic source (e.g., spinal stenosis) of leg pain
   b. Indication: subclinical stenosis. Resting ABI is normal or near normal, but the patient complains of claudication symptoms
   c. Patient preparation: as for ABI, leaving cuffs in place after baseline (resting) supine ABI is calculated
   d. Instrumentation: as for ABI, plus watch or timing device and treadmill capable of adjusted speed and grade
   e. Procedure
      1) Obtain careful history: Neurospinal problems are not usually as reproducible as true claudication (good days, bad days; pain brought on with sitting or standing as well as walking; have to lie down for relief)
      2) Obtain resting supine ABI and waveforms as above
      3) Patient walks for 5 minutes or until disabled by leg pain at standardized speed and grade on treadmill: 1.5 to 2.0 mph with grade of 10% to 12%. Note time, symptoms, and walking distance/time at end of test
      4) Record ABI on each limb every minute until pre-exercise level is obtained. Terminate test at 10 minutes after exercise
   f. Findings/interpretation
      1) Exercise normally increases flow; occlusive disease does not allow for this increase and pressures decrease with exercise
      2) Pressure reduction proportionate to degree of stenosis and recovering time
      3) Multilevel disease is additive, as in segmental examination
      4) If pressures do not decrease with exercise, suspect noncirculatory origin of leg pain
   g. Limitations: reserve test for patients who are physically able to perform exercise safely. Contraindicated for patients who have angina, known abnormal cardiac stress test, recent coronary artery bypass graft without normal postoperative stress test, significant dyspnea, uncontrolled hypertension, or unable to ambulate unassisted
   h. Complications/precautions: Patients who have unknown cardiac or pulmonary disease may experience cardiac or respiratory symptoms during testing. Be prepared to abort testing; have rescue equipment/system available. Because of the high percentage of cardiac disease, cardiac monitoring during testing is recommended
   i. Nursing implications
      1) Constant observation, monitoring recommended
      2) Rapid pressure recordings required for accuracy of results
      3) Contact referring provider if patient is not appropriate candidate for exercise
5. Pulse volume recording (PVR) (see Fig. 5-6)
   a. Purpose: Record volume changes in limb with each arterial pulsation. May be used as alternative waveform to analog waveforms or used to supplement arterial analysis

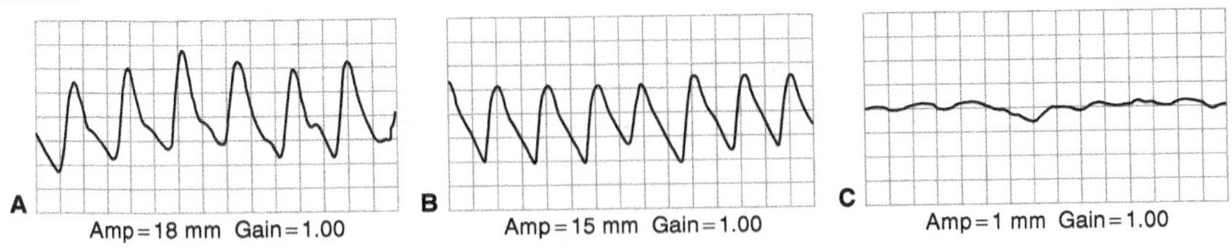

FIGURE 5-6. Pulse volume recordings. **A.** Normal. **B.** Mild arterial disease. **C.** Severe arterial disease.

b. Clinical indication: used with ABI, segmental, or toe pressure studies
c. Patient preparation: as for ABI, segmental, or toe pressure study
d. Instrumentation: air plethysmography. Pneumatic (air-filled) cuff applied to extremity, inflated to low pressure (~60 mm Hg) to ensure contact with skin and compression of venous component of flow. Volume changes in limb with each pulsation result in pressure changes within air-filled cuff. These are recorded as waveforms and analyzed for normal configuration
e. Procedure: as for ABI or segmental pressure examination. A small cushion is placed beneath heels. Large thigh cuff is placed as proximally as possible on thigh. Cuffs are inflated one at a time, to a pressure of 60 to 65 mm Hg. Volume recordings are obtained at each level for five or six cardiac cycles
f. Findings/interpretation
   1) Normal: sharp systolic peak; prominent dicrotic wave
   2) Mildly diminished: sharp systolic peak; absent dicrotic notch; downslope bowed away from baseline
   3) Moderately diminished: flattened systolic peak; upslope and downslope nearly equal; dicrotic wave absent
   4) Severely abnormal: pulse wave of very low amplitude or entirely absent; if present, equal upslope and downslope time
g. Limitations: patient must be able to lie still; tremor and motion interfere with accuracy of recording. Obesity may limit cuff placement as with segmental examination. Pain is not usually a limitation because the cuffs are not inflated above arterial systolic pressure
h. Complications/precautions: usually acceptable to perform following distal bypass graft procedure; check with surgeon as indicated
i. Nursing implications: analysis of PVR from different levels provides information regarding level or site of disease and estimate of severity of stenotic process

6. Arterial duplex scan with color Doppler of lower extremity (see Fig. 5-7)
   a. Purpose: localizing and grading stenotic lesions in the arterial system or bypass (Hodgkiss-Harlow & Bandyk, 2012) grafts in the lower extremities. Used in conjunction with ABIs, segmental pressures, or PVRs
   b. Indications
      1) Native vessels: claudication, rest pain, absent/diminished pulses, edema limiting arterial examination, cold sensitivity, identification of isolated stenotic lesions suitable for angioplasty/stent placement, suspected peripheral aneurysm with or without microemboli to foot, and documentation of peripheral flow in critically ill patient with balloon pump in place

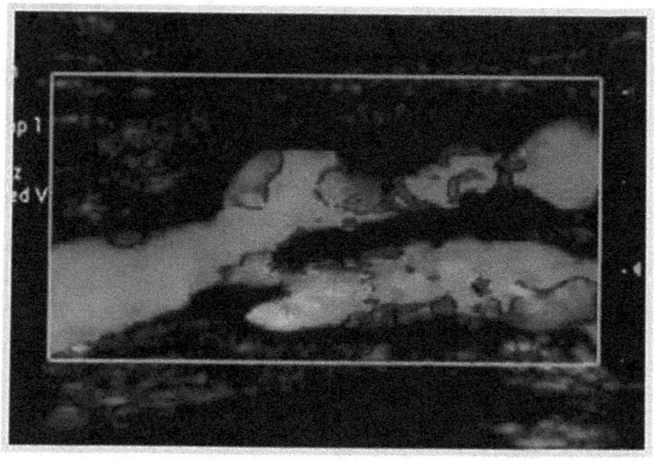

FIGURE 5-7. Arterial duplex.

2) Evaluation of bypass graft flow: Immediately postoperatively and annually for baseline evaluation; decrease in ABI value, new claudication or pain, bruit/thrill over graft
3) Evaluation of pulsatile mass—aneurysm, pseudoaneurysm, or hematoma—especially following groin cannulation for invasive procedure

c. Patient preparation
1) Explain procedure to patient
2) Remove all unnecessary clothing below waist; drape patient and keep warm
3) Position patient supine with head resting on pillow

d. Instrumentation: high-resolution duplex scanner with color flow capabilities
1) 5- to 7.5-MHz liner array probe. Low-frequency (2 to 3 MHz) probe if the aortoiliac segment is to be examined
2) Acoustic gel
3) 10-cm cuffs for ABI/brachial pressures; hand-held Doppler

e. Procedure
1) Record ABI or segmental pressures as above
2) Each vessel, common femoral artery (CFA), proximal, mid, and distal superficial femoral artery (SFA), popliteal, posterior tibial artery (PT), and dorsalis pedis artery (DP) is imaged along entire length using 2D color duplex and duplex Doppler in sagittal views. Bypass grafts are imaged in longitudinal view, including proximal and distal anastomosis and flow in native vessels
3) Color imaging is used to visualize any velocity increases that would suggest narrowing. Significant stenosis (usually ≥75%) will produce color aliasing—multiple colors mixed together combined with high-frequency signal >200 cm/sec
4) Doppler velocity samples are obtained proximal to, at, and distal to, any areas of stenosis. Doppler angle is set at 45 to 60 degrees. Smallest sample volume should be used with sample volume placed in center of vessel. Maintain Doppler angle parallel to blood flow. Obtain vessel diameter measurements
5) If no stenotic lesions are identified, velocities are recorded in the midportion of each segment

f. Findings/interpretation
   1) Normal flow: laminar pattern with highest frequency/velocity in center of lumen, lower frequencies/velocities along wall. Similar frequencies/velocities throughout vessel if unobstructed. Spectrum displayed on screen has sharp systolic peak, black "acoustic window" under peak—looks similar to analog waveform
   2) Stenotic flow: higher frequencies/velocities with more variable frequencies because of turbulence. The more stenosis, the higher the systolic frequencies and the more turbulence that is detected, especially in the segment just distal to the area of stenosis. Acoustic window becomes filled in with mixed frequency shifts ("spectral broadening")
   3) Occluded flow: dull "thump" with markedly reduced systolic flow, no diastolic flow proximal to the occlusion. At and distal to occlusion, no signal is obtained

Diameter reduction	Peak systolic velocity (PSV)
0% to 19%	Normal velocity pattern without increase in flow
20% to 49%	PSV increased >30% but <100% from normal proximal arterial segment
50% to 99%	PSV increased >100% or doubled baseline velocity (hemodynamically significant stenosis)
Occluded	No flow in imaged vessel
Waveform analysis	
0% to 19%	Triphasic; no spectral broadening
20% to 49%	Reverse component of waveform present; spectral broadening present but mild
50% to 99%	Loss of reverse component, spectral broadening, and velocity increase at stenosis; monophasic waveform and decreased systolic velocity distally
Occlusion	Monophasic, preocclusive "thump" heard proximally to stenosis; diminished velocity and monophasic waveform distally
Diameter enlargement	
Twice expected size	Suspect aneurysm; flow: often diminished velocity with midstream turbulence; thrombus seen along vessel wall
Pulsatile mass adjacent to vessel	Suspect pseudoaneurysm, may be able to identify attachment or neck, varying color flow intraluminal velocities with turbulence

g. Limitations
   1) Staples on skin may obscure imaging
   2) Time consuming

h. Complications/precautions: no adverse effects of diagnostic ultrasound have been identified
   1) Pain control measures may be needed for patients who have rest pain or postoperative pain
   2) Avoid acoustic gel in open wounds or incision line

i. Nursing implications
   1) Accurate identification and location of stenotic segments in native and conduit vessels, as well as postoperative fistula
   2) Because of time required, patients who cannot lie still may not be candidates for examination
   3) Ultrasound-guided compression of catheter-related femoral pseudoaneurysms possible with same scanning probe by manually compressing aneurysm at the point of communication with native artery. Several cycles of 10 minutes each may be needed to induce thrombosis unless pseudoaneurysm is chronic. Careful monitoring of site needed with repeat study 24 hours after compression. Monitor limb and distal pulses for evidence of change in perfusion

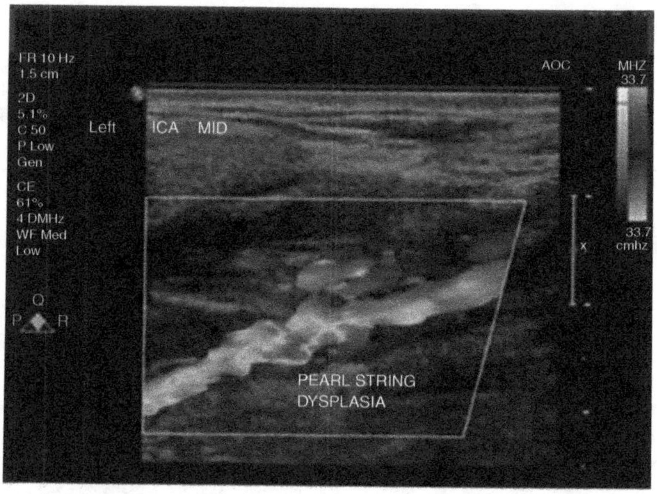

FIGURE 5-8. Carotid duplex with fibromuscular dysplasia.

7. Arterial duplex scan of extracranial arterial system (carotid, vertebrobasilar) (see Fig. 5-8)
   a. Purpose: examination of the extracranial arterial system for anatomic and physiologic evidence of arterial disease; helpful in detecting lesions amenable to operative intervention and following disease progression (Porreca, Rodriguez-Wong, & Hughes, 2012)
   b. Clinical indications
      1) Hemispheric symptoms of stroke
      2) Transient ischemic attacks; resolving ischemic neurologic deficit
      3) Amaurosis fugax or transient monocular blindness
      4) Nonhemispheric symptoms: dizziness, loss of memory, drop attacks, blurred or double vision, sudden nausea/vomiting, ataxia, or other symptoms suggestive of vertebrobasilar disease
      5) Discrepancy of brachial blood pressures of >20 mm Hg or symptoms of unilateral arm fatigue, diminished pulse, pallor, coolness, or other symptoms of subclavian steel syndrome
      6) Asymptomatic carotid bruit
      7) Intra- and postoperative surveillance of carotid endarterectomy and stent placement
      8) Evaluation for follow-up of known disease for progression
      9) Palpable pulsatile neck mass
      10) Neck trauma to assess for intimal tears (e.g., motor vehicle accident seat belt injury)
      11) Asymptomatic patient with planned cardiac bypass surgery to evaluate for comorbid carotid disease. Often surgically corrected simultaneously
   c. Patient preparation
      1) Explain procedure to patient
      2) Place patient supine with neck hyperextended (small pillow or towel roll may be used), head turned away from side to be examined. If not able to cooperate with this position, scanning may be done with patient sitting
      3) Obtain bilateral brachial blood pressures; assess for presence of carotid bruit

d. Instrumentation: high-resolution duplex scanner with color flow capabilities, 5- to 10-MHz linear array transducer, acoustic gel
e. Procedure
   1) Examiner is positioned at head of bed or at level of patient's shoulder
   2) Transducer is placed in transverse plane at base of neck, vessels identified to level of bifurcation. Color may be turned off to better image atherosclerotic plaque. Diameter reduction measurements are obtained
   3) In sagittal plane, images and duplex Doppler velocity measurements are obtained in the common, internal, and external carotid arteries
   4) If plaque is identified, velocity measurements are obtained proximal, mid, and distal to plaque formation. Highest velocity measurement used for calculation of internal carotid to common carotid ratio. Angle of insonation should be maintained as close to 60 degrees as possible
   5) Vertebral arteries are imaged in transverse and sagittal planes, imaging from the upper neck to the subclavian. Subclavian Doppler signals are also recorded
f. Findings/interpretation
   1) Images: intact intima visualized throughout common, internal, and external carotid vessels (Kingstone, Torres, & Currie, 2012)
   2) If plaque is identified, diameter reduction is measured in transverse plane by measuring with electronic calipers. Plaque is classified as homogenous (uniform composition), heterogenous (mixed composition), smooth, irregular, calcified, and ulcerated with or without thrombus.
   3) Doppler analysis
   4) Intraoperative carotid endarterectomy examination: moderate flow disturbance (peak systolic flow 125 to 140 cm/sec) with abnormal image warrants assessment with intraoperative arteriogram. Severe flow disturbance with marked spectral broadening and abnormal image warrants immediate revision
g. Limitations
   1) Requires experienced ultrasonographer and expensive scanning equipment
   2) Calcifications may obscure accuracy of diameter reduction measurements
   3) Vessel tortuosity and aberrant anatomy may limit accuracy; may confuse internal carotid artery (ICA) and external carotid artery (ECA) on imaging; need to rely on signal processing. ICA flow is low resistance (windy sound) with elevation off baseline; ECA flow is high resistance, similar to peripheral arterial signals
   4) High bifurcation under jaw limits complete evaluation
   5) Unable to examine above jaw into carotid siphon level
   6) May be difficult to identify vertebral system, especially in patient who has a thick neck or significant arthritic changes of spine
   7) Calculation of ICA/CCA ratio may be difficult in a patient who has arrhythmia, especially atrial fibrillation, because peak systolic velocities vary
   8) Occluded ICA may lead to "internalization" of ECA signal and mask diagnosis

h. Complications/precautions
   1) No adverse effects of diagnostic ultrasound
   2) Avoid excess pressure on carotid sinus during examination, which may provoke syncopal episode
   3) Patients who have sustained trauma should not undergo neck manipulation without physician clearance

i. Nursing implications
   1) Careful pretesting assessment, noting uniformity of blood pressures, neurologic status, presence of carotid bruit, and thorough history for risk factors and symptoms
   2) Comfort measures as indicated, especially in agitated patient, to ensure accuracy of results and avoid unnecessarily long examination time
   3) Correlation of test results with clinical indications, history, and physical examination; asymptomatic total occlusion is rare, but possible

8. Arterial duplex scan of renal and mesenteric arterial system and aorta (see Fig. 5-9)
   a. Purpose: anatomic and physiologic assessment of the mesenteric (splanchnic) and renal arterial systems (Neumyer, 2012)
   b. Clinical indications
      1) Abdominal bruit
      2) Unexplained weight loss
      3) Persistent postprandial nausea, vomiting, and abdominal pain
      4) Uncontrolled hypertension on antihypertensive medication therapy (suspected renovascular hypertension)
      5) Renal allograft rejection suspected
      6) Abdominal aortic aneurysm detection; identification of size and location
      7) Visualization of aortic endograft; documentation of position, patency, presence of endograft leak (Blackburn & Peterson-Kennedy, 2004; Iezzi et al., 2009)
   c. Patient preparation
      1) Fast for 6 to 8 hours before examination; preferable to perform study early in morning after overnight fast when bowel gas is at minimum

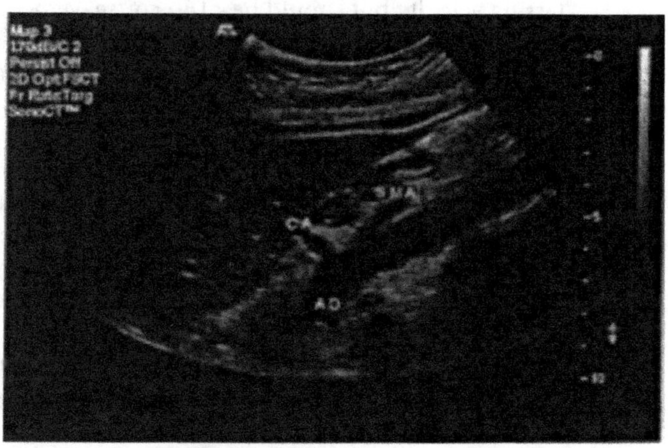

FIGURE 5-9. Normal duplex exam.

2) Supine position with head resting on pillow, slightly elevated. Will need to turn to right and left lateral decubitus position during renal examination

d. Instrumentation: high-resolution duplex scanner with color Doppler capabilities, low-frequency pulsed-Doppler probe (2 to 4 MHz), acoustic gel

e. Procedure
   1) Beginning at xyphoid process, using transverse view, identify proximal abdominal aorta; record Doppler signal in sagittal view; note any plaque or aneurysmal changes
   2) Image celiac artery and obtain Doppler signals—first branch of abdominal aorta (Roberts, Alonso, & Khatib, 2012)
   3) Image superior mesenteric artery and obtain Doppler signals—second branch of abdominal aorta just distal to celiac trunk
   4) Image and obtain signals in hepatic and splenic arteries
   5) If an enlarged inferior mesenteric artery is noted, this may suggest superior mesenteric artery (SMA) occlusive disease
   6) If scanning for suspicion of mesenteric ischemia, have patient ingest high-calorie liquid (protein shake). Repeat celiac and SMA measurements in 30 to 40 minutes
   7) If scanning for suspicion of renal artery stenosis, obtain vessel images and signals at origin (ostium), mid, and distal portions of both renal arteries, noting any plaque formations. Patient may be turned to right and left lateral decubitus positions to maximize imaging. Obtain images of each kidney, measuring pole to pole, and velocities from medulla, cortex, and renal hilum

f. Findings/interpretation
   1) Celiac signals: normally low resistance with open acoustic window in spectral wave, continuous forward flow throughout cardiac cycle. Systolic and diastolic velocities increase with protein supplement meal. Celiac systolic velocity >200 cm/sec is abnormal and indicates stenosis
   2) SMA signals: in fasting state, normally high resistance (triphasic) with early diastolic flow reversal and late diastolic forward flow. Postprandially, flow becomes low resistance because of vasodilatation of mesenteric vessels. Systolic velocity >275 to 300 cm/sec suggests stenosis of >70%. Postprandial PSV nearly doubles the fasting velocity but should be <160 cm/se. Velocities should return to baseline in 90 minutes
   3) Renal size: fairly uniform measurements of 10 cm in length. A pole-to-pole length of <9 cm or difference of 3 cm suggests stenosis or occlusion. Very small kidney length (5 to 6 cm) suggests chronic occlusion
   4) Renal signals: low-resistance pattern with continuous forward flow throughout cardiac cycle, similar to ICA or celiac. Normal PSV is <180 cm/se. Normal aorta systolic velocity is ~60 ± 15 cm/sec. Calculate peak systolic renal artery velocity/peak systolic aorta velocity ratio to obtain renal/aorta ratio. Normally, ratio is <3.5; if >3.5, stenosis is suspected
   5) Renal parenchymal signals (medulla and cortex): use highest amplitude and velocity to calculate end-diastolic/peak systolic ratio to determine parenchymal resistance. A ratio of <0.2 indicates intrinsic renal parenchymal disease (e.g., diabetic nephropathy)

6) Aorta: dilatation over twice normal size of 2 cm is indicative of aneurysmal changes; thrombus lining wall of aneurysm may be identified, as well as location and flow. Endograft surveillance should demonstrate reduction of aneurysmal sac over time; enlargement indicates endograft leak (Blackburn & Peterson-Kennedy, 2004)

g. Limitations
   1) Large body habitus
   2) Bowel gas artifact
   3) Adipose distribution
   4) Respiratory movements
   5) Unpredictable vessel course
   6) Recent abdominal surgery
   7) Requires very experienced ultrasonographer and expensive equipment
   8) Time consuming; adequate patient preparation is required
   9) Coexistent abdominal aorta may limit visualization of splanchnic and renal branches

h. Complications/precautions
   1) Patients who have true mesenteric ischemia may not tolerate high-calorie meal challenge; will cause significant pain or vomiting. Use clinical judgment
   2) Patients who have chronic obstructive pulmonary disease combined with obesity will not tolerate supine position for lengthy renal scan procedure—often 1 hour or more

i. Nursing implication
   1) Careful explanation of examination is required to ensure patient cooperation
   2) Comfort measures during lengthy examination, especially monitoring for respiratory distress as indicated by patient condition

B. Venous Examinations (see Fig. 5-10)

1. Venous duplex scan (Pellerito & Polak, 2012; Salles-Cunha & Beebe, 2001)
   a. Purpose: determine the presence and assess the location and extent of acute or chronic venous disease in the deep and superficial venous system by using ultrasound techniques
      1) Examination of choice for detection of deep vein thrombosis
      2) Visualization and localization of acute and chronic thrombosis
      3) Hemodynamic information of flow patterns in venous system
   b. Indication: evaluation of patients who have suspicion or clinical evidence of
      1) Deep venous thrombosis
      2) Postphlebitic syndrome
      3) Venous insufficiency
      4) Varicose veins
      5) Edema of the extremities of unknown etiology
      6) Mapping of greater and lesser saphenous, cephalic, and basilic veins before harvest for bypass surgery
   c. Patient preparation
      1) Explain procedure
      2) Remove all unnecessary clothing to expose extremity(ies) or area to be examined (abdomen, thorax) adequately
      3) Supine position

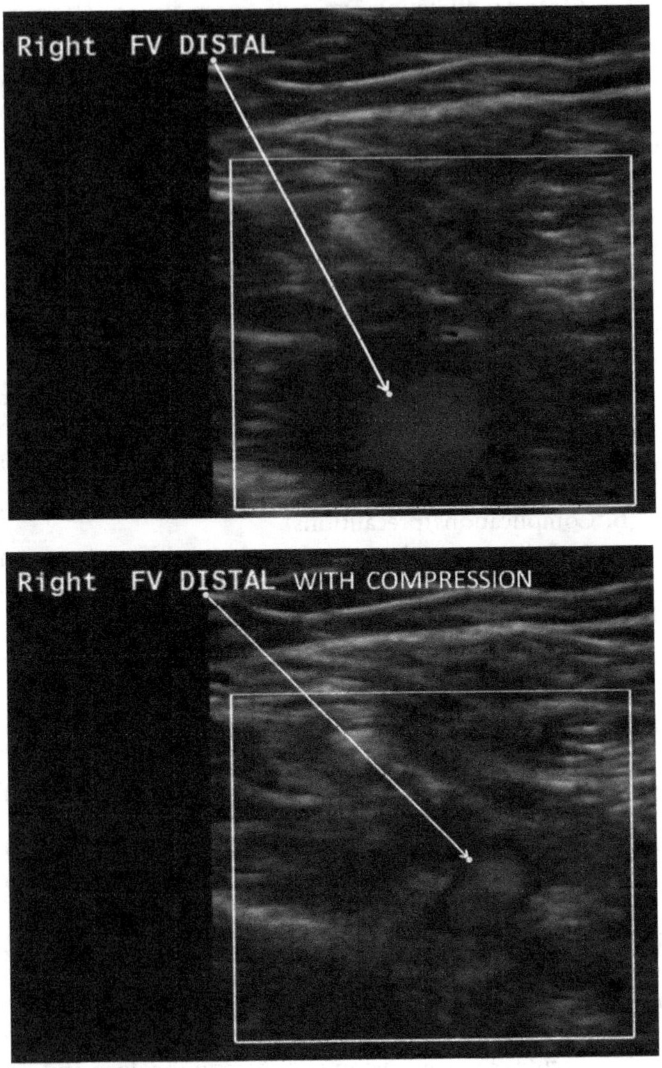

FIGURE 5-10. Normal duplex examination at the common femoral level.

4) For lower extremity examination, reverse Trendelenburg position to promote venous filling

d. Instrumentation
   1) High-resolution duplex scanner; color flow capabilities desired but not essential
   2) 5.0- to 7.5-MHz linear array transducer
   3) Acoustic gel

e. Procedure
   1) Lower extremity: with knee slightly flexed, sagittal and longitudinal (transverse) views are obtained from common femoral, superficial femoral, deep femoral (profunda), popliteal, posterior tibial, anterior tibial, and greater saphenous vein. Scan head is moved sequentially down leg, using color flow continuously if available. Gray scale used to evaluate age of thrombus, observing vessel wall echogenicity. If able, patient is placed in prone position for examination of popliteal, peroneal, soleal sinuses, and lesser saphenous vein

2) Upper extremity: with arm extended and elbow slightly flexed, sagittal and longitudinal views are obtained from jugular, subclavian, axillary, and brachial vein. Views are obtained of radial and ulnar veins from wrist to elbow. Cephalic vein is identified laterally at wrist and scanned to shoulder; basilic vein is identified medially at wrist and scanned to shoulder
3) Inferior vena cava and iliac veins: patient supine, using deep abdominal probe (2 to 3.5 MHz), scan from groin to above umbilicus in transverse and longitudinal positions, identifying bilateral common femoral and iliac veins merging to inferior vena cava below umbilicus

f. Findings/interpretation
1) Characteristics evaluated: vessel size, compressibility, flow pattern, presence/absence of thrombus
2) Normal vein: thin walls and slightly larger than corresponding artery; vein size fluctuates with respiration and increases with Valsalva maneuver. Veins collapse with external compression of probe pressure. Flowing blood seen on color flow as blue color
3) Five normal venous Doppler characteristics
   a) Spontaneity: does not require stimulation to be heard
   b) Phasicity: cyclic with respiration as inferior vena cava compressed by diaphragm and intrathoracic and intra-abdominal pressure varies with each breath
   c) Augmentation: limb compression (gentle squeeze by examiner) distal to probe causes increase in flow heard as rush of sound; seen as increased flow during imaging
   d) Competence: Valsalva maneuver/proximal compression normally results in cessation/interruption of flow signal
   e) Nonpulsatility: arterial pulsations are an abnormality; may indicate heart failure or fluid overload; do not indicate thrombosis
4) Thrombus: lack of color; blunted, absent, or continuous (nonphasic) signal; blunt or absent response to distal compression; solid speckled mass seen partially or completely filling lumen; vein partially or completely noncompressible; vessel markedly enlarged in diameter
5) Valvular incompetence: proximal compression results in reflux or retrograde flow, seen as red color; valves may be visualized as incompetent; distal compression causes bidirectional sound and augmented forward flow followed by reflux; blue color followed by red color as examiner releases squeeze (Mattos & Sumner, 2001; Pellerito & Polak, 2012)

g. Limitations
1) Obese or very muscular patient limits visualization and insonation; bowel gas limits abdominal examination
2) Problems with positioning (e.g., severe dyspnea, casts, traction)
3) Nonocclusive thrombus does not always alter flow signals; need to rely on imaging
4) Requires experienced examiner
5) Cannot rule out pulmonary embolus
6) Small vessels in calf difficult to examine; color helpful
7) Clavicle often obscures complete view of subclavian vein

8) Postoperative incisions with staples or wounds limit imaging
9) One intact valve proximal to an incompetent valve will invalidate reflux testing; difficult to generate sufficient pressure in some limbs to promote reflux

h. Complications/precautions: no adverse effects of diagnostic ultrasound identified. Other problems that may be encountered
1) Severe leg pain, infection, or wounds may not tolerate compression maneuvers
2) External compression (tumor, bone) alters venous flow; slight flexion of knee and elbow may improve flow signal
3) Anechoic thrombus: very early thrombus may not reflect echoes until more organized; rescan after several hours or the following day if suspicious
4) Acute versus chronic thrombus: often difficult to age clot because echogenicity is often similar; also difficult to identify new clot superimposed on old clot. Chronic thrombus usually shrinks with age, denser echoes, has collateral vessel, vessel size of near normal diameter
5) False aneurysms: appear as echo-filled mass, often partially clotted but with flowing blood in center of lumen; may be completely or partially compressible
6) Baker's popliteal cyst: anechoic (echo-free) fluid-filled structure in popliteal space adjacent to venous system, occasionally extends into calf; causes symptoms that mimic deep vein thrombosis (DVT); lacks color flow or signal; no connection to vascular system

i. Nursing implications
1) Pain medication; assistance with, or modification of, positioning for comfort
2) Repetitive distal compression empties venous system, allows system to refill after compressions to avoid false-positive results
3) No data to support concern that venous examination technique promotes propagation or embolization of clot

j. Venous duplex in the treatment of venous insufficiency
1) Endovascular radiofrequency ablation and thermal ablation; venous duplex is used to obtain access to the greater saphenous vein prior to the procedure (Gioviczki, Camerota, Dalsing, & Eklof, 2011)
2) Ultrasound-guided sclerotherapy, to help locate the vein prior to injection (Yamaki, Nozaki, Sakurai, Takeuchi, & Kono, 2008)

2. Plethysmography
a. Purpose: assessment of venous outflow; record volume changes in limbs by assessing, directly or indirectly, dimensional changes in response to temporary outflow obstruction or exercise (McPharlin, 2012). Several techniques include
1) Air
2) Impedance (IPG)
3) Strain gauge (SPG)
4) Photoplethysmography (PPG)

b. Indications: acute and chronic venous occlusive disease; venous insufficiency

c. Patient preparation
1) Explain procedure
2) Room must be ≥72°F for accurate testing
3) For air, IPG: patient is supine with legs elevated above heart, flexed at knee. Pneumatic cuff placed around thigh, connected to air pressure

system transducers applied to calf. IPG electrodes placed 8 to 12 cm apart around largest circumference of calf. For SPG, leg elevated off bed with gauge placed around largest circumference of calf

4) For PPG: patient sitting so that feet dangle; patient sits quietly for ≥2 minutes without talking. Phototransducer adhered to medial supramalleolar surface with double-stick tape 10 cm above malleolus, select skin with normal turgor and avoid wounds, varicosities, and areas of dense fibrosis

5) For SPG: patient sitting with both feet on floor; strain placed around calves with slight tension of gauge

d. Instrumentation (see "c")

e. Procedure

1) Air, IPG: after transducers placed, system is calibrated; pneumatic cuff inflated to approximately 60 mm Hg (above usual venous pressure) to occlude venous outflow temporarily; volume within calf increases during occlusion; recorded by transducer as increase from baseline on strip chart recorder. Cuff is deflated rapidly to allow for venous emptying, decrease in recording back to baseline

2) PPG: patient is instructed to dorsiflex and plantarflex feet rapidly 5 to 10 times to empty venous system. Tracing is recorded on strip chart to indicate decrease of venous capacity from baseline. Patient rests quietly without moving or talking while strip chart records postexercise return to baseline volume

3) SPG: patient raises and lowers heels five times. Recovery time measured on strip chart in seconds as for PPG. Cuff or tourniquet applied above gauge to occlude superficial system and test is repeated. SPG is also used for detection of DVT, similar to air or IPG

f. Findings/interpretation

1) Air, IPG: venous outflow at 3 seconds after cuff deflation is calculated and plotted on a scoring form. A positive test for DVT shows a marked decrease in outflow after cuff deflation (strip chart recording does not decrease to baseline)

2) PPG: normal recovery time after exercise is 25 seconds. If recovery occurs in <20 seconds, the test is positive for venous insufficiency that is due to reflux of flow in the venous system. A cuff can be applied above the knee and inflated to 60 mm Hg to identify superficial versus deep venous insufficiency. If recovery time normalizes with cuff inflation, superficial insufficiency is suspected. If recovery time remains abnormal before and after cuff inflation, the test is positive for deep venous insufficiency

3) SPG: normal recovery time is 12 seconds. Superficial venous incompetence is indicated by recovery of <12 seconds that normalizes with cuff or tourniquet. Deep venous insufficiency does not normalize with cuff or tourniquet. For DVT detection, results expressed as centimeters per 100 cm^3 of tissue per minute (quantitative measurement)

g. Limitations

1) For SPG or PPG, patient must be able to cooperate with ankle exercises. Calf compressions could be done manually by examiner if necessary, but this is not ideal

2) Wounds or dense fibrosis may limit PPG transducer placement

3) For IPG or air plethysmography, patient must be able to lie supine with leg above heart. Severe congestive heart failure (CHF), dyspnea, obesity, or arthritic conditions may limit cooperation

4) False-positive results: improper positioning, extrinsic compression
5) False-negative results: nonocclusive thrombus may not be detected
6) Detection of calf thrombi not possible with these methods

h. Complications/precautions
1) Capacitance outflow testing cannot be used to localize thrombus to specific site
2) Cannot be used to track progress of disease reliably

i. Nursing implications
1) Demonstration of technique for PPG and SPG may be helpful for patient before testing to aid understanding and cooperation during testing
2) Pain control may be required before air or IPG testing

III. Invasive Diagnostic Studies

A. Arteriography (Vogelzang, 2004)

1. Purpose: obtain radiographic images of various segments of arterial circulation via catheter-based injection of contrast media to outline vessel lumen
2. Indications
   a. Atherosclerotic, thrombotic, and embolic occlusions in the extremities or extracranial or intracranial circulation, visceral circulation for renovascular hypertension or ischemia
   b. Congenital abnormalities
   c. Vasculitides
   d. Ischemia related to dissection or trauma
   e. Provide anatomic detail before and after percutaneous or surgical intervention
   f. Aneurysms
   g. Vascular tumors in solid organs, such as liver or kidneys
3. Patient preparation
   a. Thorough explanation of procedure; discuss risks/benefits; obtain informed consent
   b. Laboratory evaluation
      1) Renal function: serum urea nitrogen, creatinine
      2) Bleeding tendency: prothrombin time, international normalized ration (INR), partial thromboplastin time, platelet count
   c. Assess for allergies to iodine or contrast material. May require pretreatment or cancellation for history of severe anaphylaxis
   d. Assess women of child-bearing age for pregnancy. Appropriate precautions or alternative procedure may be indicated
   e. If patient is taking metformin, hold medication for specified period of time per institution protocol (2 to 5 days). May resume 1 to 2 days after procedure (Pomposelli, 2010)
   f. Nothing by mouth (NPO) for specified period of time before examination per institution protocol (usually after midnight)
   g. Pain control and comfort measures as indicated
   h. IV access established
   i. Discontinue anticoagulants
   j. Basic monitoring: blood pressure, cardiac monitor, pulse oximetry
   k. Other monitoring devices as indicated by patient condition (e.g., urinary catheter, central venous pressure)

4. Instrumentation
   a. Iodine contrast agent
      1) High-osmolar, ionic: less expensive but more adverse effects of burning pain, allergy, and higher intravascular osmotic fluid shift (difficult to tolerate for patients who have CHF or renal failure)
      2) Low-osmolar, ionic, and nonionic: very expensive but with less pain, and therefore better images; fewer allergic reactions, lower osmotic effect on intravascular fluid shift
      3) Nonionic compounds: reduced risk of contrast-related anaphylaxis reactions (urticaria, flushing, coughing, wheezing, dyspnea, facial edema, sudden decrease in blood pressure)
   b. Transarterial catheter and guidewire
   c. Sequential imaging x-ray equipment, usually computerized digital imaging (DI) or digital subtraction angiography (DSA)
      1) DI: all structures, including bones, soft tissues, gas, and contrast, appear on same image. Motion does not affect image, but full-strength contrast is needed for adequate resolution of image
      2) DSA: Computer subtracts early images from later images in same filming sequence. Structures (bone, soft tissue) that do not change during contrast injection are canceled out or disappear. Less contrast with better resolution, but any motion limits quality of final image
   d. Team: radiologist, radiographic technologist, nurse, darkroom technician, support staff, including quality assurance coordinator
5. Procedure
   a. Patient preparation completed: adequately draped, comfort measures, monitoring equipment applied, IV access and fluid administration established, skin site for injection prepared
   b. Seldinger technique, usually of femoral artery, but may use lumbar, brachial, or axillary; needle puncture of artery followed by placement of guidewire through needle into lumen of vessel. Catheter threaded over guidewire; guidewire removed and catheter placed at desired site with fluoroscopy guidance. Catheter connected to pressure injection equipment programmed for appropriate flow rate and volume. Sequential x-ray images obtained
      1) Total contrast does not usually exceed 350 mL
      2) Heparinized flush solution constantly infused to prevent thrombosis
   c. Catheter withdrawn; pressure placed over puncture site for 15 to 20 minutes; if no bleeding, patient is transferred to recovery area or hospital room for observation. Immobility for 4 to 6 hours to prevent bleeding
6. Findings/interpretation
   a. Sites of stenosis or occlusion are identified by partial filling defect or complete lack of filling of vessel with contrast distal to occlusion
   b. Aneurysm, pseudoaneurysm, tumor or bypass grafts are identified with or without obstruction, thrombus
7. Limitations
   a. Renal impairment or history of allergy to contrast medium may limit or prevent use
      1) Absolute contraindication: anaphylaxis with previous iodine exposure
      2) Relative contraindication: renal impairment; rash with previous iodine exposure

3) Nephrotoxicity related to contrast: occurs equally with high and low-osmolar agents, even when patients are well hydrated. Need to identify patients at risk, control comorbidities (e.g., CHF) before procedure as much as possible, assure appropriate hydration with IV fluids before and during procedure, limit amount of contrast injected during imaging

b. Puncture of occluded vessel with atherosclerotic plaque limits ability to pass guidewire and catheter; alternate site needed

c. Motion and artifact limit quality of DSA images

d. Tortuosity of vessels may make catheter placement difficult. Experienced angiographer required to select appropriate catheters and guidewires, decide about selective catheterization of vessels, amount and timing of contrast injection, filming sequence and projections

e. Not useful for screening or multiple sequential studies because of cost and complication risk

8. Complications/precautions (Vogelzang, 2004)
   a. Puncture site hematoma: swelling at puncture site or loss of pulse
   b. Pseudoaneurysm: pulsatile mass over puncture site
   c. Local arterial occlusion: cool, pulseless limb
   d. Embolus: loss of distal pulse
   e. Contrast-induced allergy/anaphylaxis: urticaria, wheezing, dyspnea, cardiac arrhythmia, cardiac arrest; reactions may be immediate or delayed. Emergency equipment and personnel available
   f. Contrast-induced renal failure: anuria, oliguria
   g. Neurologic complication: aphasia, confusion, unconsciousness, hemiparesis
9. Nursing implications
   a. Careful monitoring during and after procedure for complications
   b. Postprocedure care
      1) Every 15 minutes vital signs, pulse checks, neurologic status for 1 hour, then every hour for 2 hours or as per institution protocol
      2) Assess puncture site for hematoma
      3) Bedrest for 6 hours or per institution protocol, with affected leg straight
      4) IV fluid for 6 hours
      5) Resume heparin as indicated 4 hours after procedure
      6) Resume medications and diet
      7) Assess renal function within 24 hours with serum urea nitrogen, creatinine; monitor urine output. Assess complete blood count if translumbar approach is used

B. Venography (Kamida, Kistner, Elkof, & Masuda, 2001)

1. Purpose: radiographic examination of the deep and superficial venous system to identify acute or chronic venous occlusive disease when sonographic or capacitance study is nondiagnostic
   a. Ascending venography: assessment of anatomy and patency of deep veins
   b. Descending venography: assessment of valvular competence in lower extremities
2. Indications
   a. DVT suspected but not proven by noninvasive method because of patient-related or technical limitations, especially

1) Tibial veins
2) Upper extremity veins
3) Inferior vena cava

b. Distinguish between thrombosis and extrinsic compression (e.g., renal cell carcinoma with invasion of inferior vena cava)
c. Preoperative investigation for patient who has chronic occlusive disease with severe postphlebitic syndrome contemplating venous reconstructive surgery
d. Superior vena cava syndrome
    1) Extrinsic compression from tumor or radiation effect
    2) Thrombosis of superior vena cava from indwelling catheter
e. Congenital venous anomalies

3. Patient preparation
    a. Explain procedure; obtain informed consent.
        1) Patient should understand that multiple attempts at venipuncture might be required
        2) Cannulation of pedal vein usually is painful
        3) Main complication is contrast-induced thrombophlebitis
    b. Assess for allergy to iodine contrast
    c. Hold metformin as for angiography per institution protocol
    d. Assess women of child-bearing age for pregnancy; alternative procedure indicated
    e. Clear liquids 3 to 4 hours before examination
    f. Start IV before examination
    g. Emergency equipment and personnel available
    h. Position: 45 degrees upright with leg to be examined nonweight bearing
4. Instrumentation
    a. Contrast medium
    b. Fluoroscopy equipment
    c. Digital or digital subtraction imaging equipment
    d. Team: as for arteriography
5. Procedure
    a. Pedal vein cannulated with small IV needle, preferably at lateral dorsal aspect of foot
    b. Contrast medium injected rapidly by hand
    c. Images of tibial, popliteal, femoral, and iliac veins obtained, with attempt to see contrast entering inferior vena cava
    d. For inferior or superior vena cava, cannulation done at femoral or antecubital vein level
    e. For descending venography: femoral catheterization; contrast injected with patient upright
    f. Selective venography and venous pressure monitoring may be done to evaluate the portal system or renal or hepatic veins with selective sampling of blood pressures or serum samples (e.g., evaluation of renovascular hypertension)
6. Findings/interpretation
    a. Normal ascending venogram: contrast fills the entire deep venous system without interruption or intraluminal defects
    b. Abnormal ascending venogram: thrombus is a filling defect (partial obstruction) or complete lack of filling of venous system with contrast (total occlusion)

   c. Chronic or recanalized DVT: strands within veins; parallel collateral channels or small channels within old intraluminal fibrotic thrombus
   d. Normal descending venogram: intact valves stop the flow of contrast down the leg
   e. Abnormal descending venogram: damaged or absent valves allow contrast to fill venous system in retrograde fashion to distal level

7. Limitations
   a. Painful procedure
   b. Difficult to cannulate pedal veins, especially in presence of edema, obesity, or trauma
   c. Contrast allergy may be absolute (anaphylaxis) or relative (rash) contraindication. Pretreatment with steroid therapy may be indicated to prevent or minimize reaction
   d. Often difficult to visualize proximal iliac system and subclavian system reliably
8. Complications/precautions
   a. Main complication: contrast-induced thrombophlebitis caused by endothelial injury. Prevent by flushing contrast from venous system with heparinized saline solution
   b. Allergic reaction to contrast (see Angiography)
   c. Extravasation of contrast from injection site: leads to local inflammation or skin necrosis; rare
9. Nursing implications
   a. Careful explanation of procedure to patient
   b. Appropriate comfort/pain control measures
   c. Postprocedure monitoring for local complications and thrombophlebitis
   d. If femoral vein is used, patient is maintained on bedrest for 2 hours after the procedure or per institution protocol with appropriate observation of cannulation site for hematoma, bleeding

IV. Additional Diagnostic Studies

A. Transcutaneous Oxygen Tension (Kalani, Brismar, Fagrell, Ostergren, & Jorneskog, 1999)

1. Purpose: assess tissue metabolism as a function of perfusion in the evaluation of PAD
2. Indications
   a. Evaluation of degree of ischemia in an extremity
   b. Prediction of success of ulcer healing
   c. Prediction of success of amputation site healing
   d. Identification of patients who have comorbidities and are at risk for pressure ulcer development (e.g., paraplegia, diabetes)
   e. Prediction of success of therapeutic intervention in prevention of amputation (e.g., spinal cord stimulation)
3. Patient preparation: relaxed, in supine position with access to brachial artery midway between axilla and antecubital fossa and anterolateral and posterior calf
4. Instrumentation: transcutaneous oxygen sensors (e.g., Kontron, Roche, Inc.)
5. Procedure for determining below knew amputation (BKA) healing potential
   a. After cleansing skin on arm and leg areas with alcohol pad, affix sensors with double-stick tape

b. Anterior and posterior calf monitoring sites are located 6 to 8 inches below knee overlying the anterior tibialis muscle and medial head of gastrocnemius muscle, respectively
c. Measurements are recorded after 15 minutes, by means of a sensor temperature at 44°C
d. A calf/brachial PO_2 index is calculated by use of the lesser value from the lower extremity

6. Findings/interpretation
   a. Absolute value (transcutaneous partial pressure of oxygen ($tcPO_2$)): 50% of patients with $tcPO_2$ of <20 mm Hg had primary healing of BKA wound (Kram, Appel, & Shoemaker, 1989)
   b. Calf/brachial PO_2 index
      1) ≤0.20: unsuccessful healing of BKA
      2) ≥0.20: successful healing with sensitivity, specificity, and overall accuracy of 100%, 86%, and 98%, respectively (Kram et al., 1989)
   c. No significant difference noted in $tcPO_2$ values or calf/brachial PO_2 indices between diabetics/nondiabetics, smokers/nonsmokers, trauma/peripheral vascular disease (PVD) patients. No significant difference between anterior and posterior calf readings in ultimate outcome (Kram et al., 1989)
7. Limitations
   a. Successful wound healing occurs in a significant percentage of patients with $tcPO_2$ <20 mm Hg. Use of the calf/brachial index increases predictive value of test
   b. $tcPO_2$ measurements are dependent on systemic blood flow and arterial oxygen content (determined by cardiac output, arterial PO_2, hemoglobin, temperature) which may vary significantly in the same patient from one measurement to the next; makes comparison recordings difficult unless indices are used
   c. $tcPO_2$ values do not always reflect underlying muscle oxygenation, which must be adequate for wound healing
8. Complications/precautions: none
9. Nursing implications
   a. Note changes in patient condition between recordings, especially if not calculating calf/brachial index
   b. This test may be useful when added to other clinical assessment parameters for wound healing or ulcer formation potential, but should not be relied upon solely for wound or healing assessment

B. Transcranial Doppler (TCD) (see Fig. 5-11)

1. Purpose: noninvasive evaluation of intracranial arterial anatomy and flow hemodynamics
   a. Gray scale image identifies intracranial structures
   b. Color Doppler identifies flow direction, relative velocity, and flow disturbance
   c. "TCD is an extension of the extracranial carotid duplex scan. It provides information regarding blood flow velocity of the intracranial vessels in the presence of extracranial occlusive disease. Changes observed include decreased blood flow velocity, change in direction of flow, delayed systolic upstroke, decreased pulsatility, and turbulence" (Sanders, 1998)

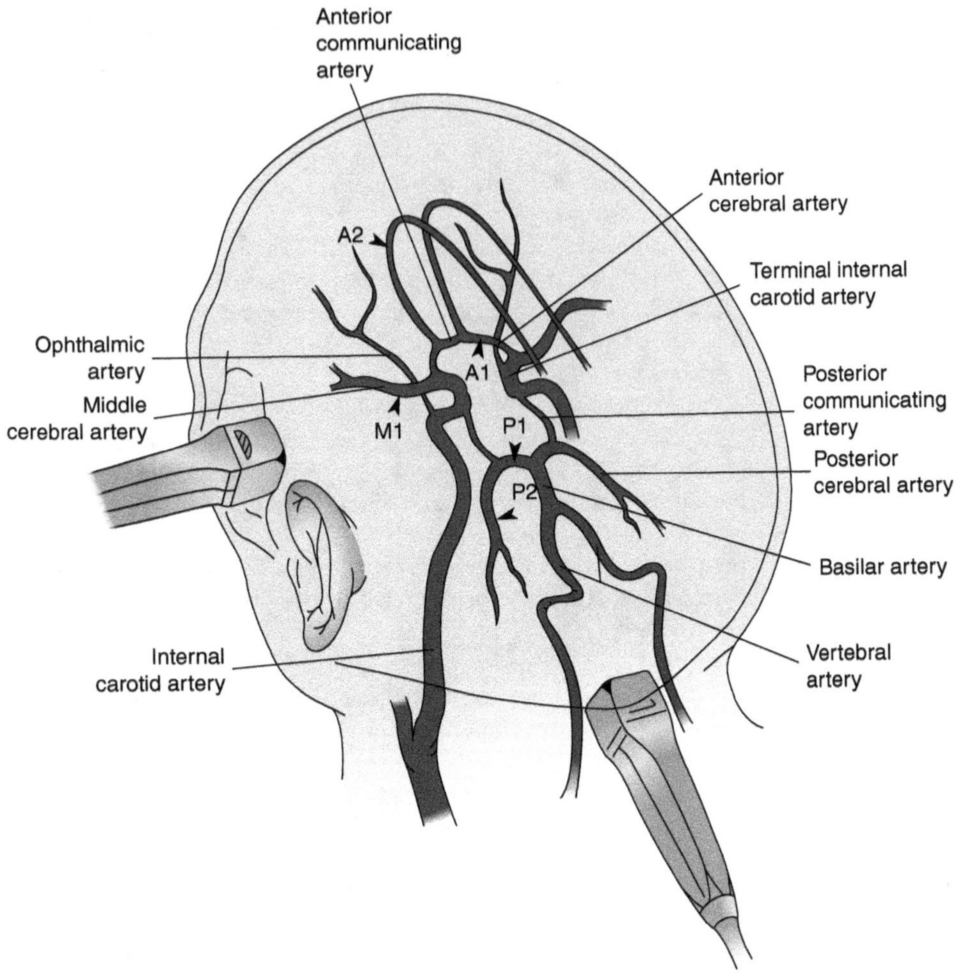

FIGURE 5-11. Diagram of normal Circle of Willis and the window used in transcranial examination.

2. Indications
   a. Intracranial stenosis
   b. Collateral circulation in patients who have ICA occlusions
   c. Vertebrobasilar insufficiency; subclavian steal syndrome
   d. Cerebral vasospasm after subarachnoid hemorrhage: onset, location, severity, and course over time
   e. Assessment of circulatory status in patients who are suspected of brain death
   f. Monitor hemodynamics in surgery (carotid endarterectomy and cardiac surgery on cardiopulmonary bypass) or with therapeutic interventions (e.g., embolization procedures)
   g. Identification of arteriovenous malformations
3. Instrumentation
   a. 2-MHz pulsed-Doppler transducer with real-time B-mode color duplex scanner
   b. Nonimaging, hand-held 2- to 3-MHz probe that provides online spectral analysis that gives time-average velocity measurements, including peak systole, mean velocity, and pulsatility index
   c. Acoustic coupling gel

4. Patient preparation
   a. Nonoperative: patient initially supine with head flat or slightly elevated, accessible for scanning at temporal and orbital regions. For foramen/occipital scanning, patient may turn to side with chin tucked toward chest or may be sitting with chin bent toward chest. Technologist sits at head of patient
   b. Intraoperative: transtemporal Doppler with standard nonimaging probe secured onto headset to allow for continuous intraoperative monitoring of middle cerebral artery (MCA)
5. Procedure: three standard "windows" (areas on skull where bone is thin enough to allow penetration by ultrasound) are used to insonate the intracranial vessels. Depth, color, and Doppler signals assist in vessel identification
   a. Temporal: when scanned in transverse plane, provides access to major vessels of Circle of Willis
      1) MCA: from terminal branches to the MCA/anterior cerebral artery (ACA) bifurcation
      2) ACA: usually the A1 segment is seen
      3) Posterior cerebral artery (PCA): P1 and P2 segments
      4) Terminal internal carotid artery
      5) Anterior communicating artery, if functional
      6) Posterior communicating artery, if functional
   b. Orbital
      1) Ophthalmic artery
      2) Carotid siphon
   c. Transforaminal (foramen magnum/occipital)
      1) Distal vertebral arteries
      2) Proximal basilar artery
   d. Submandibular: internal carotid artery insonated to obtain hemispheric ratio of PSV in MCA compared with ICA (MCA/ICA)
6. Findings/interpretation
   a. Vessel identification criteria
      1) Direction of blood flow relative to transducer
      2) Relationship to the acoustic window used: probe orientation
      3) Depth of vessel
      4) Traceability: distance that the course of the vessel can be followed
      5) Spatial relationships to other vessels
      6) Bony landmarks (used for imaging studies)
   b. Under normal conditions, mean velocities are higher in the anterior circulation (ICA) than in the posterior circulation (vertebrobasilar)
   c. MCA carries 80% of flow received by the cerebral hemispheres; the mean velocity normally is highest in the MCA, followed by the ACA, PCA, basilar, and vertebrals
   d. Intracranial cerebral artery stenosis
      1) Focal increase in velocity with associated turbulence or disturbed flow beyond stenosis
      2) Decreased velocities proximal or distal to stenosis
      3) Delayed systolic upstroke
      4) Abnormal pulsatility index
   e. MCA/ICA ratio
      1) >3.00: consistent with vasospasm
      2) 3.00 or less: consistent with hyperdynamic flow that is due to stenosis

f. Intraoperative monitoring: when the carotid artery is clamped during endarterectomy, a decrease of >65% from the preclamp value, or a decrease to zero, in mean blood flow velocity in the ipsilateral MCA is consistent with inadequate collateral flow. Carotid shunting is indicated
g. Diagnosis of vasospasm: usually occurs between days 4 and 14 after subarachnoid hemorrhage; there are three categories of vasospasm as reflected by increased velocity
   1) Mild: 120 to 140 cm/sec
   2) Moderate: 140 to 200 cm/sec
   3) Severe: >200 cm/sec
   4) Velocity elevations >250 cm/sec are associated with poor outcome
h. Reversal of flow direction indicates occlusion in another vessel segment (e.g., reversal of flow in vertebral artery indicates occlusion in ipsilateral proximal subclavian artery)

7. Limitations
   a. No temporal window: 15% of population, varies with age, sex, race. Most difficult are older women and African Americans; may be unilateral
   b. Unable to insonate 5% to 10% of patients
   c. Patient capacity to cooperate (e.g., restless, seizure, pain) may limit examination
   d. Anatomic variants occur in up to 50% of population, with most common being vessel course, size, and origin
   e. Requires high degree of technical expertise and experience; extensive learning curve for accuracy
   f. Occlusion versus technical difficulty: lack of vessel identification may be due to technical difficulty in locating vessel or total occlusion
   g. Aliasing: extremely high velocities will be elevated off the scale so that accurate measurement of peak systole is not possible
   h. Other factors that affect examination findings include age, hematocrit, hyperventilation, hypoventilation, cardiac output, and presence of extracranial carotid disease
8. Complications/precautions
   a. Recent eye surgery: orbital portion of examination may be contraindicated; need approval of ophthalmologist
9. Nursing implications
   a. Measures to promote optimal results: position, comfort measures, measures to stabilize hemodynamic and respiratory status during examination (e.g., avoidance of hypo- or hyperventilation, fever, pain control)
   b. Patient and family support during examination as needed, depending on clinical situation
   c. For patients who have high-grade stenosis of extracranial or intracranial system, monitor for signs and symptoms of cerebrovascular changes
   d. Postoperative care and assessment as indicated, especially neurologic and cranial nerve assessment/monitoring

C. CT and Spiral CT Angiography (Spiral CTA) (see Fig. 5-12)

1. Purpose: detailed identification of anatomic structures obtained by radiologic cross-sectional tomograms (slices) of structures in body cavity—head, abdomen, pelvis
   a. Major advantage over other imaging modalities: direct visualization of arterial wall and processes/structures (air, fluid, hematoma) around vessels using little radiation exposure

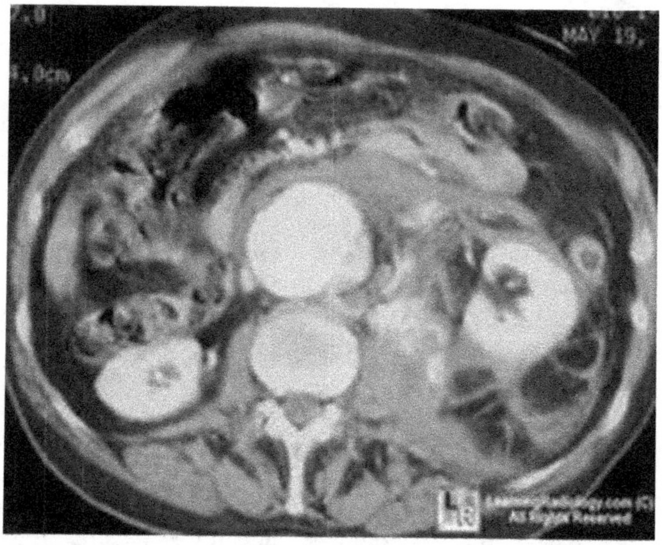

FIGURE 5-12. Computed tomography of an abdominal aortic aneurysm.

   b. Spiral CTA: overlapping slices or images allow for multiplanar reformations, 2D and three-dimensional (3D) projections of vascular structures
2. Indications
   a. Staging of aneurysms
   b. Identification of postoperative complications: graft infection, repetitive graft occlusion, hemorrhage, abscess, endoleaks (Bent, Jaskolka, Lindsay, & Tan, 2010)
   c. Guidance of biopsy procedures
   d. CTA: evaluation of Circle of Willis, carotid bifurcation, aortic arch, and abdominal vasculature for stenosis, thrombosis, aneurysmal changes, tumor encasement, dissection
      1) Pulmonary emboli and aberrancies of pulmonary vascular (i.e., coarctation, double aortic arch, right arch)
      2) Portal vein thrombosis
      3) Renal vein involvement in renal cell carcinoma
      4) Vascular encasement in pancreatic carcinoma
      5) Aberrant arterial branching in celiac and mesenteric system for presurgical planning
3. Patient preparation
   a. Explain procedure; obtain informed consent.
   b. If contrast needed, assess for iodine allergy. See precautions under "angiography"
      1) Assess for comorbidities: renal failure, diabetes, CHF
      2) Hold metformin as for angiography
      3) Assess women of child-bearing age for pregnancy; alternative procedure may be indicated
      4) Start IV line for injection of contrast for CT and spiral CTA
      5) For abdomen and pelvic CT, patient also drinks contrast preparation to illuminate bowel structures
4. Instrumentation: CT scanner (gantry) with experienced radiology team

5. Procedure
   a. Patient placed supine in circular open gantry with x-ray tube and multiple x-ray detectors
   b. Tube moves around body while emitting x-rays confined to narrow slice varying from 2 to 10 mm. Rays pass through body and are detected on opposite side by detectors
   c. High-speed computer processes images
   d. Spiral CTA: patient passes through gantry at constant velocity while x-ray rotates at constant velocity around patient; this produces a helical or spiral x-ray path around patient. Continuous data sent to computer with overlapping of slices to form 2D and 3D images
      1) CTA dependent on proper contrast delivery with delay time between injection and image acquisition of 20 to 25 seconds for head, neck, and thorax, but 50 to 70 seconds for abdomen
      2) Patient may be asked to hold breath for up to 30 seconds periodically; holding still is very important for accuracy of images
   e. CT-guided biopsy/drainage procedures: needle, catheter, or guidewire placed into fluid collections, masses to drain abscesses or obtain biopsy of deep masses
6. Findings/interpretation: identification of anatomic pathology of vascular system and surrounding structures
7. Limitations
   a. Expensive equipment requiring experienced technical support staff and radiologist who is familiar with interpretation of results
   b. Patient must be able to lie flat in gantry without moving for optimal imaging
   c. Use of contrast to enhance imaging may not be possible because of allergy
8. Complications/precautions
   a. Allergic reaction to contrast: need emergency equipment and team as for angiography/venography
   b. Critically ill patients need attendant in room: attendant requires lead apron for protection
   c. If examination is being done for suspected aneurysm, monitor closely for evidence of rupture and transport to operating room immediately if indicated
   d. If CT used to obtain biopsy or drain fluid collections, monitor for unexpected bleeding, puncture of organ, and so forth
9. Nursing implications
   a. Adequate preparation by way of IV hydration if contrast is used
   b. Monitor for adverse effects of contrast: urine output, creatinine, evidence of rash or allergic reaction
   c. Monitor for evidence of hemorrhage or sepsis if biopsy or drainage procedure is performed
   d. Sedation/pain control measures as indicated

D. Magnetic Resonance Angiography (MRA)

1. Purpose: noninvasive imaging of vascular structures in multiple projections obtained using the magnetic properties of protons in blood and adjacent tissues. When protons are excited by a pulse of radiofrequency energy, they return the signal, which is recorded and reconstructed into an image that represents proton density or emitted energy (Dolmatch,

Davros, & Grist, 1996). The rate of flow of protons within blood influences the quantity and rate of energy emission. Laminar flow is imaged most reliably by MRA; turbulence may simulate disease that is not accurate. Nevertheless, many institutions are replacing angiography with MRA technology for imaging the vascular system noninvasively, because it eliminates the need for invasive catheterization and contrast. MRA images are based on physiology of flowing blood rather than intraluminal anatomy. Functional studies that show movement of blood flow are being developed

2. Clinical indications
   a. Stenosis in carotid, thoracic, and abdominal vascular systems, including renal and mesenteric stenosis
   b. Thoracic and abdominal aneurysm
   c. Preliminary studies show promise for imaging the infrainguinal arterial system using MRA (Dolmatch et al., 1996)
3. Patient preparation
   a. Explain procedure; obtain informed consent. Patient should be aware of need to lie still while enclosed in hollow tube for several minutes, unless "open" MRI unit is used, and loud sound of magnet during procedure
   b. Evaluate for claustrophobia; medication may be indicated
   c. Remove all metals
   d. Patients with implanted metal port (Port-o-cath, Infusaport), intrauterine device, pacemakers, implanted defibrillators, implanted surgical clips, joint prosthesis, vena cava filters, or life support devices are not candidates for this examination. In most cases, metallic fillings, braces, surgical screws, staples, and pins pose no risk but may distort images
      1) Metals produce large artifacts that distort image
      2) Surgical clips in head might move during examination with MRI
      3) Force of magnet in room pulls devices toward magnet, risking harm to patient
      4) Some tattoos and permanent eyeliner may contain metallic iron oxide and could heat up during MRI
   e. Evaluate for pregnancy and notify radiologist; there is no radiation exposure risk but MRI is usually avoided in first 12 weeks
4. Instrumentation: MRI scanner (cylindrical magnet) combined with time-of-flight (TOF) or phase-contrast (PC) angiographic imaging capabilities
   a. TOF: faster imaging with better spatial resolution
   b. PC: allows visualization of smaller vessels or vessels with slower flow
   c. Gadolinium may be used as a contrast medium for selected tests. No renal toxicity or allergic problems related to use of gadolinium
5. Procedure
   a. Several scanning sequences, each lasting a few seconds up to 15 minutes, are performed to obtain cross-sectional images in several planes of various body segments
   b. Patient may communicate with staff by way of intercom
   c. If contrast is used, IV is inserted and connected to IV solution. Contrast usually is injected two thirds of the way through examination, which lasts up to 45 minutes
6. Findings/interpretation: highly detailed images of vascular system depicting normal and abnormal anatomic structures
7. Limitations
   a. Some patients with implants and so forth may not be candidates; see "patient preparation" above

b. Turbulent flow, flow through high-grade lesion, and blood flow not in alignment with imaging plane can lead to MRA images that do not depict anatomy accurately
c. Accurate grading of carotid stenosis still limited, usually overestimates; high-grade stenosis appears as complete occlusion
d. Highly pulsatile nature of aortic and pulmonic flow creates artifact in image
e. Abdominal aortic aneurysms (AAAs) with slow or turbulent flow cause signal loss and inaccurate depiction of true vessel lumen
f. Expensive equipment requires a highly skilled team of technologists and radiologist to obtain and interpret images accurately
g. Not useful for emergency procedures

8. Complications/precautions
   a. Undetected metal (e.g., bullet) may distort image or cause potential harm to patient
   b. Patient may become restless, agitated, or fearful in closed unit; movement distorts image
9. Nursing implications: careful screening to identify patients who are at risk for claustrophobia, need for pain control, removal of all metal objects. Sedation may be required

E. Intravascular Ultrasound

1. Indications: to provide high-yield structural detail with improved resolution of the arterial wall
2. Studies have been done comparing angiography to intravascular ultrasound in providing accurate arterial anatomy (Arthurs et al., 2010)
3. Data obtained only by intravascular ultrasound included plaque morphology and volume
4. Intravascular ultrasound is useful in improving long-term patency of certain lesions treated with balloon angioplasty and primary stenting (Buckley et al., 2002; Timaran et al., 2010).

TEST QUESTIONS

Review Questions/Answers/Rationale

1. The following examination provides an anatomic map of the sites of arterial stenosis and aids in planning appropriate intervention:
   a. Pulse volume recording
   b. Arteriography
   c. Plethysmography
   d. Transcutaneous oxygen testing

ANSWER: b. Arteriography outlines sites of disease by way of catheter cannulation of an artery with instillation of radio-opaque contrast medium.

2. Noninvasive diagnostic tests are based on
   a. The Doppler effect
   b. Poiseuille law
   c. Spectral analysis
   d. All of the above

ANSWER: d. All of the above. The Doppler effect is the reflection of high-frequency (ultrasound) sound from moving structures (blood cells) returning at different frequencies than originally used to generate the sound. This frequency shift is used to calculate the speed of blood flow across an area of stenosis. Poiseuille law states that the speed of blood flow will increase across an area of narrowing in a blood vessel, which results in higher frequency shifts on Doppler evaluation. Spectral analysis is used to analyze the frequency of the returning signal after it has been converted into an audible and visible waveform and serves as the basis for classification of disease.

3. Which test is used to screen the general population for the presence of peripheral artery disease?
   a. Pulse volume recording
   b. Arterial duplex ultrasound
   c. Ankle–brachial index ABI's
   d. Spiral CT scan

ANSWER: c. Ankle–brachial index is an inexpensive, noninvasive, and readily reproducible method of determining the presence of arterial stenosis in the lower extremities by calculating the variance between brachial and ankle pressures.

4. Accuracy of the ankle–brachial index may be affected by which of the following conditions:
   a. Obesity
   b. Diabetes mellitus
   c. Acute deep vein thrombosis
   d. Parkinson's tremor
   e. All of the above

ANSWER: e. All of the above. Obesity may limit appropriate cuff size selection. Patients who have diabetes mellitus may have vessel calcification that leads to artificial elevation of pressures. Extensive acute deep vein thrombosis limits arterial inflow by causing an outflow obstruction. Restlessness or tremor makes localization of pulse variable or unreliable.

5. Mr. Smith tells you that he lost the vision in one eye for approximately 5 minutes. "It was like someone pulled a shade down and lifted it back up." What test should be ordered to evaluate this complaint?
   a. Carotid duplex ultrasound
   b. Transcranial Doppler
   c. MRI of the brain
   d. All of the above

ANSWER: a. Carotid duplex ultrasound. Clinical indications for carotid duplex ultrasound include symptoms of hemispheric stroke; transient ischemic attacks; resolving ischemic neurologic deficit; amaurosis fugax; symptomatic and asymptomatic carotid bruit; palpable neck mass; and nonhemispheric symptoms, such as dizziness, loss of memory, and drop attacks.

6. Normal venous Doppler characteristics of blood flow include
   a. Spontaneity, incompetence, noncompressibility
   b. Spontaneity, phasicity, augmentation
   c. Competence, nonpulsatility, compressibility
   d. Phasicity, pulsatility, continuity

ANSWER: b. Spontaneity, phasicity, augmentation. Venous blood flow does not require stimulation to be heard (spontaneity). It is cyclic with respiration (phasicity, not continuous) and increases with compression of the limb below the level of the Doppler (augmentation).

Pulsatility is a characteristic of arterial flow. A competent venous system is manifested by interruption of flow with a Valsalva maneuver.

7. Mrs. White is scheduled for an arteriogram to plan intervention for a nonhealing diabetic foot ulcer. Which medication should be held before the test and resumed 1 to 2 days after the test?
   a. Long-acting insulin
   b. Glyburide (DiaBeta)
   c. Metformin (Glucophage)
   d. Rosiglitazone (Avandia)

ANSWER: c. Metformin. Because metformin and contrast medium are excreted renally, metformin should be held for 2 to 5 days (varies per institution protocol) before the procedure and for up to 2 days after the procedure to avoid renal impairment.

8. Mr. Renziti is a 67-year-old patient with a history of obesity, poorly controlled hypertension, one-half block claudication, and a 50 pack-year smoking habit. While bending over to remove his shoes for follow-up ankle–brachial index in the Noninvasive Vascular Lab, he complains of sudden low back pain and appears pale. Which test should be considered for urgent evaluation of his complaint?
   a. Lumbar–sacral spine x-ray
   b. Exercise ankle–brachial index
   c. Angiogram
   d. Abdominal CT scan

ANSWER: d. Abdominal CT scan. Mr. Renziti has classic risk factors for abdominal aortic aneurysm. CT scan is indicated for staging of aneurysms. The patient requires close monitoring for evidence of rupture with immediate transport to the operating room if indicated.

9. Mr. Young is hospitalized for acute dyspnea and chest pain and has multiple pulmonary emboli on pulmonary arteriography. Because he has a known allergy to heparin products, an inferior vena caval filter is placed and he initiates warfarin anticoagulation. One week later, he exhibits symptoms of left-sided weakness and aphasia. Which test should not be selected to evaluate his new symptoms?
   a. Magnetic resonance angiography
   b. CT
   c. Transcranial Doppler
   d. Carotid duplex ultrasound

ANSWER: a. Magnetic resonance angiography. The presence of a recently placed metallic device is a contraindication for magnetic resonance angiography.

10. Objective evaluation of the circulatory system is approached best with a combination of a thorough history and physical examination, use of appropriate testing modality, and
    a. A mini-mental status exam
    b. Assessment of the functional impact of disease on the patient's life
    c. Approval from the patient's third-party payment system
    d. All of the above.

ANSWER: b. Assessment of the functional impact of disease on the patient's life. A patient's functional capacity is an important factor in planning appropriate care. For example, a nonambulatory individual who has a decrease in peripheral circulation is less affected functionally by the disease than is an ambulatory individual.

Noninvasive Arterial Examinations

Test	Procedure
Ankle–brachial index (ABI)	1. Inflating blood pressure cuff to 20 mm Hg above systolic pressure, record systolic pressure as cuff is deflated using Doppler in both right and left brachial, dorsalis pedis, and posterior tibial arteries 2. If analog waveform is to be recorded, obtain tracings in all vessels prior to blood pressure recordings 3. Calculate ratio of distal pressure to proximal pressure by dividing highest distal pressures on each limb by the highest brachial pressure. Ankle Brachial Index
Segmental pressures and analog waveforms	1. After obtaining both brachial blood pressures, sequentially obtain analog waveforms and blood pressure on each segment of the lower extremities 2. All distal pressures are heard with the Doppler placed over the posterior tibial or dorsalis pedis artery, whichever is most audible 3. Calculate ABI as above for each extremity
Toe pressures	1. Obtain brachial systolic Doppler pressures as above 2. Place toe cuff around great toe of each foot, auscultate for arterial signal, and obtain waveform tracing and pressure 3. Calculate toe/brachial index
Exercise testing	1. Obtain careful history: neurospinal problems are not usually as reproducible as true claudication (good days, bad days; pain brought on with sitting or standing as well as walking; have to lie down for relief) 2. Obtain resting supine ABI and waveforms as above 3. Patient walks for 5 minutes or until disabled by leg pain at standardized speed and grade on treadmill: 1.5 to 2.0 mph with grade of 10% to 12%. Note time, symptoms, and walking distance/time at end of test 4. Record ABI on each limb every minute until pre-exercise level obtained. Terminate test at 10 minutes postexercise
Pulse volume recording (PVR)	1. As for ABI and/or segmental pressure exam 2. A small cushion is placed beneath heels 3. Large thigh cuff placed as proximally on thigh as possible 4. Cuffs are inflated sequentially, one at a time, to a pressure of 60 to 65 mm Hg. Volume recordings are obtained at each level for five to six cardiac cycles
Arterial duplex scan with color Doppler of lower extremity	1. Record ABI or segmental pressures as above 2. Each vessel (CFA, proximal, mid and distal SFA, Popliteal, PT, and DP) is imaged along entire length using 2D color duplex and duplex Doppler in sagittal views. Bypass grafts imaged in longitudinal view, including proximal and distal anastomosis and flow in native vessels 3. Color imaging is used to visualize any velocity increases that would suggest narrowing. Significant stenosis (usually 75% or more) will produce color aliasing—multiple colors mixed together combined with high-frequency signal over 200 cm/sec 4. Doppler velocity samples are obtained proximal to, at, and distal to any areas of stenosis. Doppler angle is set at 45 to 60 degrees. Smallest sample volume should be utilized with sample volume placed in center of vessel. Maintain Doppler angle parallel to blood flow. Obtain vessel diameter measurements 5. If no stenotic lesions are identified, velocities are recorded in the midportion of each segment
Arterial duplex scan of extracranial arterial system (carotid, vertebrobasilar)	1. Examiner is positioned either at head of bed or at level of patient's shoulder 2. Transducer placed in transverse plane at base of neck, vessels identified to level of bifurcation. Color may be turned off to better image atherosclerotic plaque. Diameter reduction measurements obtained 3. In sagittal plane, images and duplex Doppler velocity measurements are obtained in the common, internal, and external carotid arteries

(continued)

Noninvasive Arterial Examinations (continued)

Test	Procedure
	4. If plaque is identified, velocity measurements obtained proximal, mid, and distal to plaque formation. Highest velocity measurement used for calculation of internal carotid to common carotid ratio. Angle of insonation should be maintained as close to 60 degrees as possible 5. Vertebral arteries are imaged in transverse and sagittal planes, imaging from the upper neck to the subclavian. Subclavian Doppler signals also recorded
Arterial duplex scan of renal and mesenteric arterial system	1. Beginning at xiphoid process, using transverse view, identify proximal abdominal aorta; record Doppler signal in sagittal view; note any plaque or aneurysmal changes 2. Image celiac artery and obtain Doppler signals—first branch of abdominal aorta 3. Image superior mesenteric artery and obtain Doppler signals—second branch of abdominal aorta just distal to celiac trunk 4. Image and obtain signals in hepatic and splenic arteries 5. If an enlarged inferior mesenteric artery is noted, this may suggest SMA occlusive disease 6. If scanning for suspicion of mesenteric ischemia, have patient ingest high-calorie liquid (protein shake). Repeat celiac and SMA measurements in 30 to 40 minutes 7. If scanning for suspicion of renal artery stenosis, obtain vessel images and signals at origin (ostium), mid, and distal portions of both renal arteries, noting any plaque formations. Patient may be turned to right and left lateral decubitus positions to maximize imaging. Obtain images of each kidney, measuring pole to pole, and velocities from medulla, cortex, and renal hilum

Noninvasive Venous Examinations

Test	Procedure
Venous duplex scan	1. Lower extremity: with knee slightly flexed, sagittal and longitudinal (transverse) views are obtained from common femoral, superficial femoral, deep femoral (profunda), popliteal, posterior tibial, anterior tibial, and greater saphenous veins. Scan head is moved sequentially down leg, using color flow continuously if available. Gray scale used to evaluate age of thrombus, observing vessel wall echogenicity. If able, patient placed in prone position for examination of popliteal, peroneal, soleal sinuses, and lesser saphenous vein. 2. Upper extremity: with arm extended and elbow slightly flexed, sagittal and longitudinal views are obtained from jugular, subclavian, axillary, and brachial veins. Views then obtained from wrist to elbow of radial and ulnar veins. Cephalic vein identified laterally at wrist and scanned to shoulder; basilic vein identified medially at wrist and scanned to shoulder 3. Inferior vena cava and iliac veins: patient supine, using deep abdominal probe (2 to 3.5 MHz), scan from groin to above umbilicus in transverse and longitudinal positions, identifying bilateral common femoral and iliac veins merging to inferior vena cava below umbilicus
Plethysmography	1. Air, IPG: after transducers placed, system is calibrated; pneumatic cuff inflated to approximately 60 mm Hg (above usual venous pressure) to temporarily occlude venous outflow; volume within calf increases during occlusion; recorded by transducer as rise from baseline on strip chart recorder. Cuff is then rapidly deflated to allow for venous emptying, drop in recording back to baseline 2. PPG: patient instructed to rapidly dorsiflex and plantarflex feet 5 to 10 times to empty venous system. Tracing is recorded on strip chart to indicate fall of venous capacity from baseline. Patient rests quietly without moving or talking while strip chart records postexercise return to baseline volume

Noninvasive Venous Examinations (continued)

Test	Procedure
	3. SPG: patient raises and lowers heels five times. Recovery time measured on strip chart in seconds as for PPG. Cuff or tourniquet applied above gauge to occlude superficial system and test repeated. SPG also used for detection of DVT similar to air or IPG

Invasive Diagnostic Studies

Test	Procedure
Arteriography	1. Patient preparation completed: adequately draped, comfort measures, monitoring equipment applied, IV access and fluid administration established, skin site for injection prepared 2. Seldinger technique, usually of femoral artery, but may use lumbar, brachial, or axillary—needle puncture of artery followed by placement of guidewire through needle into lumen of vessel. Catheter threaded over guidewire; guidewire removed and catheter placed at desired site with fluoroscopy guidance. Catheter connected to pressure injection equipment programmed for appropriate flow rate and volume. Sequential x-ray images obtained • Total contrast does not usually exceed 350 ml • Heparinized flush solution constantly infused to prevent thrombosis 3. Catheter withdrawn; pressure placed over puncture site for 15 to 20 minutes; if no bleeding, patient transferred to recovery area or hospital room for observation. Immobility for 4 to 6 hours to prevent bleeding
Venography	1. Pedal vein cannulated with small intravenous needle, preferably at lateral dorsal aspect of foot 2. Contrast medium rapidly injected by hand 3. Images of tibial, popliteal, femoral, and iliac veins obtained, with attempt to see contrast entering inferior vena cava 4. For inferior or superior vena cava, cannulation done at femoral or antecubital vein level 5. For descending venography—femoral catheterization; contrast injected with patient upright 6. Selective venography and venous pressure monitoring may be done to evaluate the portal system, renal or hepatic veins with selective sampling of blood pressures or serum samples, that is, evaluation of renovascular hypertension

Additional Diagnostic Studies

Test	Procedure
Transcutaneous oxygen tension	1. Procedure for determining BKA healing potential • After cleansing skin on arm and leg areas with alcohol pad, affix sensors with double-stick tape • Anterior and posterior calf monitoring sites are located 6 to 8 inches below knee overlying the anterior tibialis muscle and medial head of gastrocnemius muscle, respectively • Measurements are recorded after 15 minutes by means of a sensor temperature at 44°C • A calf/brachial PO_2 index is calculated by use of the lesser value from the lower extremity
Transcranial Doppler (TDC)	1. Procedure: three standard "windows" (areas on skull where bone is thin enough to allow penetration by ultrasound) are used to insonate the intracranial vessels. Depth, color, and Doppler signals assist in vessel identification a. Temporal—when scanned in transverse plane, provides access to major vessels of Circle of Willis i. Middle cerebral artery (MCA)—from terminal branches to the MCA/ACA bifurcation ii. Anterior cerebral artery (ACA)—usually the A1 segment seen iii. Posterior cerebral artery (PCA)—P1 and P2 segments

(continued)

Additional Diagnostic Studies (continued)

Test	Procedure
	iv. Terminal internal carotid artery v. Anterior communicating artery (AcoA) if functional vi. Posterior communicating artery (PcoA) if functional b. Orbital i. Ophthalmic artery ii. Carotid siphon c. Transforaminal (foramen magnum/occipital) i. Distal vertebral arteries ii. Proximal basilar artery d. Submandibular—internal carotid artery insonated to obtain hemispheric ratio of peak systolic velocity in MCA compared to ICA (MCA/ICA)
Computed tomography (CAT scan) and spiral computed tomographic angiography (spiral CTA)	1. Patient placed supine in circular open gantry with x-ray tube and multiple x-ray detectors 2. Tube moves around body while emitting x-rays confined to narrow slice varying from 2 to 10 mm. Rays pass through body and are detected on opposite side by detectors 3. High-speed computer processes images 4. Spiral CTA—patient passes through gantry at constant velocity while x-ray simultaneously rotates at constant velocity around patient, thus producing helical or spiral x-ray path around patient. Continuous data sent to computer with overlapping of slices to form 2D and 3D images • CTA dependent on proper contrast delivery with delay time between injection and image acquisition of 20 to 25 seconds for head, neck, and thorax, but 50 to 70 seconds for abdomen • Patient may be asked to hold breath for up to 30 seconds periodically; holding still very important for accuracy of images 5. CT-guided biopsy/drainage procedures: needle, catheter, or guidewire placed into fluid collections, masses to drain abscesses or obtain biopsy of deep masses
Magnetic resonance angiography (MRA)	1. Several scanning sequences, each lasting a few seconds up to 15 minutes, are performed to obtain cross-sectional images in several planes of various body segments 2. Patient may communicate with staff via intercom 3. If contrast used, IV inserted and connected to intravenous solution. Contrast usually injected two thirds of the way through exam, which lasts up to 45 minutes.

REFERENCES

Arthurs, Z., Bishop, P., Feiten, L., Eagleton, M., Clair, D., & Kashop, V. (2010). Evaluation of peripheral atherosclerosis: A comparative analysis of angiography and intravascular ultrasound imaging. *Journal of Vascular Surgery, 51*(4), 933–939.

Bent, C., Jaskolka, J., Lindsay, T., & Tan, K. (2010). The use of dynamic volumetric CT angiography for the characterization of endoleaks following fenestrated EVAR. *Journal of Vascular Surgery, 51*(1), 203–206.

Blackburn, D. R., & Peterson-Kennedy, L. (2004). Noninvasive vascular testing. In V. Fahey (Ed.), *Vascular nursing* (4th ed., pp. 73–96). St. Louis, MO: Saunders.

Buckley, C., Arko, F., Lee, S., Little, D., Mamming, L., & Patterson, D. (2002). Intravascular ultrasound scanning improves long-term patency of iliac lesions treated with balloon angioplasty and primary stenting. *Journal of Vascular Surgery, 35*(2), 316–323.

Dolmatch, B., Davros, W. J., & Grist, T. M. (1996). Diagnostic angiography. In J. R. Young, J. W. Olin, & J. R. Bartholomew (Eds.), *Peripheral vascular diseases* (2nd ed., pp. 65–88). St. Louis, MO: Mosby-Year Book Inc.

Gioviczki, P., Camerota, A., Dalsing, M., & Eklof, B. (2011). The care of patients with varicose veins and associated chronic venous diseases: Clinical practice guidelines of the Society for Vascular Surgery and the American Venous Forum. *Journal of Vascular Surgery, 53*, 2S–48S.

Hodgkiss-Harlow, K., & Bandyk, D. (2012). Arterial duplex imaging of lower-extremity arteries and interventions. *Journal of Vascular Ultrasound, 36*(2), 143–151.

Iezzi, R., Bsillico, R., Giancristofara, D., Pacall, D., Cotroneo, A., & Storto, L. (2009). Contrast-enhanced ultrasound versus color duplex imaging in the follow-up of patients after endovascular abdominal aortic aneurysm repair. *Journal of Vascular Surgery, 49*(3), 552–560.

Kalani, M., Brismar, K., Fagrell, B., Ostergren, J., & Jorneskog, G. (1999). Transcutaneous oxygen tension and toe blood pressure as predictors for outcome of diabetic foot ulcers. *Diabetes Care, 22*, 147–151.

Kamida, C. B., Kistner, R. L., Elkof, B., & Masuda, E. M. (2001). Lower extremity ascending and descending phlebography. In P. Gloviczki & J. S. T. Yao (Eds.), *Handbook of venous disorders* (2nd ed., pp. 132–139). London: Arnold.

Kingstone, L., Torres, C., & Currie, G. (2012). A systematic literature review of ultrasonography for morphology and characterization of vulnerable carotid artery plaques. *Journal of Vascular Ultrasound, 36*(3), 191–198.

Kram, H. B., Appel, P. L., & Shoemaker, W. C. (1989). Multisensor transcutaneous oximetric mapping to predict below knee amputation wound healing: Use of a critical PO2. *Journal of Vascular Surgery, 9*, 796–800.

Mattos, M. A., & Sumner, D. (2001). Direct noninvasive tests (duplex scan) for the evaluation of chronic venous obstruction and valvular incompetence. In P. Gloviczki & J. S. T. Yao (Eds.), *Handbook of venous disorders* (2nd ed., pp. 120–131). London: Arnold.

McPharlin, M. (2012). Lower extremity arterial air plethysmography evaluation. *Journal of Vascular Ultrasound, 36*(2), 135–142.

Neumyer, M. (2012). Characterization of blood flow patterns in the hepatoportal, mesenteric and renal vessels by analysis of Doppler spectoral waveforms. *Journal of Vascular Ultrasound, 36*(2), 113–122.

Pellerito, J., & Polak, J. (2012). *Introduction to vascular ultrasonography* (6th ed.). Philadelphia, PA: Elsevier, Saunders.

Pomposelli, F. (2010). Arterial imaging in patients with lower extremity ischemia and diabetes mellitus. *Journal of Vascular Surgery, 52*(3), 81S–91S.

Porreca, F., Rodriguez-Wong, A., & Hughes, J. (2012). Three-dimensional reconstruction of the vessel lumen as an adjunct to the cerebrovascular duplex evaluation. *Journal Vascular Ultrasound, 36*(3), 199–204.

Ridgway, D. P. (1992). *Introduction to vascular scanning: A guide for the complete beginner*. Pasadena, CA: Appleton Davies, Inc.

Roberts, J., Alonso, C., & Khatib, Y. (2012). The role of duplex ultrasound in the detection of celiac aneurysm. *Journal of Vascular Ultrasound, 36*(3), 213–215.

Rumwell, C., & McPharlin, M. (1998). *Vascular technology: An illustrated review for the Registry Exam*. Pasadena, CA: Appleton Davies, Inc.

Salles-Cunha, S. X., & Beebe, H. G. (2001). Direct noninvasive tests (duplex scan) for the evaluation of acute venous disease. In P. Gloviczki & J. S. T. Yao (Eds.), *Handbook of venous disorders* (2nd ed., pp. 110–119). London: Arnold.

Salles-Cunha, S. X., Braga, F. A., Caiafa, J. S., Melo, L. H. A., Castro, A. A., & Pitta, G. B. B. (2012). Diastolic ankle-brachial indices as a complementary measure for peripheral arterial disease in diabetic patients. *Journal of Vascular Ultrasound, 36*(3), 205–209.

Sanders, R. C. (Ed.). (1998). *Clinical sonography: A practical guide* (3rd ed.). Philadelphia, PA: Lippincott.

Strandness, D. E. (1996). Noninvasive vascular laboratory and vascular imaging. In J. R. Young, J. W. Olin, & J. R. Bartholomew (Eds.), *Peripheral vascular diseases* (2nd ed., pp. 33–64). St. Louis, MO: Mosby-Year Book, Inc.

Timaran, C. H., Rosero, E. B., Martinez, A. E., Ilarraza, A., Modrall, J. G. & Clagett, G. P. (2010). Atherosclerotic plaque composition assessed by virtual histology intravascular ultrasound and cerebral embolization after carotid stenting. *Journal of Vascular Surgery, 52*(5), 1188-1195.

Vogelzang, R. L. (2004). Percutaneous endovascular intervention and imaging techniques. In V. Fahey (Ed.), *Vascular nursing* (4th ed., pp. 97–125). St. Louis, MO: Saunders.

Wolf, K. J., & Fobbe, F. (Eds.). (1995). *Color duplex sonography: Principles and clinical applications*. New York, NY: Thieme Medical Publishers, Inc.

Yamaki, T., Nozaki, M., Sakurai, H., Takeuchi, M., & Kono, T. (2008). Prospective randomized efficacy of ultrasound-guided foam sclerotherapy compared with liquid sclerotherapy in the treatment of varicose veins. *Journal of Vascular Surgery, 47*(3), 578–584.

CHAPTER 6

Medications Used in Patients with Peripheral Vascular Disease

Lori L. Schirmer
Renee Mosier
First Edition Authors: *Sarah E. Connelly and Marjorie Lovell*

OBJECTIVES

1. Identify medication classes used to medically manage patients with vascular disease.
2. Describe the mechanism of action for each medication discussed.
3. Discuss appropriate indications for each medication class discussed, specifically relating to vascular disease management.
4. Describe key nursing parameters for monitoring the medications discussed.

Introduction

The medical management of patients with vascular disease involves modification of known atherosclerotic risk factors to slow vascular disease progression, treatment of intermittent claudication (IC) symptoms, prevention of atherothrombotic complications, and treatment of acute thrombotic events. Several classes of medications are used to accomplish the goals of medical management, namely, antithrombotics, cholesterol-lowering medications, vasodilators, nutritional supplements, and antihypertensive agents. This chapter will focus on agents of each medication class and describe how they are used in the management of vascular disease.

Section 1: Lori L. Schirmer

Antithrombotics

Antithrombotic agents include anticoagulant, antiplatelet, and thrombolytic drugs. Each antithrombotic agent will be discussed separately since each has a specific role in vascular disease. The clinical use of dextran will also be discussed because surgeons have used the antithrombotic side effects of this agent to advantage.

Anticoagulants

Commonly used anticoagulants are as follows:

Vitamin K antagonist
- Warfarin (Coumadin)

Direct thrombin inhibitors (DTIs)
- Argatroban
- Dabigatran (Pradaxa)

Factor Xa inhibitors
- Apixaban (Eliquis)
- Edoxaban (investigational use)
- Fondaparinux (Arixtra)
- Rivaroxaban (Xarelto)

Heparins
- Unfractionated heparin (UFH)
- Low molecular weight heparin (LMWH)

Dalteparin (Fragmin)
Enoxaparin (Lovenox)
Nadroparin (Fraxiparin, Fraxiparine) not available in the United States
Tinzaparin (Innohep) not available in the US

Of these agents, warfarin, dabigatran, apixaban, and rivaroxaban are oral anticoagulants. UFH may be administered intravenously (IV) or subcutaneously (SC). LMWHs and fondaparinux are given SC for peripheral vascular disease (PVD) indications. Argatroban is administered IV.

Mechanism of Action

Warfarin, DTIs, factor Xa inhibitors, and heparins differ slightly in their mechanisms of action, but each works by inhibiting specific coagulation factors, which disrupt the coagulation pathway and ultimately prevent the formation of fibrin, the substance responsible for clot stabilization.

Warfarin

Warfarin inhibits the hepatic conversion of vitamin K epoxide back to vitamin K (Ageno et al., 2012). The result is a reduction in the amount of vitamin K that is available to activate clotting factors II, VII, IX, and X (Ageno et al., 2012). The liver ultimately slows down production of clotting factors when vitamin K is unavailable and the factors that do get synthesized are inactive. The formations of natural anticoagulant proteins C and S are also dependent on vitamin K. The inhibition of protein C (half-life, 8 to 10 hours) and S (half-life, 40 to 60 hours) occurs rapidly compared with the inhibition of clotting factor II (half-life, 60 to 100 hours) and may cause a temporary procoagulant effect within the first 5 days of therapy (Ageno et al., 2012; Haines, Witt, & Nutescu, 2008). This temporary hypercoagulable state means that many patients will receive two anticoagulants (e.g., warfarin plus an LMWH) for the first 5 days of warfarin treatment to prevent clots from forming.

The initial partial suppression of the coagulation pathway may be evident within 24 to 36 hours of therapy and is represented by small elevations in the international normalized ratio (INR). However, full anticoagulation or an antithrombotic effect (the ability to prevent or interfere with thrombi formation) occurs once the formation of all four vitamin K clotting factors has been impaired. The time to full anticoagulation onset is affected primarily by the half-lives of vitamin K clotting factors and is generally not seen until 8 to 15 days of warfarin therapy (Haines et al., 2008). Factor VII production is the first to be inhibited because its half-life is only 6 to 8 hours. Factor II, with a half-life of 60 to 100 hours, is the final coagulation factor inhibited (Haines et al., 2008).

In summary, small elevations in INR may be apparent within 24 hours and the INR may be therapeutic within 5 days; however, full anticoagulation results from the inhibition of all vitamin K clotting factors, which requires up to 15 days of warfarin therapy (Haines et al., 2008). The time to anticoagulation onset and the dose a patient will require to achieve a therapeutic INR are variable due to the following: age, liver metabolism differences determined by genetics, dietary intake of vitamin K containing foods, overall nutritional status, drug interactions, and drug metabolism (Haines et al., 2008).

Direct Thrombin Inhibitors

Argatroban and dabigatran are DTIs and work by binding directly to thrombin (factor IIa) and blocking its action. They are considered to be direct because they do not need to bind to another cofactor to be active, unlike the indirect anticoagulants heparin and LMWHs (Ageno et al., 2012; Garcia, Baglin, Weitz, & Samama, 2012). Argatroban is administered IV and dabigatran is taken orally.

Factor Xa Inhibitors

Apixaban, fondaparinux, and rivaroxaban are factor Xa inhibitors. Fondaparinux is an *indirect* inhibitor of Xa since it interacts with AT similar to heparin and LMWH (Haines et al., 2008). Apixaban and rivaroxaban are direct inhibitors of factor Xa since they bind to Xa without needing a cofactor like antithrombin (Ageno et al., 2012; Weitz, Eikelboom, & Samama, 2012). Fondaparinux is administered SC while apixaban and rivaroxaban are taken orally.

Unfractionated Heparin

UFH is a mixture of heparin molecules of different sizes. Heparin binds to and potentiates the effect of antithrombin III (AT), a natural anticoagulant. Heparin is considered an indirect anticoagulant because it needs to bind to AT to work. The heparin–AT complex binds to and inactivates thrombin (factor IIa), the coagulation factors IXa, Xa, XIa, and XIIa. The anticoagulant effect is achieved primarily through inactivation of factors IIa and X, because they are more responsive to the heparin–AT complex inhibition (Haines et al., 2008). By blocking thrombin, heparin prevents the formation of fibrin and also inhibits thrombin-induced activation of platelets (Garcia et al., 2012). Unlike warfarin, the anticoagulation effect is rapid. UFH prevents thrombi from expanding and allows the patient's thrombolytic pathway to degrade the clot. Note that with IV administration, the effect is immediate, and with SC administration, anticoagulation is apparent within 1 to 2 hours (Haines et al., 2008).

Low Molecular Weight Heparins

LMWHs are heparin fragments that are approximately one third the size of a heparin molecule. The mechanism of action of LMWHs is similar to that of UFH in that LMWHs bind to and potentiate the effect of AT. However, because the LMWHs are smaller molecules, the LMWH–AT complex is only capable of binding with and inactivating coagulation factors Xa and IIa. The anticoagulation effect is achieved primarily through factor Xa inhibition. The decreased ability of LMWH to inactivate factor IIa (thrombin) occurs because the majority of the small heparin fragments are unable to bind simultaneously to both AT and factor IIa (Garcia et al., 2012; Haines et al., 2008).

Indications and Evidence

Warfarin

Maintaining vascular surgery graft patency: The administration of long-term warfarin therapy after vascular reconstructive surgery is not recommended because the evidence that it is beneficial is weak and the risk of hemorrhagic complications is high in comparison with the small increase in long-term graft patency (Alonso-Coello et al., 2012). The American College of Chest Physicians recommends that a single antiplatelet agent (discussed below) be used alone instead of adding warfarin for long-term therapy after peripheral artery bypass graft surgery (Alonso-Coello et al., 2012).

Postoperative care (post-thrombectomy): The administration of long-term warfarin therapy may be initiated with IV heparin therapy after a thrombectomy to prevent recurrent embolism. Warfarin therapy is usually maintained for 3 months (Kearon et al., 2012; Norgren et al., 2007).

However, it should be noted that long-term (past 3 months) administration of warfarin remains controversial after thrombectomy in the absence of a proven emboli source. The American College of Cardiology Guidelines have recently changed the recommendation from supporting long-term anticoagulation with warfarin in 2008 (Sobel & Verhaeghe) to only recommending it in low or moderate bleeding risk patients in 2012 (Kearon et al.).

Cardiovascular risk reduction: Warfarin is not recommended to be added to antiplatelet therapy (discussed below) for decreasing the risk of cardiovascular ischemic events unless there is another proven indication (e.g., atrial fibrillation) for warfarin (Rooke et al., 2011).

Argatroban and Fondaparinux

Treatment of heparin-induced thrombocytopenia (HIT): HIT is an adverse reaction to heparin or LMWH that results in the formation of antibodies against the drug and can result in severe thromboembolic complications (PE, ischemic limb, stroke, etc.). The role for argatroban in patients with PVD is in treatment and prevention of thrombosis in patients who currently have antibodies to heparin (Linkins et al., 2012). Fondaparinux may be used in patients with a past history of HIT who do not currently produce antibodies but who later (during an event unrelated to the initial episode of HIT) need treatment for or prevention of thrombosis (Linkins et al., 2012).

Apixaban, Dabigatran, and Rivaroxaban

Treatment or prevention of embolism: Oral anticoagulant alternatives to warfarin are a significant advance in patient care because they do not require the laboratory monitoring and frequent adjustments in dosing that warfarin requires. A potential for concern exists however, because an agent that can be used to reverse the anticoagulant effect of these drugs does not exist currently but may be available in the future. The three oral drugs currently approved for use, apixaban, dabigatran, and rivaroxaban are indicated for the treatment of venous thromboembolism and pulmonary embolism and/or prevention of embolic stroke in atrial fibrillation (Ageno et al., 2012; Lexi-Drugs, 2013). Other indications are currently being investigated.

UFH and LMWHs

The rapid onset of action of UFH and LMWHs allows these anticoagulants to be used when an immediate anticoagulant effect is required. A lower rate of recurrence of VTE is associated with achieving therapeutic anticoagulation within the first 24 hours of IV UFH treatment (Garcia et al., 2012). LMWHs are used infrequently in the vascular surgery population primarily because there is a wealth of evidence for the use of UFH and because the elimination half-life of LMWHs is significantly greater compared with UFH. However, a few studies using LMWHs have been completed.

Acute limb ischemia: The administration of IV UFH at a full anticoagulant dose is required immediately following the diagnosis of acute limb ischemia secondary to thromboembolic arterial occlusion to prevent clot propagation and secondary arterial embolus formation. There are no trials comparing UFH to another anticoagulant for this indication and so heparin remains the standard therapy (Alonso-Coello et al., 2012; Norgren et al., 2007).

Postoperative care (post-thrombectomy/thrombolysis): A full anticoagulant dose of IV UFH should be administered to prevent embolic recurrence immediately after a thrombectomy or thrombolysis procedure for the management of acute limb ischemia. Treatment with IV UFH should be followed by warfarin for a minimum of 3 months (Ageno et al., 2012; Norgren et al., 2007).

Intraoperative anticoagulation: UFH is used routinely to prevent intravascular coagulation, stasis thrombosis, and accumulation of thrombi during vascular reconstructive procedures (Effeney, Goldstone, Chin, Krupski, & Ellis, 1981; Martin, Greenstein, Gupta, Walker, & Kester, 1994; Sobel & Verhaeghe, 2008; Thompson et al., 1996; Wakefield et al., 1994). Despite the common use of IV UFH prior to clamping arteries, vascular surgeons have not come to a consensus regarding the dose, timing, or method of administration (Wakefield et al., 1994). LMWHs have been shown to be as effective as UFH during infrainguinal bypass surgery (Samama, Gigou, & Ill, 1995; Swedenborg, Nydahl, & Egberg, 1996); however, UFH continues to be the recommended agent for intraoperative use (Sobel & Verhaeghe, 2008) (see Table 6-1).

TABLE 6-1 Antithrombotic Comparison Chart

Drug	Indication	Dose and Route	Onset (O) and Duration (D)	Monitoring Parameters	Contraindications
Warfarin (Coumadin)	Post-thrombectomy/VTE/high-risk bypass/hypercoagulable condition	A typical starting dose is 5–10 mg daily Dose is individualized for each patient to maintain INR range 2–3	O: 24–72 h D: 2–5 d, $t_{1/2}$ = 20–60 h	• PT/INR • Hemoglobin • Signs and symptoms of bleeding	• Hypersensitivity to warfarin • History of bleeding problems or tendencies • Recent trauma or surgery of eye or central nervous system • Uncontrolled hypertension • Pregnancy • Noncompliance
Argatroban	Prevention of thrombosis in HIT	Continuous IV infusion: initial rate 2 mcg/kg/min (0.5–1.2 mcg/kg/min for patients with heart failure or postcardiac surgery) Adjust using aPTT measurements and dosing nomogram	O: immediate D: $t_{1/2}$ = 39–51 min (longer in significant hepatic failure)	• aPTT • Hemoglobin • Signs and symptoms of bleeding	• Hypersensitivity to argatroban • Active major bleeding
Fondaparinux (Arixtra)	VTE prevention in history of (but not current) HIT	2.5 mg SC daily	O: rapid, peak effect 2–3 h D: $t_{1/2}$ = 17–21 h (longer in renal failure)	• Hemoglobin • Platelets • Signs and symptoms of bleeding	• Hypersensitivity to fondaparinux • Creatinine clearance <30 mL/min • Weight <50 kg • Active major bleeding • Active antibodies to heparin
UFH	Acute limb ischemia/postoperative care	Continuous IV infusion: Option 1: bolus with 5,000 units, then follow with at least 32,000 units/d Option 2: bolus with 80 units/kg, then follow with an infusion of 18 units/kg/h Adjust either regimen using q6 h aPTT measurements and a dosing nomogram	O: immediate with IV D: half-life ($t_{1/2}$) is dose dependent and nonlinear. $t_{1/2}$ = 30 min @ 25 units/kg bolus $t_{1/2}$ = 60 min @ 100 units/kg bolus $t_{1/2}$ = 150 min @ 400 units/kg bolus	• aPTT (or antiXa) • Hemoglobin • Platelets • Signs and symptoms of bleeding • Renal function (clearance declines)	• Hypersensitivity to heparin • HIT or severe thrombocytopenia • Active major bleeding

TABLE 6-1 Antithrombotic Comparison Chart (continued)

Drug	Indication	Dose and Route	Onset (O) and Duration (D)	Monitoring Parameters	Contraindications
	Intraoperative	100–150 units/kg IV before cross-clamps applied, followed by additional doses of 50 units/kg every 45–50 min		• ACT	
LMWH: enoxaparin (Lovenox)	Intraoperative	0.75 mg/kg IV before cross-clamps applied, followed by 0.75 mg/kg SC q12 h beginning 8 h after IV bolus	O: immediate with IV D: $t_{1/2}$ is not dose dependent $T_{1/2}$ = 4.5–7 h	• antiXa • Hemoglobin • Platelets • Signs and symptoms of bleeding • Renal function (clearance declines)	• Hypersensitivity to enoxaparin, heparin, or pork products • HIT • Active major bleeding
Dalteparin (Fragmin)	Intraoperative	70 units/kg IV before cross-clamps applied	O: immediate with IV D: $t_{1/2}$ is not dose dependent $T_{1/2}$ = 2–5 h	• antiXa • Hemoglobin • Platelets • Signs and symptoms of bleeding • Renal function (clearance declines)	• Hypersensitivity to dalteparin, heparin, or pork products • HIT • Active major bleeding

HIT, heparin-induced thrombocytopenia.
Sources: Garcia et al. (2012), Lexi-Drugs™ (2013), Samama et al. (1995), and Swedenborg et al. (1996).

Antiplatelet Drugs

The available and commonly used antiplatelet drugs are as follows:

- Aspirin
- Clopidogrel (Plavix)
- Ticlopidine (Ticlid)
- Dipyridamole and aspirin (Aggrenox)
- Ticagrelor (Brilinta)—recommended only for coronary patients

Patients with PVD are at high risk for cardiovascular ischemic events. Studies with PVD patients have shown that approximately 50% have symptoms of coronary artery disease (CAD) (or electrocardiographic abnormality); 90% have abnormalities on coronary angiography; and 40% have duplex evidence of carotid artery disease (Tierney, Fennessy, & Hayes, 2000). When all relevant and current trials are summarized, it appears that approximately 60% of PVD patients will have significant atherosclerosis of the cardiac or cerebral arteries (Norgren et al., 2007). The risk of death with symptomatic PVD is approximately 30% and 50% within 5 and 10 years, respectively. The primary cause of death is related to myocardial infarction (40% to 60%) or stroke (10% to 20%) (Norgren et al., 2007). The overall mortality rate among PVD patients, which is caused by a cardiovascular event, is estimated to occur in approximately 80% of cases (Aronow & Ahn, 1994; Dormandy et al., 1989; Hertzer et al., 1984). The primary role of antiplatelet therapy is to reduce a patient's risk of experiencing a cardiovascular ischemic event (myocardial infarction, stroke, or transient ischemic attack) (Hiatt, 2001; Norgren et al., 2007; Tierney et al., 2000).

Mechanism of Action

Aspirin

Aspirin irreversibly inhibits the cyclooxygenase (COX) enzyme and thereby prevents the conversion of arachidonic acid to various prostaglandins. Two types of COX enzymes exist: COX-1, which is located predominately within platelets, and COX-2, which is expressed within tissues in response to an inflammatory reaction. The COX-1 enzyme is more sensitive to aspirin inhibition, and it is this enzyme, which is responsible for the production of the prostaglandin thromboxane A2, that causes vasoconstriction and stimulation of platelet aggregation. Low doses (30 to 100 mg) of aspirin are effective at inhibiting COX-1 but are less effective against COX-2. Thus, to prevent platelet aggregation, clinicians may use low doses of aspirin to achieve an adequate response with less gastrointestinal and bleeding adverse effects (Eikelboom, Hirsh, Spencer, Baglin, & Weitz, 2012).

Clopidogrel and Ticlopidine

Clopidogrel and ticlopidine are thienopyridine derivatives, and both are ADP-receptor antagonists. Clopidogrel and ticlopidine are first activated through the cytochrome P450-dependant pathway and subsequently bound with and irreversibly alter receptor P2Y(12) on the surface of platelets. The irreversible change to this receptor antagonizes ADP from binding to platelets and thereby prevents subsequent ADP-mediated platelet aggregation (Eikelboom et al., 2012). The inhibition of ADP platelet aggregation in turn inhibits platelet aggregation induced by other agonists such as thromboxane A2, platelet-activating factor, collagen, and low concentrations of thrombin. However, this additional effect may not be clinically significant (Eikelboom et al., 2012).

Ticlopidine use is associated with significant blood toxicities including neutropenia, thrombocytopenia, and aplastic anemia; therefore, its use is generally reserved for those who cannot take aspirin or clopidogrel (Lexi-Drugs, 2013; Sobel & Verhaeghe, 2008) and is rarely prescribed.

Dipyridamole

Dipyridamole is an agent with vasodilator and antiplatelet actions. Dipyridamole causes accumulation of cyclic AMP (cAMP) within platelets and this leads to platelet inhibition. There are two proposed mechanisms for this buildup of cAMP. One is the inhibition of the enzyme (cyclic nucleotide phosphodiesterase) that degrades cAMP. The second mechanism is blockade of platelet uptake of adenosine which further contributes to increased cAMP. The vasodilator properties may then result from the direct stimulation of prostaglandin I2 synthesis and protection against its degradation (Eikelboom et al., 2012).

Dipyridamole alone has not produced favorable clinical results. However, a modified-release dipyridamole in combination with low-dose aspirin (Aggrenox) has been shown to significantly reduce the risk of stroke in patients who had previously experienced a cerebral ischemic event compared with patients who received aspirin alone (Eikelboom et al., 2012).

Ticagrelor

Ticagrelor is a non-thienopyridine (ADP) receptor antagonist that inhibits platelet aggregation. "Tricagrelor completely inhibits ADP-induced platelet inhibition ex vivo through reversible binding reversibly to the P2Y12 receptors" (Jennings, 2010). Tricagrelor does not require metabolic activation in order to inhibit platelets.

Indications

Aspirin

To reduce peripheral vascular graft occlusion in patients with prior bypass surgery
To reduce the need for peripheral arterial surgery
To reduce the risk of cardiovascular ischemic events

Clopidogrel and Ticlopidine

To reduce peripheral vascular graft occlusion in patients with prior bypass surgery
To reduce the risk of cardiovascular ischemic events

Dipyridamole and Aspirin

To reduce peripheral vascular graft occlusion in patients with prior bypass surgery. [Note that the dose of aspirin in the combination product Aggrenox is 25 mg and may not be adequate to prevent recurrent myocardial infarctions or angina attacks (Lexi-Drugs, 2013.)

Ticagrelor

Ticagrelor is indicated to reduce the rate of thrombotic cardiovascular events in patients with acute coronary syndrome (ACS) (unstable angina, non-ST elevation myocardial infarction, or ST elevation myocardial infarction (Wallentin et al., 2010). Ticagrelor should be used in combination with aspirin.

Evidence

Prevention of Arterial Graft Occlusion

Aspirin and dipyridamole: A metaanalysis conducted by Tangelder, Lawson, Algra, and Eikelboom (1999) of five randomized controlled trials (Donaldson et al., 1985; Goldman, & McCollum, 1984; Green, Roedersheimer, & DeWeese, 1982; Kohler et al., 1984; McCollum, Alexander, Kenchington, Franks, & Greenhalgh, 1991) demonstrated a pooled overall treatment effect favoring the use of aspirin and dipyridamole for preventing graft occlusion. Only one of the five studies examined the use of aspirin alone compared with placebo (Green et al., 1982). The pooled relative risk (RR) across the five trials for bypass occlusion was 0.78 (95% CI, 0.64% to 0.95%) or a risk reduction of approximately 22% (Tangelder et al., 1999). A review performed by the Antiplatelet Trialists' Collaboration (ATC) group (ATC, 1994) supported the findings of Tangelder et al. (1999). The ATC group concluded that antiplatelet therapy with aspirin significantly improved vascular graft patency in 3,226 patients with PVD who were treated with bypass surgery (saphenous vein or prosthetic graft) or peripheral angioplasty (ATC, 1994). There was a statistically significant 43% proportional reduction in vascular graft occlusion, from 25% in the control group to 16% in the antiplatelet group (ATC, 1994). Despite these positive results, caution should be exercised when interpreting the findings because the trials following the bypass procedures were small (a total of 423 patients in the active group and 393 patients in the control group) and of a relatively short duration (1-year follow-up). Ultimately the question of whether or not there is sufficient evidence of value of using aspirin with dipyridamole to prevent graft occlusion is somewhat irrelevant since all patients with symptomatic PVD who do not have a contraindication are recommended to take aspirin for the prevention of cardiovascular ischemic events (Alonso-Coello et al., 2012; Sobel & Verhaeghe, 2008).

Ticlopidine: A single clinical study currently supports the use of ticlopidine for the prevention of bypass occlusion in PAD patients undergoing infrainguinal surgery. Becquemin (1997) randomized 243 patients who underwent femoropopliteal or femorotibial saphenous vein bypass graft to either ticlopidine or placebo and followed them for an average of 2 years. Cumulative graft patency rate at 2 years' follow-up was 82% and 63% for the ticlopidine and placebo groups, respectively (Becquemin, 1997). Despite the clinical evidence, which supports the benefits of ticlopidine on late peripheral bypass occlusion, the use of ticlopidine has been discouraged because of the risk of hematologic side effects (Eikelboom et al., 2012).

Clopidogrel: Evidence to support the use of clopidogrel after peripheral arterial bypass surgery is limited. The CASPAR trial evaluated clopidogrel plus aspirin versus aspirin alone in patients after below knee bypass grafting (Belch & Dormandy, 2010). There was no significant difference in the composite primary outcome of graft occlusion, amputation, or death in the overall patient population, but there was a significant benefit of the addition of clopidogrel to aspirin in the subgroup that had a prosthetic graft (Belch & Dormandy, 2010). The combination of clopidogrel and aspirin is now recommended for 1 year (the average follow-up time in the study) after bypass surgery in those with a prosthetic graft (Alonso-Coello et al., 2012).

Reducing Risk for Peripheral Arterial Surgery

Aspirin: The Physicians' Health Study (Goldhaber et al., 1992) was designed as a primary prevention trial for patients who had no history of myocardial infarction, stroke, or transient cerebral ischemia. Treatment with aspirin, 325 mg every other day, produced a significant reduction in the need for peripheral arterial surgery (RR of peripheral artery surgery in the aspirin arm was 0.54, $p < 0.03$). The study, however, showed no difference between aspirin and placebo treatment in the prevention of IC (Goldhaber et al., 1992).

Prevention of Cardiovascular Events

Antiplatelets (aspirin and dipyridamole): The ATC group demonstrated that in patients who are at a higher risk for experiencing vascular events (i.e., those with a history of unstable angina, acute myocardial infarction, prior myocardial infarction, stroke, or transient ischemic attack, and patients with other evidence of vascular disease such as PVD), antiplatelet therapy significantly reduced the odds ratio of experiencing a myocardial infarction, stroke, or subsequent death from a vascular event by 27%. When patients with PVD were examined separately (those with IC, peripheral grafts, or peripheral angioplasty), the benefit of antiplatelet treatment was similar in magnitude but was nonsignificant (ATC, 1994).

While the evidence supporting aspirin for secondary prevention of cardiovascular events is clear in those with symptomatic PVD, it is unclear and controversial if those without symptoms (and therefore in need of primary prevention) benefit from aspirin. The Antithrombotic Trialists' Collaboration attempted to answer the question of primary prevention benefit in asymptomatic patients with PVD (Baigent et al., 2009). In their metaanalysis of trials with low-dose aspirin they found a significant reduction of nonfatal MI (0.18% vs. 0.23% per year, $p < 0.0001$), a nonsignificant difference in stroke rates, and a nonsignificant difference in vascular mortality (Baigent et al., 2009). There was also a significant increase in major gastrointestinal and extracranial bleeding (0.10% vs. 0.07% per year, $p < 0.0001$) that tempers the benefit of a reduced risk of MI (Baigent et al., 2009) in those without symptoms of PVD. The latest ACCP clinical practice guidelines recommend aspirin 75 to 100 mg daily in asymptomatic PVD (Alonso-Coello et al., 2012). The American College of Cardiology Foundation and American Heart Association (ACCF/AHA) practice guideline for peripheral artery disease has not recommended aspirin due to "usefulness not well established" in asymptomatic patients using the same evidence (Rooke et al., 2011). The TASC II (Trans-Atlantic inter-Society Consensus) document for management of peripheral artery disease has taken a neutral stance on the question with their recommendation that aspirin "can be considered" in those without symptoms (Norgren et al., 2007).

Aspirin versus clopidogrel: The study clopidogrel versus aspirin in patients at risk of ischemic events (CAPRIE Steering Committee, 1996) directly compared the effects of aspirin and clopidogrel in reducing the risk of ischemic events in patients who had recent myocardial infarctions, ischemic strokes, or PVD. Overall, clopidogrel was found to be significantly more effective in reducing the combined endpoint of ischemic stroke, myocardial infarction, and death from a vascular cause (RR reduction 8.7%, $p < 0.043$). When PVD patients were examined separately, clopidogrel reduced the average ischemic event rate significantly more compared with aspirin, 4.86% and 3.71%, respectively (RR reduction 23.8%, $p < 0.0028$) (CAPRIE Steering Committee, 1996).

Aspirin versus clopidogrel and ticlopidine: A review of the Cochrane database for studies using ticlopidine and clopidogrel versus aspirin in high-risk vascular patients determined that ticlopidine and clopidogrel reduced the odds of stroke, myocardial infarction, and vascular death by approximately 9% compared with aspirin therapy. Although ticlopidine and clopidogrel therapy were shown to be significantly more effective than aspirin in preventing vascular events, the magnitude of this benefit was small and must be weighed against adverse effects and cost. Ticlopidine usage has diminished and is discouraged because the risks of complications, such as neutropenia and thrombocytopenia, are significant compared with clopidogrel or aspirin therapy. Clopidogrel use is associated with a greater incidence of diarrhea and skin rash and is significantly more expensive than aspirin. Aspirin is associated with more gastrointestinal intolerance and bleeding (Hankey, Sudlow, & Dunbabin, 2000).

Ticagrelor: The PLATelet inhibition and patient Outcomes (PLATO) trial showed Ticagrelor to be more effective than clopidogrel for the continuous prevention of ischemic events, stent thrombosis, and death in the acute and long-term treatment of patients with ACS with no change in the overall risk of major bleeding (Wallentin et al., 2010). Ticagrelor was approved by the FDA in July 2011. However, there is no data on its use in patients with peripheral artery disease.

Summary

Aspirin or clopidogrel may be used long term in patients after bypass graft surgery to maintain patency. Patients who have a prosthetic graft are recommended to take *both* aspirin and clopidogrel for the first year after surgery (Alonso-Coello et al., 2012).

Aspirin remains the drug of choice for cardiovascular risk reduction though clopidogrel is an alternative that can be used in symptomatic patients. Although clinical trials have demonstrated clopidogrel to be more effective in reducing cardiovascular events in patients with PVD, the magnitude of this benefit is small, and the cost of clopidogrel is significantly more compared with aspirin (Hankey et al., 2000).

Ticlopidine therapy has dropped out of favor for clinical use because it is associated with a greater incidence of neutropenia and thrombocytopenia (Eikelboom et al., 2012; Hankey et al., 2000).

The combination product dipyridamole and aspirin is not recommended for the prevention of cardiovascular events in patients with PVD. However, it is an appropriate and effective therapy for secondary stroke prevention in patients who have failed aspirin therapy (Lexi-Drugs, 2013).

Unless there is a contraindication to aspirin therapy, every patient with symptomatic PVD should be taking aspirin (the majority of patients) or clopidogrel (those who have an allergy or intolerance to aspirin or who have an unusually low bleeding risk). Some patients with asymptomatic PVD will be candidates for aspirin for primary prevention. After surgical intervention and placement of a prosthetic graft, patients should be considered for both aspirin and clopidogrel for 1 year and then continue one of the two drugs long term (Alonso-Coello et al., 2012; Norgren et al., 2007; Rooke et al., 2011) (see Table 6-2).

Thrombolytics

The thrombolytics that have been used in vascular surgery include the following:

Streptokinase (SK) (Streptase)
Urokinase (UK) (Abbokinase—retired brand name, may return to market as Kinlytic in the future)
Alteplase (recombinant tissue plasminogen activator [rt-PA], Activase)
Reteplase (Retavase)
Tenecteplase (TNKase)

TABLE 6-2 Antiplatelet Comparison Chart

Drug	Indication	Dose	Onset (O) and Duration (D)	Monitoring Parameters	Contraindications
Aspirin	Cardiovascular risk reduction/ arterial graft patency	75–325 mg daily	O: immediate release tablet: peak levels 30–40 min, inhibition of platelet function evident after 1 h Enteric-coated tablet: peak levels 3–4 h D: drug $t_{1/2}$ = 15–20 min. However, platelet inhibition lasts for the lifetime of the platelet	• Gastrointestinal adverse events (bleeding, ulcer, dyspepsia) • Complete blood count (monitor for rare hematologic side effects) • Signs and symptoms of bleeding	• Hypersensitivity to aspirin or other NSAIDs • Use with caution: asthma, rhinitis, or nasal polyps • Bleeding disorders • Active peptic ulcer
Clopidogrel (Plavix)	Cardiovascular risk reduction/ arterial graft patency	75 mg daily	O: inhibition of platelet function detected on second day of therapy D: drug $t_{1/2}$ = 6 h but platelet function does not return to normal for 7–10 d after last dose	Signs and symptoms of bleeding	• Hypersensitivity to clopidogrel • Active major bleeding
Ticlopidine* (Ticlid)	Cardiovascular risk reduction	250 mg twice daily	O: 6 h D: $t_{1/2}$ = 24–36 h after a single dose and up to 96 h after 2 wks of therapy	• Complete blood count with differential q2 wks for first 3 mos of therapy • Liver function tests if liver dysfunction is suspected • Signs and symptoms of bleeding	• Hypersensitivity to ticlopidine • Active major bleeding • Severe liver impairment • Hematopoietic disorders (neutropenia, thrombocytopenia, aplastic anemia, or TTP)
Dipyridamole and aspirin (Aggrenox)	Arterial graft patency	200/25 mg twice daily	Dipyridamole: O: peak levels within 1.5–2 h D: $t_{1/2}$ = 10 h However, platelet inhibition lasts for the lifetime of the platelet due to the aspirin	Dipyridamole: • Blood pressure • Signs and symptoms of bleeding	• Hypersensitivity to aspirin or dipyridamole • Use with caution: asthma, rhinitis, or nasal polyps • Bleeding disorders • Active peptic ulcer

NSAIDs, nonsteroidal anti-inflammatory drugs; TTP, thrombotic thrombocytopenic purpura.
*use has generally been replaced by newer, less toxic drugs including clopidogrel
Source: Eikelboom et al. (2012), Goldhaber et al. (1992), Lexi-Drugs™ (2013), and Rooke et al. (2011).

Streptokinase is no longer manufactured and will not be discussed in detail. Urokinase is not currently available since Abbokinase is no longer manufactured and Kinlytic is not yet FDA approved. The use of urokinase will be discussed here because it may become available in the future. The thrombolytics currently available do not have FDA-approved uses for vascular disease indications with the exception of alteplase for treatment of PE or stroke but off-label use is common.

Mechanism of Action

Refer to Table 6-3, Thrombolytic Comparison Chart.

Indications

Thrombolytic drugs may be used intravenously as in treatment of acute MI or acute ischemic stroke. Thrombolytics are used more commonly in patients with PVD in catheter-directed thrombolysis or

TABLE 6-3 Thrombolytic Comparison Chart

Drug	Mechanism of Action	Indication	Dose (for ~70 kg Adult)	Duration
Urokinase	Directly activates the conversion of plasminogen to plasmin. Plasmin degrades fibrin and other procoagulant plasma proteins	Acute limb ischemia	Catheter directed: 250,000 International Units bolus, then 4,000 International Units/min for 4 h, then 2,000 International Units/min for a maximum of 48 h[a]	$T_{1/2}$ = 6.4–18.8 min, but effect may last over 4 h
		Arteriovenous graft occlusion	Catheter directed: 250,000 International Units, then overnight infusion 240,000 International Units/h if minimal improvement with initial bolus[a]	
Alteplase (Activase)	Recombinant human tissue plasminogen activator (rt-PA)	Acute limb ischemia	Catheter directed: 0.5–2.5 mg/h for extended infusions (>12 h) OR 0.05 mg/kg/h up to 12 h or until maximum of 100 mg is administered[a]	$T_{1/2}$ ~ 5 min, about 80% of drug cleared within 10 min
		Arteriovenous graft occlusion	Catheter directed: 2 mg[a]	
Reteplase (Retavase)	Same as alteplase but with a longer half-life due to change in size of protein structure	Acute limb ischemia	Catheter directed: 2 units bolus, then 0.5–1 unit/h (do not exceed a total maximum of 20 units)[a]	$T_{1/2}$ = 13–16 min
		Arteriovenous graft occlusion	Catheter directed: 1 unit[a]	
Tenecteplase (TNKase)	Same as alteplase but with a longer half-life due to changes in amino acids in protein structure	Acute limb ischemia	Catheter directed: 0.25–0.5 mg/h. Stop infusion if arteriograms do not show improvement[a]	Biphasic elimination: initial $t_{1/2}$ = 20–24 min, terminal $t_{1/2}$ = 90–130 min
		Arteriovenous graft occlusion	Catheter directed: 1 mg[a]	

[a]These doses are not FDA approved but are based on case reports and other clinical use data.
Note: Monitoring is the same for all thrombolytics on this table: hemoglobin, aPTT, fibrinogen, platelet count, signs and symptoms of bleeding, blood pressure.
Source: Lew and Weaver (2010) and Lexi-Drugs™ (2013).

TABLE 6-4 Contraindications to Thrombolysis

Absolute	Relative
1. Active internal bleeding 2. Recent (within 2 mos) cerebrovascular accident, trauma, or intracranial or intraspinal surgery 3. Known intracranial neoplasm 4. Severe uncontrollable hypertension 5. Uncontrollable clotting disorders 6. Previous severe allergic reactions to the thrombolytic agent	1. Recent (within 10 d) operative or obstetric procedures, biopsy or procedure in a location that is not compressible, gastrointestinal bleeding, or trauma, including cardiopulmonary resuscitation 2. Left heart thrombus 3. Subacute bacterial endocarditis 4. Severe liver or kidney disease 5. Diabetic hemorrhagic retinopathy 6. Acute pancreatitis 7. Pregnancy 8. Any other condition in which bleeding constitutes a significant hazard or would be particularly difficult to manage because of its location

Source: Lew and Weaver (2010).

with mechanical thrombectomy. Heparin is often used concurrently to prevent thrombus propagation (Lew & Weaver, 2010). Table 6-4 indicates the contraindications to thrombolytic therapy that help to determine whether a patient is a candidate for thrombolysis.

Contraindications and Complications of Thrombolytic Therapy

Contraindications to thrombolytic therapy and potential risk of adverse events must first be evaluated prior to initiating therapy. The major concern with thrombolytic use is the risk of hemorrhage. A comparative bleeding risk rate between thrombolytics with peripheral administration is limited; however, available trials have demonstrated that UK and rt-PA have similar bleeding complications and that SK is associated with more hemorrhagic complications in comparison with rt-PA. A collected series of patients enrolled in the British Thrombolysis Study Group showed the incidence of hemorrhagic and ischemic stroke to be 2.3% (27 of 1,157 patients) (Dawson et al., 1996). Most bleeding complications during the administration of thrombolytic therapy occur at the site of the catheter puncture (arterial or venous) and may be controlled with local pressure, by increasing the catheter size, sheath placement around the catheter, or a surgical stitch. Although bleeding at other sites is less frequent, retroperitoneal, intra-abdominal, or gastrointestinal bleeding may also occur. The dose of thrombolytic may be higher in PE, DVT, and acute limb ischemia and lower in arteriovenous graft occlusion. Higher doses tend to be associated with more bleeding complications. The true incidence of bleeding complications is unknown due to inconsistencies in how bleeding is defined (Lew & Weaver, 2010) (see Table 6-4).

Evidence

Acute Limb Ischemia/Graft Occlusion

The Surgery vs. Thrombolysis for the Ischemic Lower Extremity (STILE) trial compared open surgical therapy with catheter-directed rt-PA or UK in patients with up to 6 months of symptoms (Weaver et al., 1994). The study was stopped early due to adverse primary outcomes in the thrombolysis group compared to the surgical group. However, a subgroup analysis showed that in patients with symptoms lasting less than 14 days there was a statistically significant lower 6-month amputation rate with thrombolytics than with surgery (11% vs. 30%, respectively) (Weaver et al., 1994). The Thrombolysis or Peripheral Arterial Surgery (TOPAS) trial enrolled patients with less than 14 days of symptomatic arterial or bypass graft occlusion and randomized them to open surgery versus catheter-directed UK (Ouriel, Veith, & Sasahara, 1998). After 12 months of follow-up, there were similar amputation-free survival and mortality rates. In the thrombolysis treatment group, 40% of the patients avoided surgery but at the expense of an increase in major bleeding rates (5.5% in surgical group vs. 12.5% in UK group) (Ouriel et al., 1998). Based on these two trials, the ACCP practice guidelines recommended intraarterial thrombolytic therapy for less than 14 days of symptoms provided that patients are at low risk for complications (myonecrosis and ischemic nerve damage) due to time delays inherent in this method (Sobel & Verhaeghe, 2008).

Metaanalyses have been performed to compare the benefits and risks of surgery with thrombolysis for the treatment of lower limb ischemia (Berridge, Kessel, & Robertson, 2002). The study by Berridge et al. (2002) included five randomized controlled trials (1,283 participants) that compared thrombolysis with surgical intervention for acute limb ischemia. There was no significant difference in limb salvage or death at 30 days, 6 months, or 1 year after initial surgery or thrombolysis. The metaanalysis also determined that the hemorrhage complications after thrombolysis were significantly greater than surgical intervention (Berridge et al., 2002). After a re-review of the evidence above and including this metaanalysis, the latest ACCP guidelines recommend surgery over thrombolysis (Alonso-Coello et al., 2012).

Summary

SK and UK are no longer available for clinical use because they have been discontinued by the manufacturer. None of the rt-PA products are FDA approved for treatment of acute limb ischemia but some evidence for dosing exists (see Table 6-4).

Despite the recent controversy, thrombolysis remains a viable therapeutic option because it has the theoretical advantage of reduced risk of myointimal injury after catheter-directed thrombectomy and uncovering underlying lesions and the ability to visualize run-off vessels (Norgren et al., 2007).

Dextran

In the past, dextran was used primarily as a plasma volume expander; however, significant bleeding complications were associated with its use. Bleeding effects have been linked to dextran interfering with fibrin polymerization, which causes enhanced fibrinolysis. Factor VIII and von Willebrand's factor are also decreased in the presence of dextran. Lastly, dextran absorbs to platelet surfaces to prevent platelet aggregation. Interestingly, clinicians have attempted to use the adverse bleeding effects of dextran to advantage, and as a result, dextran has been used and studied for its antithrombotic effect though it is not FDA approved for this indication (Gortier et al., 2006).

For the purpose of treating vascular patients, dextran has been used pre- and postoperatively to prevent thrombotic complications in carotid endarterectomy (Roseborough & Perler, 2010). Lennard et al. (1999) determined that 3 hours of monitored dextran 40 infusion was as effective as 6 hours of monitoring. An infusion of 10% dextran 40 decreased the emboli detected by transcranial Doppler ultrasonography as follows: 46% fewer embolic signal counts in the dextran group after 1 hour postoperatively and 64% fewer after 2 to 3 hours postoperatively (Levi et al., 2001). A larger study ($n = 600$) used a fixed rate of dextran 40 at 20 mL/hour and cost-effectively decreased stroke rates from 4% to 0.2% (Hayes et al., 2000).

Section 2: Renee Mosier

Cholesterol-Lowering Medications

Anitschkow (1913) first recognized the association between hypercholesterolemia and atherosclerosis approximately 80 years ago (Anitschkow, 1913), and numerous clinical trials have since been performed. It is now accepted that elevated low-density lipoprotein (LDL) ("bad cholesterol") and low high-density lipoprotein (HDL) ("good cholesterol") levels are strongly correlated with increased risks of coronary events (Grundy et al., 1993). The National Cholesterol Educational Program Adult Treatment Panel III has clearly identified LDL reduction as the primary focus of cholesterol-lowering therapy, with increasing HDL as an important secondary focus (Grundy et al., 1993).

Five classes of cholesterol-lowering medications are commonly used to manage hypercholesterolemia:

- 3-Hydroxy-3-methylglutaryl-coenzyme A (HMG-CoA) reductase inhibitors (statins)
- Fibrinic acid derivatives (fibrates)
- Bile acid–binding resins
- Niacin
- Cholesterol absorption inhibitors

Each class affects the various types of cholesterol differently. For example, fibrates are most effective at lowering triglyceride levels, whereas statins are the drugs of choice to decrease LDL cholesterol (Sisson & Tisdel, 2001). With the adoption of the ATP III guidelines in 2004, a new emphasis was placed on the treatment of individuals having specific risk factors and an increased 10-year risk for the development of coronary heart disease (CHD), rather than just those with active CHD. The primary focus of hyperlipidemia treatment remains on lowering LDL cholesterol levels with more stringent treatment thresholds adopted (ATP III). With the publication of the Heart Protection Study (Heart Protection Study Collaborative Group, 2002), investigators have confirmed that patients at high risk for developing CAD (e.g., those with PVD, cerebral vascular disease, diabetes) do experience significant benefits from statin therapy designed to lower LDL concentrations. Newer American College of Cardiology/American Heart Association (ACC/AHA) guidelines released in November 2013 support atherosclerotic cardiovascular disease risk reduction with statin therapy, though makes no recommendation for or against specific LDL or non-HDL targets (Stone et al., 2013). Newer guidelines agreed with previous studies that mortality from all causes and from CHD was significantly reduced with fixed dose simvastatin therapy, compared with placebo (Heart Protection Study Collaborative Group, 2002). Given the wealth of evidence showing the ability of statins to reduce cardiovascular mortality and morbidity through LDL-lowering effects, they are considered the cholesterol drug of choice in patients with PVD (Dormandy & Rutherford, 2000; Heart Protection Study Collaborative Group, 2002; Stone et al., 2013).

Fibrinic acid derivatives and bile acid–binding resins are used but are second-line agents added to statin therapy to raise HDL concentrations or provide additional triglyceride-lowering effects. Niacin (nicotinic acid or vitamin B3) is effective for raising HDL levels. However, because this agent is contraindicated for use in diabetes and is otherwise poorly tolerated (because of potent vasodilating properties), it is not commonly used in patients with PVD.

HMG-CoA Reductase Inhibitors (Statins)

- Simvastatin (Zocor)
- Lovastatin (Mevacor, Altocor)
- Pravastatin (Lipostat, Pravachol)
- Atorvastatin (Lipitor)
- Fluvastatin (Lescol)
- Rosuvastatin (Crestor)
- Pitavastatin (Livalo)

Mechanism of Action

All statins competitively inhibit HMG-CoA reductase, an enzyme involved in cholesterol and other sterol synthesis (Chong, Seeger, & Franklin, 2001). Statins directly inhibit cholesterol synthesis in the liver and peripheral tissues and induce the synthesis of LDL receptors on cell membranes of the liver to remove LDL cholesterol. The ATP III guidelines summarized the class effects of statins and found that on average, statins will decrease LDL by 18% to 55%, increase HDL by 5% to 15%, and decrease triglycerides by 7% to 30% (ATP III), making them the agent of choice for most patients with elevated LDL levels. 2013 ACC/AHS Blood Cholesterol Guideline (Stone et al., 2013) reviewed percent reductions in LDL for a specific statin and dose. High-intensity therapy on average lowers LDL by >50% (atorvastatin 40 to 80 mg or rosuvastatin 20 to 40 mg daily). Moderate-intensity therapy lowers LDL by approximately 30% to 50% (atorvastatin 10 to 20 mg, rosuvastatin 5 to 10 mg, simvastatin 20 to 40 mg, pravastatin 40 to 80 mg, lovastatin 40 mg daily, pitavastatin 2 to 4 mg, or fluvastatin 40 mg twice daily.) Low-intensity therapy lowers LDL on average <30% (simvastatin 10 mg, pravastatin 10 to 20 mg, lovastatin 20 mg, fluvastatin 20 to 40 mg, or pitavastatin 1 mg daily).

Indication

- To decrease cardiovascular events
- Arterial plaque stabilization

Fibrinic Acid Resins (Fibrates)

- Clofibrate (Atromid-S)
- Fenofibrate (Tricor, Lofiba, Lipidil Supra, Fenogal, Lipantil, Supralip)
- Gemfibrozil (Lopid)
- Fenofibric Acid (Fibricor, Trilipix)—active metabolite of fenofibrate

Mechanism of Action

Fibrates increase HDL concentrations and decrease very low density lipoprotein (VLDL) (the precursor to LDL), yet the mechanism of action is not completely understood. Evidence suggests that the antiatherosclerotic effects of fibrates are achieved through a combination of pharmacologic actions.

1. Enhanced catabolism of triglyceride-rich lipoproteins (TGRLs) through lipoproteinlipase (LPL) stimulation and/or hepatic lipase activity (Gotto & Pownall, 1998)
2. Activation of transcription factors for peroxisome proliferator–activated receptor-a (a hormone receptor that controls several genes) that decreases apolipoprotein (apo)C-3production, which in turn decreases VLDL secretion from the liver (Gotto & Pownall, 1998; Sisson & Tisdel, 2001)
3. Activation of transcription factors for peroxisome proliferator–activated receptor-a that, in turn, promotes apoAI and apoAII synthesis. The result is increased HDL production
4. Activation of peroxisome proliferator–activated receptors and nuclear transcription factors that upregulate LPL transcription (Gotto and Pownall, 1998)

Bile Acid Sequestrants

- Cholestyramine (Questran, QuestranLight, Locholest, Prevalite)
- Colestipol (Colestid)
- Celesevelam (WelChol)

Mechanism of Action

Both cholestyramine and colestipol are anion exchange resins. They exert cholesterol-lowering effects by binding to bile (a cholesterol-rich substance) in the gut, which in turn increases fecal elimination of bile salts and disrupts the enterohepatic cholesterol circulation, an important metabolic pathway for lipids and lipoproteins. Daily intestinal bile salt loss increases from 1 to 3 g/day. A decrease in bile reabsorption increases intrahepatic cholesterol for bile acid production and increases LDL removal from the plasma.

Niacin (Nicotinic Acid, Vitamin B3)

Niacin is a water-soluble vitamin B complex and is available over the counter in immediate release formulations and by prescription in high-dose, extended release formulations.

Mechanism of Action

Only recently has research been able to uncover the mechanisms of action of niacin which are varied and complex. Historically, scientists thought that niacin worked primarily by inhibiting fatty acid release from adipose tissue. We now also understand that niacin plays a role in inhibiting synthesis and increasing metabolism of fatty acids in the liver. With fatty acids being a main substrate for triglyceride production, triglyceride levels are significantly impacted (Kamanna & Kashyap, 2008; Morgan, Carey, Lincoff, & Capuzzi, 2004). Following the chain of lipid synthesis, decreased triglycerides result in decreased VDLD and thus slightly decreased LDL.

Niacin has also been found to downregulate the catabolism of HDL, thereby increasing the half-life of HDL particles and thus the overall serum concentration of HDL. These HDL particles seem to remain functional throughout their extended lives and continue the transport of LDL to the liver for breakdown, yet another way that niacin has a minor impact on decreasing LDL levels (Kamanna & Kashyap, 2008; Morgan et al., 2004).

The ATP III guidelines indicate that at doses of 1 to 3 g daily niacin can expectedly decrease LDL 5% to 25%, increase HDL 15% to 35%, and decrease triglycerides 20% to 50%.

Cholesterol Absorption Inhibitors

- Ezetimibe (Zetia)

Mechanism of Action

Approved by the FDA in 2001, ezetimibe is the first in this class of medications. It works locally at the brush border of the small intestine inhibiting absorption of dietary cholesterol. A clinical study of 18 patients showed that ezetimibe inhibited intestinal cholesterol absorption by 54% compared to placebo. With decreased uptake of cholesterol from the intestines, the liver shifts to increasing uptake from the blood to maintain cholesterol stores and LDL cholesterol is thereby decreased (Ezetimibe Prescribing Information, 2013).

Ezetimibe is approved for use as monotherapy, or in combination with a statin or fenofibrate. When added to statin therapy, ezetimibe has been shown to lower LDL cholesterol by 12 to 15 points more than statin therapy alone and also has a slight impact on lower triglycerides and increasing HDL. The addition of ezetimibe to fenofibrate therapy was shown to lower LDL by an additional 14 points (Ezetimibe Prescribing Information, 2013).

Medications Used to Treat Intermittent Claudication

The following medications are used to treat symptoms of IC:

- Pentoxifylline (Trental)
- Cilostazol (Pletal)

Mechanism of Action

Pentoxifylline has several pharmacologic actions. First, in a dose-related fashion, pentoxifylline decreases blood viscosity and increases erythrocyte flexibility. Second, pentoxifylline inhibits platelet aggregation, and as a result, blood flow. Thus oxygenation is improved throughout the atherosclerotic microvasculature (Tjon & Riemann, 2001; Trental Package Information, 2013).

Cilostazol is a phosphodiesterase inhibitor that, like pentoxifylline, has antiplatelet properties and has vasodilatory properties. It exhibits beneficial lipid effects (15% reduction in triglycerides and 10% increase in HDL) and has vascular antiproliferative properties (Dawson, Cutler, & Meissner, 1998; Reilly & Mohler, 2001; Tjon & Riemann, 2001).

Evidence

Pentoxifylline

- There is an unpredictable increase in claudication distance and maximum walking distance (Radack & Deck, 1991; Radack & Wyderski, 1990).

- Many clinical trials have been performed; however, they are small studies, the endpoints were variable, and data on patient smoking habits and IC symptoms prior to enrollment were lacking (Tjon & Riemann, 2001).
- Metaanalyses of pentoxifylline trials have demonstrated a significant but small improvement in the absolute claudication distance (Hood, Moher, & Barber, 1996).
- The clinical significance of the small benefits seen in trials has been questioned (Radack & Deck, 1991; Radack & Wyderski, 1990).
- Patients with symptoms for greater than 1 year, moderately severe ischemia, and ABI <0.8 are most likely to benefit from therapy (Lindgarde et al., 1989).
- The American College of Chest Physicians recommends against the use of pentoxifylline for the treatment of patients with peripheral artery disease because benefits according to current evidence are conflicting and weak (Clagett et al., 2004).

Cilostazol

- Three randomized, placebo control trials have evaluated the efficacy of cilostazol (50 or 100 mg twice daily) on absolute walking distance or pain-free walking distance (Beebe, Dawson, & Cutler, 1999; Dawson et al., 1998; Money et al., 1998). All studies demonstrated significant improvements in both outcomes for patients treated with cilostazol.
- One randomized clinical control trial designed to compare cilostazol, pentoxifylline, and placebo demonstrated that cilostazol is significantly more effective in improving absolute claudication distance than pentoxifylline (350 m for cilostazol vs. 308 m for pentoxifylline, $p = 0.0005$). Initial claudication distance was also more significant at the end of the 24-week trial for patients treated with cilostazol. No difference in quality of life was observed (Dawson et al., 2000).
- The American College of Chest Physicians recommends that cilostazol may be used for patients with disabling IC who do not respond to risk factor modification and exercise therapy and who are not surgical or catheter-based intervention candidates (Clagett et al., 2004).

Summary

Cilostazol is the agent of choice for the management of IC symptoms in patients with disabling symptoms. Pentoxifylline is not likely to provide any relief of IC symptoms. However, before either agent is initiated, underlying causes of PVD, risk factor management, and exercise therapy must be addressed (see Table 6-5, Comparison chart of pentoxifylline and cilostazol).

Vasodilators

Vasodilators were commonly used in the early 1980s to increase perfusion to occluded blood vessels. However, clinical trials have demonstrated that these agents have no benefit in the management of IC symptoms and have the potential for aggravating symptoms (Coffman, 1979; Solomon, Ramsay, Yeo, Darnell, & Morris-Jones, 1991; Spence et al., 1993). The vasodilatory effects are minimal in diseased vessels because the vessels are already maximally dilated, and dilation occurs only in other areas of the body. The shunting of blood away from diseased to well-perfused vessels results in a "steal" phenomenon and can worsen IC symptoms (Dormandy & Rutherford, 2000; Hiatt, 2001). Vasodilators are not contraindicated in patients with PVD; however, vasodilators are no longer used to specifically manage IC symptoms.

Nutritional Supplements

Homocysteine is a sulfur-containing amino acid metabolite, which if not metabolized, can be toxic to the endothelial layer of the arterial wall, causing oxidation of LDL, thrombosis, and the inhibition of nitric oxide, which results in vasoconstriction and the enhancement of smooth muscle proliferation. Thus, hyperhomocysteinemia is viewed as an independent risk factor for

TABLE 6-5 Comparison Chart of Pentoxifylline and Cilostazol

Drug	Dose	Indication	Contraindications	Precautions
Pentoxifylline (Trental)	400 mg three times a day with meals	Intermittent claudication	Should not be used in persons with recent cerebral and/or retinal hemorrhage or in persons who have previously exhibited intolerance to this or methylxanthines such as caffeine, theophylline, and theobromine	Persons with concurrent CAD and cerebrovascular disease have had occasional reports of angina, hypotension, and arrhythmia Small decrease in BP observed when taking pentoxifylline plus nifidipine or captopril, BP should be monitored and antihypertensive agents decreased as needed Persons on warfarin should have more frequent monitoring of prothrombin time Persons with other risk factors complicated by hemorrhage (recent surgery, peptic ulceration, cerebral and/or retinal bleeding should have periodic exams for bleeding including H & H May increase theophylline level, monitor blood levels
Cilostazol (Pletal)	100 mg twice daily 30 min before or 2 h after a meal with a full glass of water Reduced dose considered when taking concomitantly with CYP3A4 or CYP2C19 inhibitors	Intermittent claudication	Should not be used in persons with congestive heart failure of any severity Should not be used in persons with hemostatic disorders or active pathologic bleeding such as peptic ulcer or intracranial bleeding	Rare cases of thrombocytopenia or leukopenia progressing to agranulocytosis when not immediately discontinued (but reversible), follow CBC Use caution when used with clopidogrel, check bleeding times

CAD, coronary artery disease; BP, blood pressure; H & H, hemoglobin & hematocrit; CBC, complete blood count.
Source: Drugs.com (2013a, 2013b).

atherosclerosis. Normal homocysteine levels are 5 to 15 mmol/L. Because vitamins B6, B12, and folic acid are necessary in the metabolism of homocysteine, studies have shown that supplementing these vitamins can help metabolize homocysteine. Recommended doses of these supplements are as follows: B12 (cobalamin), 0.6 to 1.2 mg/day; B6 (pyridoxine), 2 mg/day; and folic acid, 1 to 5 mg/day (Robertson, Iemolo, Stabler, Allen, & Spence, 2005).

Blood Pressure Agents

Hypertension is another important, modifiable cardiovascular risk factor for patients with PVD (Hiatt, 2001). The vascular TASC working group recognizes hypertension as a modifiable risk factor and recommends the following Joint National Committee on Prevention, Detection, Evaluation, and Treatment of High Blood Pressure (JNC) guidelines for hypertension management (Chobanian et al., 2003; Dormandy & Rutherford, 2000). Tight blood pressure control appears to be equally important to the agent used (Neal, MacMahon, & Chapman, 2000). The target blood pressure goal recommended for PVD patients generally is <140/90 mm Hg (Chobanian et al., 2003). Treatment of hypertension in PVD patients has been shown to reduce the risk of MI, stroke, heart failure, and death (Olin, 2003). However, antihypertensive drug treatment is ineffective in relieving the symptoms of PVD, and vasodilating antihypertensive agents do no improve walking distance or symptoms of claudication (Chobanian et al., 2003). Some patients will even experience an increase in the severity of PVD symptoms with decreased blood pressure; however, therapy should not be discontinued (Dormandy & Rutherford, 2000). The worsening effect that many antihypertensives have on symptoms of PVD may be due to (1) inability of maximally dilated diseased vessels to dilate further during exercise; (2) redistribution of flow caused by the creation of a "steal" phenomenon where blood flow increases in nondiseased vascular beds at the expense of diseased beds; or (3) alteration of pressure–flow relationships distal to the occluded areas by BP reduction (Chobanian et al., 2003).

The risk of cardiovascular mortality and morbidity in patients with hypertension is determined by blood pressure level and underlying comorbidities (e.g., hyperlipidemia and smoking). Prompt pharmacologic management should be considered in conjunction with lifestyle modifications (decreased weight and increased physical activity) (Chobanian et al., 2003). There have been no class-specific benefits demonstrated for antihypertensive medications in PVD patients; therefore, medication selection should be made on the basis of other compelling indications and adherence to guidelines (Chobanian et al., 2003).

Several classes of medications are available for hypertension management as follows:

- Angiotensin-converting enzyme inhibitors (ACEI)
- Angiotensin receptor blockers (ARB)
- β-Blockers (BBs)
- Calcium channel blockers (CCBs)
- Diuretics
- Arteriole and venodilators
- α-Adrenergic blockers
- Renin inhibitors

Randomized controlled trials have clearly demonstrated that certain agents are associated with improved cardiovascular outcomes in certain patient populations (Chobanian et al., 2003; Feldman et al., 1999). See Chapter 8, Table 8-6. Because PVD patients often have a variety of comorbidities, several agents are available to manage hypertension, and it is common to use one or more different classes of antihypertensive medications. However, the roles of ACEI and BB will be discussed in detail because they are likely to have the greatest impact on PVD patients with multiple cardiovascular risk factors. Because α-blockers and vasodilators are not commonly used for the management of chronic hypertension, they will not be discussed.

ACEI

- Ramipril (Altace, Tritace)
- Quinapril (Accupril)
- Enalapril (Vasotec, Innovace, Ednyt)
- Lisinopril (Prinivil, Zestril, Carace)
- Fosinopril (Monopril, Staril)
- Captopril (Capoten, Acepril, Kaplon, Tensopril)
- Benazepril (Lotensin)
- Cilazapril (Inhibace)
- Perindopril (Coversyl, Aceon)

- Trandolapril (Mavik, Odrik, Gopten)
- Moexipril (Univasc)

Mechanism of Action

ACEI drugs specifically inhibit the angiotensin-converting enzyme, which converts angiotensin I to angiotensin II. Angiotensin II has two primary actions that increase blood pressure. First, it is a potent vasoconstrictor that increases peripheral vascular resistance, and second, it stimulates aldosterone secretion that causes increased water and sodium retention. By inhibiting the production of angiotensin II, ACEI agents are able to decrease peripheral vascular resistance and prevent increased water and sodium retention. Angiotensin-converting enzyme is also responsible for the breakdown of a vasoactive substance called bradykinin (Komajda & Wimart, 2000). Thus, ACEI agents decrease blood pressure through two pathways:

1. Inhibition of angiotensin II production
2. Inhibition of bradykinin breakdown

Evidence for ACEI in PVD

The ACEI agents are likely to be the drugs of choice in patients with PVD. This is primarily because of the results of the Heart Outcomes Prevention Evaluation (HOPE) study (Yusuf et al., 2000). It is interesting that cardiovascular benefits seen in this trial were independent of the blood pressure–lowering effects of ramipril. The key findings pertinent to PVD patients are summarized immediately below:

HOPE study: This trial enrolled 4,051 patients with PVD (with or without hypertension) and demonstrated that patients receiving ramipril experienced the combined endpoint of myocardial infarction, stroke, or death from cardiovascular causes significantly less frequently than patients assigned to placebo did. This trial also demonstrated that ramipril had the ability to reduce the incidence of complications related to diabetes as well as new cases of diabetes. Overall, patients enrolled in the ramipril group experienced a significant reduction in stroke, CHD, major cardiovascular events, and cardiovascular death (20% to 30%) compared with patients in the placebo arm (Yusuf et al., 2000). Thus, ACEI agents have become a mainstay of PVD drug therapy.

Contraindications for Use of ACEI

1. Hypersensitivity to ACEI
2. History of angioedema related to ACEI
3. Acute renal failure
4. Pregnancy

Monitoring Parameters

1. Hypersensitivity reactions
2. Cough
3. Serum potassium
4. Serum creatinine
5. Liver function

β-Blockers (Oral Formulations)

- Acebutolol (Sectral)
- Atenolol (Tenormin)
- Bisoprolol (Zebeta)
- Carvedilol (Coreg, Corge CR)
- Labetalol (Normodyne, Trandate)
- Metoprolol (Lopressor, Toprol XL)
- Nadolol (Corgard)

- Propranolol (Inderal, Inderal LA, Pronol)
- Timolol (Betimol, Blocadren, Istalol)

Mechanism of Action

The pharmacologic action of BBs is divided into the following categories:

- Nonselective BB with intrinsic sympathomimetic activity (ISA)
- β1-Selective BB with ISA
- Nonselective BB without ISA
- β1-Selective BB without ISA

All drugs in this class competitively antagonize the effects of catecholamines at bad renoreceptors, but the affinity for β1 and β2 receptors varies among these drugs. In general, selective β1-blockers preferentially inhibit β1-adrenoreceptors found in cardiac muscle. This type of β blockade antagonizes catecholamine stimulation, causing the heart rate, contractility, and output to decrease. Preferential β1 blockade, however, is not 100% selective. At high normal doses, the degree of β2 blockade of adrenoreceptors in the bronchial and vascular musculature increases. An elevated degree of β2 blockade generally is not desired because bronchospasm can result, particularly in sensitive patients (asthmatics). Nonselective BBs have approximately equal affinity for both β1 and β2 receptors. BBs also antagonize adrenoreceptors located in the kidney to inhibit renin release (substance that promotes water retention and vasoconstriction) and to inhibit the vasomotor centers (Hoffman, 1998).

Several BBs act as partial agonists, meaning they are able to partially stimulate adrenoreceptors but not to the same degree as full agonists such as epinephrine (Hoffman, 1998). ISA is not a desirable pharmacologic effect in patients who have previously experienced a myocardial infarction. The use of non-ISA BB is associated with decreased reinfarction and reduced incidence of sudden cardiac death (Chobanian et al., 2003). Note that partial agonist activity may be required in patients with asthma or those who develop symptomatic bradycardia (Hoffman, 1998).

Evidence for β-Blockers in PVD

In the past, BBs were believed to have a negative effect on IC symptoms. Evidence supporting this notion arose from case reports of patients who experienced an increase in claudication and decreased lower limb blood flow (Hiatt, 2001). However, metaanalysis and review of several randomized controlled trials, on several occasions, did not demonstrate a decreased walking distance, increased pain, or decreased calf blood flow in patients taking BBs. Despite the absence of any large, double blind trials, it is now recommended that clinicians could use BBs safely in mild to moderate IC in the absence of other contraindications (Paravastu, Mendonca, & DaSilva, 2008; Radack & Deck, 1991; Radack & Wyderski, 1990). However, caution should still be used when PVD is severe, such as in critical limb ischemia (Dormandy & Rutherford, 2000; Heintzen & Strauer, 1994).

Independent of blood pressure–lowering effects, the use of BBs during the perioperative period of vascular surgery has been associated with a reduction in postoperative cardiovascular events, particularly in high-risk surgical patients. Noncardiac surgery generally carries a 2% to 5% risk of myocardial events, and the risk increases up to 30% in patients undergoing vascular surgery (Lee, 1999; Lee et al., 1999; Poldermans et al., 1999). Poldermans et al. (1999) have demonstrated that bisoprolol reduced the perioperative incidence of death and nonfatal myocardial infarctions by 0.1% in high-risk patients undergoing vascular surgery compared with patients who received standard care (Poldermans et al., 1999). This trial was stopped early because the interim analysis revealed that patients experienced a 90% lower rate of death and nonfatal myocardial infarctions in the bisoprolol arm (Poldermans et al., 1999). At 2 years after vascular surgery, the randomized controlled trial published by Mangano, Layug, Wallace, and Toteo (1996) showed a relative reduction in all-cause mortality of approximately 55% with perioperative atenolol use (up to 7 days of active treatment) (Mangano et al., 1996). Despite the positive results, BB therapy carries the risk of bradycardia and bronchospasm and the potential to experience withdrawal effects with short-term and sudden removal of therapy. Evidence for BB use is limited to patients at higher risks of experiencing cardiovascular events postoperatively. The effectiveness of BBs on patients with aortic stenosis or unstable or severe cardiovascular symptoms remains unknown (Auerbach, 2001). These theories have been heavily scrutinized and confirmed since these early findings in the late 1990s. More recent corroboration for the use of BBs preoperatively has been provided by large retrospective studies and guidelines have been updated recommending the continuation of BBs preoperatively for any patient taking these medications already as well as initiation of BB therapy perioperatively for high-risk cardiac patients (Lindenauer et al., 2005).

Summary

BBs are effective antihypertensive agents used in PVD patients to reduce the long-term and perioperative risks of cardiovascular events in high-risk patients undergoing vascular surgery.

Contraindications

1. Sinus bradycardia
2. Second- or third-degree heart block
3. Right ventricular failure secondary to pulmonary hypertension
4. Cardiogenic shock
5. Anesthesia with agents that produce myocardial depression
6. Bronchospastic disease—B1-selective BBs are preferred in this patient population
7. Diabetes

Monitoring Parameters

1. Heart rate
2. Atrioventricular block
3. Bronchospasm

Calcium Channel Blockers

Dihydropyridines

- Amlodipine (Norvasc)
- Felodipine (Plendil, Renedil)
- Isradipine (Dynacirc)
- Nicardipine (Cardene)
- Nifedipine (Adalat-XL, Procardia, Apo-Nifed-PA)
- Nisoldipine (Sular)

Non-Dihydropyridines

- Diltiazem (Tiazac, Cardizem)
- Verapamil (IsoptinIsoptin SR, Chronovera)

Mechanism of Action

All drugs in this class competitively inhibit the influx of calcium into cardiac and smooth muscle cells. The resulting effect is decreased force of myocardial and smooth muscle contractions and decreased conduction velocity in cardiac and smooth muscles. Clinically, the effect produced with CCB use is decreased heart rate and contractility as well as pronounced peripheral vasodilation. Thus, CCB therapy has a place in the management of heart failure and/or hypertensive patients. Non-dihydropyridines have a greater affinity for myocardial calcium receptors, whereas the dihydropyridines preferentially affect smooth muscle calcium receptors. Vasodilation, which may be a desired clinical effect for PVD patients, is more pronounced with dihydropyridines, whereas there is decreased cardiac contractility and rate with non-dihydropyridines.

Contraindications

1. Hypersensitivity
2. Extreme bradycardia
3. Second- or third-degree heart block or sick sinus syndrome
4. Cardiogenic shock—relative contraindication
5. Severe CHF or severe left ventricular dysfunction, unless patient is experiencing supraventricular tachycardia
6. Patients prone to excessive hypotension
7. Aortic stenosis

Monitoring Parameters

1. Heart rate
2. Atrioventricular block
3. Cardiovascular side effects: pedal edema, flushing, palpitations, angina, CHF
4. Central nervous system effects—dizziness, paresthesia

Diuretics

Thiazide Diuretics

- Hydrochlorothiazide (HydroDiuril, Microzide)
- Chlorothiazide (Diuril)
- Chlorthalidone (Thalitone, Hygroton)
- Indapamide (Lozol, Natramid, Natrilix, Lozide)
- Metolazone (Zaroxolyn, MykroxMetenix-5)

Loop Diuretics

- Bumetanide (Bumex)
- Furosemide (Lasix, Froop, Frusid)
- Ethacrynate acid
- Torsemide (Demadex)

Potassium-Sparing Diuretics

- Amiloride (Midamor)
- Spironolactone (Aldactone, Laractone, Spiretic)
- Triamterene (Dyrenium)

Osmotic Diuretics

- Mannitol (Osmitrol, Resectisol)

Mechanism of Action

Thiazides

Thiazide diuretics inhibit reabsorption of sodium and chloride in the distal convoluted renal tubule to promote sodium and water loss and are generally considered first-line therapy for hypertension (Chobanian et al., 2003).

Loop Diuretics

The primary site of action for all loop diuretics is the ascending loop of Henle, where sodium reabsorption is inhibited to promote water loss. Sodium reabsorption is also inhibited in the distal and proximal renal tubules. Loop diuretics generally increase sodium excretion more than thiazide diuretics and thus are used more commonly for heart failure patients. Loop diuretics also have a greater efficacy than thiazide diuretics in patients with severe renal insufficiency (Pharmacists Letter # 250214).

Potassium-Sparing Diuretics

True to their name, potassium-sparing diuretics increase sodium excretion without secondary increased excretion of potassium as is seen with thiazide and loop diuretics. The potassium-sparing diuretic spironolactone competes competitively for aldosterone-dependent sodium–potassium exchange sites within the distal renal tubule to increase sodium and water reabsorption while preventing potassium loss. Amiloride and triamterene work independently from aldosterone. Both disrupt sodium for potassium exchange within the distal convoluted renal tubule and collecting duct of the nephron by inhibiting the sodium–potassium ATPase pump. Sodium excretion is increased while potassium excretion is not.

Osmotic Diuretics

The site of action for mannitol is the proximal and descending limb of the loop of Henle, the permeable sections for water movement. When an osmotic agent, such as mannitol, passes through these points, increased water pressure results within the renal tubules to promote water excretion.

REFERENCES

Ageno, W., Gallus, A. S., Wittkowsky, A., Crowther, M., Hylek, E. M., & Palareti, G. (2012). Oral anticoagulant therapy: Antithrombotic Therapy and Prevention of Thrombosis, 9th ed: American College of Chest Physicians Evidenced-Based Clinical Practice Guidelines. *Chest, 141*(2 Suppl.), e44S–e88S.

Alonso-Coello, P., Bellmunt, S., McGorrian, C., Anand, S. S., Guzman, R., Criqui, M. H., ... Spencer, F. A. (2012). Antithrombotic therapy in peripheral artery disease: Antithrombotic Therapy and Prevention of Thrombosis, 9th ed: American College of Chest Physicians Evidenced-Based Clinical Practice Guidelines. *Chest, 141*(2 Suppl.), e669S–e690S.

Anitschkow, N. (1913). Uber die Veranderungen der Kaninchenaorta bei experimenteller Cholesterinsteatose. *Beitrage zur Pathologie, 56*, 379–404.

Antiplatelet Trialists' Collaboration. (1994). Collaborative overview of randomized trials of antiplatelet therapy II: Maintenance of vascular graft or arterial patency by antiplatelet therapy. *British Medical Journal, 308*(6922), 159–168.

Aronow, W. S., & Ahn, C. (1994). Prevalence of coexistence of coronary artery disease, peripheral arterial disease, and atherothrombotic brain infarction in men and women > or = 62 years of age. *American Journal of Cardiology, 74*(1), 64–65.

Auerbach, A. D. (2001). *Beta-blockers and reduction of perioperative cardiac events.* Retrieved from http://www.ahcpr.gov/clinic/ptsafety/chap25.htm

Baigent, C., Blackwell, L., Collins, R., Emberson, J., Godwin, J., Peto, R., ... Zanchetti, A. (2009). Aspirin in the primary and secondary prevention of vascular disease: Collaborative meta-analysis of individual participant data from randomized trials. *Lancet, 373*(9676), 1849–1860.

Becquemin, J. P. (1997). Effect of ticlopidine on the long-term patency of saphenous-vein bypass grafts in the legs. Etude de la Ticlopidine apres Pontage Femoro-Poplite and the Association Universitaire de Recherche en Chirurgie. *New England Journal of Medicine, 337*(24), 1726–1731.

Beebe, H. G., Dawson, D. L., & Cutler, B. S. (1999). A new pharmacological treatment for intermittent claudication: Results of a randomized, multicenter trial. *Archives of Internal Medicine, 159*(17), 2041–2050.

Belch, J. J. F., & Dormandy, J. (2010). Results of the randomized, placebo-controlled clopidogrel and acetylsalicylic acid in bypass surgery for peripheral arterial disease (CASPAR) trial. *Journal of Vascular Surgery, 52*(4), 825–833.

Berridge, D. C., Kessel, D., & Robertson, I. (2002). Surgery versus thrombolysis for initial management of acute limb ischaemia. *Cochrane Database of Systemic Review,* (3), CD002784.

CAPRIE Steering Committee. (1996). A randomised, blinded, trial of clopidogrel versus aspirin in patients at risk of ischaemic events. *Lancet, 348*(9038), 1329–1339.

Chobanian, A. V., Bakris, G. L., Black, H. R., Cushman, W. C., Green, L. A., Izzo, J. L., Jr., ... Roccella, E. J. (2003). The Seventh Report of the Joint National Committee on Prevention, Detection, Evaluation, and Treatment of High Blood Pressure: The JNC 7 report. *Journal of the American Medical Association, 289*(19), 2560–2572.

Chong, P. H., Seeger, J. D., & Franklin, C. (2001). Clinically relevant differences between the statins: Implications for therapeutic selection. *American Journal of Medicine, 111*(5), 390–400.

Clagett, G. P., Sobel, M., Jackson, M. R., Lip, G. Y., Tangelder, M., & Verhaeghe, R. (2004). Antithrombotic therapy in peripheral arterial occlusive disease: The Seventh ACCP Conference on Antithrombotic and Thrombolytic Therapy. *Chest, 126*(Suppl. 3), S609–S626.

Coffman, J. D. (1979). Drug therapy: Vasodilator drugs in peripheral vascular disease. *New England Journal of Medicine, 300*(13), 713–717.

Dawson, D. L., Cutler, B. S., Hiatt, W. R., Hobson, R. W, II, Martin, J. D., Bortey, E. B., ... Strandness, D. E., Jr. (2000). A comparison of cilostazol and pentoxifylline for treating intermittent claudication. *American Journal of Medicine, 109*(7), 523–530.

Dawson, D. L., Cutler, B. S., & Meissner, M. H. (1998). Cilostazol has beneficial effects in treatment of intermittent claudication: Results from a multicenter, randomized, prospective, double-blind trial. *Circulation, 98*(7), 678–686.

Dawson, K., Armon, A., Brauthwaile, B., Galland, R., Kendrick, R., Downes, M., ... Hamilton, G. (1996). Stroke during intra-arterial thrombolysis: A survey of experience in the UK. *British Journal of Surgery, 83*, 568.

Donaldson, D. R., Salter, M. C. P., Kester, R. C., Rajah, S. M., Hall, T. J., Sreeharan, N., & Crow, M. J. (1985). The influence of platelet inhibition on the patency of femoro-popliteal dacron bypass grafts. *Vascular and Endovascular Surgery, 19*, 224–230.

Dormandy, J., Mahir, M., Ascady, G., Balsano, F., DeLeeuw, P., Blombery, P., ... Deutshinoff, A. (1989). Fate of the patient with chronic leg ischaemia: A review article. *Journal of Cardiovascular Surgery (Torino), 30*(1), 50–57.

Dormandy, J. A., & Rutherford, R. B. (2000). Management of peripheral arterial disease (PAD). TASC Working Group. TransAtlantic Inter-Society Consensus (TASC), *Journal of Vascular Surgery, 31*(1 Pt 2), S1–S296.

Drugs.com. (2013a, December 1). Drug information online regarding cilostazol. Retrieved from http://www.drugs.com/pro/pletal.html

Drugs.com. (2013b, December 1). Drug information online regarding pentoxifylline. Retrieved from http://www.drugs.com/pro/trental.html

Effeney, D. J., Goldstone, J., Chin, D., Krupski, W. C., & Ellis, R. J. (1981). Intraoperative anticoagulation in cardiovascular surgery. *Surgery, 90*(6), 1068–1074.

Eikelboom, J. W., Hirsh, J., Spencer, F. A., Baglin, T. P., & Weitz, J. I. (2012). Antiplatelet drugs: Antithrombotic Therapy and Prevention of Thrombosis, 9th ed: American College of Chest Physicians Evidenced-Based Clinical Practice Guidelines. *Chest, 141*(2 Suppl.), e89SS–e119S.

Ezetimibe Prescribing Information. (2013, January 15). Retrieved from http://www.rxlist.com/zetia-side-effects-drug-center.htm.

Feldman, R. D., Campbell, N., Larochelle, P., Bolli, P., Burgess, E. D., Carruthers, S. G., ... Zarnke, K. B. (1999). 1999 Canadian recommendations for the management of hypertension. *Canadian Medical Association Journal, 161*(12), S1–S17.

Garcia, D. A., Baglin, T. P., Weitz, J. I., & Samama, M. M. (2012). Parenteral anticoagulants: Antithrombotic Therapy and Prevention of Thrombosis, 9th ed: American College of Chest Physicians Evidenced-Based Clinical Practice Guidelines. *Chest, 141*(2 Suppl.), e24S–e43S.

Goldhaber, S. Z., Manson, J. E., Stampfer, M. J., LaMotte, F., Rosner, B., Buring, J. E., & Hennekens, C. H. (1992). Low-dose aspirin and subsequent peripheral arterial surgery in the Physicians' Health Study. *Lancet, 340*(8812), 143–145.

Goldman, M. D., & McCollum, C. N. (1984). A prospective randomized study to examine the effect of aspirin plus dipyridamole on the patency of prosthetic femoro-popliteal grafts. *Vascular and Endovascular Surgery, 18*, 217–221.

Gortier, D., Maloney, S., Rutland, R., Westvik, T., Muto, A., Kudo, F. A., & Dardik, A. (2006). Adjunctive pharmacologic use in carotid endarterectomy: A review. *Vascular, 14*(2), 93–102.

Gotto, A. M., & Pownall, H. J. (1998). *Manual of lipid disorders: Reducing the risk for coronary heart disease* (2nd ed., pp. 292–328). Philadelphia, PA: Lippincott Williams & Wilkins.

Green, R. M., Roedersheimer, L. R., & DeWeese, J. A. (1982). Effects of aspirin and dipyridamole on expanded polytetrafluoroethylene graft patency. *Surgery, 92*(6), 1016–1026.

Grundy, S. M., Bilheimer, D., Chait, A., Clark, L. T., Denke, M., Havel, R. J., ... Quint-Adler, L. (1993). Summary of the second report of the National Cholesterol Education Program (NCEP) Expert Panel on detection, Evaluation, and Treatment of High Blood Cholesterol in Adults (Adult Treatment Panel II). *Journal of the American Medical Association, 269*(23), 3015–3023.

Haines, S. T., Witt, D. M., & Nutescu, E. A. (2008). Venous thromboembolism. In J. T. Dipiro, R. L. Talbert, G. C. Yee, G. R. Matzke, B. G. Wells, & L. M. Posey (Eds.), *Pharmacotherapy: A pathophysiologic approach* (8th ed., pp. 331–371). New York, NY: McGraw Hill.

Hankey, G. J., Sudlow, C. L., & Dunbabin, D. W. (2000). Thienopyridine derivatives (ticlopidine, clopidogrel) versus aspirin for preventing stroke and other serious vascular events in high vascular risk patients. *Cochrane Database Systematic Reviews*, (2), CD001246.

Hayes, P. D., Lloyd, A. J., Lennard, N., Wolstenholme, J. L., London, N. J., Bell, P. R., & Naylor, A. R. (2000). Transcranial Doppler-directed dextran-40 therapy is a cost-effective method of preventing carotid thrombosis after carotid endarterectomy. *European Journal of Vascular and Endovascular Surgery, 19*(1), 56–61.

Heart Protection Study Collaborative Group. (2002). MRC/BHF heart protection study of cholesterol lowering with simvastatin in 20,536 high-risk individuals: A randomised placebo-controlled trial. *Lancet, 360*(9326), 7–22.

Heintzen, M. P., & Strauer, B. E. (1994). Peripheral vascular effects of beta-blockers. *European Heart Journal, 15*(Suppl. C), 2–7.

Hertzer, N. R., Beven, E. G., Young, J. R., O'Hara, P. J., Ruschhaupt, W. F., III, Graor, R. A., … Maljovec, L. C. (1984). Coronary artery disease in peripheral vascular patients. A classification of 1000 coronary angiograms and results of surgical management. *Annals of Surgery, 199*(2), 223–233.

Hiatt, W. R. (2001). Medical treatment of peripheral arterial disease and claudication. *New England Journal of Medicine, 344*(21), 1608–1621.

Hoffman, B. (1998). Adrenoceptor antagonist drugs. In B. G. Katzung (Ed.), *Basic and clinical pharmacology* (7th ed., pp. 136–151). Stamford, CT: Appleton and Lange.

Hood, S. C., Moher, D., & Barber, G. G. (1996). Management of intermittent claudication with pentoxifylline: Meta-analysis of randomized controlled trials. *Canadian Medical Association Journal, 155*(8), 1053–1059.

Jennings, D. L. (2010). Ticagrelor: An oral, non-thienopyridine P2Y12 receptor antagonist for the treatment of acute coronary syndromes. Retrieved from http://formularyjournal.modernmedicine.com/formulary-journal/news/clinical/clinical-pharmacology/ticagrelor-oral-non-thienopyridine-p2y12-recep

Kamanna, V. S., & Kashyap, M. L. (2008). Mechanism of action of niacin. *American Journal of Cardiology, 101*(8A), 20B–26B.

Kearon, C., Akl, E. A., Comerota, A. J., Prandoni, P., Bounameaux, H., Goldhaber, S. Z., … Kahn, S. R. (2012). Antithrombotic therapy for VTE disease: Antithrombotic Therapy and Prevention of Thrombosis, 9th ed: American College of Chest Physicians Evidenced-Based Clinical Practice Guidelines. *Chest, 141*(2 Suppl.), e419S–e494S.

Kohler, T. R., Kaufman, J. L., Kacoyanis, G., Clowes, A., Donaldson, M. C., Kelly, E., … Mannick, J. A. (1984). Effect of aspirin and dipyridamole on the patency of lower extremity bypass grafts. *Surgery, 96*(3), 462–466.

Komajda, M., & Wimart, M. C. (2000). Angiotensin converting enzyme inhibition: From viper to patient. *Heart (British Cardiac Society), 84*(Suppl. 1), S11–S14.

Lee, T. H. (1999). Reducing cardiac risk in noncardiac surgery. *New England Journal of Medicine, 341*(24), 1838–1840.

Lee, T. H., Marcantonio, E. R., Mangione, C. M., Thomas, E. J., Polanczyk, C. A., Cook, E. F., … Goldman, L. (1999). Derivation and prospective validation of a simple index for prediction of cardiac risk of major noncardiac surgery. *Circulation, 100*(10), 1043–1049.

Lennard, N., Smith, J. L., Hayes, P., Evans, D. H., Abbott, R. J., London, N. J., … Naylor, A. R. (1999). Transcranial Doppler directed dextran therapy in the prevention of carotid thrombosis: Three hour monitoring is as effective as six hours. *European Journal of Vascular and Endovascular Surgery, 17*(4), 301–305.

Levi, C. R., Stork, J. L., Chambers, B. R., Abbott, A. L., Cameron, H. M., Peeters, A., … Donnan, G. A. (2001). Dextran reduces embolic signals after carotid endarterectomy. *Annals of Neurology, 50*(4), 544–547.

Lew, W. K., & Weaver, F. A. (2010). Thrombolytic agents. In J. L. Cronenwett & K. W. Johnston (Eds.), *Rutherford's vascular surgery* (7th ed., pp. 556–570). Philadelphia, PA: Saunders Elsevier.

Lexi-Drugs™. (2013, July 19). Retrieved from http://www.lexi.com/home/newdrugs/

Lindenauer, P. K., Pekow, P., Wang, K., Dheeresh, M. S., Mamidi, D. K., Gutierrez, B., & Benjamin, E. M. (2005). Perioperative beta-blocker therapy and mortality after major noncardiac surgery. *New England Journal of Medicine, 353*, 349–361.

Lindgärde, F., Jelnes, R., Björkman, H., Adielsson, G., Kjellström, T., Palmquist, I., & Stavenow, L. (1989). Conservative drug treatment in patients with moderately severe chronic occlusive peripheral arterial disease. *Circulation, 80*(6), 1549–1556.

Linkins, L., Dans, A. L., Moores, L. K., Bona, R., Davidson, B. L., Schulman, S., & Crowther, M. (2012). Treatment and prevention of heparin-induced thrombocytopenia: Antithrombotic Therapy and Prevention of Thrombosis, 9th ed: American College of Chest Physicians Evidenced-Based Clinical Practice Guidelines. *Chest, 141*(2 Suppl.), e495S–e530S.

Mangano, D. T., Layug, E. L., Wallace, A., & Toteo, I. (1996). Effect of atenolol on mortality and cardiovascular morbidity after noncardiac surgery. *New England Journal of Medicine, 335*(23), 1713–1721.

Martin, P., Greenstein, D., Gupta, N. K., Walker, D. R., & Kester, R. C. (1994). Systemic heparinization during peripheral vascular surgery: Thromboelastographic, activated coagulation time, and heparin titration monitoring. *Journal of Cardiothoracic and Vascular Anesthesia, 8*(2), 150–152.

McCollum, C., Alexander, C., Kenchington, G., Franks, P. J., & Greenhalgh, R. (1991). Antiplatelet drugs in femoropopliteal vein bypasses: A multicenter trial. *Journal of Vascular Surgery, 13*(1), 150–161.

Money, S. R., Herd, J. A., Isaacsohn, J. L., Davidson, M., Cutler, B., Heckman, J., & Forbes, W. P. (1998). Effect of cilostazol on walking distances in patients with intermittent claudication caused by peripheral vascular disease. *Journal of Vascular Surgery, 27*(2), 267–274.

Morgan, J. M., Carey, C. M., Lincoff, A., & Capuzzi, D. M. (2004). The effects of niacin on lipoprotein subclass distribution. *Preventive Cardiology, 7*(4), 182–187.

Neal, B., MacMahon, S., & Chapman, N. (2000). Effects of ACE inhibitors, calcium antagonists, and other blood-pressure-lowering drugs: Results of prospectively designed overviews of randomised trials. *Lancet, 356*(9246), 1955–1964.

Norgren, L., Hiatt, W. R., Dormandy, M. R., Nehler, M. R., Harris, K. A., & Fowkes, F. G. R. (2007). Inter-society consensus for the management of peripheral arterial disease (TASC II). *Journal of Vascular Surgery, 45*(Suppl.), s5–s67.

Olin, J. W. (2003). Treatment of hypertensive patients with peripheral arterial disease. In J. L. Izzo, Jr & H. R. Black (Eds.), *Hypertension primer: The essentials of high blood pressure– Basic science, population science, and clinical management* (pp. 467–469). Philadelphia, PA: Lippincott, Williams & Wilkins.

Ouriel, K., Veith, F. J., & Sasahara, A. A. (1998). A comparison of recombinant urokinase with vascular surgery as initial treatment for acute arterial occlusion of the legs. *New England Journal of Medicine, 338*, 1105–1111.

Paravastu, S. C., Mendonca, D., & DaSilva, A. (2008). Betablockers for peripheral arterial disease. *Cochrane Database Systematic Reviews*, (4), CD005508.

Pharmacist's Letter #250214 (2013, January 25). Comparison of commonly used diuretics. Retrieved from http://pharmacistsletter.therapeuticresearch.com/pl

Poldermans, D., Boersma, E., Bax, J. J., Thomson, I. R., van de Ven, L. L. M., Blankensteijn, J. D., ... van Urk, H. (1999). The effect of bisoprolol on perioperative mortality and myocardial infarction in high-risk patients undergoing vascular surgery. *New England Journal of Medicine, 341*(24), 1789–1794.

Radack, K., & Deck, C. (1991). Beta-adrenergic blocker therapy does not worsen intermittent claudication in subjects with peripheral arterial disease: A meta-analysis of randomized controlled trials. *Archives of Internal Medicine, 151*(9), 1769–1776.

Radack, K., & Wyderski, R. J. (1990). Conservative management of intermittent claudication. *Annals of Internal Medicine, 113*(2), 135–146.

Reilly, M. P, & Mohler, E. R., III (2001). Cilostazol: Treatment of intermittent claudication. *Annals of Pharmacotherapy, 35*(1), 48–56.

Robertson, J., Iemolo, F., Stabler, S. P., Allen, R. H., & Spence, J. D. (2005). Vitamin B12, homocysteine and carotid plaque in the era of folic acid fortification of enriched cereal grain products. *Canadian Medical Association Journal, 7*, 1569–1573.

Rooke, T. W., Hirsch, A. T., Misra, S., Sidawy, A. N., Beckman, J. A., Findeiss, L. K., ... Zierler, R. E. (2011). ACCF/AHA focused update of the guideline for the management of patients with peripheral artery disease (updating the 2005 guideline): A report of the American College of Cardiology Foundation/American Heart Association Task Force on Practice Guidelines. *Journal of the American College of Cardiology, 58*, 2020–2045.

Roseborough, G. S., & Perler, B. A. (2010). Carotid artery disease: Endarterectomy. In J. L. Cronenwett & K. W. Johnston (Eds.), *Rutherford's vascular surgery* (7th ed., pp. 1443–1468). Philadelphia, PA: Saunders Elsevier.

Samama, C. M., Gigou, F., & Ill, P. (1995). Low-molecular-weight heparin vs. unfractionated heparin in femorodistal reconstructive surgery: A multicenter open randomized study. Enoxart Study Group. *Annals of Vascular Surgery, 9*(Suppl.), S45–S53.

Sisson, E. M., & Tisdel, K. A. (2001). Hyperlipidemias. In B. A. Mueller, K. E. Bertch, T. E. Dunsworths, et al. (Eds.), *Pharmacotherapy self-assessment program, Cardiovascular I module* (4th ed., pp. 45–83). Kansas City, MO: American College of Clinical Pharmacy.

Sobel, M., & Verhaeghe, R. (2008). Antithrombotic therapy for peripheral artery occlusive disease: American College of Chest Physicians Evidenced-Based Clinical Practice Guidelines (8th edition). *Chest, 133*(6 Suppl.), 815S–843S.

Solomon, S. A., Ramsay, L. E., Yeo, W. W., Darnell, L., & Morris-Jones, W. (1991). Beta blockade and intermittent claudication: Placebo controlled trial of atenolol and nifedipine and their combination. *British Medical Journal, 303*(6810), 1100–1104.

Spence, J. D., Arnold, J. M. O., Munoz, C. E., Viswanatha, A., Huff, M., DeRose, G., & Harris, K. (1993). Angiotensin-converting enzyme inhibition with cilazapril does not improve blood flow, walking time, or plasma lipids in patients with intermittent claudication. *Journal of Vascular Medicine and Biology, 4*, 23–27.

Stone, N. J., Robinson, J., Lichtenstein, A. H., Bairey Merz, C. N., Blum, C. B., Eckel, R. H., ... Wilson, P. W. F. (2013). 2013 ACC/AHA Guideline on the Treatment of Blood Cholesterol to Reduce Atherosclerotic Cardiovascular Risk in Adults: A report of the American College of Cardiology/American Heart Association Task Force on Practice Guidelines. *Circulation*. Published online November 12, 2013. Retrieved from http://circ.ahajournals.org/content/early/2013/11/11/01.cir.0000437738.63853.7a.citation

Swedenborg, J., Nydahl, S., & Egberg, N. (1996). Low molecular mass heparin instead of unfractionated heparin during infrainguinal bypass surgery. *European Journal of Vascular and Endovascular Surgery, 11*(1), 59–64.

Tangelder, M. J., Lawson, J. A., Algra, A., & Eikelboom, B. C. (1999). Systematic review of randomized controlled trials of aspirin and oral anticoagulants in the prevention of graft occlusion and ischemic events after infrainguinal bypass surgery. *Journal of Vascular Surgery, 30*(4), 701–709.

Thompson, J. F., Mullee, M. A., Bell, P. R., Campbell, W. B., Chant, A. D., Darke, S. G., ... Clyne, C. A. (1996). Intraoperative heparinisation, blood loss and myocardial infarction during aortic aneurysm surgery: A Joint Vascular Research Group study. *European Journal of Vascular and Endovascular Surgery, 12*(1), 86–90.

Tierney, S., Fennessy, F., & Hayes, D. B. (2000). ABC of arterial and vascular disease: Secondary prevention of peripheral vascular disease. *British Medical Journal, 320*(7244), 1262–1265.

Tjon, J. A., & Riemann, L. E. (2001). Treatment of intermittent claudication with pentoxifylline and cilostazol. *American Journal of Health-System Pharmacy, 58*(6), 485–493.

Trental Package Information. (2013, January 15). Retrieved from http://products.sanofi.us/trental/trental.pdf

Wakefield, T. W., Lindblad, B., Stanley, T. J., Nichol, B. J., Stanley, J. C., Berggvist, D., ... Bergentz, S. E. (1994). Heparin and protamine use in peripheral vascular surgery: A comparison between surgeons of the Society for Vascular

Surgery and the European Society for Vascular Surgery. *European Journal of Vascular and Endovascular Surgery, 8*(2), 193–198.

Wallentin, L., James, S., Storey, R. F., Armstrong, M., Barratt, B. J., Horrow, J., ... Becker, R. C. (2010). Effect of CYP2C19 and ABCB1 single nucleotide polymorphisms on outcomes of treatment with ticagrelor versus clopidogrel for acute coronary syndromes: A genetic substudy of the PLATO trial. *Lancet, 376*(9749), 1320–1328. doi:10.1016/S0140-6736(10)61274-3

Weaver, F. A., Comerota, A. J., Youngblood, M., Froehlich, J., Hosking, J. D., & Papanicolaou, G. (1994). Results of a prospective randomized trial evaluating surgery versus thrombolysis for ischemia of the lower extremity: The STILE trial. *Annals of Surgery, 220*(3), 251–268.

Weitz, J. I., Eikelboom, J. W., & Samama, M. M. (2012). New antithrombotic drugs: Antithrombotic Therapy and Prevention of Thrombosis, 9th ed: American College of Chest Physicians Evidenced-Based Clinical Practice Guidelines. *Chest, 141*(2 Suppl.), e120S–e151S.

Yusuf, S., Sleight, P., Pogue, J., Bosch, J., Davies, R., & Dagenais, G. (2000). Effects of an angiotensin-converting-enzyme inhibitor, ramipril, on cardiovascular events in high-risk patients. *New England Journal of Medicine, 342*(3), 145–153.

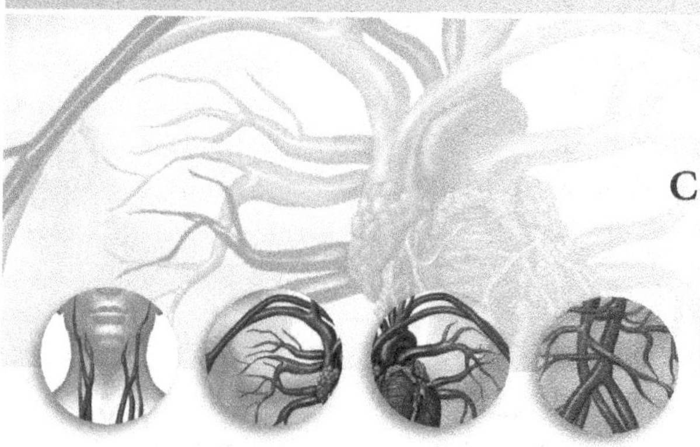

CHAPTER 7

Teaching and Learning Principles

Marjorie Lovell

OBJECTIVES

1. Understand the theories of motivation and learning.
2. Identify the principles of effective teaching and learning.
3. Discuss adult and patient education principles.
4. Discuss barriers to effective communication and learning.
5. Describe the different learning styles.

Introduction

Learning is an ongoing and life-long process. People learn within social and cultural contexts, independently and through interaction with others. This chapter will focus on the vascular patient as the adult learner and will discuss ways to achieve effective patient education. Patient education is often the key to helping patients fully benefit from their care, with the nonoperative management, and during and after a hospital stay. The goal of patient education has changed from telling the patient the best actions to take, to now assisting patients in learning about their health care to improve their own health. This view of health education requires more communication between patients and healthcare providers.

Education will help patients understand their condition, how to effectively use any medications or medical equipment required, and how to perform any necessary self-care. It must be ongoing, interactive, and consistent with the patients' plan of care, comprehension, educational level, and needs for continuity of care.

I. Learning and Motivation

A. Theories (Theories that explain behavior change can be applied as guidelines for patient education; these theories come from the disciplines of sociology, psychology, adult education, communication, and organizational development)

1. Health belief model—behavior of individual's health action dependant upon
   a. Belief of risk of developing a specific condition
   b. Belief that condition will have serious effect on life (Janz & Becker, 1984)

c. Belief that behavior change outweighs barriers to action (Goeppinger & Lorig, 1996)

2. Transtheoretical model
   a. Intentional change requires movement through distinct motivational changes over period of time
   b. Five-stage process or continuum related to person's readiness to change
      1) Precontemplation—little interest in changing specific behavior
      2) Contemplation—thinking about changing specific behavior
      3) Preparation for action—considering attempts to change behavior
      4) Action—actively working toward changing behavior
      5) Maintenance—changes to behavior minimized
3. Social cognitive theory
   a. Behavior modeling learned through environmental reinforcements (Bandura, 1991)
   b. Individuals most likely to model behavior observed by others they identify with
4. Theory of reasoned action
   a. Effects of attitudes toward behavioral intentions (DeBono, 1993)
   b. Individual may require family members and friends to agree with changed behavior

B. Principles of Motivation (Principles of Motivation, 2013)

1. The environment can be used to focus patient attention on what needs to be learned
2. Incentives motivate learning
3. Internal motivation is longer lasting and more self-directive than is external motivation
4. Learning is most effective when an individual is ready to learn, that is, when one wants to know something
5. Motivation is enhanced by the way in which the instructional material is organized

C. Learning Behavior Classifications—There are three domains of learning educational activities: cognitive, affective, and psychomotor

1. Cognitive: includes knowledge, intellectual abilities, and information; six levels within this domain (Benjamin, Bloom, Mesia, & Krathwohl, 1964)
   a. Knowledge: recalling information (e.g., list, describes, defines, arrange, repeat)
   b. Comprehension: lowest level of understanding (e.g., describe, explain, locate, discuss, report)
   c. Application: use of information in concrete situations (e.g., apply, demonstrate, solve, show)
   d. Analysis: ability to break down material into parts so it is easily understood (e.g., analyze, arrange, explain, diagrams, compare)
   e. Synthesis: putting elements together to make a whole (e.g., combine, plan, categorizes, modifies)
   f. Evaluation: ability to make judgments about value of ideas or materials (e.g., assess, compare, summarize, measure, test)

2. Affective: includes feelings, emotions, and attitudes; five categories within this domain
   a. Receiving—awareness, willingness to hear, selected attention (asks, chooses, names)
   b. Responding—attends and reacts to particular phenomenon (e.g., answers, greets, discusses, reports)
   c. Valuing—accepting, commitment to a value (e.g., completes, demonstrates, initiates, selects)
   d. Organization—organizes values into priorities (e.g., arranges, combines, organizes, integrates)
   e. Characterization—internalizing values—has value system that controls behavior (e.g., discriminates, acts, displays, practices)
3. Psychomotor: includes physical movement, coordination, and motor skills. Seven categories within this domain (Simpson, 1972)
   a. Perception—ability to use sensory cues to guide motor activity (e.g., chooses, describes, relates, selects)
   b. Set—readiness to act (e.g., begins, displays, moves, shows, states)
   c. Guided response—learning a skill, imitation (e.g., copies, traces, follows, responds)
   d. Complex overt response—skilful performance of motor acts that involve complex movements (e.g., assembles, builds, dismantles, calibrates)
   e. Adaptation—skills are well developed and can adapt to new problems (e.g., adapts, alters, changes, varies)
   f. Orientation—creates new movement skills to a specific situation or problem (e.g., combines, designs, creates, constructs)

D. Andragogy and Pedagogy

1. Andragogy: art and science of teaching adults; the six key principles include
   a. Adults are autonomous
   b. Adults are relevancy orientated—must have "need to know"
   c. Adults have a lifetime of experience and knowledge
   d. Adults must be shown respect in an environment conducive to learning
   e. Adults' learning shifts from subject-centeredness to problem-centeredness
   f. Adults are motivated by external and internal factors (Knowles, 1984)
2. Pedagogy: art and science of teaching children and youth
   a. Teacher or parent assumes responsibility for what is learned
   b. Knowledge acquired is for application when appropriate

II. Patient Education

A. Patient Education—Acquisition of a skill or knowledge by practice, study, or instruction that should provide the patient with the knowledge needed for maintenance and promotion of optimal health and illness prevention (Davis, 1995)

B. Goals and Objectives

1. Improve knowledge and awareness of vascular disease
2. Increase compliance to management of vascular disease

3. Develop skills to manage care
4. Family-centered care

C. Principles (Bartlett, 1999)

1. Relevant to patients needs
2. Adapt teaching to patients' level of readiness, past experience, culture, and understanding
3. Involve patient in learning process by goal setting and progress evaluation
4. Create environment conducive to learning with trust, respect, and acceptance
5. Provide opportunities for demonstration of information and skills

D. Needs Assessment

1. Physical condition
2. Knowledge and understanding of disease and management
3. Demographics (age, family status, employment status education)
4. Stage of life development
5. Means of social support
6. Cultural beliefs
7. Learning style preferences
8. Spiritual beliefs
9. Educational preferences

E. Planning

1. Goal setting
2. Content
   a. Specific to patient needs
   b. Guidelines

F. Implementation

1. Instructional methods
   a. One-on-one discussion
   b. Group instruction
   c. Preparatory instruction
   d. Demonstration
2. Activities
   a. Lecture
   b. Discussion
   c. Demonstration
   d. Role play
3. Tools—enforces teaching by using a variety of tools to capture learning styles (auditory, visual, and psychomotor)
   a. Printed materials
   b. Audiotapes
   c. Videotapes
   d. CDs
   e. Flipcharts
   f. Physical models
   g. Posters
   h. Internet

G. Evaluation—Confirms teaching is effective and appropriate to meet individual needs (Fenwick & Parsons, 1999)

1. Methods (Kilpatrick, 1998)
   a. Level 1—learner's reactions--how did you like it
   b. Level 2a—modification of attitudes
      Level 2b—acquisition of knowledge or increase in skill
   c. Level 3—change in behavior
   d. Level 4—change with benefits to patient (improve quality of life)
2. Tools
   a. Interviews
   b. Surveys
   c. Questionnaires
   d. Observations

III. Barriers to Patient Education (Beagley, 2011)

A. Physiological

1. Age
2. Health

B. Cognitive

1. Language development
2. Reading level
3. Processing skills
4. Learning style
5. Prior knowledge

C. Affective

1. Motivation to learn
2. Interests
3. Attitude toward learning
4. Anxiety level
5. Cultural/spiritual beliefs
6. Side effect of medication
7. Environment

D. Social

1. Relationship with peers, staff, or family
2. Feelings toward authority
3. Socioeconomic background
4. Ethnic background

IV. Strategies for Patient Education

A. Involve Patient in Goal Setting

B. Assess Learning Style of Patient

C. Move from Simple to Complex Ideas

D. Repetition

E. Support and Encouragement

V. Limitations of Education in Vascular Disease

A. Patient Factors

1. Lack of knowledge
2. Poor access to medical system
3. Financial
4. Social
5. Geographical

B. Disease Factors

1. Unmanageable disease

REVIEW QUESTIONS

1. Learning the signs and symptoms of vascular disease is an example of which domain of learning?
   a. Affective
   b. Cognitive
   c. Psychomotor
   d. Behavioral
2. All of the following are barriers to patient education except
   a. Age
   b. Sex
   c. Learning style
   d. Language
3. This type of learner does well by demonstrating the action taught:
   a. Visual
   b. Kinesthetic
   c. Auditory
   d. Cognitive
4. Which of the following strategies would be best to demonstrate ace wrapping?
   a. Lecture
   b. Role playing
   c. Demonstration with return demonstration
   d. Instructional booklet
5. This theory reflects intentional change through distinct motivational changes over a period of time:
   a. Health belief model
   b. Social cognitive theory
   c. Theory of reasoned action
   d. Transtheoretical model

ANSWERS

1. b. Cognitive.
2. b. Sex.
3. b. Kinesthetic.
4. c. Demonstration with return demonstration.
5. d. Transtheoretical model.

REFERENCES

Bandura, A. (1991). Social cognitive theory of moral thought and action. In W. M. Kurtines & J. L. Gerwitz (Eds.), *Handbook of moral behavior and development* (Vol.1, pp. 45–103). Hillsdale, NJ: Erlbaum.

Bartlett, E. (1999). At last a definition of patient education. *Patient Education and Counseling, 7*, 323–324.

Beagley, L. (2011). Educating patients: Understanding barriers, learning styles, and teaching techniques. *Journal of PeriAnesthesia Nursing, 26*(5), 331–337.

Benjamin, S., Bloom, B., Mesia, B., & Krathwohl, D. R. (1964). *Taxonomy of educational objectives (Two vols: The affective domain & the cognitive domain)*. New York, NY: David McKay.

Davis, S. M. (1995). An investigation into nurses' understanding of health education and health promotion within a neuro-rehabilitation setting. *Journal of Advanced Nursing, 21*(5), 951–955.

DeBono, K. G. (1993). Individual differences in predicting behavioral intentions from attitude and subjective norm. *The Journal of Social Psychology, 133*(6), 825–832.

Fenwick, T., & Parsons, J. (1999). *The art of evaluation: A handbook for educators and trainers.* Toronto, ON: Thompson Educational Publishing.

Goeppinger, L., & Lorig, K. (1996). What we know about what works: One rationale, two models, three theories. In K. Lorig (Ed.), *Patient education: A practical approach* (pp. 195–224). Thousand Oaks, CA: Sage Publications.

Janz, N. K., & Becker, M. H. (1984). The health belief model: A decade later. *Education Quarterly, 11*, 1–47.

Kilpatrick, D. L. (1998). *Evaluating training programs, the four levels* (2nd ed.). San Francisco, CA: Berrett-Koehler.

Knowles, M. (1984). *Andragogy in action: Applying modern principles of adult learning.* San Francisco, CA: Jossey-Boss.

Principles of Motivation. (2013, July 21). Retrieved from http://www2.honolulu.hawaii.edu/facdev/guidebk/teachtip/m-files/m-motiva.htm

Simpson, E. (1972). *The classification of educational objectives in the psychomotor domain: The psychomotor domain* (Vol. 3). Washington, DC: Gryphon House.

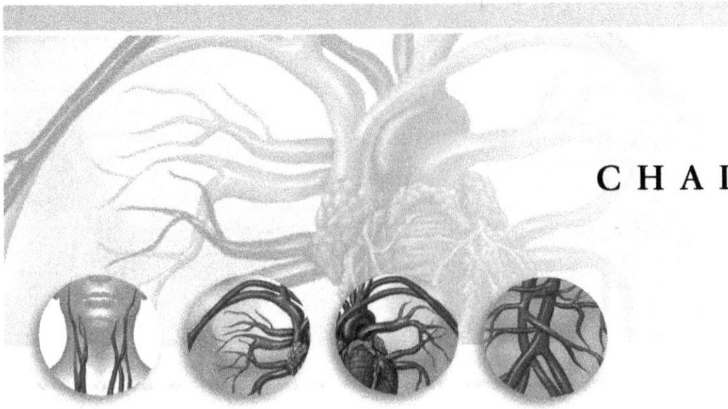

CHAPTER 8

Vascular Medicine and Rehabilitation

Debra Kohlman-Trigoboff

First Edition Authors: *Debra Kohlman-Trigoboff, Mitzi Ekers, and Cynthia Christensen*

OBJECTIVES

1. Identify risk factors associated with development of atherosclerosis.
2. Describe elements of a comprehensive treatment plan for management of hypertension, dyslipidemia, diabetes, and smoking cessation.
3. Explain the role of exercise in the management of peripheral artery disease (PAD) risk factors and claudication symptoms.
4. List the components of each phase of a structured PAD Rehabilitation Program (PRP), including strategies for in-patient education, as well as outpatient assessment, physical reconditioning, education, and evaluation methods.

Introduction

Atherosclerosis is a systemic disease affecting the peripheral, coronary, and cerebral circulation resulting in myocardial infarction (MI), stroke, amputation, renal failure, pain, and death. PAD coexisting with other cardiovascular diseases are seen as follows: patients with symptomatic PAD are more likely to have symptomatic coronary artery disease (CAD) in the form of angina, PAD may be a stronger predictor of concurrent cerebrovascular (CVD) risk than is CAD, 11% of patients with CAD have cerebrovascular disease (CVD), while 9% have abdominal aortic aneurysms. PAD affects over 8.3 million people in the United States affecting 5% to 10% of adults over age 40, with over 4 million people being symptomatic with intermittent claudication (Go, Mozaffarian et al., 2013; Smith et al., 2006). Even though PAD is a marker for systemic atherosclerosis, it often goes unrecognized or is ineffectively treated (Hirsch et al., 2006; Rosamond et al., 2008). Many clinicians fail to understand the serious impact of PAD on the functional capacity, quality of life, and overall mortality of those it affects. The presence of PAD has been identified as an independent risk factor of mortality, posing a 3 to 10 times greater risk of cardiac events or death (Hirsch et al., 2006). Major risk factors for vascular disease are smoking, diabetes, dyslipidemia, and hypertension.

- Smoking appears to be the single most important modifiable risk factor for PAD and its progression toward ischemic events (Hennrikus et al., 2010). The diagnosis of PAD is made a decade earlier in smokers, and intermittent claudication is three times more common in smokers than in nonsmokers (Fiore et al., 2008).

- Diabetes accelerates atherosclerosis 200% to 400%. Diabetics have a fourfold increased risk of developing PAD or intermittent claudication. Diabetic patients have a sevenfold higher rate of amputations than those without the disease (American Diabetes Association [ADA], 2013). Elevated hemoglobin A1C is an established predictor for developing atherosclerosis (ADA, 2013; Gerstein et al., 2003).
- Dyslipidemia indicates elevated levels of total cholesterol, low-density lipoprotein (LDL), and triglycerides or lower levels of high-density lipoprotein (HDL), all of which increase the likelihood of cardiovascular disease (Grundy et al., 2002; Hirsh et al., 2006). However, new ACC/AHA guidelines focus on statin therapy to lower LDL according to patients' atherosclerotic cardiovascular risk (Stone et al., 2013).
- Hypertension is a constant and independent risk factor for vascular disease (Chobanian et al., 2003). Individuals with hypertension have about a twofold increased risk of developing claudication, and the risk of stroke, heart attack, abdominal aortic aneurysm expansion, kidney disease, and death from uncontrolled hypertension is magnified in individuals with PAD (Chobanian et al., 2003). Antihypertensive therapy must be directed at both the reduction of blood pressure as well as improved endothelial function and arterial compliance (Chobanian et al., 2003). In the Heart Outcomes Prevention Evaluation (HOPE) study, patients with symptomatic PAD who received ramipril had a 25% risk reduction of MI, stroke, or vascular death (Yusuf et al., 2000).

The successful long-term management of PAD is enhanced by a medical management program that may delay disease progression, decrease morbidity and mortality, and improve quality of life. The vascular healthcare team, the patients, and the patients' families should develop a partnership to help negotiate the steps involved in these major lifestyle changes. An ideal resource for this partnership is a well-designed PRP which includes exercise and cardiovascular risk factor management.

I. Comprehensive Vascular Medical Therapeutic Approach

A. Purpose: To recognize and treat preventable vascular disease risk factors to reduce disease incidence and complications

B. Smoking and Peripheral Artery Disease

1. Incidence
   a. In 2011, an estimated 19.0% (43.8 million) US adults were current cigarette smokers (Agaku, King, & Dube, 2012)
   b. Deaths resulting from cigarette smoking: over 400,000 accounting for about 20% of cardiovascular deaths (Benowitz, 2003)
   c. Approximately 443,000 US adults die from smoking-related illnesses each year (Agaku et al., 2012; U.S. Department of Health and Human Services, 2010)
   d. The Framingham study: 78% of cases of intermittent claudication could be contributed to smoking (Tendera et al., 2011)
2. Cigarette smoking accelerates atherosclerosis; increases risk of ischemic and thrombotic events (US Dept HHS, 2010)
   a. Endothelial dysfunction occurs from a reduction in nitric oxide resulting in impaired vasodilatation
   b. Carbon monoxide
      1) Reduces the capacity of hemoglobin to carry oxygen
      2) Impairs release of oxygen to body tissues
      3) Results in a state of relative hypoxemia

TABLE 8-1 Benefits of Smoking Cessation

Short-Term Benefits	Long-Term Benefits
Blood pressure returns to pre-smoking levels within 20 min	Lung function improves up to 30% within 2–3 mos
Carbon monoxide levels drop within hours	Risk of coronary heart disease is reduced by 50% after 1 yr
Money is saved each day by not buying cigarettes	Risk of stroke is similar to that of a nonsmoker within 5–15 yrs
Sense of smell and taste improve within days	Patient enjoys increased self-esteem as a result of quitting smoking
Patient earns greater self-respect because of a real sense of accomplishment in quitting	

Source: Adapted from *The surgeon general's report: How tobacco smoke causes disease: the biology and behavioral basis for smoking-attributable disease* (U.S. Department of Health and Human Services (2010).

c. Increased blood viscosity: increases risk of thrombosis
   1) Polycythemia develops as a reaction to induced hypoxemia
   2) Fibrinogen levels also increase, contributing to increased viscosity

d. Smoking induces a chronic inflammatory state
   1) Evidenced by increased blood levels of C-reactive protein
   2) Chronic inflammation is one theory of athrogenesis

e. Nicotine
   1) Increases the heart rate and transiently increases blood pressure
   2) Adds to the injury theory of athrogenesis

f. The gas and tar phases of tobacco smoke
   1) Contain many reactive oxidizing species which enhance the free radical load of smokers
   2) Results in increased oxidation of fatty acids and athrogenicity of LDL cholesterol (Benowitz, 2003)

3. Benefits of smoking cessation (see Table 8-1)
4. Smoking cessation: four crucial factors

a. Make the decision to quit: patient more likely to quit if
   1) Believes he could get a tobacco-related disease
   2) Knows someone who has health problems related to smoking
   3) Believes the benefits of quitting outweigh the benefits of smoking

b. Setting a quit date
   1) Pick a date and mark it on the calendar
   2) Tell friends and family about quit day
   3) Stock up on oral substitutes such as sugar-free gum and candy, carrot sticks

c. Decide on a plan
   1) Obtain nicotine replacement if desired
   2) Sign up for a class, set up a support system

d. Develop a maintenance plan
   1) Review reasons for quitting
   2) Develop alternatives to smoking: increase activity, find alternate stress relievers
   3) Don't worry about weight gain. Even without special attempts to diet, weight gain usually less than 10 pounds; more dangerous to continue smoking (AHA, 2010)

5. Symptoms of withdrawal
   a. Depression
   b. Feelings of frustration and anger
   c. Irritability
   d. Insomnia
   e. Trouble concentrating
   f. Restlessness
   g. Headache
   h. Tiredness
   i. Increased appetite (AHA, 2010)
6. Techniques available to assist with smoking cessation
   a. According to the 2005 PAD guidelines and Zwar et al. (2011), individuals with lower extremity PAD who smoke cigarettes or use tobacco should be advised by their clinicians to stop smoking at each clinic visit. These patients should be offered comprehensive smoking cessation interventions (behavioral modifications, nicotine replacement therapy, or bupropion)
   b. Five components of effective smoking cessation (Five A's) (Fiore et al., 2008)
      1) Ask
      2) Assess
      3) Advise
      4) Assist
      5) Arrange follow-up
   c. Nicotine replacement products and medications
      1) Nicotine: drug found naturally in tobacco; as addictive as heroin or cocaine (National Institute on Drug Abuse, 2012)
      2) When smokers try to quit or cut back, the absence of nicotine leads to withdrawal symptoms
      3) Pharmacological interventions such as nicotine replacement therapy and bupropion achieve 1-year smoking cessation rates of approximately 16% and 30%, respectively (Hirsch et al., 2006)
      4) Medications helpful for successful smoking cessation and control of withdrawal (see Table 8-2)
   d. Telephone "Quit lines"
      1) Quit lines link smokers to counselors; help develop a plan for each person and help avoid common mistakes that may hurt a quit attempt
      2) Convenient and accessible
      3) People who use telephone counseling quit at twice the rate of those who do not get this type of help (AHA, 2010)
   e. Self-help materials are the most common type of counseling but have not been found to be effective (Benowitz, 2003)
   f. Both individual and group counseling have been found to increase rates of cessation (Benowitz, 2003)
   g. Other tools for smoking cessation include
      1) Hypnosis (useful for some people)
      2) Acupuncture (no strong evidence to support effectiveness)
      3) Filter to reduce tar and nicotine (not effective, as studies show smokers tend to smoke more with filters)
      4) Over-the-counter products that change the taste of tobacco, combinations of vitamins (have little scientific evidence to support their claims) (AHA, 2010)

TABLE 8-2 Medications Used for Smoking Cessation (Rennard, Rigotti, & Doughton, 2013)

Name	Form	Dose	Length of Use	Cautions	Side Effects
Bupropion, sustained release	Zyban or Wellbutrin (prescription only)	150 mg in morning for 3 d, then 150 mg twice a day	Begin 1–2 wks before quit date, then 7–12 wks	Seizure, eating disorder	Insomnia, dry mouth
Varenicline	Chanitx (prescription only)	0.5 mg PO once daily on days 1–3, then 0.5 mg PO twice daily on days 4–7, and finally 1 mg PO twice daily on day 8 until end of treatment	12–24 wks	Depression	Nausea, suicidal ideation, anxiety, lethargy
Nicotine gum	Nicorette, Nicorette DS, Nicorette Mint, Nicorette Orange (OTC only)	Up to 24 pieces/d; 25 cigs/d 3 2 mg $25 cigs/d 3 4 mg	Up to 12 wks	Temporomandibular joint (TMJ) disorder	Sore mouth, dyspepsia
Nicotine patch	Nicoderm CQ (OTC only), generic/house brand patches (OTC and prescription) Nicotrol (OTC only)	21 mg/24 h; 14 mg/24 h; 7 mg/24 h; 15 mg/16 h	4 wks; then 2 wks; then 2 wks 8 wks		Local skin reaction
Nicotine nasal spray	Nicotrol NS (prescription only)	8–40 doses/d	3–6 mo	Dependency	Nasal irritation
Nicotine inhaler	Nicotrol inhaler (prescription only)	6–16 cartridges/d	Up to 6 mo		Mouth/throat irritation

7. Regardless of technique used, certain information increases the chances of success
   a. Thinking about the times of the day one is likely to smoke and plan distraction for those times; helps to start these distractions before one actually quits smoking
   b. Social support in the form of caring, concern, and encouragement; this can come from healthcare providers, family, friends, and other community members (Rennard, Rigotti, & Doughton, 2013)

C. Antiplatelet and Antithrombotic Strategies (see Chapter 6, Medications Used in Patients with Peripheral Vascular Disease for full discussion)

1. Platelet aggregation starts with vascular trauma such as atherectomy, angioplasty, stent, surgery, hyperhomocysteinemia, smoking, external trauma, and burns
2. Platelet activation involves
   a. Adhesion to the site of injury to the exposed collagen in the subendothelial layer
   b. Release of intracellular granules containing chemical mediators
   c. Aggregation of the other platelets caused by the chemical mediators, which forms a plug (Rooke et al., 2011)
3. Types of antiplatelet medications (Alberts et al., 2009)
   a. Acetylsalicylic acid (aspirin)
   b. Thienopyridines
      1) Clopidogrel
      2) Ticlopidine
      3) Prasugrel
   c. Ticagrelor
   d. Dipyridamole
4. Goal of antiplatelet therapy: to reduce the risk of MI, stroke, or vascular death in individuals with atherosclerotic lower extremity PAD (Rooke et al., 2011)
   a. Individuals with symptomatic lower extremity PAD
      1) Intermittent claudication
      2) Critical limb ischemia
      3) Prior lower extremity revascularization (endovascular or surgical)
      4) Prior amputation for lower extremity ischemia
   b. In asymptomatic individuals with an ABI <0.90
      1) Use in asymptomatic individuals with borderline abnormal ABI, defined as 0.91 to 0.99, not well established
5. Dual antiplatelet therapy (DAT): ASA + plavix may be considered to reduce the risk of cardiovascular (CV) events in patients with symptomatic atherosclerotic lower extremity PAD who are at high perceived CV risk (Rooke et al., 2011)
6. Oral anticoagulation therapy with warfarin is not indicated to reduce the risk of adverse CV ischemic events in individuals with atherosclerotic lower extremity PAD (Rooke et al., 2011)

D. Dyslipidemia Strategies

1. Body lipids: building blocks of fats (Galton, 2003; Jellinger et al., 2012).
   a. In animals, lipids are spheres of oil stored for energy
      1) Surface: phospholipid, free cholesterol, protein
      2) Core: triglycerides and cholesterol
      3) Triglycerides: fatty acid molecules contained in fats of both animals and plants
      4) Difficult to transport in blood because of insolubility
   b. Bound to proteins (albumin) and transported as lipoproteins
      1) Complex aggregates of protein and lipid molecules transporting triglycerides and cholesterol from the intestines for use in peripheral tissues

2) Categorized into five types according to size and density, and whether they carry cholesterol or triglycerides
3) Cholesterol-carrying lipoproteins
   a) Low density (LDL): "bad," mostly cholesterol; lesions arise from transport and retention of plasma LDL through endothelium layer into subendothelial space, where LDL is then oxidized and initiates an inflammatory response; arterial wall becomes a scavenger for more LDL
      - Apolipoprotein is a protein that binds to fats (lipids) forming lipoproteins. The lipoproteins then transport dietary fats through the bloodstream
      - Apolipoprotein measurements (especially apolipoprotein B (apoB)) in several studies significantly predicted coronary heart disease (CHD) death, independently of conventional lipids and other cardiovascular risk factors (smoking, hypertension dyslipidemia, diabetes, and C-reactive protein). Sierra-Johnson et al. (2009) also found that the predictive ability of apoB alone to detect CHD death is better than any of the routine clinical lipid measurements
   b) High density (HDL): "good," mostly protein, large molecules that remove cholesterol from walls of arteries and transport to liver; prevent oxidation of LDL (antioxidant). High levels (over 60 mg/dL) are as important as low levels of LDL in prevention of disease
4) Triglyceride-carrying lipoproteins
   a) Intermediate (IDL) and very low density (VLDL)
   b) Chylomicrons: largest in size, lowest in density
   c) Interact with HDL to cause fall in HDL as triglycerides rise
   d) Also associated with arterial wall inflammation and thrombosis
5) Lipoprotein (a)
   a) Size and density between LDL and HDL
   b) Carry a protein that may deter the body's ability to dissolve blood clots
   c) Under investigation as either a marker or cause for arterial disease
   d) Usually inherited; does not respond to diet/exercise
   e) Older women and African Americans more at risk
6) Remnant lipoproteins: byproducts of chylomicrons and/or VLDLs; may be marker of arterial disease when cholesterol is normal

c. Two forms of metabolism of cholesterol and lipoproteins: endogenous and exogenous
   1) Endogenous pathway: handles cholesterol produced by liver and chylomicron remnants that result from digestion of fat; chylomicron remnants converted in liver to VLDL, IDL, and LDL
   2) Exogenous pathway: fats from diet absorbed in gut, incorporated into chylomicron particles made from triglycerides and apolipoproteins that are soluble in blood; chylomicrons are broken down by enzyme, lipoprotein lipase in capillaries, taken to liver where they enter endogenous pathway of lipid metabolism or are excreted through bile acids

d. Cholesterol sources
   1) Dietary fats
   2) Two thirds manufactured by liver
   3) Production stimulated by saturated fat—animal products, meat, dairy

e. Cholesterol, an essential nutrient for
    1) Repair of cell membrane (biogenesis)
    2) Manufacturing vitamin D on skin's surface
    3) Production of hormones (estrogen, testosterone)
    4) Steroid synthesis
    5) Formation of bile acids (Jellinger et al., 2012)

f. Normal values for healthy people
    1) Total cholesterol: 180 to 200 mg/dL
    2) LDL, 130 mg/dL (70 mg/dL for individuals with atherosclerosis or diabetes mellitus)
    3) HDL, 40 mg/dL (the higher, the better); for each 4-mg/dL decline, there is a 10% increase in cardiovascular disease
    4) Triglycerides, 150 mg/dL or less

g. LDL particle size (LDL-P) (Jellinger et al., 2012)
    1) The small and dense LDL particle is thought to be atherogenic. However, researchers have found that compared to LDL or non-HDL assessments, the number of LDL particles is a more sensitive indicator of CAD risk
    2) Patients who have therapeutic LDL concentration on the standard lipid panel may still have a large number of circulating atherogenic LDL particles
    3) LDL-P values: low = <1,000 nmol/L; borderline = 1,300 to –1,599 nmol/L; high = >2,000 nmol/L
    4) Testing for particle size can be expensive and may not be needed since triglyceride levels >120 mg/dL and low HDL levels (<40 mg/dL in men, <50 mg/dL in women) are usually associated with small, dense LDL particles

2. Dyslipidemia
    a. Defined as either elevated levels of total cholesterol, LDL, and triglycerides or lower levels of HDL
    b. Fat transport: complicated system of proteins, enzymes, and receptors evolved to optimize transport and delivery of fat to peripheral tissue; when system breaks down, common disorders of lipid transport (dyslipidemia) and lipid storage (atherosclerosis) occur (Galton, 2003)
        1) All abnormalities increase likelihood of cardiovascular disease (Grundy et al., 2002)
        2) 50% of atherosclerosis deaths related to lipid disorders
    c. Independent risk factor for vascular disease; when controlled, can lead to decreased development and progression of atherosclerotic plaque (Jellinger et al., 2012)

3. Role of dyslipidemia in atherosclerosis (Jellinger et al., 2012)
    a. Evolution of atherosclerotic plaque is lifelong; a fatty streak in aorta evident by autopsy as early as age 10
    b. Leading theory: injury to arterial endothelium followed by infiltration of lipids
    c. Inflammation occurs after endothelial injury, making endothelium prothrombotic and susceptible to monocyte migration to the subendothelial or intimal space
    d. Monocytes differentiate to macrophages that promote lipid oxidation and uptake; eventually become lipid-laden foam cells that characterize fatty streak

e. Smooth muscle cells may proliferate over the early atherosclerotic lesion or fatty streak and create a fibrous cap
f. Bang, Saver, Liebeskind, Pineda, and Ovbiagele (2008) found that patients with high cholesterol had an increased thrombotic potential compared with patients who had normal cholesterol
    1) When aggressive cholesterol management achieved, evidence of decreased platelet thrombus formation seen
    2) Increased thrombotic potential can accelerate the atherosclerotic process
    3) Management of dyslipidemia should include some form of antiplatelet therapy

4. Dyslipidemia categories: Classification of dyslipidemias according to etiology can help clarify origin and management of lipid disorders (Galton, 2003)
    a. Inherited: genetic predisposition to have an elevation in either triglycerides or cholesterol by defect of LDL receptor, lipase, or apolipoprotein
    b. Acquired: elevation of cholesterol, triglycerides, or both
        1) Elevated cholesterol caused by hypothyroidism, chronic renal failure, cholestatis, diabetes mellitus, anorexia nervosa, biliary cirrhosis
        2) Elevated triglycerides caused by diabetes mellitus, alcoholism, obesity, and diet
        3) Elevated cholesterol and triglycerides cause by obesity, insulin resistance, nephritic syndrome, alcoholism, hypothyroidism, oral estrogen treatment, pregnancy, Cushing's syndrome, or drugs such as steroids, thiazides, or beta-blockers (BBs)
5. Screening for dyslipidemia risk assessment (Galton, 2003; Jellinger et al., 2012)
    a. Modifiable risk factors—personal habits: smoking, exercise tolerance, alcohol, diet and occupation, obesity (BMI >30)
    b. Current medications
    c. Family history of dyslipidemia and evidence of atherosclerosis (e.g., MI, claudication, or stroke)
    d. Other medical comorbidities, especially PAD and cerebral or cardiac vascular disease, hypertension, diabetes mellitus
    e. Nonmodifiable risk factors; age (men <55; women <65), sex (higher risk in men than women until menopause), early menopause, positive family history
6. Diseases associated with dyslipidemia (Galton, 2003; Jellinger et al., 2012)
    a. See above for acquired dyslipidemias
    b. Multiple myeloma: abnormal gamma globulins secreted interfere with clearance of lipids from bloodstream
    c. Metabolic syndrome (syndrome X): collection of health risks that increase likelihood of CAD, stroke, DM; characterized by central obesity, atherogenic dyslipidemia (high triglycerides plus low HDL), hypertension >130/85, insulin resistance, prothrombotic state (high fibrinogen), and proinflammatory state (elevated high-sensitivity C-reactive protein). Caused by obesity, inactivity, genetic factors predisposing to insulin resistance; 70 to 80 million Americans
7. Medications that interfere with lipids (Galton, 2003)
    a. Diuretics: thiazides and spironolactone (increase both cholesterol and triglycerides)
    b. BBs (increase triglycerides and decrease HDL)
    c. Sympatholytics: prazosin or clonidine (decrease cholesterol)

8. ACC/AHA Cardiovascular Risk (Goff et al., 2013)
   a. Calculation of risk of atherosclerotic cardiovascular disease (ASCVD) (10 years and lifetime risk). Those with 10-year risk of ASCVD ≥7.5%—need aggressive treatment
   b. Assess risk factors every 4 to 6 years in patients 20 to 79 years of age
   c. Variables
      1) Sex
      2) Age
      3) Race (African American or Caucasian and all others)
      4) TC
      5) HDL
      6) Systolic blood pressure (SBP)
      7) Treatment for HTN
      8) DM
      9) Smoking
   d. Formula http://my.americanheart.org/professional/StatementsGuidelines/PreventionGuidelines/Prevention-Guidelines_UCM_457698_SubHomePage.jsp
9. ACC/AHA guideline on the treatment of blood cholesterol to reduce atherosclerotic cardiovascular risk in adults (Stone et al., 2013)
   a. Evidence no longer supports specific LDL or HDL treatment targets
   b. Focuses on statin therapy to provide acceptable reduction in cardiovascular risk
   c. Devised four statin benefit groups treated by either high-intensity or moderate-intensity statin therapy
   d. Atherosclerotic cardiovascular disease (ASCVD): Defined as acute coronary syndrome (ACS), history of MI, stable or unstable angina (USA), CAD, vascular disease, history of transient ischemic attack (TIA) or stroke (CVA) thought vascular in origin
   e. Statin therapy goals
      1) High-intensity-lowering LCL-C by ≥50%
      2) Moderate-intensity-lowering LDL-C by 30% to <50%
   f. Four statin benefit groups
      1) Patients with ASCVD
      2) LDL ≥190 mg/dL
      3) DM ages 40 to 79 with LDL 70 to 189 mg/dL without ASCVD
      4) No ASCVD or DM and LDL 70 to 189 mg/dL with 10-year ASCVD of ≥7.5%
   g. Types of statin therapy
      1) High-intensity statin therapy
         a) Population
            - >21 and ≤75 years with ASCVD
            - LDL-C ≥190 mg/dL
            - DM (I or II) ages 40 to 75 years with and estimated cardiovascular risk score ≥7.5%
         b) Medications: goal: lower LDL-C >50%
            - Atorvastatin 40 to 80 mg
            - Rosuvastatin 20 to 40 mg
      2) Moderate-intensity statin therapy
         a) Population
            - >75 years with ASCVD or not a candidate for high-intensity statin

- LDL-C ≥190 mg/dL and not a candidate for high-intensity statin
- DM (I or II) ages 40 to 75 years

b) Medications: goal: lower LDL-C 30% to <50%

- Atorvastatin 10 to 20 mg
- Rosuvastatin 5 to 10 mg
- Simvastatin 20 to 40 mg
- Pravastatin 40 to 80 mg
- Lovastatin 40 mg
- Fluvastatin XL 80 mg
- Fluvastatin 40 mg BID
- Pitavastatin 2 to 4 mg

3) Low-intensity statin therapy

a) Medications: goal: lower LDL-C <30%

- Simvastatin 10 mg
- Pravastatin 10 to 20 mg
- Lovastatin 20 mg
- Fluvastatin 20 to 40 mg
- Pitavastatin 1 mg

10. Lifestyle modification, the foundation for ASCVD risk factor reduction (Stone et al., 2013), includes

a. Heart healthy diet

1) Diet often neglected in advent of drug therapy despite recommendations (Jellinger et al., 2012; Kreisberg & Oberman, 2003)

a) Patients would rather take pill; providers see diet as ineffective/unimportant

b) Diet control allows lower drug dosage; minimizes adverse side effect potential

c) Lipid-lowering diet also aids control of other risk factors: hypertension, obesity, diabetes

2) General principles of lipid-lowering diet (Galton, 2003; Jellinger et al., 2012)

a) Decrease total and saturated fat intake

b) Increase high protein

c) Increase complex carbohydrates

d) Increase fruit and vegetables

e) Decrease dietary cholesterol

f) Moderately decrease sodium intake

3) Goals of dietary treatment of dyslipidemia: lower ingested fat content and reduce operation of metabolic pathways that increase circulating LDL and triglycerides (Grundy et al., 2002; Jellinger et al., 2012). See Table 8-3 for recommended dietary goals

a) Saturated fatty acids found in high-fat dairy products, meats, tropical oils, and hard shortening increase LDL levels

b) *Trans*-fatty acids found in hydrogenated vegetable oils increase LDL and triglycerides and lower HDL

c) Substituting unsaturated fat for saturated fat improves cardiovascular risk and may improve insulin sensitivity

d) Exercise combined with diet can decrease triglycerides and increase HDL levels and will increase HDL levels with incremental advances in energy expenditure

e) Disadvantage: high carbohydrate intake may raise triglycerides and lower HDL (Jellinger et al., 2012)

TABLE 8-3 ATP III Diet Guidelines

Saturated fat	<7% calories/d
Polyunsaturated fat	Up to 10% calories/d
Monounsaturated fat	Up to 20% calories/d
Total fat	20–25% calories/d
Carbohydrates	50–60% calories/d
Fiber	20–30 g/d
Proteins	15% calories/d
Cholesterol	<200 mg/d

4) Regular exercise: 30 to 45 minutes, in sessions performed at least three to five times per week (raises HDL, lowers triglycerides; inactivity is independent risk factor)
5) Maintain healthy weight (weight loss: improves insulin sensitivity and serum glucose uptake, lessens DM risk; lowers LDL)
6) Avoid tobacco products (smoking cessation: 30% increase in HDL)

11. Medication therapy (see also Chapter 6, Medications Used in Patients with Peripheral Vascular Disease)
   a. Statins (Galton, 2003; Jellinger et al., 2012; Mihaylova et al., 2012; Stone et al., 2013)
      1) Also known as HMGCoA (hydroxymethylglutaryl coenzyme A) reductase inhibitors
      2) Directly inhibit cholesterol synthesis in the liver and peripheral tissues, as well as induces the synthesis of LDL receptors on cell membranes of the liver to remove LDL cholesterol
      3) Most powerful agent for LDL lowering: 20% to 60% depending on medication used
      4) Other benefits
         a) Anti-inflammatory effects (pravastatin)
         b) Stabilize the atherosclerotic plaque (by decreasing smooth muscle cell proliferation)
         c) Alter vasomotor responsiveness and their antithrombotic effects (influencing platelet aggregation)
         d) Recommended to be the first line of treatment in diabetic patients and those with increased triglycerides
      5) Optimal dosing schedule: after the evening meal so that the synthesis of the liver is inhibited overnight
      6) Examples of statins: atorvastatin (Lipitor), fluvastatin (Lescol), lovastatin (Mevacor), pravastatin (Lipostat), rosuvastatin (Crestor), simvastatin (Zocor)
      7) Caution in patients with liver and renal dysfunction, pregnancy, or a high alcohol intake
      8) Side effects of statins include reversible myositis; can ultimately lead to severe myopathy with rhabdomyolysis if drug is not discontinued
         a) Individuals at higher risk for myopathy/rhabdomyolysis have
            - Advanced age (>65 years)
            - Hypothyroidism
            - Renal insufficiency

b) CPK will become elevated
c) Crestor revised their labeling following an investigation by the FDA for myopathy and renal failure. Recommend starting patient on lowest dose initially
d) Dietary caution: grapefruit juice interferes with activity; 4 oz. of juice or 1/2 grapefruit is acceptable
e) Drug–drug interaction: atorvastatin may impair antiplatelet activity of clopidogrel
   - The proposed mechanism is competitive inhibition of CYP450 3A4 enzymatic activity, which is responsible for the conversion of clopidogrel to its active metabolite
   - Pravastatin (Pravachol), fluvastatin (Lescol), and rosuvastatin (Crestor) are not metabolized by CYP450 3A4 and are theoretically not expected to interact with clopidogrel

b. Nonstatin dyslipidemic medications: Research controlled trials show that nonstatin therapies do not provide acceptable ASCVD risk reduction benefits compared to their potential for adverse effects in the routine prevention of ASCVD (Stone et al., 2013)
   1) Nicotinates (Galton, 2003; Jellinger et al., 2012)
      a) Potent antilipolytic agents that inhibit the release of free fatty acids from adipose tissue, thus reducing the flux of free fatty acids to the liver
      b) Niacin has been shown to reduce LDL and triglycerides and to increase HDL
      c) Contraindications: chronic liver disease, arterial bleeding, and peptic ulcer disease
      d) Side effects
         - Skin flushing, dizziness, and palpitations; aspirin 30 minutes prior to niacin may decrease flushing
         - Increasing insulin resistance in diabetics
         - Increasing serum homocysteine
         - Increasing uric acid levels
      e) Examples of nicotinates
         - Nicotinic acid (niacin)
         - Advicor (lovastatin/niacin)
         - Niaspan, Slo-Niacin, Niacin SR, Niacor
   2) Fibrates (Galton, 2003; Jellinger et al., 2012)
      a) Aid in lowering triglycerides and increasing HDL
      b) Bind to peroxisomal proliferator–activated nuclear receptors to form transcription factors that regulate genes to drive fat utilization
      c) Contraindications
         - Hepatic or renal dysfunction
         - Primary biliary cirrhosis
         - Pre-existing gallbladder disease
      d) Side effects (rare)
         - Skin rashes
         - Bone marrow dysplasias
         - Gallstones
         - Myositis
         - Use with caution when combined with statins (statin doses should be reduced 25% to 50%) because of the increased risk of rhabdomyolysis

e) Examples of fibrates
- Clofibrate (Atromid)
- Bezafibrate (Bezalip)
- Fenofibrate (Tricor, procetophen)
- Gemfibrozil (Lopid)
- Ciprofibrate (Modalim)

3) Bile acid resins (Galton, 2003; Jellinger et al., 2012)

a) Bind bile acids in the small intestines and interrupt the circulation of bile in the liver, promoting its excretion in the feces

b) Without reabsorption of bile, there is an increased intracellular conversion of cholesterol to bile acids, ultimately leading to an increased catabolism of LDL particles

c) Contraindications
- Biliary obstruction
- Familial dysbetalipoproteinemia (triglycerides >500 mg/dL)

d) Side effects
- Increase in triglycerides
- Constipation, back pain, fatigue, cough
- Interference with the absorption of fat-soluble vitamins and some medications
- Bile acid resins are not directly absorbed into the body; systemic side effects do not occur

e) Examples
- Colestyramine (Questran)
- Colestipol (Colestid)
- May use in combination with statins or nicotinic acid but not fibrates (drug interaction)

4) Cholesterol absorption inhibitors (Jellinger et al., 2012; Kreisberg & Oberman, 2003)

a) A new class of dyslipidemic medication

b) Interferes with the absorption of cholesterol secreted in the bile and enterohepatic circulation

c) Zetia (Ezetimibe) is the only drug in this class available

d) Should be used adjunctively in patients whose LDL reduction is suboptimal

e) Cardiovascular end points of the effects of Zetia are yet unknown

f) A recent study Vytorin (Zetia/Simvastatin) vs. Simvastatin did not reduce carotid intima-media thickness. More research needs to be done (Kastelein et al., 2008)

12. Special considerations

a. Diabetics (ADA, 2013; Faxon et al., 2004)

1) Dyslipidemia commonly associated with type II diabetes; believed to be a major source of increased risk of vascular events

2) Diabetic patients tend to produce small, dense LDL that is more vulnerable to oxidation; LDL particles of diabetics contain more triglycerides than those of nondiabetics

3) According to the ATP, other mechanisms in diabetics that promote vascular disease are glycation of arterial wall proteins, change in arterial cellular function, promotion of thrombogenesis, and enhancement of LDL oxidation

4) 19% of poorly controlled diabetics have hypertriglyceridemia and low HDL levels; insulin deficiency leads to the impairment in clearance of plasma triglycerides
5) Because of the magnitude of the problem, dyslipidemia must be managed aggressively in diabetics; most recent American Diabetes Association guidelines recommend lipid-lowering therapy initiated in patients with type II diabetes and LDL levels ≥100 mg/dL

b. Women
1) Elevated triglyceride levels recognized as an independent predictor of CHD risk, especially in women and in patients with impaired glucose metabolism (Faxon et al., 2004)
2) Triglyceride levels are a more sensitive predictor of CHD risk in women than in men, and high triglyceride levels lead to greater atherogenic LDL particles and lower HDL levels; however, clinical trials on the vascular outcome of lowering triglycerides in women are lacking (Jellinger et al., 2012)
3) Postmenopausal women (Faxon et al., 2004)
a) Increased risk of ASCVD thought attributable to the loss of the "protective" effect of estrogen
b) Often gain weight and decrease their physical activity; when combined with the lower estrogen levels, can lead to increased lipids levels (Hsia et al., 2004)
c) Should have aggressive lipid-lowering therapy to include diet, exercise, and if necessary medication to lower their cholesterol levels
4) Women have increased regression of vascular plaques/lesions and similar improvement in survival as men on statin therapy

c. Elderly (Jellinger et al., 2012)
1) Providers may be reluctant to prescribe drug therapy for elderly patients; may feel patients have a short life span ahead or that their atherosclerosis is irreversible
2) Research controlled trials support continuing statins beyond 75 years of age in persons who are already taking and tolerating these drugs. More research data support the use of moderate-intensity statin therapy for secondary prevention in individuals with clinical ASCVD >75 years of age. However, there is less to support starting high-intensity statin therapy for secondary prevention in individuals >75 years (Stone et al., 2013)
3) Considerations in using lipid-lowering drugs in the elderly
a) Resins usually cause constipation, already an issue with most elderly
b) Renal function: most cases of myopathy with the use of statins associated with renal insufficiency
c) Fibrates can increase the risk of gall stones
d) Nicotinic acid: dry mouth and dry skin, along with flushing

d. Renal insufficiency (Jellinger et al., 2012)
1) Increased risk of cardiovascular events in patients with renal insufficiency and end-stage renal disease
2) Despite this increased risk, drug therapy for dyslipidemia in renal-diseased patients revealed a 28% reduction in major cardiovascular events

13. Summary
    a. Dyslipidemia indicates elevated levels of total cholesterol, LDL, and triglycerides or lower levels of HDL, all of which increase the likelihood of cardiovascular disease
    b. When associated with other vascular risk factors such as hypertension, smoking, diabetes, and a family history of vascular problems, dyslipidemia is a substantial risk factor for the progression of vascular disease
    c. Evidence no longer supports specific LDL or HDL treatment targets. Guidelines now focus on statin therapy to provide acceptable reduction in cardiovascular risk
    d. Risk factors for atherosclerosis are the target for therapeutic intervention and the method of risk assessment in the prevention of atherosclerotic vascular disease
    e. Modification of dyslipidemias through diet, exercise, and/or drug therapy can decrease the progression of atherosclerosis, decrease cardiovascular events, increase atherosclerotic plaque stability, and decrease hyperthrombotic potentials in vascular patients

E. Hypertension Management (see Table 8-4)

1. Effects of elevated blood pressure, or Hypertension (HTN) (Chobanian et al., 2003)
    a. One of the four major factors that contribute to the development of atherosclerosis and is an independent risk factor for cardiovascular disease. Hypertension is a risk factor for
        1) CAD
        2) Heart failure (HF)
        3) Stroke (CVA) or TIA
        4) PAD
        5) Chronic kidney disease (CKD)
        6) Aortic regurgitation (AR/AI)
        7) Atrial fibrillation/flutter
    b. Incidence
        1) Statistics: 81.5% of those with hypertension are aware they have it; 74.9% are being treated for HTN; 52.5% are under control (Go, Bauman et al., 2013)
        2) Hypertension affects approximately 26.4% of the worldwide population and is the leading chronic risk factor for mortality, causing 13.5% of all deaths (Brook et al., 2013)

TABLE 8-4 Stages of Hypertension (Chobanian et al., 2003; Go, Bauman et al., 2013)

BP Classification	SBP (mm Hg)	DBP (mm Hg)	Treatment
Normal	<120	and <80	
Pre-HTN	120–139	or 80–89	Lifestyle modification
Stage I	140–159	or 90–99	Lifestyle modification, consider diuretic recheck in 3 mos
Stage II	≥160	or ≥100	Lifestyle modifications and 2 HTN meds: • Thiazide and ACEI, ARB, or CCB • Or consider ACEI and CCB *Recheck in 2–4 wks*

3) Onset between ages 20 to 50 years. Increases with advancing age
4) Men > risk for hypertension than women until age 55 years
   a) Men and women at equal risk ages 55 to 74 years
   b) Women are at greater risk at age >74 years
5) African American patients and Caucasian patients in Southeastern United States have greater prevalence of HTN and higher mortality from stroke compared to the rest of United States
6) African American patients develop HTN at a younger age and have more severe HTN; leading to 1.3 times rate of nonfatal stroke, 1.8 times rate of fatal stroke, 1.5 times rate of heart disease mortality, and 5 times rate of end-stage renal disease

2. Identifiable (secondary) causes of hypertension (Chobanian et al., 2003)
   a. Primary aldosteronism
   b. Renovascular disease
   c. Sleep apnea—83% of patients were found to have >10 episodes of apnea/hour
   d. Drug-induced/related
   e. CKD
   f. Pheochromocytoma
   g. Thyroid or parathyroid disease
   h. Cushing's syndrome or steroid therapy
   i. Coarctation of the aorta
3. Primary hypertension
   a. No known/obvious cause
   b. Most common form of hypertension
   c. Based on average of two or more properly measured, seated BP readings on each of two or more office visits
   d. Classification of blood pressure for adults over 18 (Chobanian et al., 2003)
4. Diagnostic evaluation (Chobanian et al., 2003; Cifkova et al., 2003)
   a. In addition to identifying the causes of hypertension, provider should assess for risk factors and comorbidities
   b. Cardiovascular-focused complete history and physical needed to assess for target organ damage (TOD)
      1) Left ventricular hypertrophy
      2) MI, angina, congestive heart failure (CHF)
      3) Carotid artery disease (ultrasound evidence of arterial wall thickening [carotid IMT (intima-media thickness) ≥0.9 mm] or atherosclerotic plaque)
      4) Renal insufficiency (slight increase in serum creatinine [men 1.3 to 1.5, women 1.2 to 1.4 mg/dL]), microalbumin (30 to 100 mg/24 hours)
      5) Diabetic nephropathy
      6) Cerebrovascular accident (CVA), cerebral hemorrhage, TIA
      7) Increase in abdominal aortic aneurysm diameter
      8) PAD: lower extremity arterial disease (intermittent claudication or critical ischemia)
      9) Advanced retinopathy
   c. Laboratory tests recommended prior to antihypertensive therapy (Daniel, Kelsberg, & Jankowski, 2005; Lookinland & Beckstrand, 2003)
      1) Hematocrit
      2) Blood chemistries (potassium, calcium, creatinine/glomerular filtration rate [GFR])

3) Fasting glucose, HDL, LDL, and triglycerides
4) EKG
5) Urinalysis to include microalbuminurea
6) Drug screen if history is suggestive of substance abuse

5. Indication for hypertension treatment (James et al., 2013)
   a. The Eighth Joint National Committee on the Prevention, Detection, Evaluation, and Treatment of High Blood Pressure (JNC-8) is based on evidence-based studies of hypertension in patients with CAD, diabetes, PAD, HF, prior stroke, CKD, smokers, representatives of both sexes and all races with sample sizes of each study of at least 100. Rather than defining hypertension and prehypertension as in JNC-7, JNC-8 defines the threshold for treating hypertension
   b. Lifestyle modifications of healthy diet, weight control, and regular exercise should always be initiated prior to starting any antihypertensive medications; see Table 8-5
      1) Goals (Lichtenstein et al., 2006; Stone et al., 2013)
         a) Consume an overall healthy diet
         b) Aim for a healthy body weight
         c) Aim for LDL reduction in those with high ASCVD risk
         d) Aim for a normal blood pressure
         e) Aim for a normal blood glucose level
         f) Be physically active
         g) Avoid use of and exposure to tobacco products
      2) Benefits of lifestyle modification
      3) In alternative approaches to lowering blood pressure, the strongest evidence support using aerobic and/or dynamic resistance exercising as an adjunctive treatment of HTN (Brook et al., 2013)
   c. Blood pressure goals
      According to the JNC-8 guidelines (James et al., 2013), the blood pressure goal for those individuals 60 or older should be 150/90 or less. In those individuals 30 to 59 years of age, the diastolic blood pressure goal

TABLE 8-5 Lifestyle Modifications to Reduce Hypertension (Chobanian et al., 2003; Go, Bauman et al., 2013)

Modification	Recommendation	Decrease SBP
Weight reduction	BMI 18.5–24.9	5–20 mm Hg/10 kg
DASH: *D*ietary *A*pproaches to *S*top *H*ypertension	Rich in K^+ and Ca: • Low-fat dairy • ↑fruits & vegetables • ↓salt • ↓total fat	8–14 mm Hg
Sodium restriction	• No more than 2,400 mg sodium/d; • Reduction of sodium intake to 1,500 mg/d is associated with even greater reduction in BP • Reduce intake by at least 1,000 mg/d since that will lower BP, even if the desired daily sodium intake is not achieved	2–8 mm Hg
Physical activity	30 min/d brisk	4–9 mm Hg
Moderation of alcohol	2 drinks (e.g., 24 oz beer, 10 oz wine, or 3 oz 80-proof whiskey)/d (men) 1 drink/d (women)	2–4 mm Hg

is 90 mm Hg or less. While there are no research controlled trials indicating optimal SBP in the 30- to 59-year-old age group, expert opinion recommends SBP 140 mm Hg or less

d. Treatment recommendations
   1) If not at goal after lifestyle modification, an antihypertensive medication should be started (James et al., 2013)
   2) Based on the evidence-based studies, four classes of hypertension medications are recommended: thiazide diuretics, calcium channel blockers (CCBs), angiotensin converting enzyme inhibitor (ACEi), and angiotensin receptor blockers (ARBs). All of these classes of medications showed comparable outcomes in all cardiovascular patient groups except in HF patients, in whom thiazide diuretics worked best as the initial hypertensive medication. Antihypertensive medications from other antihypertensive medication classes (e.g., beta- and alpha-blockers, vasodilators) did not demonstrate sufficient evidence to be recommended as one of the four evidence-based antihypertension classes
      a) James et al. (2013) reported that in one study, BBs used as the initial hypertensive treatment showed worsening cardiovascular morbidity (MI or stroke) compared to ARBs
      b) In another study, alpha-blockers used as the initial hypertensive treatment showed worsening cerebrovascular and HF outcomes compared to using thiazide diuretics as the initial hypertension treatment
   3) Stage 1—should start treatment with a diuretic—The European HTN guidelines recommend diuretics, BBs, CCBs, ACEi are suitable for the initial therapy for HTN management (Jennings & Touyz, 2013)
   4) Stage 2—will likely need a two-drug combination, for example, diuretic with an ACEi, ARBs, CCBs or BBs. Using two-drug therapy for stage II hypertensive patients showed more rapid achievement of target BP and was found to be the main contributor to the estimated risk reduction (23% reduction in CV events and all-cause mortality) (Gradman et al., 2013)
   5) Treatment recommendations
      a) James et al. (2013) recommends that the initial hypertensive treatment medication in the non-black population be a thiazide diuretic, CCB, ACEi, or ARB, while the initial hypertension treatment for black patients is either a thiazide diuretic or CCB since studies showed that blacks who were initially treated for HTN with an ACEi showed a 51% higher stroke rate than those treated initially with CCB
      b) Those patients with CKD (of any age) should be on either an ACEi or ARB to preserve renal function
   6) Treatment titration
      a) James et al. (2013) recommends the following method of hypertension medication titration. If blood pressure not at goal after 1 month of initiating an antihypertensive medication, increase the dose of the medication or add a second antihypertensive medication. After maximizing the doses of both antihypertensive medications and the patient's BP is not at goal, a third antihypertensive medication should be added

TABLE 8-6 Guideline for Compelling Indications for Drug Classes for Hypertension (Go, Bauman et al., 2013)

Indication	Thiazide	BB	ACEi	ARB	CCB	Aldos Antag
SHF	√	√	√	√		√
DHF	√	√	√	√		√
DM	√	√	√	√	√	
CVA	√		√			
CKD			√	√		
CAD/post MI		√	√			

KEY: SHF, systolic heart failure; DHF, diastolic heart failure; MI, myocardial infarction; DM, diabetes; CVA, stroke; CKD, chronic kidney disease; CAD, coronary artery disease; BB, beta-blocker; ACEI, ACE inhibitor; ARB, angiotensin receptor blocker; CCB, calcium channel blocker; Aldos Antag, aldosterone antagonist.

b) These guidelines cautioned to never use ACEi and ARB together

c) If BP not at goal after maximizing the third antihypertensive or if patient has a reaction to one of the four classes of antihypertensive medications recommended, then the provider should start an antihypertensive medication from one of the classes of antihypertensive medications with less evidence-based recommendations (e.g., BBs, alpha-blockers). See Table 8-6 for Compelling Indications for Other Classes of Hypertensive Medications

d) Some researchers suggested starting an antihypertensive medication with two combined HTN medications as the initial treatment when the SBP is greater than 160 mm Hg or the DBP exceeds 100 mm Hg

6. Medications
   a. Diuretics: basis of antihypertensive management
      1) Thiazide-type diuretics should be initial line of therapy for most patients
      2) Proven to prevent cardiovascular complications of hypertension. Diuretics also enhance the efficacy of other antihypertensive medications. Recent data suggests that use of diuretics such as chlorthalidone and indapamide show a better reduction of cardiovascular mortality in patients with hypertension (Chobanian et al., 2003; Jennings & Touyz, 2013; Roush, Holford, & Guddati, 2012)
      3) Mechanism of action
         a) Sodium and water mobilization from arterial wall → ↓ blood volume and cardiac output
         b) Changes in electrolyte composition of intra-arteriolar walls: Na, K, Mg, Ca alterations decrease vascular response to pressor substances and increase response to depressor substances
         c) Direct smooth muscle relaxation
         d) Examples of diuretics
            Chlorothiazide (Diuril), hydrochlorothiazide (HCTZ), metolazone (Zaroxolyn)
         e) Side effects
            Low Na, K, Mg; hyperuricemia, hyperglycemia, dyslipidemia; muscle cramps, dizziness, HA; sexual dysfunction
      4) Because hypertension is a disease of the endothelium, treatment should be directed at improving the vascular biology and function

a) ACEis, CCBs, ARBs improve endothelial dysfunction, lower blood pressure, and arterial compliance (Lookinland & Beckstrand, 2003)

b. ACEis/ARBs (Chobanian et al., 2003; Lookinland & Beckstrand, 2003)
   1) Mechanism of action
      a) Inhibition of renin–angiotensin–aldosterone
      b) Inhibit bradykinin degradation
      c) Stimulate vasodilating prostaglandin synthesis
      d) Reduce sympathetic nervous system activity
      e) Most effective on younger white patients
      f) Less effective on African Americans and elderly
      g) Drug of choice for DM—delay progression to ESRD
   2) Examples of ACEis
      Benazepril (Lotensin), captopril (Capoten), enalapril (Vasotec), fosinopril (Monopril), lisinopril (Prinivil, Zestril), moexipril (Univasc), perindopril(Aceon), quinapril (Accupril) ramipril (Altace), trandolapril (Mavik)
   3) Examples of ARBs
      Candesartan (Atacand), eprosartan (Tevetan), irbesartan (Avapro), telmisartan (Mycardis), valsartan (Diovan), losartan (Cozaar)
   4) Side effects
      a) Cough occurs in 5% to 15%
      b) Severe hypotension
      c) May worsen RI with bilateral RAS
      d) Hyperkalemia if intrinsic renal disease

c. CCBs
   1) Mechanism of action
      a) Peripheral vasodilatation with less reflex tachycardia
      b) Effective in all groups and grades of HTN: preferred for African Americans
   2) Examples
      Norvasc (amlodipine), Plendil (felodipine), Cardizem, Cardizem CD, Cardizem SR, Dilacor XR, Diltia XT, Tiazac (diltiazem), Calan, Calan SR, Covera-HS, Isoptin, Isoptin SR, Verelan, Verelan PM (verapamil), Adalat Adalat CC Procardia, Procardia XL (nifedipine), Cardene, Cardene SR (nicardipine), Sular (nisoldipine), Vascor (bepridil)
   3) Side effects
      a) Negative ionotropic effect—may worsen HF
      b) May depress AV conduction and sinus node automaticity, especially if used with BBs
      c) Flushing, palpitations, HA, peripheral edema

d. BBs (Kertai et al., 2003)
   1) Especially useful in patients with tachycardia
   2) Decrease morbidity and mortality in patient undergoing major vascular surgery when used in the perioperative period
   3) Used with caution in patients with asthma, reactive airway disease, or heart bock
   4) Mechanism of action
      a) Decrease heart rate and cardiac output
      b) Decrease renin release
      c) May increase systemic vascular resistance

d) Indicated for patients with MI, angina, migraine, anxiety
e) Types
- Beta1—cardioselective
- Beta2—bronchi, vessels

5) Examples
Betapace (sotalol), Blocadren (timolol), Brevibloc (esmolol), Cartrol (carteolol), Coreg (carvedilol), Corgard (nadolol), Inderal (propranolol), Inderal-LA (propranolol), Kerlone (betaxolol), Levatol (penbutolol), Lopressor (metoprolol), Normodyne (labetalol), Sectral (acebutolol), Tenormin (atenolol), Toprol-XL (metoprolol), Trandate (labetalol), Visken (pindolol), Zebeta (bisoprolol)

6) Side effects
a) Bradycardia, AV conduction defects, LV failure, asthma symptoms, nasal congestion, hypoglycemia, Raynaud's, depression, fatigue, confusion, impotence, ↑ TG, ↓ HDL
b) Contraindicated: bronchospasm, HF, hypoglycemia

7. Resistant hypertension
a. Definition: receiving ≥3 different classes of antihypertensive therapy, one of which is a diuretic and the maximum dose for all other CV medications (Symplicity, 2011)
b. Causes (Chobanian et al., 2003; He et al., 2002)
1) Improper blood pressure measurements
2) Renovascular hypertension (renal artery stenosis)
3) Insufficient treatment of other causes of secondary hypertension
4) Inadequate diuretic therapy
5) Excess sodium intake
6) Medication misuse—inadequate doses, drug actions and interactions, over-the-counter drugs (i.e., ibuprofen, pseudoephedrine), and herbal supplements
7) Excessive alcohol intake
8) Continued cigarette smoking
c. Treatment
1) Percutaneous, catheter-based renal sympathetic denervation is done to disrupt renal afferent and efferent nerves using radiofrequency ablation
2) Showed a 33/11 mm Hg reduction in 6 months office BP after treatment
3) Durability of procedure is unknown (Symplicity, 2011)

8. Application to vascular patients (Chobanian et al., 2003)
a. PAD is equivalent in risk to ischemic heart disease
b. Any class of antihypertensives can be used in most patients with arterial disease
c. Other risk factors should also be managed aggressively
1) Diabetes
a) Hypertension is twice as common in diabetics as nondiabetics (ADA, 2013)
b) Requires more precision in control of hypertension because of greater risk for the development of cardiovascular events
c) Benefits: can decrease the development of both macrovascular and microvascular disease (Berlowitz et al., 2003)
d) Regardless of the antihypertensive drug chosen, diabetic patients seem to benefit more from blood pressure control than nondiabetics (Berlowitz et al., 2003)

e) Thiazide diuretics, BBs, ARBs, ACEis, and CCBs all reduce cardiovascular disease and stroke in diabetics (Chobanian et al., 2003; Lookinland & Beckstrand, 2003)
f) ACEis: renoprotective and reducing acute coronary events
g) BBs may be associated with decreased glucose tolerance, but may be more beneficial to diabetics than ACEis in decreasing hypertension
h) Diabetics often require multidrug therapy to control their hypertension
i) Microalbumin: tested in all type I and type II diabetics as an indication for antihypertensive treatment, especially when using angiotensin receptor blocking agents
j) Hypertension is more poorly controlled in diabetics, perhaps because the healthcare providers are more focused on controlling their diabetes (Berlowitz et al., 2003)
k) Diabetes + HTN: increased prevalence of sexual dysfunction (ADA, 2013)
l) Diabetics often obese; complicates control of hypertension, especially if obstructive sleep apnea present (Berlowitz et al., 2003)
m) Hypertension poorly identified in obese patients; require larger blood pressure cuffs to accurately measure pressure (Berlowitz et al., 2003)

2) Elderly
a) Response to medications changes with aging (Lookinland & Beckstrand, 2003)
b) Diuretics can lead to dehydration, electrolyte imbalance, and hypotension in the elderly (Lookinland & Beckstrand, 2003)
c) Blood pressure control should be gradual, particularly in frail patients; electrolytes should be monitored regularly (Cifkova et al., 2003)
d) Blood pressure measurements should be done in erect posture to evaluate for postural effects (Cifkova et al., 2003)
e) BP goal for those individuals 60 or older should be 150/90 or less (James et al., 2013).

3) African Americans (Lookinland & Beckstrand, 2003)
a) Higher prevalence of hypertension and levels of TOD
- 50% higher mortality from cardiac events
- 80% higher stroke mortality rate
- Six times higher risk for end-stage renal disease

b) May have a higher rate of hypertension due to
- Endothelial dysfunction from reduced bradykinin and nitric oxide
- Higher levels of intracellular calcium stores
- Low circulating rennin with excessive levels of angiotensin II
- Abnormal sympathetic nervous activation
- Higher levels of obesity, especially in women

c) All classes of antihypertensives lower blood pressure in this population; CCBs and diuretics are considered first drugs of choice for African Americans (Chobanian et al., 2003)

d. Summary
1) Hypertension, the leading cause of morbidity and mortality worldwide, is a modifiable risk factor for atherosclerosis

2) Lifestyle modification and hypertension control have a strong association
   a) Modifications in weight loss; decreased sodium intake and increased potassium intake have been shown to be beneficial in HTN control
   b) Alcohol and smoking consumption has been associated with lower percentages in persons with controlled blood pressure
   c) An opportune time to assist in encouraging lifestyle modification in vascular patients may be more receptive in making this change, following a vascular procedure
3) Antihypertensive therapy must be directed at both the reduction of blood pressure and improved endothelial function and arterial compliance; improved cardiovascular outcomes will result from the improved structure and function of the vasculature.
4) Because one of the triggers in the development of atherosclerosis is hypertension, control of this risk factor will decrease the expression of vascular disease

F. Diabetes

1. Prevalence: 18.8 million persons with physician-diagnosed diabetes in United States (Diabetes Statistics, 2013). Increases with age; 10.9 million, or 26.9% of all people ≥65 years of age (Diabetes Statistics, 2013)
2. Syndrome defined by abnormal metabolism of carbohydrates, fats, and proteins
   a. Includes hyperglycemia, large vessel disease, microvascular disease, retinopathy, and neuropathy (ADA, 2013)
   b. Insulin resistance and hyperinsulinemia affect the vascular endothelium, coagulation and fibrinolytic systems, and blood lipids (ADA, 2013)
   c. Hyperglycemia decreases endothelium-mediated vascular reactivity, activates protein kinase C, increases production of vasoconstrictors, and leads to glycosylation of proteins and production of advanced glycation end products
   d. Advanced glycosylation end products contribute to atherosclerotic plaque progression by
      1) Stimulating foam cell formation
      2) Augmenting platelet aggregation
      3) Enhancing chemotaxis of monocytes
      4) Increasing production of growth factors and cytokines
      5) Stimulating vascular smooth muscle cell proliferation
      6) Increasing binding and deposition of LDL in the arterial wall
      7) Enhancing mural fibrosis (ADA, 2013)
3. Two forms of vascular disease in diabetics
   a. Microvascular: endothelial proliferative changes in arterioles with thickening of basement membrane of capillaries
      1) Nephropathy: 10% to 21%; peaks at 25 years after onset persistent albuminuria, decreased GFR, hypertension, increased mortality for cardiovascular disease (ADA, 2013; Diabetic Neuropathies, 2013); 43% of new ESRD cases related to diabetes
      2) Retinopathy: leading cause of blindness in people 20 to 74 years; two types are nonproliferative (background retinopathy vessels leak fluid, causing swelling and deposits with macular edema) and proliferative (retinal ischemia leads to neovascularization, affects central and peripheral vision; neovascular glaucoma occurs when new vessels form on iris [diabetic retinopathy])

TABLE 8-7 Diabetic Neuropathies, Locations, and Symptoms (Diabetic Neuropathies, 2013)

Types of Diabetic Neuropathies	Location	Symptoms
Peripheral neuropathy	Toes Feet Legs Hands Arms	Numbness, insensitivity to pain or temperature Sensitivity to touch Loss of balance or coordination Sharp pains or cramps Tingling, burning sensation Foot deformities, changes in gait
Autonomic neuropathy	Heart, blood vessels Urinary tract Sex organs Sweat glands Eyes Digestive system	Orthostasis, constipation or diarrhea, dysphagia Gastroparesis; can cause vomiting, bloating, poor food absorption resulting in malnutrition, and hypoglycemia as the stomach emptying is unpredictable affecting blood glucose levels Decreased bladder emptying, urinary incontinence, increased urinary infections Decreased sexual response in men and women, erectile dysfunction Profuse sweating at night or while eating, difficulty with night driving
Proximal neuropathy, also called lumbosacral plexas neuropathy, femoral neuropathy, or diabetic amyotrophy	Thighs Hips Buttocks	Pain in thighs, hips, or buttocks or legs, usually on one side of the body Causes weakness in the legs manifested by the inability to go from a sitting to a standing position without assistance
Focal neuropathy—painful and unpredictable; occurs most often in older people	Eyes Facial muscles Ears Pelvis and lower back Thighs Abdomen	Sudden weakness of one nerve or group of nerves causing muscle weakness or pain Examples: inability to focus the eye, double vision, aching behind one eye, Bell's palsy, severe pain in lower back or pelvis, pain in the front of a thigh; pain in chest, stomach or flank; pain on lateral calf or medial foot

3) Neuropathy; causes fall into five categories: metabolic-microvessel hypoxic, immune-vasculitic, compression and repetitive injury, repeated hypoglycemia, and ischemia (ADA, 2013; Diabetic Neuropathies, 2013) (see Table 8-7)

b. Macrovascular: atherosclerosis and arteriosclerosis
   1) Influenced by all other risk factors for vascular disease
   2) Rapid progression in multiple organ systems (ADA, 2013)

4. Diagnosis
   a. American Diabetes Association guidelines for the diagnosis of diabetes mellitus (ADA, 2013)
      1) Symptoms of diabetes plus casual plasma glucose concentration ≥200 mg/dL (11.1 mmol/L)
      2) Fasting plasma glucose ≥126 mg/dL (7.0 mmol/L). Fasting is defined as no caloric intake for at least 8 hours
      3) 2 hours postload glucose ≥200 mg/dL (11.1 mmol/L) during a glucose tolerance test

b. Hemoglobin A1C
   1) A form of hemoglobin used to identify the average plasma glucose concentration over 2 to 3 months
   2) Goal is <7% (Qaseem et al., 2007)

c. Testing for diabetes (ADA, 2013): consider in adults with BMI ≥25 kg/m^2 at least 45 years of age who have additional risk factors
   1) Physical inactivity
   2) First-degree relative with DM
   3) High-risk race (African American, Latino, Native American, Asian)
   4) Women who have delivered a baby weighing ≥9 lbs
   5) HTN (≥140/90)
   6) HDL cholesterol ≤35 mg/dL and or TG ≥250 mg/dL
   7) A1C ≥5.7%
   8) History of cardiovascular disease

5. Treatment (ADA, 2013)
   a. Manage hypertension in patients with diabetes
      1) After 3 months of lifestyle modifications, if systolic BP is 130 to 139 or diastolic BP is 80 to 89, initiate drug therapy
      2) When BP is more than 20/10 to 30/10 mm Hg above goal, initiating HTN therapy with two medications, one of which should be ACEi
      3) If microalbuminuria is present, start ACEi. If intolerant to ACEi, start ARB
      4) For patients with diabetes and hypertension, the target blood pressure should be based on the JNC-8 recommendations noted above
   b. Dyslipidemia and diabetes
      1) Moderate statin therapy (goal of 30% to <50% reduction in LDL-C) DM (I or II) in ages 40 to 79 with LDL 70 to 189 mg/dL without ASCVD
      2) High statin therapy (goal of ≥50% reduction in LDL-C) DM (I or II) and LDL 70 to 189 mg/dL with 10-year ASCVD of ≥7.5% (Stone et al., 2013)
   c. Drug therapy for primary/secondary prevention of cardiovascular disease in diabetics
      1) ACEis should be prescribed to patients with diabetes age ≥55 years with one or more cardiovascular factors (total cholesterol >200 mg/dL, HDL cholesterol <40 mg/dL, hypertension, microalbuminuria, or current smoking) or a history of cardiovascular disease (CAD, stroke, or PAD) to prevent renal insufficiency
      2) Patients with diabetes ≥40 years old should be treated with at least 81 mg/day aspirin unless contraindicated
      3) BBs are recommended for patients with diabetes with a history of MI
      4) Those diabetics with CKD (of any age) should be on either an ACEi or ARB to preserve renal function (James et al., 2013)
   d. Management of diabetes (ADA, 2013)
      1) Metformin is recommended as the first-line glucose-lowering drug in overweight patients with type II diabetes, especially for those with BMI >35 kg/m^2, age <60 years, and women with prior gestational diabetes
      2) Following failure to achieve goals on monotherapy, more than one medication is recommended
      3) The treatment goal for HbA1c is <7%. A1c ≤7% has been shown to reduce microvascular complications of DM and is associated with long-term reduction in microvascular disease

4) Continued monitoring of microalbumin is optional in people with diabetes and established microalbuminuria, who are on an ACEi or ARB
5) All diabetics should have a foot screening that includes a monofilament test. Patients with an abnormal monofilament test are at a high risk for lower limb complications

e. Summary
1) Diabetes is a syndrome defined by abnormal metabolism of carbohydrates, fats, and proteins
2) The two forms of vascular disease in diabetics is microvascular and macrovascular disease
3) Hemaglobin A1C measures compliance to therapy over a 2- to 3-month period
4) ACEis are recommended in diabetics with microalbuminuria

G. Estrogen Replacement Therapies

1. The Heart and Estrogen/Progestin Replacement Study (HERS), Women' Health Initiative
   a. Failed to demonstrate protection against PAD or coronary events with use of estrogen replacement (Hulley & Grady, 2004)
   b. Estrogen plus progestin study showed an approximate 31% increase in total stroke risk compared to placebo (Wassertheil-Smoller et al., 2003)
2. The North American Menopause Society (NAMS) Hormone Therapy Advisory Panel recommendation: hormone therapy be used at "the lowest effective dose and time consistent with treatment goals"

H. Exercise

1. Benefits
   a. Reduces the incidence of CHD and PAD
   b. Increases muscle size and strength
   c. Increases bone density
   d. Increases maximal exercise and endurance capacity
   e. Increases cardiac dimensions and stroke volume, plasma volume
   f. Increases insulin sensitivity
   g. Increases HDL cholesterol
   h. Decreases plasma triglyceride concentration
   i. Improves symptoms of intermittent claudication (Thompson, 2003)
   j. Causes vasodilation which lowers blood pressure
2. The beneficial effects of exercise may take 1 to 2 weeks to appear (Murphy et al., 2012) but may be lost within days
3. CDC recommendation: Amount of exercise needed to reduce cardiovascular disease is 30 minutes of moderately intense physical activity on most to all days of the week (Thompson, 2003)
4. The most impressive increases in maximal exercise capacity from training occur in patients with intermittent claudication
   a. Summary data from 21 studies using exercise training as therapy for claudication showed the average walking distance increased by 179% to the onset of pain and 122% to maximal pain (Thompson, 2003)
   b. Improvement was greatest in studies that trained subjects to the point of maximal tolerated pain, continued for more than 6 months, and used walking as the type of exercise

c. Results are better than those reported for most pharmacologic or surgical treatments (Thompson, 2003)
d. The CLEVER (2012) showed that there were greater walking gains from "supervised exercise" than stenting in proximal PAD (Murphy et al., 2012)

II. PAD Rehabilitation Program (PRP) (Ekers & Hirsch, 2004)

A. Goal of PRP

1. Help patients gain control over their disease
   a. Avoid debilitating consequences of the disease
   b. Improve physical function
   c. Requires major lifestyle changes
      1) Difficult for patients to make these changes on their own
      2) Structured, supervised program increases success
      3) Employs a biopsychosocial approach
2. Benefits of exercise (Gardner & Afaq, 2008; Giada et al., 2008; Oka, 2006)
   a. Improved walking capacity (increased walking speed, distance, duration, and decreased symptoms)
   b. Improved quality of life
   c. Biological changes
      1) Increased endothelium-dependent vasodilation
      2) Increased capillary density
      3) Increased extraction of oxygen by the ischemic muscle
      4) Improved endothelial function
      5) Reduction in markers of chronic inflammation
      6) Improved cardiac conditioning
      7) Reduction in atherosclerotic risk factors

B. Objectives of the PRP

1. Provide patients with a sound knowledge base of vascular disease and treatment
2. Help patients discover their personal goals and motivation to take action
3. Partner with patients to develop a personalized action plan

C. PRP Model: Modeled after Cardiac Rehabilitation Programs

1. Limited by lack of reimbursement
2. CPT code 93668 (American Medical Association [AMA], 2012); for phase II component of PRP
   a. Series of sessions lasting 45 to 60 minutes per session
   b. Involves use of either a motorized treadmill or track
   c. Patients walk to achieve symptom-limited claudication
   d. Each session supervised by a nurse or exercise physiologist
   e. Adjust workload to patient's claudication threshold and other cardiovascular limitations
   f. Development of angina symptoms, new arrhythmias, or patient's inability to progress may require further physician review; physician services are reported separately under appropriate level evaluation/management (E/M) code

3. Phase I: inpatient program
   a. For patients hospitalized for revascularization intervention
   b. Initiate education about PAD
      1) Etiology of the disease process, symptoms, risk factors, and type of revascularization procedure the patient had
      2) Increase patient awareness of circulatory system and the signs and symptoms to report to healthcare provider (recurrent claudication, rest pain, problems with wound healing, etc.)
      3) Safe care at home (incision care, meticulous care of feet, activity, nutrition during recovery, etc.)
      4) Remind patients they are not "cured" by this revascularization procedure and must make lifestyle changes to maintain circulation and keep the disease in check
      5) Start now with simple walking program, smoking cessation tips, diet changes, medications that may have been added to their regimen (for cholesterol, blood pressure, antiplatelet or anticoagulation therapy, etc.)
      6) Introduce the idea of participating in a structured PRP and provide referral information
4. Phase II: outpatient program
   a. Components: initial and ongoing assessments, regular physical reconditioning sessions, and in-depth education
      1) Exercise training for PAD patients should involve three training sessions per week comprising 45 minutes of intermittent treadmill walking in a supervised environment for a time period of 20 weeks or more (Bulmer & Coombes, 2004)
      2) Success depends on integration of the PRP information/techniques into the patient's daily home routine
      3) Requires frequent evaluations, continuous encouragement, consistent reinforcement of information
      4) Arm ergometry may be an alternative form or exercise therapy for lower extremity claudicants. Dynamic arm exercise training has been shown in a pilot study to show greater improvement in maximal walking distance and pain-free walking distance compared to treadmill exercise program or a combination of the two (Treat-Jacobson, Bronas, & Leon, 2009).
   b. Assessment
      1) Cardiac assessment through exercise/pharmacologic stress test
         a) Determines clinical significance of any cardiac disease
         b) Evaluates relative risk of entering an exercise program
         c) Documents patient's exercise capacity
         d) Information used to calculate the personal exercise prescription
      2) Treadmill walking assessment
         a) On admission into program, evaluates initial severity claudication
         b) On completion of program, evaluates effectiveness of PRP interventions
         c) Measures onset of claudication, the intermittent claudication distance (ICD), and absolute claudication distance (ACD)
         d) Graded treadmill protocols at fixed speed 2 mph: Hiatt protocol 3.5% incremental increases in grade every 3 minutes (Hiatt, Nawaz, Regensteiner, & Hossack, 1988); Gardner-Skinner protocol 2.0% incremental increases every 2 minutes (Treesak, Kasemsup, Treat-Jacobson, Nyman, & Hirsch, 2004)

e) Possible to evaluate coronary ischemic symptoms at the same time with EKG monitoring

3) Functional status assessment
   a) Determines impact of claudication on patient's ability to perform daily activities
   b) Assessment tools: Walking Impairment Questionnaire (Nicolaï et al., 2009)
4) Quality of life assessment—Medical Outcomes Study SF-36 (Regensteiner et al., 2008) to evaluate the impact of PAD on general health, mental health, social function, and vitality domains
5) Atherosclerosis risk factor assessment. Smoking, diabetes, hypertension, dyslipidemia, estrogen replacement, antiplatelet strategies, sedentary lifestyle
6) Assessment of patient's goals and expectations of the PRP
   a) Long-term goals (3 to 6 months) are important
   b) Short-term goals appear more achievable, encourage patients to start immediately, and serve as early determinants of progress

c. Physical reconditioning at the rehabilitation center
   1) Cornerstone of phase II of PRP
   2) Optimal results achieved with minimum of 24 weeks of therapy (Treesak et al., 2004)
   3) Individualized exercise prescription: includes recommended time and intensity of exercise with a variety of equipment and target heart rate
   4) Key elements of exercise sessions are gradual warm-up, aerobic conditioning, and sufficient cool-down
   5) Walking provides best exercise for improving claudication
      a) Walk to point of near-maximal pain
      b) Continue on calf-sparing equipment such as arm ergometry, stationary bikes, stairs, rowing machines
   6) Alternate back and forth from treadmill to other equipment; prevents boredom, provides total body fitness training
   7) Record tolerance for each modality; include heart rate, onset of claudication, total exercise time, level of perceived difficulty
   8) Goal is 35 to 40 minutes of discontinuous aerobic exercise per session
   9) Continuously evaluate claudication symptoms
      a) Continue to increase with walking
      b) Reach a tolerable level and stay there
      c) Diminish with continued exercise

d. Home exercise programs: Exercise therapy is a highly efficacious and cost-effective approach that can significantly improve functional outcomes. Medically supervised exercise programs have been shown to improve ambulatory function; however, home-based exercise programs can elicit similar improvements (McDermott et al., 2013)
   1) Goal: to establish a life-long exercise habit
   2) Essential to incorporate exercise into the daily routine at home for long-term compliance/maintenance
   3) Clinician and patient develop plan together; initiate home program during phase II of PRP
   4) Walking should remain as major component; strive to walk every day, working up to 30 to 45 min/day

5) Explore community walking options: mall-waling programs, parks, community and senior citizen centers, YMCA, etc.
6) Keep a home exercise log; review weekly with rehab staff
7) Explore exercise motives with patients for greater long-term success
   a) Body motives: look better, healthier body
   b) Psychological motives: feel better, increased self-esteem
   c) Social motives: exercise partners, social event

e. Education
   1) Knowledge of the disease process and prognosis may provide additional motivation to modify behavior
   2) Formal setting: classroom lectures; open to community to improve visibility of the rehabilitation program and increase awareness of PAD
   3) Informal settings: during exercise sessions; use of bulletin boards, DVD or videos and audio tapes, internet resources, individual counseling
   4) Topics: anatomy/physiology of cardiovascular system, pathophysiology, symptoms (include PAD, cardiac and stroke symptoms), risk factors, and treatment (as discussed earlier in this chapter)

f. Progress evaluations
   1) Ongoing evaluations during daily exercise sessions
   2) Midpoint evaluations important to overall program success
   3) Treadmill walking test, progress with risk factor modification, home exercise efforts, goals for last half of program
   4) Final evaluation: treadmill walking, risk factor control, functional status using Walking Impairment Questionnaire or PAD Physical Activity
   5) Recall questionnaire, quality of life assessment (SF-36), compliance with home exercise program

5. Phase III: maintenance program
   a. Continue at a rehab center with less supervision
   b. Continue exercising on their own at home
   c. Consider bringing patients back to rehab center every 3 to 6 months for evaluations to keep them on track
6. Summary
   a. PRPs proven safe, beneficial, and cost-effective
      1) Improved pain-free walking distance and maximum walking distance by 97% to 179% over baseline distances (Cheetham et al., 2004; Falcone et al., 2003)
      2) PRPs are cost-effective (Treesak et al., 2004)
   b. Trend toward improved risk factor modification and long-term compliance with exercise after participation in a PRP (Menard et al., 2004)

CASE STUDY

J.W. is a 63-year-old Caucasian female who presents to the office for evaluation of her elevated blood pressure. Her last visit has shown her blood pressure to be 140/89. Past medical history includes diabetes type II, PVD with intermittent claudication, tobacco abuse, hypercholesterolemia, hypertension, and obesity. She has two-block claudication. She used to play tennis but can no longer do so because of leg pain. She enjoys exercise and is very motivated to get back to playing tennis. She has gained 25 pounds over the past 18 months mostly because of her exercise limitations. Current medications include Metformin 500 mg twice daily, Cilostazol 100 mg twice daily, Ramipril 5 mg, Atorvastatin 20 mg, multivitamin, and vitamin E. Her assessment today reveals the following: VS 98.4–82–16, blood pressure 138/87. Heart: regular rate and rhythm; lungs: clear to auscultation; bowel sounds × 4 with soft, nontender abdomen; no peripheral edema, pedal skin intact. Vascular assessment: no carotid bruit.

Normal aorta on palpation. Strong femoral pulses but no palpable distal pulses; biphasic Doppler signals at the PT and DP bilaterally. ABIs 0.75 on the right, 0.66 on the left. Laboratory tests performed include a basic metabolic panel with results within normal limits; HgbA1C of 6.2%; lipid panel with total cholesterol of 120, triglycerides of 223, LDL of 90, HDL of 22.

REVIEW QUESTIONS

1. J.W. tells you she would like to quit smoking and would like a medication to help her. What would you recommend?
2. J.W. says she has heard she should take clopridogrel for her PAD instead of cilostazol. Explain the difference in these two medications.
3. What are the combined effects of clopridogrel and atorvastatin?
4. J.W. has several risk factors for PAD. What medication could be added to reduce her risk of an ischemic event, keeping in mind that she pays for all her medications?
5. Along with macrovascular changes, diabetes can cause microvascular changes resulting in what three major disease processes?
6. What are the initial treatment options for J.W.?
7. How can her elevated triglycerides be managed?
8. Can we say that her hypertension is controlled?
9. What are the benefits of managing her hypertension?
10. J.W. elects to try a PAD rehabilitation program. She is reluctant to walk on the treadmill in the PRP because of her leg pain. She asks whether using the stationary bike, arm ergometer, and rowing machine is just as good to help her claudication. How would you answer her?

ANSWERS

1. Would include a discussion of bupropion and nicotine replacement medications such as nicotine gum, patch, inhaler, or spray (Benowitz, 2003).
2. Clopridogrel is an antiplatelet medication, important for patients with PAD to prevent platelets from clumping together and blocking off an already narrowed artery. Important to prevent strokes and cardiac events. It will not improve her claudication symptoms. Cilostazol is specifically designed to improve claudication symptoms through its vasodilating effects. It also has some antiplatelet effects, though not as much as clopridogrel. Patients can be on both if their healthcare provider deems them necessary.
3. Atorvastatin may impair the antiplatelet activity of clopridogrel. J.W.'s statin drug could be changed to lovastatin or simvastatin to prevent this.
4. Aspirin 81 mg is recommended to reduce the risk of an ischemic event. Even though clopidogrel was found to be more effective, the benefit over aspirin is small and the cost is significantly more.
5. Nephropathy, retinopathy, and neuropathy (ADA, 2013).
6. Home walking program or structured vascular rehab program; dietary counseling to assist with weight, lipid, and diabetes and hypertension management.
7. Elevated TG levels are an independent predictor in women for heart disease and in patients with impaired glucose tolerance. Encourage her to avoid low carbohydrate diets as these diets tend to cause elevated TG levels. Her healthcare provider may consider cautious addition of either niacin (may elevate fasting blood glucose) or one of the fibrate medication (close monitoring of liver function required).

8. No. Blood pressure must be monitored for three office visits, in sitting position, and with the appropriate blood pressure cuff to determine average blood pressure. Blood pressure diuretics may also enhance the efficacy of the ACE inhibitor that she is taking.
9. Keeping the blood pressure under control will decrease the progression of atherosclerosis, decrease the incidence of target organ damage (MI, renal failure, carotid stenosis), and decrease morbidity and mortality.
10. To improve claudication symptoms, she really needs exercise that uses the calf muscle. Walking has been shown to be the best exercise at relieving claudication. Other exercise modalities are important to improve total body fitness and maintain cardiopulmonary benefits.

REFERENCES

Agaku, I., King, B., & Dube, S. R. (2012). Current cigarette smoking among adults—United States, 2011. *Morbidity and Mortality Weekly Report, 61*(44), 889–894. Retrieved from http://www.cdc.gov/mmwr/preview/mmwrhtml/mm6144a2.htm, accessed February 21, 2013.

Alberts, M. J., Bhatt, D. L., Mas, J.-L., Ohman, E. M., Hirsch, A. T., Röther, J.,... Steg, G. (2009). Three-year follow-up and event rates in the international REduction of Atherosclerosis for Continued Health Registry. *European Heart Journal, 30*(19), 2318–2326.

American Diabetes Association (ADA). (2013). Standards of medical care in diabetes. *Diabetes Care, 36*(1), S11–S66.

American Heart Association-Quit Smoking. Retrieved from http://www.heart.org/HEARTORG/GettingHealthy/QuitSmoking/QuittingSmoking/Medicines-To-Help-You-Quit-Smoking_UCM_307921_Article.jsp, accessed October 16, 2010.

American Medical Association (AMA). (2012). *CPT 2013 standard edition (current procedural terminology (standard))*. Chicago, IL: American Medical Association.

Bang, O. Y., Saver, J. L., Liebeskind, D. S., Pineda, S., & Ovbiagele, B. (2008). Association of serum lipid indices with large artery atherosclerotic stroke. *Neurology, 70*(11), 841–847.

Benowitz, N. L. (2003). Smoking and smoking cessation. In E. Braunwald & L. Goldman (Eds.), *Primary cardiology* (pp. 329–336). Philadelphia, PA: W.B. Saunders.

Berlowitz, D. R., Ash, A. S., Hickey, E. C., Glickman, M., Friedman, R., & Kader, B. (2003). Hypertension management in patients with diabetes: The need for more aggressive therapy. *Diabetes Care, 26*(2), 355–359.

Brook, R. D., Appel, L. J., Rubinfire, M., Ogedegbe, G., Bisognano, J. D., Elliott, W. J.,... Rajagopalen, S. (2013). Beyond medications and diet: Alternative approaches for lowering blood pressure. *Hypertension, 61*, 1360–1383. doi:10.1161/HYP.0b013e318293645f

Bulmer, A. C., & Coombes, J. S. (2004). Optimizing exercise training in peripheral arterial disease. *Sports Medicine, 34*(14), 983–1003.

Cheetham, D. R., Burgess, L., Ellis, M., Williams, A., Greenhalgh, R. M., & Davies, A. H. (2004). Does supervised exercise offer adjuvant benefit over exercise advice alone for the treatment of intermittent claudication? A randomized trial. *European Journal of Vascular and Endovascular Surgery, 27*(1), 17–23.

Chobanian, A. V., Bakris, G. L., Black, H. R., Cushman, W. C., Green, L. A., Izzo, J. L., Jr.,... Roccella, E. J. (2003). The seventh report of the Joint National Committee on Prevention, Detection, Evaluation, and Treatment of High Blood Pressure. *Hypertension, 42*, 1206–1252. doi:10.1161/01.HYP.0000107251.49515.c2

Cifkova, R., Erdine, S., Fagard, R., Farsang, C., Heagerty, A. M., Kiowski, W.,... Zanchetti, A. (2003). Practice guidelines for primary care physicians: 2003 ESH/ES hypertension guidelines. *Journal of Hypertension, 21*(10), 1779–1786.

Daniel, B., Kelsberg, G., & Jankowski, T. (2005). Clinical inquiries. What is the initial work-up in the diagnosis of hypertension? *The Journal of Family Practice, 54*(9), 809–810, 812.

Diabetes Statistics. (2013). Retrieved from http://www.diabetes.org/diabetes-basics/statistics/ accessed September 2, 2013.

Diabetic Neuropathies. (2013). The nerve damage of diabetes. Retrieved from http://diabetes.niddk.nih.gov/dm/pubs/neuropathies/index.htm, accessed September 2, 2013.

Ekers, M. A., & Hirsch, A. T. (2004). Vascular medicine and peripheral arterial disease rehabilitation. In V. Fahey (Ed.), *Vascular nursing* (4th ed., pp. 187–213). Philadelphia, PA: W.B. Saunders.

Falcone, R. A., Hirsch, A. T., Regensteiner, J. G., Treat-Jacobsen, D., Williams, M. A., Hiatt, W. R., & Stewart, K. J. (2003). Peripheral arterial disease rehabilitation: A review. *Journal of Cardiopulmonary Rehabilitation, 23*(3), 170–175.

Faxon, D., Fuster, V., Libby, P., Beckman, J. A., Hiatt, W. R., Thompson, R. W.,... Loscalzo, J. (2004). Atherosclerotic Vascular Disease Conference: Writing Group III: Pathophysiology. *Circulation, 109*(21), 2617–2625. doi:10.1161/01.CIR.0000128520.37674.EF

Fiore, M. C., Jaén, C. R., Baker, T. B., Bailey, W. C., Benowitz, N. L., Curry, S. J.,... Wewers, M. E. (2008). *Treating tobacco use and dependence: 2008 update. Clinical Practice Guideline.* Rockville, MD: U.S. Department of Health and Human Services. Public Health Service. Retrieved from http://www.ncbi.nlm.nih.gov/books/NBK63952/, accessed November 29, 2013.

Galton, D. (2003). *Dyslipidaemia.* New York: Gower Medical Publishing.

Gardner, A. W., & Afaq, A. (2008) Management of lower extremity peripheral arterial disease. *Journal of Cardiopulmonary Rehabilitation and Prevention, 28,* 349–357. doi:10.1097/HCR.0b013e31818c3b96

Gerstein, H. C., Anand, S., Yi, Q. L., Vuksan, V., Lonn, E., Teo, K.,...Yusuf, S. (2003). The relationship between dysglycemia and atherosclerosis in South Asian, Chinese, and European individuals in Canada: A randomly sampled cross-sectional study. *Diabetes Care, 26,* 144–149. doi:10.2337/diacare.26.1.144

Giada, F., Biffi, A., Agostoni, P., Anedda, A., Belardinelli, R., Carlon, R.,...Zeppilli, P. (2008) Exercise prescription for the prevention and treatment of cardiovascular diseases: Part II. *Journal of Cardiovascular Medicine, 9*(6), 641–652. doi:10.2459/JCM.0b013e3282f7ca96

Go, A. S., Bauman, M. A., King, S. M. C., Fonarow, G. C., Lawrence, W., Williams, K. A., & Sanchez, E. (2013). An effective approach to high blood pressure control: A science advisory from the American Heart Association, the American College of Cardiology, and the Centers for Disease Control and Prevention. *Hypertension.* Published online before print November 15, 2013. Retrieved from http://hyper.ahajournals.org/content/early/2013/11/14/HYP.0000000000000003, accessed November 29, 2013.

Go, A. S., Mozaffarian, D., Roger, V. L., Benjamin, E. J., Berry, J. D., Borden, W. B.,...Turner, M. B. (2013). Heart disease and stroke statistics – 2013 report: A report from the American Heart Association. *Circulation, 127,* e6–e245. doi:10.1161/CIR.0b013e31828124ad

Goff, D. C., Lloyd-Jones, D. M., Bennett, G., Coady, S., D'Agostino, R. B., Sr., Gibbons, R.,...Wilson, P. W. F. (2013). 2013 ACC/AHA Guideline on the Assessment of Cardiovascular Risk: A report of the American College of Cardiology/American Heart Association Task Force on Practice Guidelines. *Circulation.* Published online before print November 12, 2013. Retrieved from http://circ.ahajournals.org/content/early/2013/11/11/01.cir.0000437741.48606.98, accessed November 29, 2013.

Gradman, A. H., Parisé, H., Lefebvre, P., Falvey, H., Lafeuille, M.-H., & Duh, M. S. (2013). Initial combination therapy reduces the risk of cardiovascular events in hypertensive patients. *Hypertension, 61*(2), 309–318. doi:10.1161/HYPERTENSIONAHA.112.201566

Grundy, S. M., Becker, D., Clark, L. T., Cooper, R. S., Denke, M. A., Howard, W. J.,...Van Horn, L. (2002). The Third Report of the National Cholesterol Education Program (NCEP) Expert Panel on Detection, Evaluation, and Treatment of High Blood Cholesterol in Adults (Adult Treatment Panel III) final report. *Circulation, 106*(25), 3143–3421.

He, J., Muntner, P., Chen, J., Roccella, E. J., Streiffer, R. H., & Whelton, P. K. (2002). Factors associated with hypertension in the general population of the United States. *Archives of Internal Medicine, 162*(9), 1051–1058.

Hennrikus, D., Joseph, A. M., Lando, H. A., Duval, S., Ukestad, L., Kodl, M., & Hirsch, A. T. (2010). Effectiveness of a smoking cessation program for peripheral artery disease patients: A randomized controlled trial. *Journal of the American College of Cardiology, 25,* 2105–2112. doi:10.1016/j.jacc.2010.07.031

Hiatt, W. R., Nawaz, D., Regensteiner, J. G., & Hossack, K. F. (1988). The evaluation of exercise performance in patients with peripheral vascular disease. *Journal of Cardiopulmonary Rehabilitation, 12,* 525–532.

Hirsch, A. T., Haskal, Z. J., Hertzer, N. R., Bakal, C. W., Creager, M. A., Halperin, J. L.,...White, R. A. (2006). ACC/AHA 2005 Practice Guidelines for the Management of Patients with Peripheral Arterial Disease (lower extremity, renal, mesenteric, and abdominal aortic): A collaborative report from the American Association for Vascular Surgery/Society for Vascular Surgery, Society for Cardiovascular Angiography and Interventions, Society for Vascular Medicine and Biology, Society of Interventional Radiology, and the American College of Cardiology/American Heart Association (ACC/AHA) Task Force on Practice Guidelines. *Circulation, 113*(11), e463–e654.

Hsia, J., Criqui, M. H., Rodabough, R. J., Langer, R. D., Resnick, H. E., Phillips, L. S.,...Kotchen, J. M. (2004). Estrogen plus progestin and the risk of peripheral arterial disease. *Circulation, 109,* 620–626.

Hulley, S. B., & Grady, D. (2004). The WHI estrogen-alone trial do things look any better? *Journal of the American Medical Association, 291,* 1769–1771.

James, P. A., Oparil, S., Carter, B. L., Cushman, W. C., Dennison-Himmelfarb, C., Handler, J.,...Oritz, E. (2013). 2014 Evidence-based guideline for the management of high blood pressure in adults. Report from the panel members appointed to the Eighth Joint National Committee (JNC 8). *Journal of the American Medical Association,* Published online December 18, 2013. doi:10.1001/jama.2013.284427. Retrieved from http://jama.jamanetwork.com/article.aspx?articleid = 1791497, accessed December 28, 2013.

Jellinger, P. S., Smith, D. A., Mehta, A. E., Ganda, O., Handelsman, Y., Rodbard, H. W.,...Seibel, J. A. (2012). American Association of Clinical Endocrinologists' guidelines for dyslipidemia and the prevention of atherosclerosis. *Endocrine Practice, 18*(Suppl. 1), 1–78.

Jennings, G. L., & Touyz, R. M. (2013). Hypertension guidelines: More challenges highlighted by Europe. *Hypertension.* Published online August 19, 2013. Retrieved from http://hyper.ahajournals.org/content/early/2013/08/19/HYPERTENSIONAHA.113.02034.citation, accessed November 29, 2013.

Kastelein, J. J. P., Akdim, F., Stroes, E. S. G., Zwinderman, A. H., Bots, M. L., Stalenhoef, A. F. H.,...de Groot, E. (2008). Simvastatin with or without ezetimibe in familial hypercholesterolemia. *The New England Journal of Medicine, 358,* 1431–1443. doi:10.1056/NEJMoa0800742

Kertai, M. D., Boersma, E., Bax, J. J., Thomson, I. R., Cramer, M. J., van de Ven, L. L. M.,... Poldermans, D. (2003). Optimizing long-term cardiac management after major vascular surgery: Role of beta-blocker therapy, clinical characteristics, and dobutamine stress echocardiography to optimize long-term cardiac management after major vascular surgery. *Archives of Internal Medicine, 163*(18), 2230–2235. doi:10.1001/archinte.163.18.2230

Kreisberg, R., & Oberman, A. (2003). Medical management of hyperlipidemia/dyslipidemia. *Journal of Clinical Endocrinology and Metabolism, 88*(6), 2445–2461.

Lichtenstein, A. H., Appel, L. J., Brands, M., Carnethan, M., Daniels, S., Franch, H. A.,... Wylie-Rosett, J. (2006). Diet and lifestyle recommendations revision 2006: A scientific statement from the American Heart Association Nutrition Committee. *Circulation, 114*(1), 82–96.

Lookinland, S., & Beckstrand, R. L. (2003). Evidence-based treatment of hypertension. *Advance for Nurse Practitioners, 11*, 32–39.

McDermott, M. M., Lui, K., Guralnik, J. M., Criqui, M. H., Spring, B., Tian, L.,... Rejeski, W. J. (2013). Home-based walking exercise intervention in peripheral artery disease: A randomized clinical trial. *Journal of the American Medical Association, 310*(1), 57–65.

Menard, J. R., Smith, H. E., Riebe, D., Braun, C. M., Blissmer, B., & Patterson, R. B. (2004). Long term results of peripheral arterial disease rehabilitation. *Journal of Vascular Surgery, 39*(6), 1186–1192.

Mihaylova, B., Emberson, J., Blackwell, L., Keech, A., Simes, J., Barnes, E. H.,... Baigent, C. (2012). The effects of lowering LDL cholesterol with statin therapy in people at low risk of vascular disease: Meta-analysis of individual data from 27 randomized trials. *Lancet, 380*(9841), 581–590. doi:10.1016/S0140-6736(12)60367-5

Murphy, T. P., Cutlip, D. E., Regensteiner, J. G., Mohler, E. R., Cohen, D. J., Reynolds, M. R.,... Hirsch, A. T. (2012). Supervised exercise versus primary stenting for claudication resulting from aortoiliac peripheral artery disease: Six-month outcomes from the Claudication: Exercise Versus Endoluminal Revascularization (CLEVER) study. *Circulation, 125*(1), 130–139.

National Institute on Drug Abuse (NIDA). (2012). Research report series: Tobacco addiction. Retrieved from http://www.drugabuse.gov/publications/research-reports/tobacco-addiction, accessed August 26, 2012.

Nicolaï, S. P., Kruidenier, L. M., Rouwet, E. V., Graffius, K., Prins, M. H., & Teijink, J. A. (2009) The walking impairment questionnaire: An effective tool to assess the effect of treatment in patients with intermittent claudication. *Journal of Vascular Surgery, 50*(1), 89–94. doi:10.1016/j.jvs.2008.12.073

Oka, R. (2006). Peripheral arterial disease in older adults: Management of cardiovascular disease risk factors. *Journal of Cardiovascular Nursing, 21*(5 Suppl. 1), S15–S20.

Qaseem, A., Vijan, S., Snow, V., Cross, J. T., Weiss, K. B., & Owens, D. K. (2007). Glycemic control and type 2 diabetes mellitus: The optimal hemoglobin A1 c targets. A guidance statement from the American College of Physicians. *Annals of Internal Medicine, 147*(6), 417–422.

Regensteiner, J. G., Hiatt, W. R., Coll, J. R., Criqui, M. H., Treat-Jacobson, D., McDermott, M. M., & Hirsch, A. T. (2008). The impact of peripheral arterial disease on health-related quality of life in the Peripheral Arterial Disease Awareness, Risk, and Treatment: New Resources for Survival (PARTNERS) Program. *Vascular Medicine, 13*(1), 15–24.

Rennard, S., Rigotti, N., & Daughton, D. (2013). Pharmacotherapy for smoking cessation in adults. *Up to Date.* Retrieved from http://www.uptodate.com/contents/pharmacotherapy-for-smoking-cessation-in-adults, accessed August 23, 2013

Rooke, T. W., Hirsch, A. T., Misra, S., Sidaway, A. N., Beckman, J. A., Findeiss, L. K.,... Zierler, R. E. (2011). 2011 ACCF/AHA Focused Update of the Guideline for the Management of Patients with Peripheral Artery Disease (updating the 2005 guideline). *Circulation, 124*, 2020–2045. doi:10.1161/CIR.0b013e31822e80c3

Rosamond, W., Flegal, K., Furie, K., Go, A., Greenlund, K., Haase, N.,... Hong, Y. (2008). Heart disease and stroke statistics–2008 update: A report from the American Heart Association Statistics Committee and Stroke Statistics Subcommittee. *Circulation, 117*(4), e25–e146.

Roush, G. C., Holford, T. R., & Guddati, A. K. (2012). Chlorthalidone compared with hydrochlorothiazide in reducing cardiovascular events: Systematic review and network meta-analyses. *Hypertension, 59*, 1110–1117.

Sierra-Johnson, J., Fisher, R. M., Romero-Corral, A., Somers, V. K., Lopez-Jimenez, F., hrvik, J.,... Hamsten, A. (2009). Concentration of apolipoprotein B is comparable with the apolipoprotein B/apolipoprotein A-I ratio and better than routine clinical lipid measurements in predicting coronary heart disease mortality: Findings from a multi-ethnic US population. *European Heart Journal, 30*, 710–717.

Smith, S. C., Allen, J., Blair, S. N., Bonow, R. O., Brass, L. M., Fonarow, G. C.,... Taubert, K. A. (2006). AHA/ACC Guidelines for Secondary Prevention for Patients with Coronary and Other Atherosclerotic Vascular Disease: 2006 update. *Journal of the American College of Cardiology, 47*, 2130–2139. doi:10.1016/j.jacc.2006.04.026

Stone, N. J., Robinson, J., Lichtenstein, A. H., Bairey Merz, C. N., Blum, C. B., Eckel, R. H.,... Wilson, P. W. F. (2013). 2013 ACC/AHA Guideline on the Treatment of Blood Cholesterol to Reduce Atherosclerotic Cardiovascular Risk in Adults: A report of the American College of Cardiology/American Heart Association Task Force on Practice Guidelines. *Circulation*. Published online November 12, 2013. Retrieved from http://circ.ahajournals.org/content/early/2013/11/11/01.cir.0000437738.63853.7a.citation, accessed November 18, 2013

Symplicity HTN-1 Investigators. (2011). Catheter-based renal sympathetic denervation for resistant hypertension: Durability of blood pressure reduction out to 24 months. *Hypertension, 57*, 911–917.

Tendera, M., Aboyans, V., Bartelink, M.-L., Baumgartner, I., Clément, D., Collet, J.-P., . . . Zeller, T. (2011). ESC Guidelines on the diagnosis and treatment of peripheral artery diseases: Document covering atherosclerotic disease of extracranial carotid and vertebral, mesenteric, renal, upper and lower extremity arteries. The Task Force on the Diagnosis and Treatment of Peripheral Artery Diseases of the European Society of Cardiology (ESC). *European Heart Journal, 32*(22), 2851–2906.

Thompson, P. D. (2003). Exercise and heart disease. In E. Braunwald & L. Goldman (Eds.), *Primary cardiology* (pp. 337–347). Philadelphia, PA: Saunders.

Treat-Jacobson, D., Bronas, U. G., & Leon, A. S. (2009). Efficacy of arm-ergometry versus treadmill exercise training to improve walking distance in patients with claudication. *Vascular Medicine, 14*(3), 203–213.

Treesak, C., Kasemsup, V., Treat-Jacobson, D., Nyman, J. A., & Hirsch, A. T. (2004). Cost effectiveness of exercise training to improve claudication symptoms in patients with peripheral arterial disease. *Vascular Medicine, 9*(4), 279–285.

U.S. Department of Health and Human Services. (2010). *How tobacco smoke causes disease: The biology and behavioral basis for smoking-attributable disease: A report of the surgeon general.* Atlanta, GA: U.S. Department of Health and Human Services, Centers for Disease Control and Prevention, National Center for Chronic Disease Prevention and Health Promotion, Office on Smoking and Health.

Wassertheil-Smoller, S., Hendrix, S. L., Limacher, M., Heiss, G., Kooperberg, C., Baird, A., . . . Mysiw, W. J. (2003). Effect of estrogen plus progestin on stroke in postmenopausal women. *Journal of the American Medical Association, 289*, 2673–2684.

Yusuf, S., Sleight, P., Pogue, J., Bosch, J., Davies, R., & Dagenais, G. (2000). Effects of an angiotensin-converting-enzyme inhibitor, ramipril, on cardiovascular events in high-risk patients. *New England Journal of Medicine, 342*(3), 145–153.

Zwar, N., Richmond, R., Borland, R., Peters, M., Litt, J., Bell, J., . . . Ferretter, I. (2011). *Supporting smoking cessation: A guide for health professionals.* Melbourne, VIC: The Royal Australian College of General Practitioners. Retrieved from http://www.treatobacco.net/en/uploads/documents/Treatment%20Guidelines/Australia%20treatment%20guidelines%20in%20English%202011.pdf, accessed August 23, 2013.

RELEVANT WEBSITES

SMOKING CESSATION

American Cancer Society: www.cancer.org
American Heart Association: www.americanheart.org
American Lung Association: www.lungusa.org
Office on Smoking and Health Centers for Disease Control and Prevention: www.cdc.gov/tobacco
Smoking Quitline: www.smokefree.gov
National Cancer Institute: http://www.cancer.gov/cancertopics/smoking
National Heart, Lung, and Blood Institute: www.nhlbi.nih.gov
National Institutes of Health-Local Smoking Cessation Resources: http://www.nlm.nih.gov/medlineplus/golocal/topicmap_1359.html
National Institutes of Health-Clinical Trials on Smoking Cessation:
http://clinicaltrials.gov/search/open/condition=%22Smoking+Cessation%22
National Institute on Aging Information Center: www.nia.nih.gov
National Network of Tobacco Cessation Quitlines: www.naquitline.org
Nicotine Anonymous: www.nicotine-anonymous.org

DYSLIPIDEMIA

American Association of Clinical Endocrinologists' Guidelines for Dyslipidemia and the prevention of atherosclerosis. (2012) Jellinger et al. https://www.aace.com/files/lipid-guidelines.pdf
AHA Guidelines for Primary Prevention of Cardiovascular Disease and Stroke 2002: http://circ.ahajournals.org/cgi/content/full/106/3/388

Vascular Disease Foundation: www.vdf.org
Vascular Web: www.vascularweb.org
Heart Protection Study: www.lipidsonline.org
Management of Lipids/Diabetes: www.nice.org.uk
American Heart Association: http://my.americanheart.org/professional/StatementsGuidelines/Statements-Guidelines_UCM_316885_SubHomePage.jsp
ACC/AHA Cardiovascular Risk Calculator: http://my.americanheart.org/professional/StatementsGuidelines/PreventionGuidelines/Prevention-Guidelines_UCM_457698_SubHomePage.jsp
2013 ACC/AHA Guideline on the Treatment of Blood Cholesterol: http://circ.ahajournals.org/content/early/2013/11/11/01.cir.0000437738.63853.7a

HYPERTENSION

American Heart Association: www.heart.org/HEARTORG/Conditions/HighBloodPressure/High-Blood-Pressure_UCM_002020_SubHomePage.jsp
NIH Guidelines: www.nhlbi.nih.gov/guidelines/index.htm
http://www.webmd.com/hypertension-high-blood-pressure/guide/hypertension-support-resources
CDC: http://www.cdc.gov/bloodpressure/materials_for_patients.htm
CDC: http://www.cdc.gov/bloodpressure/other_resources.htm
8th Joint National Committee Hypertension Guidelines: http://jama.jamanetwork.com/article.aspx?articleid=1791497

DIABETES

Complications of Diabetes: www.diabetes.org.uk
American Chronic Pain Association (ACPA): www.theacpa.org
National Chronic Pain Outreach Association (NCPOA): www.chronicpain.org
American Diabetes Association: www.diabetes.org
National Institute of Dental and Craniofacial Research (NIDCR): www.nidr.nih.gov
Juvenile Diabetes Research Foundation International: www.jdrf.org
American Podiatric Medical Association: www.apma.org
Centers for Disease Control and Prevention: www.cdc.gov/diabetes
Lower Extremity Amputation Prevention Program: www.hrsa.gov/leap/
National Diabetes Education Program: ndep.nih.gov/
National Digestive Diseases Information Clearinghouse: www.niddk.nih.gov/health/digest/nddic.htm
National Institute of Neurological Disorders and Stroke: www.ninds.nih.gov
National Kidney and Urologic Diseases Information Clearinghouse: kidney.niddk.nih.gov/
Pedorthic Footwear Association: www.pedorthics.org

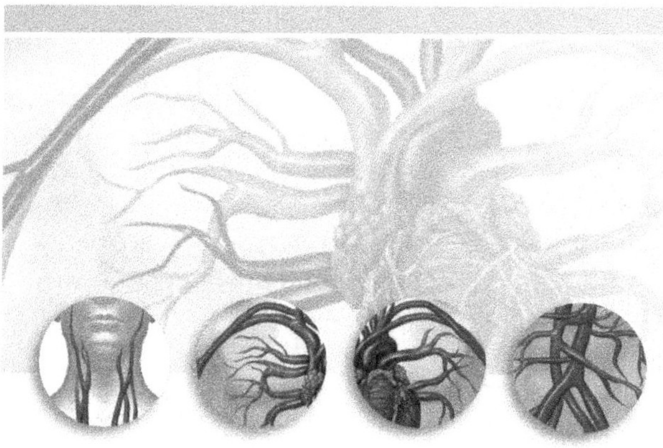

CHAPTER 9

Lower Extremity Arterial Disease

Mary Sieggreen
M. Eileen Walsh
First Edition Author: *Roberta Ronayne; combined with Arterial Ulcers by Mary Sieggreen*

OBJECTIVES

1. Identify risk factors for the development of lower extremity peripheral artery disease (PAD).
2. Discuss preventive measures for acute and chronic PAD.
3. Describe the etiology of arterial ulcers and the differential characteristics of arterial ulcers.
4. Identify subjective and objective assessment data related to PAD and arterial ulcers.
5. Compare tests and procedures used in the evaluation and diagnosis of PAD of the lower extremity.
6. Describe medical and surgical treatment options for individuals with PAD of the lower extremities.
7. Identify interventions to treat arterial ulcers, including aggravating and alleviating factors for arterial ulcers.
8. Discuss nursing interventions related to patient teaching, health promotion, disease prevention, preoperative care, postoperative care, and home care.

Introduction and Overview

Peripheral artery disease (PAD), commonly referred to as arterial occlusive disease, results from an acute or chronic occlusion that causes narrowing of arteries, resulting in decreased blood flow (ischemia) to the lower extremities. Symptoms of occlusion are intermittent claudication which is typically described as a muscle cramp or ache with activity, rest pain, and ulceration. Atherosclerosis is the underlying process that precipitates the onset and progression of PAD. Individuals with PAD may have other systemic atherosclerotic problems such as coronary artery disease, cerebrovascular disease, and renal insufficiency. Other comorbidities include chronic renal failure and chronic obstructive pulmonary disease (Aponte, 2011; Creager & Libby, 2011; Hirsch et al., 2007).

The incidence of PAD increases with age. There is a higher prevalence in males and those over 70 years of age. The true incidence of chronic disease, however, is difficult to determine as many people are asymptomatic and others fail to report symptoms as they attribute these symptoms to the normal aging process. Other individuals tolerate the disease by modifying contributing lifestyle risk factors (Hirsch et al., 2007; Verma, Prasad, Elkadi, & Chi, 2011).

Atherosclerotic disease tends to occur in a symmetric fashion by respective segments of the arterial tree: aortoiliac, femoropopliteal, and tibial-peroneal disease. The signs and symptoms of chronic disease occur over time as this allows for the development of collateral vessels around the obstruction. Although PAD is not a leading cause of death, it significantly impacts quality of life, mobility, and limb loss (Collins et al., 2011). Mortality is primarily due to coexisting health problems (Gandhi, Weinberg, Margey, & Jaff, 2011; Jaffery et al., 2009).

Acute arterial occlusion results from a sudden interruption of blood supply. Critical limb ischemia can develop within hours and threaten both limb and life. With acute arterial occlusion, hemodynamic and metabolic consequences are more severe than with chronic disease (Jaffery et al., 2009; Muir, 2009).

Arterial ulcers usually occur at the most distal end of the arterial tree. Arterial ulcers are also called ischemic ulcers because they are caused by diminished arterial blood flow to the tissues. Ulcers may be the result of a precipitating event such as a trauma injury which fails to heal. Arterial occlusive disease including atherosclerosis, arterial vasospasm, or arterial inflammatory disease may be the underlying cause of ischemia. These ulcers are painful and debilitating. There may be substantial loss of tissue and in severe situations can be limb threatening (Holtman & Gahtan, 2008).

I. Anatomy

A. Arterial Wall—Arteries are composed of three histologic and functional layers: intima, media, and adventitia

1. Intima
   a. Innermost layer lining the lumen of the arterial wall
   b. Single layer of endothelial cells providing smooth lining
   c. Separated from the media by the internal elastic membrane
   d. Receives nutrients from the arterial lumen by diffusion
2. Media
   a. Middle layer of thick smooth muscle cells, collagen, and elastic fibers
   b. Regulates vessel diameter by dilation and constriction
   c. Inner area receives nutrients from the arterial lumen by diffusion; outer area receives nutrients from the vasa vasorum, the small blood vessels that penetrate the arterial wall
   d. Separated from the adventitia by an external elastic membrane
3. Adventitia
   a. Outermost layer of the artery
   b. Composed of connective tissue, collagen, and elastic fibers
   c. Provides majority of strength to the arterial wall and maintains its shape
   d. Receives nutrients from the vasa vasorum, the small blood vessels that penetrate the arterial wall

B. Arteries of the Lower Extremity (see Figure 9-1)

1. Distal aorta branches into the internal and external common iliac arteries
   a. Internal iliac artery (also called the hypogastric artery) enters the pelvic cavity and divides into branches that supply
      1) Pelvic viscera (urinary bladder, uterus, vagina, and rectum)
      2) Muscles of the gluteal and lumbar regions
      3) Walls of the pelvis
      4) External genitalia
      5) Middle region of thigh

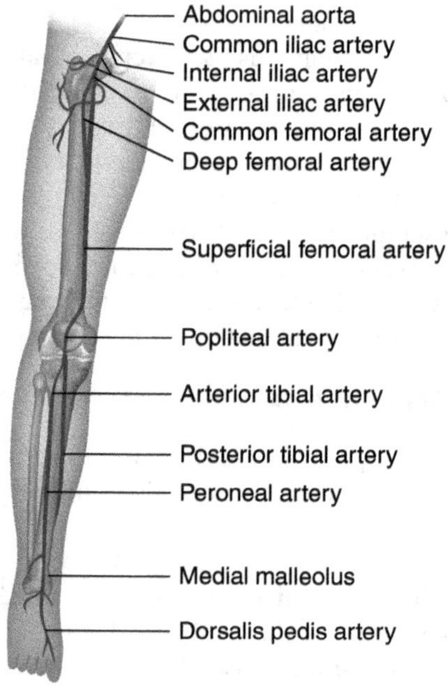

FIGURE 9-1. Lower extremity arterial anatomy.

b. External iliac arteries pass under the inguinal ligament and divide into the common femoral artery upon entering the thigh, supply the muscles and skin of the lower abdominal wall which branches into
   1) Superficial femoral artery
   2) Deep femoral or profunda femoris artery: supplies muscles of the thigh
   3) Popliteal artery: arises from the superficial femoral artery as it passes through the adductor hiatus in the distal thigh. Divides into
      a) Anterior tibial artery, lies between the tibia and fibula; supplies muscles and skin in the front of the leg; becomes the dorsalis pedis artery at the ankle joint
      b) Posterior tibial artery, continues down the back of the leg into the ankle; divides into the medial and lateral planter arteries to supply the sole of the foot and form the plantar arch
      c) Peroneal artery, supplies structures in the lateral aspect of the leg

II. Pathophysiology

The underlying etiology of arterial disease is varied. A prolonged decrease in blood flow may result in acute or chronic ischemia of the skin, muscles, nerves, and tissues

A. Acute Arterial Occlusion/Acute Limb Ischemia

1. Sudden decrease or worsening in limb perfusion causing a potential threat to loss of limb
2. Collateral arteries are usually absent
3. Critical ischemia develops within hours and is associated with the following conditions

a. Irreversible hypoxia to skeletal muscle or peripheral nerves occurs within 4 to 6 hours
b. Skin and subcutaneous tissue remain viable for longer periods of time due to differences in tissue tolerance to ischemia

4. Outcome depends on duration of tissue ischemia, site of obstruction, extent of thrombus propagation, adequacy of collateral circulation, and hemodynamic state of the patient
5. Signs and symptoms occur distal to the area of obstruction and vary depending on the level and severity of obstruction and adequacy of circulation
6. Paralysis is a late sign which indicates that the limb already has necrotic muscle and will not regain function. Often an amputation of the limb is needed

B. Chronic Arterial Occlusive Disease

1. Ischemia alters perfusion to the lower extremity; compensatory mechanisms initiated to counteract the ischemia include
   a. Vasodilation
   b. Development of collateral circulation
   c. Anaerobic metabolism to meet tissue needs
2. Atherosclerosis (Carroll, 2008). See Figure 9-2
   a. The most common cause of diminished arterial blood flow
   b. Characterized by the local accumulation of lipids, hemorrhage, fibrous tissue, and calcium deposits
   c. Exact cause of atherosclerosis is not known; it can begin to develop during childhood
      1) Fatty streak formation: appears as thin yellow lines and spots, slightly raised on the intima of the artery; reversible at this stage
      2) Fibrous plaques: more permanent lesions consisting of a lipid core surrounded by a capsule of elastic and collagenous tissue; causes loss of elasticity; occurs at arterial bifurcations

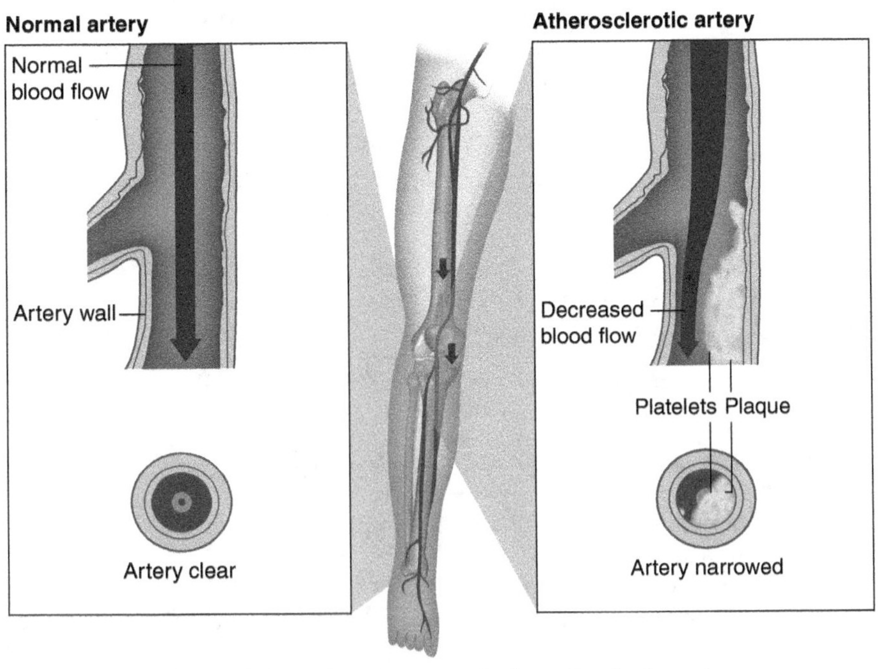

FIGURE 9-2. Normal artery and atherosclerosis of an artery.

3) Complicated lesions resulting in necrosis of the plaque and surface ulceration

d. Risk factors include age, gender, family history, smoking, diabetes, hypertension, dyslipidemia, sedentary life style, obesity, and stress

C. Arterial or Ischemic Ulcers

1. Usually the most distal end of the arterial tree
2. Occur most often in the lower extremities although they may be found at the tips of the fingers in vasospastic arterial disorders
3. Common complication of arterial occlusive disease
4. High prevalence among elderly, smokers, those with end stage renal disease, diabetes, and collagen vascular disease
5. Nonhealing foot ulcer may be the first indication that an individual has atherosclerosis
6. Altered healing occurs due to inadequate blood perfusion to the tissue. The increase in local metabolic needs for ulcer healing cannot be met

III. Etiology or Precipitating Factors

A. Acute Arterial Occlusion/Acute Limb Ischemia Results from

1. Thrombosis
   a. Obstruction from local factors such as thrombosis of narrowed atherosclerotic artery or popliteal aneurysms
   b. Obstruction from systemic factors due to decreased cardiac output from heart failure, dysrhythmias or shock, and hematologic abnormalities
2. Embolus (Chan & Cheng, 2011)
   a. Fragments of a thrombus migrate to another area; may be atheromatous plaque or tumor
   b. Commonly lodge at bifurcations of major arteries particularly in the lower extremities (aorta, femoral, iliac, popliteal) or areas where vessel suddenly tapers or branches
      1) Saddle embolus: embolus that lodges at bifurcation of aorta
      2) 50% of emboli lodge at the common femoral bifurcation
      3) 5% to 30% emboli lodge in distal aorta and iliac arteries
   c. Source of embolus
      1) Cardiac: atrial fibrillation, myocardial infarction, cardioversion, atrial myxoma, mitral stenosis, mural thrombus from myocardial infarction
      2) Noncardiac: originate from proximal atherosclerosis, such as ulcerated aortic atheroma or an aneurysm
3. Trauma
   a. Musculoskeletal injuries: fractures (femur, tibial plateau), dislocations
   b. Crushing/penetrating injuries
   c. Intimal disruption with subsequent thrombosis
   d. Laceration or transection of artery
   e. Iatrogenic trauma from percutaneous catheters used for diagnostic or therapeutic procedures

B. Chronic Arterial Occlusion from

1. Atherosclerosis
2. Arteritis
3. Vasospastic disorders
4. Fibromuscular dysplasia

IV. Assessment

Clinical manifestations of arterial occlusive disease develop below or distal to the site of obstruction. The primary factors determining the clinical presentation of lower extremity arterial diseases include the site of obstruction, onset (acute or chronic), collateral circulation, adequacy of distal arteries, and hemodynamic state (O'Connor & Ingram, 2011)

A. Risk Factors and Primary Prevention

1. Nonmodifiable (Muir, 2009; Na, Wang, Kirsner, & Federman, 2011; Oka, 2006; Treat-Jacobson & Walsh, 2003)
   a. Age: prevalence increases with age in males and females; increasing age >70
   b. Gender: more common in men and postmenopausal women
   c. Family history: increased predisposition if positive family history for PAD or any associated concomitant disease/risk factors
2. Modifiable
   a. Smoking (Verma et al., 2011)
      1) PAD occurs 8 to 10 years earlier in smokers than in nonsmokers
      2) Nicotine causes vasospasm, arterial constriction, endothelial injury, alteration of platelets, increased blood viscosity, and increases blood pressure
      3) Smoking cessation is associated with a rapid decline in the incidence of intermittent claudication
   b. Diabetes (Chou et al., 2008; Schaper et al., 2012)
      1) Increases risk of PAD two- to fourfold; PAD is twice as common in diabetics compared with nondiabetics; and develops at an earlier age
      2) Impairs arterial wound healing
      3) Increases risk for infection and gangrene
      4) Causes peripheral neuropathy
   c. Dyslipidemia—secondary to atherosclerosis; see Chapter 8, Vascular Medicine and Rehabilitation
   d. Hypertension—secondary to atherosclerosis; blood pressure increases as blood flows through narrowed vessels
   e. Coronary artery disease—increases mortality caused by myocardial ischemia
   f. Obesity
   g. Sedentary lifestyle—increases incidence of other risk factors
   h. Hyperhomocysteinemia

B. Patient History—Acute Arterial Occlusion/Acute Limb Ischemia

1. Subjective findings
   a. Chief complaint: sudden onset of the six P's; not all need to be present (see Table 9-1)

TABLE 9-1 The Classic 6 P's: Signs and Symptoms of Acute Arterial Occlusion

Pain—severe and constant, may be masked as a result of sensory deficits
Pallor—pale, yellowish tone to extremity below site of occlusion; extremity quickly appears waxy due to complete emptying and vasospasm of the arterial circulation
Pulselessness—absence of a pulse
Poikilothermia—coolness
Paresthesia—unusual or unexplained tingling, pricking, or burning sensation of skin. A sign indicating potential irreversibility. Caused by reduced blood supply to distal nerve fibers. Proprioception and light touch are lost early
Paralysis—loss of voluntary movement, a sign indicating potential irreversibility

b. Compartment syndrome/reperfusion injury: swelling within the osteofascial compartments of the limb, which causes increased intracompartmental pressure, resulting in decreased vascular perfusion; see Table 9-2
c. Metabolic complications: acidosis, hyperkalemia, and renal failure secondary to myoglobinuria

2. Objective findings
   a. Past history of cardiac disease including dysrhythmias or myocardial infarction
   b. Previous history of peripheral vascular disease, thrombosis
   c. Recent episode of hypotension

C. Patient History—Chronic Arterial Occlusive Disease

1. Subjective findings
   a. Chief complaint: intermittent claudication or ache involving the hip, buttocks, thigh, and calf with activity; frequently described as cramping, fatigue, or tired; may be unilateral or bilateral; may also present with atypical leg pain (McDermott et al., 2010)
      1) Induced by exercise (e.g., walking a predictable distance) and relieved by short periods of rest
      2) Often mistaken as a normal consequence of aging, an orthopedic problem, or sciatic nerve
      3) Distance walked before onset of pain is usually consistent, thus it is called reproducible. The shorter the distance walked, the more severe the disease process
   b. Rest pain
      1) Occurs with severe disease with extremity resting in a horizontal position
      2) Usually confined to the forefoot and metatarsal head (toes)

TABLE 9-2 Signs and Symptoms of Compartment Syndrome

Pain disproportional to injury
Tenderness and tenseness of compartment
Pain on passive stretching
Decreased muscle strength within compartment
Decreased simple touch perception
Decreased sensation of nerves in compartment
Pulses: may be normal or diminished; absent in late stages

3) Pain is aggravated by elevation
4) Partial or total relief is obtained by dangling the legs over the side of the bed, which increases arterial pressure due to gravity but may lead to edema
5) Associated with limb-threatening ischemia because blood flow is insufficient to meet even minimal metabolic requirements
6) Associated with gangrene and ulcers that do not heal
7) Coolness of the foot and/or limb
8) May require amputation

2. Objective findings
   a. Positive history of atherosclerosis such as coronary artery disease, cerebrovascular disease, and renovascular disease
   b. Positive family history of atherosclerosis, diabetes, hypertension, dyslipidemia
   c. Decreased functional ability to perform activities of daily living

D. Physical Examination—Clinical manifestations of disease vary depending on level and severity of obstruction and adequacy of collateral circulation. during each phase of assessment one limb should be compared to the other

1. Inspection
   a. Skin color changes
      1) Pallor on elevating limb 30 to 40 degrees
      2) Dependent rubor: deep red color when limb in dependent position. Color change reflects oxygen saturation and blood flow in capillary venous plexus of skin
   b. Temperature changes: coolness distal to site of occlusion
   c. Trophic changes: hair loss on affected limb; thin, smooth shiny skin; thick brittle toes nails, tapering toes; skin breakdown, ulceration, and gangrene due to nutritional changes
   d. Size and symmetry of both limbs for muscle atrophy, edema, presence of scars from previous surgery, and absence of limb
   e. Decreased capillary refill
   f. Edema usually absent; if present, may be related to dependence
   g. Arterial ulcers
      1) Color of surrounding skin and ulcer base is usually pale, increasing with elevation
      2) The skin surrounding the ulcer is shiny and smooth and appears taut, especially if the arterial disease is chronic
      3) Loss of hair occurs in conditions of chronic ischemia but an ulcer may be caused by arterial insufficiency even with hair present
      4) Gangrene may be present in the ulcer bed or in the surrounding skin
      5) Blue or purple patches of skin may indicate new ischemic areas that will soon become black
      6) Moist dead tissue may be present in the wound bed. This can be yellow or grey
      7) Ulcer characteristics are as follows
         a) Arterial ulcer location is at the distal end of the arterial tree. Ulcers are commonly found between and on the tips of toes,

around the ankle, over the malleolus, or on the foot over the phalangeal heads, or at an area of trauma
b) Arterial ulcer wound bed is usually dry and may be desiccated unless there is an infection present
c) Arterial ulcer size depends on the precipitating factors. It may be small and punched-out looking or may cover a large area resulting from trauma. A nonhealing surgical incision in an ischemic limb may be considered an arterial ulcer

2. Palpation
   a. Assess: femoral, popliteal, posterior tibial, dorsalis pedis pulse for presence and quality (present, diminished, or absent)
   b. Use Doppler to determine if signals are present
   c. Posterior tibial and dorsalis pedis pulses may be absent due to congenital anatomic variation
   d. Pedal pulses may be present with intermittent claudication but disappear with exercise
   e. Temperature
      1) Use back of hand to assess skin temperature in limbs
      2) Temperature demarcation may be felt at the skeletal segment distal to the site of arterial occlusion
      3) Asymmetric coolness is suggestive of arterial insufficiency; symmetric coolness indicates vasoconstriction or aortic obstruction
   f. Arterial ulcer
      1) Skin around the ulcer may feel cooler than skin on other parts of body
      2) Palpate the surrounding tissue for induration indicating cellulitis
      3) Palpate pulses
      4) Palpate the wound bed for tunneling or undermining. A soft boggy wound base indicated deeper necrotic tissue and possible infection with liquefaction of soft tissue necrosis
3. Auscultation
   a. Assess femoral and iliac arteries for bruit which is the sound associated with turbulent blood flood
   b. Bruit may help to localize the stenosis and differentiate between iliac and superficial femoral artery disease
      1) Auscultate using bell of stethoscope
      2) Higher pitch indicates more severe occlusion
      3) Superficial femoral artery stenosis may be present when the superficial femoral artery is compressed with the stethoscope

E. Considerations Across the Life Span

1. Young adulthood: occlusive atherosclerosis usually not seen in youth although underlying pathologic changes have begun. Provide education about modifiable risk factors and influence on disease progression
2. Pregnancy: medical and surgical management may need to be altered during pregnancy
3. Elderly: PAD is more prevalent during the later years of life and significantly affects quality of life. Recognition of pain may be complicated by physical or cognitive impairments, ongoing drug therapy, or social isolation. Self-care may be hampered by loss of vision

V. Pertinent Diagnostic Testing

A. Laboratory Tests

1. Routine electrolytes; blood urea nitrogen and creatinine—determine if renal insufficiency
2. Complete blood count
3. Electrocardiogram
4. PTT, PT/INR, platelets, fibrinogen—determine if coagulation disorder; potential for thrombus formation
5. Lipid panel, including total cholesterol, HDL, triglycerides, and LDL—determine dyslipidemia
6. Blood sugar and glycosylated hemoglobin levels—determine if diabetes

B. Noninvasive Diagnostic Test (Azam & Carman, 2011; Harrison, Lin, Blakley, & Tanaka, 2011; Owen & Roditi, 2011)

1. Ankle–brachial pressure index (ABI) (Mohler & Giri, 2008).
   a. Provides objective data on perfusion or arterial blood to lower extremities
   b. Portable, can be done at bedside
   c. Ankle systolic pressure is normally equal to or slightly higher than brachial systolic pressure; a decrease in pressure indicates arterial stenosis
   d. Assess ankle pressure at the dorsalis and posterior tibial arteries
   e. Divide the highest ankle pressure by the highest brachial pressure
   f. Any decrease in pressure indicates impaired arterial flow
      1) Normal—1.40 to 0.90
      2) Abnormal <0.90
      3) >1.40 noncompressible vessels
2. Toe systolic pressure index (TSPI) (Mohler & Giri, 2008)
   a. Appropriate for diabetics: 5% to 10% of diabetics have incompressible arteries
   b. Helps predict healing of toe and forefoot wounds and amputation sites
   c. Measurements taken at the great toe to assess arterial flow to the pedal or digital arteries
   d. Normal ≥60 mm Hg; reduced >30, <60 mm Hg; ischemic <30 mm Hg
3. Treadmill exercise testing
   a. Provides functional assessment of walking distance
   b. Determines initial claudication time or distance and absolute claudication time or distance, sometimes called peak walking time or distance
   c. Comparison of pre- to postexercise ABI provides objective information
4. Duplex ultrasonography
   a. Provides detailed images of stenosis, occlusion, and arterial diameter
   b. Provides hemodynamic information to assist in grading severity of stenosis
   c. Aids in decisions regarding treatment plan and options
   d. Assists with vein mapping if surgical revascularization is needed
5. Pulse volume recordings
   a. Assists in locating the site of occlusion in the common femoral, popliteal, dorsalis pedis, and posterior tibial arteries
   b. Requires segmental limb pressures to quantify arterial flow
      1) Pressures taken at dorsalis pedis, posterior tibial arteries, thigh, popliteal segment

        2) Highest brachial pressure is used for comparison
        3) Systolic pressure in leg is normally equal to or slightly higher than the systolic arm pressure
        4) Systolic pressure drops proportionally to severity of disease
            a) Ratio changes within a 0.15 range are considered within normal limits

6. Transcutaneous partial tension of oxygen ($TCPO_2$)
    a. Measures oxygen quality in microcirculation
    b. Measures effectiveness of interventions
    c. Helps to determine level of amputation

C. Invasive Tests

1. Arteriography
    a. Assess arterial anatomy; depicts aorta, iliac, femoral, popliteal, and tibial artery segments
    b. Identifies location and extent of arterial obstruction
    c. Provides information on status of runoff vessels
    d. Common femoral artery is the most common access site
    e. Performed before endovascular procedures (transluminal angioplasty) or operative procedure and in patients who have suspected graft occlusion or pseudoaneurysm
    f. Associated with complications
2. Digital subtraction angiography (DSA)
    a. Used to predict success of bypass grafting
    b. Provides information about the best site for proximal inflow and distal outflow and the presence of distal runoff to support a graft
3. Magnetic resonance angiography (MRA)
    a. Is based on MRI mechanisms and techniques
    b. Visualizes vasculature of lower extremities without contrast media
    c. May be used in combination with ultrasound
4. Computed tomography (CT)
    a. Provides accurate staging of abdominal aortic aneurysm, postoperative problems (graft infection, graft occlusion, hemorrhage, and abscess)
    b. Allows direct depiction of the arterial wall; accurately defines processes and structures around vessel wall that indicate disease
    c. May require the use of contrast medium

D. Special Procedures—Based on patient presentation, health history, and planned intervention

VI. Medical Management (see Chapter 8, Vascular Medicine and Rehabilitation)

Treatment is based on severity of symptoms and overall medical condition of the patient

Most patients with chronic PAD can be managed conservatively with an exercise program, modification of risk factors, and pharmacologic therapy to treat symptoms and associated concomitant diseases (Aronow, 2010; Catapano et al., 2011; Paravastu, Mendonca, & Da Silva, 2008; Treat-Jacobson & Walsh, 2003)

A. Chronic PAD

1. Risk factor reduction: smoking, diabetes, cholesterol levels, high blood pressure, sedentary lifestyle, control of other diseases
2. Walking Program (Collins et al., 2011).
    a. Helps control disease, improve quality of life, and pain-free total walking distance
    b. Improves oxygen uptake and use by muscle
    c. Promotes development of collateral arteries
        1) Collateral arteries are preexisting pathways that enlarge when flow through a parallel major artery is reduced; they are smaller, longer, and more numerous than the major arteries they replace
        2) Resistance through collateral vessels is greater than through normal artery, which limits the increase in flow occurring with exercise
3. Vascular rehabilitation program (Gardner & Afaq, 2008; Murphy et al., 2012)
    a. Structured exercise program specific to improving symptoms of intermittent claudication
    b. Incorporates techniques for physical reconditioning, education, and risk factor modification
    c. Patient advised to walk to the limit of discomfort, stop and resume walking
    d. Promotes development of collateral vessels in the affected leg
    e. Minimum three times a week
    f. Gradual increase in exercise duration and intensity based on symptoms
4. Protecting skin
    a. Use foot device to protect feet and toes, provide warmth resulting in vasodilation and increases circulation to extremities
    b. Prevent bed linens from causing pressure
    c. Use gauze between toes to prevent skin-to-skin contact
    d. Use gauze between toes with ulcers that may have exudate
5. Pain management
    a. Stop activity and rest
    b. Avoid elevating limb
    c. Take prescribed analgesia
6. Medications: few medications have demonstrated efficacy in adequately designed, placebo-controlled trials
    a. Hemorrheologic agents: pentoxifylline (Trental)
        1) Increases erythrocyte flexibility; reduces blood viscosity and increases volume of oxygenated blood to ischemic muscle; inhibits platelet aggregation
        2) Therapeutic effects occur after 4 to 8 weeks of therapy (400 mg t.i.d) with meals
        3) Current research has found a limited decrease in pain associated with intermittent claudication and does not support the widespread use of this drug
    b. Cilostazol (Pletal) (100 mg b.i.d) (Robless, Mikhailidis & Stansby, 2008)
        1) Has antiplatelet and vasodilator effects
        2) Acts directly on vascular smooth muscle
        3) Increases pain-free walking distance
        4) May increase HDL and decrease triglyceride levels

5) Long-term effects and risks are not established
6) Contraindicated in patients with heart failure

c. Antiplatelets: acetylsalicylic acid (Aspirin) and clopidogrel (Plavix)
   1) Reduce platelet aggregation and thrombus formation
   2) Reduce risk of cardiovascular morbidity and mortality associated with myocardial infarction, stroke, and vascular death
   3) May reduce rate of vascular graft occlusion
d. Other medications
   1) Vasodilators: do not increase blood flow to an ischemic limb or to exercising muscles
   2) Vascular endothelial growth factor: experimental
   3) Vitamin E: insufficient evidence

VII. Surgical Management

A. Management of Acute Ischemia

Factors to be considered in choosing an intervention include location and anatomy of lesion, duration of acute limb ischemia, type of clot, patient-related risks, surgery-related risks, and contraindications to thrombolysis

1. Bed rest
2. Anticoagulation
   a. Alters viscosity of blood and potentiates blood flow through narrowed vessels
   b. Prevents propagation of thrombus distal and proximal to occlusion; proliferation of new emboli
   c. Delay in initiation of therapy or inadequate treatment may result in limb loss, damage to vital organs, or death
   d. Types
      1) Intravenous heparin (unfractionated)—systemic heparinization with a fixed-dose bolus (5,000 to 10,000 U boluses) or weight-based dosing (80 U/kg) followed by continuous drip to maintain the APPT ratio between 1.5 and 2.5 times the control. Requires frequent and consistent monitoring of APTT levels
      2) Parenteral
         a) Subcutaneous heparin: has a slower, erratic absorption; is less precise than Intravenous administration; usually administered b.i.d
         b) Low molecular weight heparin derivatives
            - Less risk of bleeding complications with comparable anticoagulation affects than heparin
            - Administered subcutaneously
            - Does not require laboratory monitoring
      3) Oral anticoagulation: warfarin (Coumadin)
         a) Good for long-term anticoagulation
         b) Requires frequent monitoring of INR/PT levels
         c) Requires dosage adjustments
3. Thrombolytic therapy: for example, alteplase, streptokinase, and t-PA (tissue plasminogen activators) (Lipsitz & Kim, 2008)
   a. May be used alone or in conjunction with surgical intervention to treat recently formed arterial and bypass graft occlusions

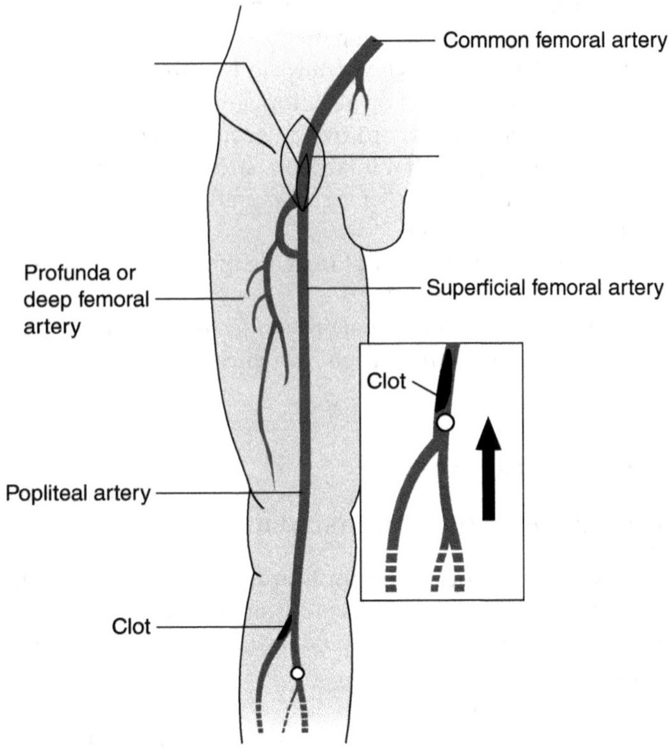

FIGURE 9-3. Thrombectomy/embolectomy of leg.

   b. Interventional angiography used to inject thrombolytics into failed grafts
   c. Associated with a higher frequency of hemorrhagic complications
   d. Contraindicated in patients who had a recent surgery or stroke and patients who have severe uncontrolled hypertension
4. Surgery
   a. Embolectomy, see Figure 9-3
      1) Extraction of embolus using an embolectomy catheter with balloon at tip
      2) When tip is beyond obstruction, balloon is inflated, and catheter and embolus are withdrawn
      3) Can be done with local anesthesia
      4) May require use of heparin and warfarin (Coumadin) postoperatively
   b. Thrombectomy
      1) Used to remove an arterial thrombus
      2) Can be used to remove an arterial thrombus within a graft
5. Complications—compartment syndrome (see Table 9-2)

B. Chronic Arterial Disease

The purpose of surgery is to restore and/or maintain limb viability, which leads to improved quality of life and decreased pain

1. Indications for lower extremity bypass surgery
   a. Disabling claudication that severely limits lifestyle and/or occupational activity
   b. Limb-threatening ischemia
   c. Nonhealing ulcers, tissue gangrene

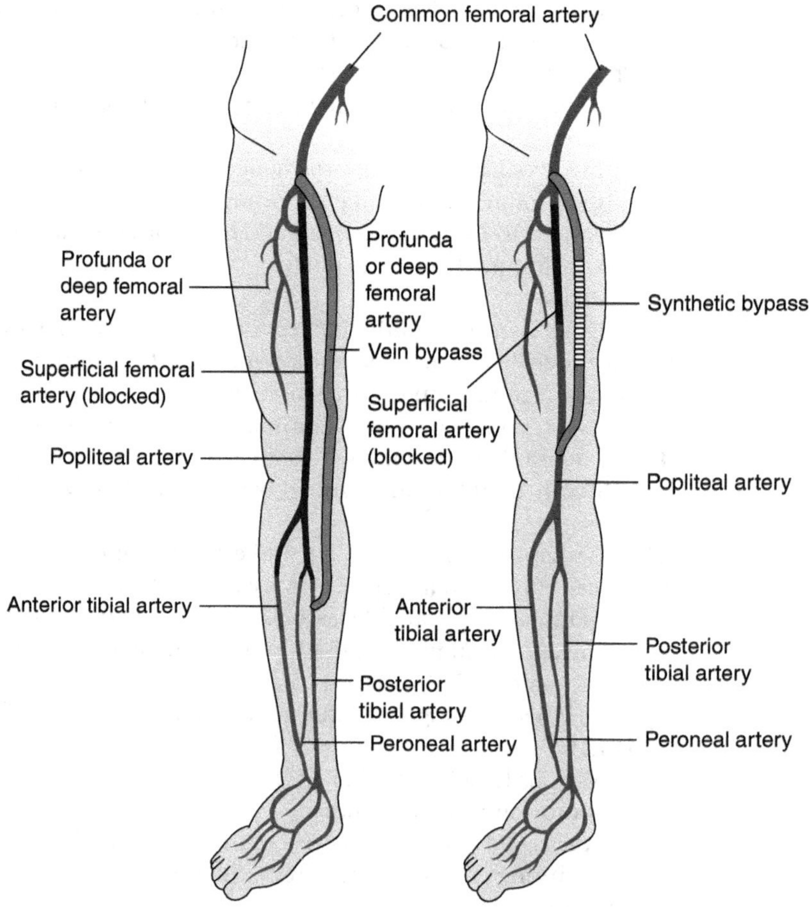

FIGURE 9-4. Examples of types of lower extremity bypasses.

2. Surgical procedures, see Figure 9-4
   a. Choice of surgical procedures depends on level of disease
   b. Bypass material determined by best proximal site for inflow and the best possible site for outflow
   c. Generally, the proximal anastomosis is sewn to the common femoral artery
   d. Distal end is anastomosed to the most cephalad portion of the leg that allows unobstructed blood flow to the foot
   e. Most common point of arterial occlusion in the leg is the lower portion of the superficial femoral artery as it passes through the medial adductor muscles just above the knee
   f. Procedure choice determined by level of arterial disease. Common surgical procedures include
      1) Aortofemoral/bifemoral bypass: indicated in aortoiliac occlusive disease
      2) Femoral-popliteal bypass: femoral artery bypass is sewn to the popliteal artery (above or below the knee) or to one of the tibial arteries, depending on degree of popliteal disease
      3) Extra-anatomic bypasses (axillo-popliteal, axillobifemoral, femorofemoral crossover)
         a) Indicated for high-risk patients with or at risk for limb loss, groin infection, multiple abdominal adhesions, previous scarring, multiple failed standard bypass procedures

b) Involves extensive subcutaneous tunneling using a synthetic polytetrafluoroethylene (PTFE) graft
4) Profundaplasty
a) Indicated for repair of stenotic profunda femoris (deep femoral) artery
b) Involves use of vein or prosthetic material to widen the lumen of the profunda after endarterectomy
5) Endarterectomy: removal of an atheromatous obstruction through an incision made into the artery

3. Graft materials
a. Autologous vein (nonsynthetic): less prone to infection; have superior patency over PTFE grafts due to biologically active endothelium which makes autogenous vein less thrombogenic. The quality of vein can affect the outcome of surgery. Commonly used veins include
1) Greater saphenous: long with sufficient diameter for use as a bypass; primarily used for infrainguinal bypasses; may be used in situ or reversed
2) Lesser saphenous: thin walled and extends from ankle to knee
3) Arms veins (cephalic, basilic): very thin walled; used if lower extremity veins are not available; associated with a high risk of aneurisms, prone to intimal fibrosis; used in tibial and peroneal bypass
b. Synthetic grafts (PTFE, Dacron)
1) Used when autologous grafts are unavailable or of insufficient length
a) Various lengths and diameters
b) Sturdy and easy to handle
c) Associated with a greater risk of ischemic complications frequently requiring emergency limb revascularization
c. Other materials
1) Human umbilical vein: associated with a high incidence of aneurysmal degeneration
2) Composite grafts (prosthetic vein): a combination graft consisting of autologous vein and prosthetic material

4. Surgical techniques
a. Reverse greater saphenous vein
1) Vein is long enough and of sufficient diameter to be used for any bypass
2) Vein is removed from its natural anatomic position and is reversed to allow unobstructed blood flow through vein valves
3) Small end of vein is sewn to a larger portion of artery; larger end is sewn to smaller portion of artery
b. In situ saphenous vein
1) Maintain vein in normal position, but remove valves using a valvulotome
2) No size disparity

5. Long-term graft patency and success of bypass grafts are influenced by (Wann-Hansson, Hallberg, Klevsgard, & Andersson, 2008)
a. Indication for surgery
b. Choice of bypass material or graft
c. Anatomic and hemodynamic characteristic of inflow artery, site of distal anastomosis, and associated outflow
d. Distal arterial anatomy

   e. Risk factors such as diabetes and smoking
   f. Use of anticoagulants
   g. Primary or secondary procedures
   h. Progression of atherosclerosis
   i. Development of fibromuscular dysplasia
6. Other surgical procedures
   a. Lumbar sympathectomy: surgical or chemical (neurolytic block): indicated in situations where there is nonreconstructible disease complicated by rest pain and tissue loss, thromboangiitis obliterans, or vasospasm; may temporarily increase lower extremity blood flow; evidence to support use is insufficient
   b. Amputation
      1) Goal: to preserve as much of the extremity as possible to ensure optimal rehabilitation potential
      2) Indications: extensive gangrene, infection, osteomyelitis, unreconstructable arterial occlusive disease
      3) Ideal site for amputation is the lowest level that will heal
7. Endovascular procedures (Chan & Cheng, 2011)
   a. Percutaneous transluminal angioplasty (PTA)
      1) Increases arterial lumen size by compressing atherosclerotic plaque against the vessel wall using a balloon or by removing atherosclerotic plaque mechanically (atherectomy and laser)
      2) Preferred treatment for localized stenosis and occlusions of the aortoiliac, femoropopliteal, and tibial arteries; may be used in conjunction with surgery
      3) Technique: similar to that used for arteriography; arterial puncture is larger than in arteriography
      4) Complications: may include distal embolization, arterial dissection, arterial thrombosis
   b. Stenting
      1) Endoluminal metallic devices that buttress the vessel wall and prevent closure
      2) May be balloon-expanded or self-expanding; arterial insertion similar to angioplasty
      3) Complications: may include distal embolization, arterial dissection, arterial thrombosis, occlusion at insertion site, hematoma, or false aneurysm

C. Wound Management

1. Debridement is appropriate when there is adequate blood supply to heal the wound. Methods of debridement include
   a. Sharp debridement with a scalpel at the bedside or in the operating room
   b. Autolytic debridement, providing a moist wound environment that promotes self-debridement
   c. Chemical debridement, using a chemical agent
2. Debridement is contraindicated without adequate blood supply to heal the wound
3. Dry gangrene is best kept dry to avoid an opportunistic organism from infecting the wound bed
4. Infected arterial wounds must be treated with appropriate systemic antibiotics

5. Infections associated with arterial wounds include cellulitis or lymphangitis of the surrounding tissue. There may be purulence in the wound from infected necrotic tissue
6. Wound cultures are done if the offending organism is unknown
7. The best way to obtain a wound culture is by tissue biopsy of nearby inflamed tissue. Caution should be used if the tissue is ischemic so as not to cause another ulcer
8. Osteomyelitis should be considered if the ulcer is over a bony prominence especially if the ulcer is chronic or the bone is exposed. An x-ray is obtained to identify bone involvement
9. Select dressings based on the goal for the ulcer
   a. Before revascularization: dry dressings
      1) Protect the wound from the environment and organisms
      2) Should be kept over eschar and around gangrenous toes
      3) Protect surrounding tissue from trauma
      4) Should avoid tape to the skin
   b. After revascularization: moist dressings
      1) Include moist saline gauze, hydrocolloids, impregnated gel gauze, or any commercial dressing that provides a moist environment for the wound
      2) Should avoid maceration of surrounding skin
10. Care of the peri-ulcer intact skin consists of
    a. Moisturizing dry skin
    b. Avoiding moisture between toes or over eschar

VIII. Nursing Management (Lovell, Myers, Forbes, Dresser, & Weiss, 2011; Sieggreen, 2006; Treat-Jacobson & Walsh, 2003; Widener, 2011)

A. Risk for Ineffective Peripheral Tissue Perfusion Related to decreased blood flow secondary to progressive arterial occlusive disease, graft thrombosis, compartment syndrome, or inadequate anticoagulation

1. Expected patient outcomes
   a. Maintain adequate tissue perfusion to involved extremities
   b. Warm, dry skin with normal pedal pulses, color, temperature, sensory and motor function, and capillary refill
2. Nursing interventions
   a. Assess (inspect, palpate, auscultate) peripheral circulation
   b. Promote factors that improve arterial flow
      1) Position extremity to optimize circulation
      2) Encourage passive and active range of motion exercises
      3) Provide warmth and avoid prolonged exposure to cold
   c. Prevent vasoconstriction
      1) Promote proper foot care
      2) Avoid constrictive clothing around leg or over any graft site
   d. Reduce risk of trauma
      1) Promote proper foot care
      2) Change patient's position as appropriate
      3) Instruct patient to avoid crossing legs
      4) Minimize external pressure points

3. Evaluation
   a. Adequate tissue perfusion is maintained; and tissue remains intact
   b. Skin is warm and dry

B. Impaired Tissue Integrity Related to decreased blood flow and nutrients to tissue secondary to arterial occlusive disease, arteriosclerosis, pressure, trauma, infection, multiple surgical procedures, and altered nutritional status

1. Expected outcomes
   a. Maintain intact skin surfaces with healed wounds, adequate temperature, sensation, hydration, perspiration, color, hair growth, and free from infection
   b. Resolution of drainage
   c. Tissue will heal and/or remain intact
   d. Ulcer complications will be avoided or minimized
2. Nursing interventions
   a. Monitor skin or wound decreased perfusion, breakdown by
      1) Assessing pain, swelling, erythema, drainage
      2) Monitor skin for breakdown, infection including low-grade fever, elevated white cell count, graft exposure
   b. Eliminate/reduce contributing factors
      1) Avoid using tape directly on the skin
      2) Use appropriate therapeutic pressure reducing products
   c. Monitor nutritional status
      1) Assess weight, serum proteins (albumin, transferrin, prealbumin)
      2) Prevent mechanical, thermal, and chemical injury
   d. Follow strict aseptic technique during wound care and dressing changes. Institute measures to increase blood flow to ulcer
      1) Protect limb from injury
      2) Protect from pressure
      3) Avoid extreme temperatures
      4) Protect surrounding skin
      5) Cleanse the wound with a nontoxic agent
      6) Remove necrotic tissue as indicated
      7) Provide a moist wound environment for cellular migration
3. Evaluation
   a. Skin health is maintained
   b. Measures to protect tissue/wound are initiated and maintained

C. Acute Pain/Chronic Pain Related to surgical incision, presence of arterial ulcers, arterial occlusive disease

1. Expected outcomes
   a. Reports satisfaction with pain symptom control
   b. Recognizes factors that precipitate the onset and/or exacerbate pain
2. Nursing interventions
   a. Perform pain assessment: identify location, characteristics, onset, duration, frequency, quality, intensity, and precipitating factors
   b. Observe for nonverbal cues
   c. Consider cultural influences on pain response
   d. Assess impact of pain on quality of life

e. Manage pain effectively
   1) Minimize environmental factors that precipitate and/or exacerbate pain
   2) Administer analgesics and consider nonpharmacological interventions
f. Evaluate effectiveness of interventions using a pain assessment tool
g. Instruct to request/take analgesics as needed before pain is severe
h. Collaborate with physician in terms of pain management

3. Evaluation
   a. Decreased pain reported
   b. Precipitating factors are recognized promptly

D. Activity Intolerance Related to decreased peripheral circulation, surgery, pain

1. Expected outcomes
   a. Maintain or improve activity level
   b. Able to perform usual activities of daily living
2. Nursing interventions
   a. Assess prior levels of activity, muscle strength, and tolerance
   b. Assist patient in prioritizing activities to accommodate energy levels
   c. Encourage alternating rest and activity patterns
   d. Determine adequacy of sleep
   e. Promote gradual increased in activity
3. Evaluation
   a. Reports ability to perform activities of daily living
   b. Improvement in activity tolerance and muscle strength

E. Risk for Neurovascular Dysfunction

1. Expected outcome
   a. No evidence of neurovascular dysfunction (compartment syndrome)
   b. Recognize factors that contribute to compartment syndrome
2. Nursing interventions
   a. Assess foot and leg for motor and sensory function, pain out of proportion to procedure
   b. Monitor leg for hematoma, tense calf, swelling
   c. Check laboratory values: myoglobin
   d. Check urine for myoglobinuria
   e. Observe for red blood cells in urine
   f. Monitor for hyperkalemia and acidosis
3. Evaluation
   a. Absence of compartment syndrome
   b. Preservation of motor and sensory function in lower extremity

IX. Patient Teaching

A. Disease Prevention/Health Promotion Secondary Prevention

B. Recognition and Avoidance of Risk Factors

1. Smoking cessation
2. Management of coexisting health problems: diabetes, hypertension
3. Consider dietary consult for lipid management and weight control

C. Injury Prevention and Foot Care: Need for lifelong observation of the foot at risk

D. Signs and Symptoms of Infection: Acute occlusion, graft failure

E. Wound/Incision Care

F. Medication Management: Purpose, dosage, side effects

G. Antibiotic Prophylaxis: With synthetic bypass grafts need for antibiotic before invasive procedures

H. Home Walking Program and/or Vascular Rehabilitation Program

CASE STUDIES

CASE STUDY 1

Mr. Jones, a 79-year-old white male was diagnosed with PAD in his left leg 5 years ago. Recent diagnostic studies indicate multiple atherosclerotic lesions in the femoral-popliteal region; his left leg ankle–brachial index (ABI) is 0.45. His other medical conditions include diabetes, hypertension, coronary artery disease, and a 45-year history of smoking. Mr. Jones underwent a triple coronary artery bypass surgery (saphenous vein and prosthetic material) 15 years ago. Over the past 2 weeks, Mr. Jones has experienced increasing rest pain in his left foot, particularly at night, which is partly relieved by sitting upright in reclining chair. Analgesics have not provided pain relief. Mr. Jones is admitted to the hospital for a femoral to below knee popliteal bypass using a synthetic graft material.

REVIEW QUESTIONS

1. What factors contribute to the development of his arterial occlusive disease?
2. What is the significance of an ABI of 0.45? Should we add a right ABI?
3. What are potential postoperative complications?
4. What are potential complications after reperfusion?
5. What are key elements in the teaching plan?

ANSWERS/RATIONALE

1. Age, diabetes, hypertension, smoking history, coronary artery disease (systemic atherosclerosis).
2. Indicative of severe ischemia.
3. Graft thrombosis, hemorrhage, infection, edema, compartment syndrome.
   On postoperative day 2, the nurse caring for Mr. Jones is unable to palpate pulses or auscultate Doppler signals in the dorsalis pedis artery. The left foot is cooler to touch than the right and is becoming increasingly pale and mottled. The nurse suspects Mr. Jones is experiencing an acute arterial occlusion of the operative limb and notifies the physician immediately.
   Mr. Jones underwent an embolectomy.
4. Compartment syndrome or swelling of skeletal muscle—high pressure within the compartments of the leg can result in nerve injury, muscle cell necrosis, and occlusion of the tibial vessels or the synthetic graft. Treatment of compartment includes a fasciotomy—to allow for expansion of the edematous muscle and decompression of compartment and relief of pressure.

5. Key elements of the teaching plan include the following:
   a. Assess for presence of foot pulses
   b. Avoid vasoconstriction—do not cross legs, no smoking
   c. Look for signs and symptoms of graft failure, infection, acute occlusion
   d. Perform meticulous foot care—avoid mechanical, thermal, and chemical injury
   e. Engage in regular exercise
   f. Manage other risk factors: hypertension, diabetes
   g. State need for prophylactic antibiotic coverage before invasive tests, procedures, or extensive dental work

CASE STUDY 2

Mr. First, a 64-year-old black male, presents with an ulcer on the tip of his right great toe. He has been cared for by his family physician for a number of years. He has hypertension and is a noninsulin-dependent diabetic. He has progressive claudication, limiting his walking ability to half a block. Mr. First smokes half a pack of cigarette a day and has been trying to quit. He states his job stress has kept him from stopping entirely.

Laboratory studies reveal a normal creatinine and cholesterol; blood glucose is 130 mg/dL. Blood pressure is 130/68. ABI results are falsely elevated due to his diabetes; toe–brachial indices are 0.4 Right and 0.6 Left.

An arteriogram is performed based on the understanding that an operation may be considered. He has stenosis at the right iliac artery and right common femoral artery. The surgeon suggests a percutaneous angioplasty with stent placement.

Mr. First arrives for the procedure and states a pain score of 9 out of 10. The ulcer is dry.

REVIEW QUESTIONS

1. What is the best local treatment for Mr. First's ulcer prior to his angioplasty?
   a. Dry dressing
   b. Wet to dry dressing
   c. Hydrocolloid
   d. Debridement
2. Which of the following are characteristics of arterial ulcers?
   a. Beefy red base
   b. Copious drainage
   c. Punched-out look
   d. Numb borders
3. What is the most important treatment for an arterial ulcer?
   a. Moist dressings
   b. Increased blood flow
   c. Leg elevation
   d. Antibiotics
4. Where are arterial ulcers most likely to be found?
   a. Fingers
   b. Medial ankle
   c. Foot
   d. Groin
5. Rest pain is
   a. Pain relieved by rest
   b. Pain with leg elevation
   c. Unrelieved claudication
   d. Constant pain

ANSWERS/RATIONALE

1. **a.** The ulcer should be kept dry until the revascularization procedure is completed.
2. **c.** All of the other answers are incorrect. Usually arterial ulcers have a definite border. They may be of the shape of whatever caused the injury if trauma precipitates the ulcer.
3. **b.** All arterial ulcers are ischemic. Nothing will stimulate healing until there is adequate blood flow.
4. **c.** Although ischemic ulcers can occur anywhere, the most common area is the foot because atherosclerosis of the arteries which lead to the lower extremities is most often the cause.
5. **b.** With leg elevation, perfusion is diminished, causing ischemic pain.

REFERENCES

Aponte, J. (2011). The prevalence of asymptomatic and symptomatic peripheral arterial disease and peripheral arterial disease risk factors in the US population. *Holistic Nursing, 25*(3), 147–161.

Aronow, W. S. (2010). Treating intermittent claudication caused by peripheral arterial disease. *Annals of Long Term Care, 18*(12), 29–30.

Azam, S. M., & Carman, T. L. (2011). Diagnostic approach to peripheral arterial disease. *Cardiology Clinics, 29*(3), 319–329.

Carroll, R. (2008). Vascular structure and function. In J. M. Black & J. Hokanson Hawks (Eds.), *Medical-surgical nursing: Clinical management for positive outcomes* (8th ed., pp. 1271–1278). Philadelphia, PA: Saunders.

Catapano, A. L., Reiner, Z., DeBacker, G., Graham, I., Taskinen, M. R., Wiklund, O., … Wood, D. (2011). ECS/EAS Guidelines for the management of dyslipidaemias. The Task Force for the Management of Dyslipidemias of the European Society of Cardiology (ESC) and the European Atherosclerosis Society (EAS). *Atherosclerosis, 217*(1), 3–46.

Chan, Y. C., & Cheng, S. W. (2011). Drug-eluting stents and balloons in peripheral arterial disease: Evidence so far. *International Journal of Clinical Practice, 65*(6), 664–668.

Chou, C. K., Weng, S. W., Chang, H. W., Chen, C. Y., Su, S. C., & Liu, R. T. (2008). Analysis of traditional and nontraditional risk factors for peripheral arterial disease in elderly type 2 diabetic patients in Taiwan. *Diabetes Research & Clinical Practice, 81*(3), 331–337.

Collins, T. C., Lunos, S., Carlson, T., Henderson, K., Lightbourne, M., Nelson, B., & Hodges, J. S. (2011). Effects of a home-based walking intervention on mobility and quality of life in people with diabetes and peripheral arterial disease: A randomized controlled trial. *Diabetes Care, 34*(10), 2174–2179.

Creager, M., & Libby, P. (2011). Peripheral arterial disease. In R. Bonow, D. Mann, D. Zipes, & P. Libby (Eds.), *Braunwald's heart disease–A textbook of cardiovascular medicine* (9th ed., pp. 1338–1356). Philadelphia, PA: Saunders.

Gandhi, S., Weinberg, I., Margey, R., & Jaff, M. R. (2011). Comprehensive medical management of peripheral arterial disease. *Progress in Cardiovascular Diseases, 54*(1), 2–13.

Gardner, A. W., & Afaq, Z. (2008). Management of lower extremity peripheral arterial disease. *Journal of Cardiopulmonary Rehabilitation & Prevention, 28*(6), 349–357.

Harrison, M. L., Lin, H. F., Blakley, D. W., & Tanaka, H. (2011). Preliminary assessment of an automatic screening device for peripheral arterial disease using ankle-brachial and toe-brachial indices. *Blood Pressure Monitoring, 16*(3), 138–141.

Hirsch, A. T., Murphy, T. P., Lovell, M. B., Twillman, G., Treat-Jacobson, D., Harwood, E. M., … Criqui, M. H. (2007). Gaps in public knowledge of peripheral arterial disease: The first national PAD public awareness survey. *Circulation, 116*(18), 2086–2094.

Holtman, D. A., & Gahtan, V. (2008). Peripheral arterial perfusion: Is it adequate for wound healing? *Wounds: A Compendium of Clinical Research & Practice, 20*(8), 230–235.

Jaffery, Z., Greenbaum, A. B., Siddiqui, M. F., Mahendraker, N., Gupta, V., Mokkala, V., … McCord, J. (2009). Predictors of mortality in patients with lower extremity peripheral arterial disease: 5-year follow-up. *Journal of Interventional Cardiology, 22*(6), 564–570.

Lipsitz, E. C., & Kim, S. (2008). Antithrombotic therapy in peripheral arterial disease. *Cardiology Clinics, 26*(2), 289–298.

Lovell, M., Myers, K., Forbes, T. L., Dresser, G., & Weiss, E. (2011). Peripheral arterial disease: Application of the chronic care model. *Journal of Vascular Nursing, 29*(4), 147–152.

McDermott, M. M., Ferrucci, L., Liu, K., Guralnik, J. M., Tian, L., Liao, Y., & Criqui, M. H. (2010). Leg symptom categories and rates of mobility decline in peripheral arterial disease. *Journal of the American Geriatrics Society, 58*(7), 1256–1262.

Mohler, E., III, & Giri, J. (2008). Management of peripheral arterial disease patients: Comparing the ACC/AHA and TASC-II guidelines. *Current Medical Research & Opinion, 24*(9), 2509–2522.

Muir, R. L. (2009). Peripheral arterial disease: Pathophysiology, risk factors, diagnosis, treatment, and prevention. *Journal of Vascular Nursing, 27*(2), 26–30.

Murphy, T. P., Cutlip, D. E., Regensteiner, J. G., Mohler, E. R., Cohen, D. J., Reynolds, M. R., ... Hirsch, A. T. (2012). Supervised exercise versus primary stenting for claudication resulting from aortoiliac peripheral artery disease: Six-month outcomes from the Claudication: Exercise Versus Endoluminal Revascularization (CLEVER) Study. *Circulation, 125*(1), 130–139.

Na, C. R., Wang, S., Kirsner, R. S., & Federman, D. G. (2011). The elderly and peripheral arterial disease. *Clinical Geriatrics, 19*(7), 41–46.

O'Connor, I., & Ingram, C. (2011). Screening for peripheral arterial disease: A real chance to improve patient care. *Primary Care Cardiovascular Journal, 4*(2), 85–87.

Oka, R. K. (2006). Peripheral arterial disease in older adults: Management of cardiovascular disease risk factors. *Journal of Cardiovascular Nursing, 21*(5 Suppl. 1), S15–S20.

Owen, A. R., & Roditi, G. H. (2011). Peripheral arterial disease: The evolving role of non-invasive imaging. *Postgraduate Medical Journal, 87*(1025), 189–198.

Paravastu, S. C., Mendonca, D., & Da Silva, A. (2008). Beta blockers for peripheral arterial disease. *Cochrane Database of Systematic Reviews*, (4), CD005508. doi:10.1002/14651858.CD00508.pub2

Robless, P., Mikhailidis, D. P., & Stansby, G. P. (2008). Cilostazol for peripheral arterial disease. *Cochrane Database of Systematic Reviews*, (1), CD003748

Schaper, N. C., Andros, G., Apelqvist, J., Bakker, K., Lammer, J., Lepantalo, M., ... Hinchliffe, R. J. (2012). Diagnosis and treatment of peripheral arterial disease in diabetic patients with a foot ulcer. A progress report of the International Working Group on the Diabetic Foot. *Diabetes/Metabolism Research & Reviews, 28*, 218–224.

Sieggreen, M. (2006). A contemporary approach to peripheral arterial disease. *Nurse Practitioner, 31*(7), 14.

Treat-Jacobson, D., & Walsh, M. E. (2003). Treating patients with peripheral arterial disease and claudication. *Journal of Vascular Nursing, 21*(1), 5–16.

Verma, A., Prasad, A., Elkadi, G. H., & Chi, Y.-W. (2011). Peripheral arterial disease: Evaluation, risk factor modification, and medical management. *Journal of Clinical Outcomes Management, 18*(2), 74–84.

Wann-Hansson, C., Hallberg, I. R., Klevsgard, R., & Andersson, E. (2008). The long-term experience of living with peripheral arterial disease and the recovery following revascularisation: A qualitative study. *International Journal of Nursing Studies, 45*(4), 552–561.

Widener, J. M. (2011). Peripheral arterial disease and disability from NHANES 2001–2004 data. *Journal of Vascular Nursing, 29*(3), 104–112.

SUGGESTED READINGS

Black, J. (2008). Management of clients with vascular disorders. In J.M. Black & J. Hokanson Hawks (Eds.), *Medical-surgical nursing: Clinical management for positive outcomes* (8th ed., pp. 1509–1545). Philadelphia, PA: Saunders.

Brazziel, T. G., Cox, L., Drury, C., & Guerra, M. (2011). Stopping the wave of PAD. *Nurse Practitioner, 36*(11), 28–33.

Crowther, R. G., Leicht, A. S., Spinks, W. L., Sangla, K., Quigley, F., & Golledge, J. (2012). Effects of a 6-month exercise program pilot study on walking economy, peak physiological characteristics, and walking performance in patients with peripheral arterial disease. *Vascular Health & Risk Management, 8*, 225–232.

deJong, A. (2010). Clinical applications. Peripheral arterial disease: Impact on lifestyle and rehabilitation opportunities. *American College of Sports Medicine Health & Fitness Journal, 14*(2), 42–44.

Hamburg, N. M., & Balady, G. J. (2011). Exercise rehabilitation in peripheral artery disease: Functional impact and mechanisms of benefits. *Circulation, 123*(1), 87–97.

Jude, E. B., Wleftheriadou, I., & Tentolouris, N. (2010). Peripheral arterial disease in diabetes–a review. *Diabetic Medicine, 27*(1), 4–14.

Khattri, S. (2009). Treadmill exercise or resistance training in patients with peripheral arterial disease.*Journal of the American Medical Association, 301*(2), 165–174.

Kruidenier, L. M., Nicolaï, S. P., Rouwet, E. V., Peters, R. J., Prins, M. H., & Teijink, J. A. (2011). Additional supervised exercise therapy after a percutaneous vascular intervention for peripheral arterial disease: A randomized clinical trial. *Journal of Vascular & Interventional Radiology, 22*(7), 961–968.

Lane, D. A., & Lip, G. Y. (2009). Treatment of hypertension in peripheral arterial disease. *Cochrane Database of Systematic Reviews*, (4), CD003075. doi:10.1002/14651858.CD003075.pub2

Mannava, K., & Money, S. R. (2007). Current management of peripheral arterial occlusive disease: A review of pharmacologic agents and other interventions. *American Journal of Cardiovascular Drugs, 7*(1), 59–66.

McDermott, M. M., Ades, P., Guralnik, J. M., Dyer, A., Ferrucci, L., Liu, K., ... Criqui, M. H. (2009). Treadmill exercise and resistance training in patients with peripheral arterial disease with and without intermittent claudication: A randomized controlled trial. *Journal of the American Medical Association, 301*(2), 165–174.

Mukherjee, D., & Cho, L. (2009). Peripheral arterial disease: Considerations in risks, diagnosis, and treatment. *Journal of the National Medical Association, 101*(10), 999–1008.

Nelson, E. A., & Bradley, M. D. (2009).Dressings and topical agents for arterial ulcers. *Cochrane Database of Systematic Reviews,* (1), CD001836. doi:10.1002/14651858.CD001836.pub2

Osinbowale, O. O., & Milani, R. V. (2011). Benefits of exercise therapy in peripheral arterial disease. *Progress in Cardiovascular Diseases, 53*(6), 447–453.

Palfreyman, S. (2007). Vascular disease. A handbook for nurses. *Journal of Advanced Nursing, 57*(4), 459.

Parmenter, B. J., Raymond, J., & Singh, F. (2010). The effect of exercise on haemodynamics in intermittent claudication: A systematic review of randomized controlled trials. *Sports Medicine, 40*(5), 433–447.

Rooke, T. W., Hirsch, A. T., Misra, S., Sidawy, A. N., Beckman, J. A., Findeiss, L. K., … Zierler, R. E. (2011). 2011 ACCF/AHA focused update of the guideline for the management of patients with peripheral artery disease: A report of the American College of Cardiology Foundation/American Heart Association Task Force on Practice Guidelines. *Journal of American College of Cardiology, 58*(19), 220–245.

Shigematsu, H., Sapoval, M., White, C., White, J., Clement, D., Creager, M., … Rosenfield, K. (2007). Inter-Society Consensus for the Management of Peripheral Arterial Disease (TASCII). *European Journal of Vascular and Endovascular Surgery, 33*(Suppl. 1), S1–S75.

Shishebor, M. (2011). The importance of functional status in the management of peripheral arterial disease. *Journal of the American College of Cardiology, 57*(23), 2365–2367.

Sieggreen, M. (2008). Assessment of the vascular system. In J.M. Black & J. Hokanson Hawks (Eds.), *Medical-surgical nursing: Clinical management for positive outcomes* (8th ed., pp. 1475–1487). Philadelphia, PA: Saunders.

Sorace, P., Ronai, P., & Churilla, J. (2010). Peripheral arterial disease: Exercise is medicine. *American College of Sports Medicine Health & Fitness Journal, 14*(1), 23–29.

Treat-Jacobson, D., Henly, S. J., Bronas, U. G., Leon, A. S., & Henly, G. A. (2011). The pain trajectory during treadmill testing in peripheral artery disease. *Nursing Research, 60,* S38–S49.

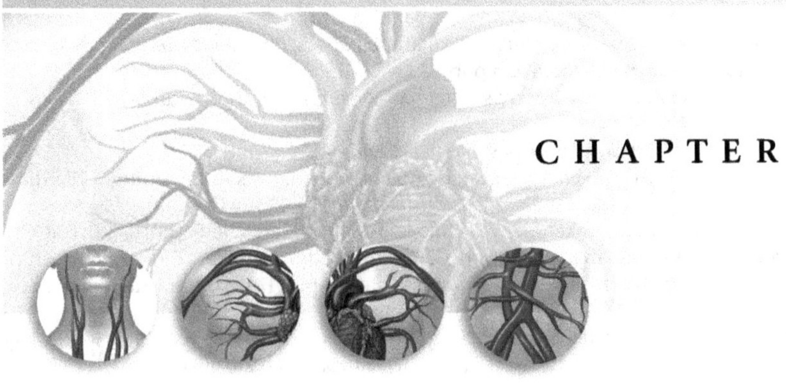

CHAPTER 10

Upper Extremity Arterial Occlusive Disease

Phyllis Gordon
Nancy Shebel
First Edition Author: *Theresa Glessner*

OBJECTIVES

1. Identify etiology and precipitating factors that lead to upper extremity occlusive disease.
2. Discuss physical examination findings pertinent to upper extremity occlusive disease.
3. List pertinent diagnostic tests related to the diagnosis of upper extremity occlusive disease.
4. Discuss medical and surgical management techniques for restoration of blood flow in patients with upper extremity disease.

Introduction

Upper extremity arterial occlusive disease is much less common than lower extremity disease (Eskandari, 2012). Although upper extremity ischemia is less prevalent that lower extremity ischemia, upper extremity impairment can be significantly devastating to those patients affected by its sequelae. Humans depend more on their upper extremities to carry out the activities of daily life than their lower extremities; therefore, a lower extremity amputation can be less debilitating than an upper extremity amputation. Although only about 5% to 10% of all embolic events involve the upper extremities, prompt diagnosis and treatment of upper extremity ischemia is paramount for limb salvage (Soloway, 2013).

I. Anatomy (see Chapter 3, Anatomy and Physiology of the Vascular System)

A. Subclavian Artery

1. Major blood supply of the upper extremities
2. As it passes over the first rib, it becomes the axillary artery

B. Axillary Artery

1. 15 cm long
2. Six major branches which serve as collaterals for the shoulder girdle

C. Brachial Artery

1. Extends from lower border of the teres muscle to its bifurcation at the head of the radius
2. Branches into the radial, ulnar, and interosseous arteries at the antecubital fossa

D. Radial and Ulnar Arteries (Mowlavi, 2012)

1. Supply most of the hand circulation
2. Supply palmar arch which supplies the fingers via the digital arteries; incomplete palmar arch supplied by the radial artery only is present in 20%

II. Pathophysiology

A. Vasculitis Fibromuscular Dysplasia and Atherosclerosis produce symptoms by narrowing or occlusion of the arterial lumen (Eskandari, Rowe, & Pearce, 2012; Mitchell & Schoen, 2010)

1. Atherosclerosis: local accumulation of lipids, initially seen as fatty streaks that progressively develop fibrous plaque and local hemorrhage, and ulceration that involve the intima with calcification of the media and loss of arterial wall elasticity. Similar to lower extremity disease (see Chapter 9, Lower Extremity Arterial Disease)
   a. Diameter reduction of 50% or a cross-sectional area reduction of 70% represents a hemodynamically significant lesion (Mowlavi, 2012)
   b. Lesions cause a pressure drop across the stenosis and exercise-induced fatigue in which demand for blood flow exceeds supply
   c. Cool extremity and decreased peripheral pulses are manifested by intermittent claudication or pain with arm use
2. Vasculitic and inflammatory arteritis disorders: severe, chronic inflammatory process of the vessel wall with cellular infiltrates and eventual necrosis (Mitchell & Schoen, 2010)
   a. Large group of systemic diseases; pathologic changes vary depending on disorder; underlying cause is unknown
   b. Involvement of upper extremities is rare
   c. Vascular lesions caused by deposits of fibrin or complement; infiltration by inflammatory cells and fibrous obliteration of the vessel
   d. Inflammation may involve entire vessel wall or only some of the layers which results in diffuse or focal changes
   e. When a vessel is destroyed by the inflammatory process, vasculitis is termed "necrotizing"
   f. Buerger disease (thromboangiitis obliterans) (see Chapter 16, Buerger Disease). Inflammation progresses to all layers of the artery; lumen contains thrombus with fibroblasts and giant cells and is associated with young male smokers (Arkkila, 2006; Espinoza, 2009). The intima, media, and adventitia have varying amounts of thickening and inflammatory changes
3. Fibromuscular dysplasia (FMD) (Rice & Armstrong, 2009)
   a. Has been found in all peripheral arteries; it occurs rarely in the upper extremity, it is more common in internal carotid artery, but may affect the vertebral arteries

   b. Long areas of smooth narrowing, intimal hyperplasia (not the usual "string of beads" as in renal FMD) with subtypes of either intimal, medial, or perimedial dysplasia; intimal hyperplasia most common
   c. Usually asymptomatic but can lead to focal stenosis and dilation, may cause a variance in blood pressure between limbs, or ischemia
   d. Limited data; seems to affect women more than men
   e. Diagnosed by angiogram (Eskandari et al., 2012)
   f. Treatment reserved for symptomatic patients
4. Vasospastic disorders (e.g., Raynaud disease): symptoms of pallor alternating with cyanosis and hyperemia of the fingers are related to episodic vasospasm (see Chapter 17, Raynaud Phenomenon)

B. Acute Arterial occlusion caused by embolus, thrombus, or trauma causes tissue perfusion to drop below a critical threshold level, which in turn causes persistent pain and tissue necrosis

1. Limb pressure <30 mm Hg
2. No Doppler signal in the digital vessels (Eskandari et al., 2012)

C. Neurovascular compression of neurovascular bundle supplying the upper extremity and/or compression of the subclavian vasculature (arterial or venous) is referred to as thoracic outlet syndrome (see Chapter 18, Thoracic Outlet Syndrome)

D. Aneurysms of Axillosubclavian Systems and Distal Arteries in the forearm or hand (Magishi, Izumi, & Shimizu, 2010)

1. Rare; data limited but have common features
2. Rupture rare, but usually fatal when rupture occurs
3. Depending on size, rate of expansion, and location of aneurysm, may have symptoms of nerve, tracheal, esophageal, or venous compression
4. Treated to prevent distal embolization and thrombosis. Most threatening aspect of aneurysms is the tendency for emboli or thrombus to cause end-organ ischemia and infarction

E. Congenital or Acquired Arteriovenous Fistulae or Malformations; direct communication between an artery and vein tend to enlarge over time

1. Congenital malformations; several types of lesions
   a. Arteriovenous fistulae
   b. Tumor-like growths (e.g., hemangiomas: arterial, venous, capillary, or mixed; also termed cavernous hemangioma)
   c. Angiodysplasias: various forms of abnormal growth of vessels
   d. Benign and malignant tumors: hemangiosarcomas, lymphosarcomas, and any large vessel tumors
2. Acquired arteriovenous fistulae: hemodialysis fistulae or trauma, including iatrogenic injuries (see Chapter 15, Vascular Access)

F. Degenerative Arteriopathies: Congenital or Acquired

1. Abnormalities in collagen or elastic tissue of vessel wall
2. May result in aneurysm formation or dissection of arteries in upper extremity (e.g., Marfan syndrome)

III. Etiology/Precipitating Factors

A. Emboli/Thrombus: thromboemboli of the upper extremity can occur from a variety of sources (Mowlavi, 2012; Weinberg, 2011); however, Licht, Balezantis, Wolff, Baudier, and Røder (2004) found that in 37% of acute ischemic cases, the cause was unknown

1. Most often originate from the heart or great vessels
2. Site can be left atrium, as in atrial fibrillation, or from injured ventricular endothelium after myocardial infarction
3. Other cardiac conditions predisposing to emboli: cardiomyopathy, congestive heart failure (CHF), rheumatic valvular disease, cardioversion, prosthetic valves, cardiac surgery or catheterization, vegetations associated with endocarditis and atrial myxoma
4. May be precipitated by progressive arterial atherosclerosis similar to lower extremity disease
5. Other noncardiac etiologies of emboli: aneurysm of ascending aorta, arch, subclavian artery, complicated aortic plaques, sepsis, peripherally inserted arterial lines, or percutaneous procedures

B. Atherosclerosis

1. Similar etiology to lower extremity or cerebrovascular atherosclerosis
2. Exact cause remains undefined but related to known risk factors: smoking, hypertension, hyperlipidemia, sedentary life style, obesity, diabetes mellitus, age, male gender, and heredity
3. Considerably less common than in lower extremities (Eskandari, 2012)
4. Confined predominantly to the origins of the vessels
5. Lesions may be stenotic or occlusive
6. Symptomatic upper extremity arterial occlusive disease is present in less than 5% due to the abundant collateral network and the infrequency of atherosclerosis in the upper extremity (Eskandari, 2012). Upper extremity claudication may manifest as tired, heavy or painful limb, with or without cyanosis of digits (see IV Assessment, C. Patient History, 1. Subjective findings)
7. Most common site of occlusion is the left subclavian artery, causing a subclavian steal
   a. Blood flow to arm is maintained via reversal of flow through left vertebral artery
   b. Right vertebral flow enters Circle of Willis; blood is directed to basilar artery and then into vertebral on left
   c. Patients seldom have cerebral symptoms (vertigo, visual disturbances or drop attacks) unless there is co-existing carotid stenosis
   d. Collateral flow to left arm usually limits ischemic symptoms but patients are at risk for embolization to digits

C. Traumatic Vessel Wall Injury: leading cause of upper extremity ischemia

1. Result of acute trauma or repetitive motion trauma: penetrating or blunt injuries, crush injuries, frostbite, procedures that require an arterial puncture
   a. Penetrating injuries: gunshot or knife wounds, lacerations
   b. Blunt injuries: clavicular fractures, shoulder or elbow dislocations, humeral fractures
   c. Crutches: prolonged use may lead to axillary artery trauma, thrombosis, or aneurysm formation

2. Acute traumatic vessel injuries need to be rapidly diagnosed and treated to prevent limb loss or death secondary to hemorrhage (Higgin & McClinton, 2010)
   a. Compartment syndrome: elevated intracompartmental pressures caused by acute swelling within osteofascial compartments in response to sudden injury or reperfusion following intervention (see Chapter 9, Lower Extremity Arterial Disease)
3. Chronic vibration trauma secondary to prolonged use of vibratory tools (e.g., jackhammer or chainsaw) (Eskandari et al., 2012)
   a. Pathologic changes in small arteries: hypertrophy of the intima and media, smooth muscle cells, sympathetic overactivity, and endothelial damage (Shepherd, 2005)
   b. Increased blood viscosity (reason unclear)
   c. Changes result in vessel narrowing, lumen obstruction, vasospasm, and thrombosis
   d. Similar small vessel problems are also seen in typists, piano players, baseball and hockey players, or any occupation or hobby that requires excessive use of hands
4. Hypothenar hammer syndrome: use of heel of hand to hammer, push, or twist objects leads to ulnar artery thrombosis or aneurysm formation with embolization and ischemia of digits (Mowlavi, 2012; Nitecki, Anekstein, Karram, Peer, & Bass, 2008)
5. Iatrogenic trauma to subclavian, axillary, brachial, or radial artery during diagnostic or therapeutic interventions (Soloway, 2013)
   a. Arterial thrombosis, hemorrhage, or embolization may result
   b. Cardiac catheterization by way of the brachial artery is common if patient has significant lower extremity atherosclerosis
   c. Bleeding into axilla following arteriography may lead to nerve compression
   d. May result from cannulation of the radial or brachial artery in the presence of an incomplete palmar arch
   e. Hand ischemia caused by dialysis access grafts: surgical injury, embolization, pseudoaneurysm formation, infection or mycotic aneurysm at anastomosis sites
6. Post-traumatic pain syndrome and neuropathies (Gradl & Rommel, 2007)
   a. Reflex sympathetic dystrophy (RSD) and post-traumatic pain syndrome
      1) Severe pain syndrome following trauma, often with peripheral nerve injury and/or ischemia as inciting event. Exact cause may be difficult to identify
      2) Three stages of RSD (symptoms vary and do not always progress):
         a) Acute stage: burning, redness, swelling, sweating, and extreme tenderness; reversible; may resolve spontaneously
         b) Dystrophic stage: coolness, cyanosis, brawny edema, continuous pain
         c) Atrophic stage: increased severity of pain affecting other limbs or body areas, skin atrophy, muscle wasting, digital ulcerations, advanced demineralization of bones with joint contractures and ankylosis
      3) Mimics nerve entrapments, Raynaud syndrome, arterial ischemia, thoracic outlet syndrome
      4) May respond to sympathetic nerve block, antidepressants (amitriptyline) or antiseizure medication (gabapentin)

b. Ischemic monomelic neuropathy: rare; pain syndrome associated with acute ischemic injury to arm manifested as "multiple axon-loss mononeuropathies distally in the limb without muscle necrosis" (Andary, Mahal, & O'Conner, 2011)
   1) Most often seen in diabetic renal failure patients after insertion of hemodialysis graft
   2) Symptoms: numbness, dysesthesias, burning continuous pain with mild motor weakness and loss of coordination; symptoms persist even after correction of cause for ischemia

D. Inflammatory or Immune Arteritis (see Pathophysiology)

1. Classified according to small, medium, or large vessel involvement
2. Small vessel arteritis (Mitchell & Schoen, 2010)
   a. Etiology thought to be autoimmunity for most disorders
   b. Frequently associated with rheumatoid disorders (e.g., systemic lupus erythematosus, rheumatoid arthritis, dermatomyositis, mixed connective tissue disorders, scleroderma)
   c. Erythema nodosum or hypersensitivity angiitis may develop spontaneously or be related to other systemic disorders
   d. Medications or circulating factors such as cryoglobulins, hepatitis A or B antigens, or tumor antigens may precipitate vasculitis manifested by arterial thickening, connective tissue swelling, and vascular occlusion
   e. Skin and joints most often involved; fingers and hands most often affected but entire limb may be symptomatic
   f. Signs and symptoms: urticaria, rashes, livedo, purpura, Raynaud phenomenon, hemorrhage, infarction, ulceration, gangrene
3. Medium vessel arteritis (Mitchell & Schoen, 2010)
   a. Polyarteritis nodosa: idiopathic and autoimmune focal, transmural inflammation of small and medium vessels which may lead to necrosis, thrombosis, and aneurysm formation; predominately affects renal and visceral vessels such as hepatic and mesenteric circulation; affects older patients; affects males twice as often as females (Mitchell & Schoen, 2010)
   b. Other diseases which rarely affect upper extremity: Wegener granulomatosis, Kawasaki disease, Churg–Strauss syndrome cause necrosis and gangrene of skin and may be associated with neuropathy
4. Large vessel and giant cell arteritis (Mitchell & Schoen, 2010)
   a. Takayasu arteritis: focal granulomatous and nongranulomatous inflammation involving entire vessel wall thickness with disruption of elastic fibers; usually involves aorta and branches; both stenoses and aneurysms common, subclavian artery most common site of stenosis; affects younger (<40 years) Asian women with 6:1 female:male ratio (Roberts, Rossmann, & Ahmed, 2011)
   b. Temporal or systemic giant cell arteritis: similar pathology to Takayasu but generally less severe; most commonly involves branches of carotid but can affect any vessel; usually affects women >50 years (Mowlavi, 2012; Ramachandran & Ramachandran, 2012)
   c. Usual symptoms: arm claudication, rest pain, skin breakdown; aneurysm of brachiocephalic vessels
   d. Other conditions: Behcet syndrome, Cogan syndrome, relapsing polychondritis, and other arthropathies

E. Buerger Disease (Thromboangiitis Obliterans): disease entity with features of severe atherosclerosis and inflammatory changes of distal vessels (Arkkila, 2006; Higgin & McClinton, 2010) (see II, Pathophysiology, and Chapter 16, Buerger Disease)

1. Initially affects small and medium vessels, then large vessels, as well as veins and nerves
2. Rarely has systemic manifestations; only affects blood vessels of extremities
3. Superficial thrombophlebitis and venous changes usually only involve lower extremities
4. Clinical features of atherosclerosis but more severe; gangrene with amputation (both surgical and auto-amputation) of digits, hands, and arms not unusual
5. Cause is unknown but tobacco use plays a critical role
6. Affects predominately young men of 35 years or below

F. Aneurysms (Menard & Belkin, 2009)

1. Relatively rare
2. Brachiocephalic: atherosclerosis, trauma or infection
   a. Prior to antibiotics, mycotic aneurysms related to syphilis were the most common type; now source of infection is IV drug use or infected arterial puncture
   b. Less common etiologies: FMD, medial degeneration, arteritis, congenital
3. Axillosubclavian: etiology predominately from atherosclerotic changes or traumatic injury, especially first rib trauma; remainder related to lesser causes
   a. Chronic injury from cervical rib or fibrous band at thoracic outlet
   b. Improper crutch use
   c. Aberrant right subclavian artery
   d. Other less common etiologies: FMD, arteritis, infection, medial degeneration, arteritis, congenital anomalies
   e. 30% to 50% of patients with axillary aneurysms have other associated aneurysms
4. Other distal sites: rare and related to trauma, infection, or dialysis access

G. Genetic Degenerative Arteriopathies result from an imbalance of elastin and the lack of collagen in the vessel walls as the aneurysm grows (Mitchell & Schoen, 2010)

1. Marfan syndrome
   a. High incidence of aortic dilatation, dissection, and rupture; high mortality without early surgical intervention
   b. Aneurysms of proximal major upper extremity vessels may occur
2. Ehlers–Danlos syndrome: rare; arteries occlude by rupture with thrombosis or aneurysm with embolization; affects younger patients; diagnosed by clinical presentation involving skin, eyes, and musculoskeletal defects
3. Pseudoxanthoma elasticum: rare; chronic occlusion of the forearm, thigh, and calf arteries with skin changes

H. Hypercoagulable State (see Chapter 19, Superficial Thrombophlebitis and Deep Vein Thrombosis)

1. Most commonly an inherited disorder that causes intravascular coagulopathy (Factor V Leiden mutation or prothrombin gene mutation) or

dysproteinemia (Protein C or S); also problematic for patients with thrombocytosis or polycythemia (Mitchell, 2010)

2. May have history of DVT or other manifestations of clotting disorder
3. Increased risk in patients with malignancy; cause uncertain

IV. Assessment

A. Risk Factors (usually related to risk of inflammation and/or thrombus production)

1. Personal history of atrial fibrillation, CHF, recent myocardial infarction, recent cardiac surgical intervention
2. Recent arterial diagnostic or monitoring procedure
3. History of atherosclerosis, previous graft problems, or infections
4. Cardiac valve prosthesis
5. Social history of injection of drugs
6. Occupational history of repetitive trauma to the hand by blunt or vibratory mechanisms or high-risk occupations for limb trauma (e.g., farmer or lumberjack)
7. Risk factors for atherosclerosis: tobacco use, hypertension, diabetes, lipid disorders, male gender, advancing age, heredity, obesity
8. Sensitivity to cold, familial history of connective tissue disorders or hypercoagulable disorders
9. Hemodialysis with upper extremity arteriovenous fistula
10. Personal history of irradiation

B. Primary Prevention

1. Smoking cessation
2. Blood pressure and lipid control
3. Public education
   a. Awareness of risk factors
   b. Promotion of a healthy lifestyle; weight management, exercise
   c. Risks of occupational exposure to blunt or vibratory mechanisms of trauma
4. Professional college education: appropriate technique for arterial puncture and care of catheters, as well as cannulation of dialysis access grafts
5. Assess for presence of risk factors
6. Familial coagulation studies if positive family history

C. Patient History

1. Subjective findings: influenced by level and severity of stenosis and occlusion and presence of arterial collaterals
   a. Claudication: arm fatigue, pain or cramping with exercise
   b. Rest pain involving the hand or digits
   c. Color changes in arm or hand
   d. Acute or chronic arm pain
   e. Arm and/or hand feel cold intermittently or continuously
   f. History of trauma
2. Objective findings
   a. Fever
   b. Unequal blood pressures in arms

   c. Signs of trauma to arm or hand
   d. Family history of hypercoagulable state
   e. Recent MI, CHF, coronary or valve surgery
   f. Medication history: use of vasoconstrictors, ergot alkaloids, dopamine
3. Social history
   a. Occupation: repetitive lifting, use of vibratory equipment, high risk for traumatic injury
   b. Tobacco use: duration, amount per day, type
   c. Illicit drug use
   d. Social support system and living situation, especially if at risk for amputation

D. Physical Examination

1. Inspection of affected upper extremity
   a. Skin: cool, mottled, blanching, erythema or purple discoloration of arms and or fingers; fingers may have ulcerative lesions or gangrene; punctate lesions on fingertips; tight, shiny, or atrophic skin on fingers and arms
   b. Cardiovascular: prominent arm veins, supra- or infraclavicular pulsatile mass; if there is trauma bleeding will be observed and must be controlled
   c. Neuro: loss of sensation and movement in affected extremity
   d. Upper extremity: muscle atrophy, swelling, or edema
   e. Measurement of upper arm circumferences
2. Palpation of the upper extremity
   a. Pulses in the carotid, axillary, brachial, radial, and ulnar arteries should be palpated; assess for pulsatile mass or enlarging hematoma over vessel
   b. Note pulse strength, tortuosity of the vessel, and any aneurysmal dilation of the artery
   c. An Allen test will indicate patency of the palmar arch: radial and ulnar arteries are compressed while patient clenches fist to empty blood from hand; hand is opened and appears pale and mottled. If palmar arch patent, release of pressure over one vessel restores normal color immediately; if radial artery diseased, color does not return until ulnar artery released; if ulnar artery diseased, color returns when radial artery released
   d. Adson maneuver (loss of radial pulse upon abduction and external rotation of the upper extremity and/or rotation of the head to the ipsilateral side) for thoracic outlet obstruction. Maybe used in assessing for thoracic outlet syndrome; however, not a strong indicator (see Chapter 18, Thoracic Outlet Syndrome) (Eskandari et al., 2012)
   e. Presence and amount of edema
   f. Skin color, temperature, capillary refill of the digits
   g. Tight, swollen upper extremity may be an indication of compartment syndrome; compartment pressure may need to be measured
3. Auscultation
   a. Blood pressure measurements in both upper extremities
   b. Should be performed over the subclavian, axillary, and brachial arteries to reveal bruits which indicate areas of stenosis (Eskandari et al., 2012)
   c. Cardiac: murmur, rub, arrhythmia
   d. Pulmonary: breath sounds; rales, diminished lung sounds, pleural friction rub
   e. Dialysis grafts: presence of appropriate bruit

4. Complete physical examination (especially cardiac and lower extremity) to assess for presence of systemic atherosclerosis, infection, or inflammatory disease as indicated

E. Considerations Across the Lifespan

1. Young adulthood: contact sports, illicit drug injection, congenital anomalies, cardiomyopathy, CHF
2. Women of childbearing age: hypercoagulable disorder, cardiac arrhythmias, illicit drug use, planned pregnancy if using warfarin for anticoagulation, pregnancy-induced CHF or cardiomyopathy, increase in autoimmune diseases in this age group
3. Elderly: cardiac arrhythmias, subtherapeutic warfarin doses secondary to poor nutritional status or multiple drug interactions, trauma from falls, incidence of atherosclerosis increases with advancing age (Eskandari et al., 2012)

V. Pertinent Diagnostic Testing

A. Laboratory Tests

1. Chest x-ray
   a. Important to identify enlarged heart, heart failure
   b. Prominent lung markings
   c. Atelectasis, infiltrates or effusions associated with CHF
   d. Bony structure anomalies or injuries causing vascular compression
2. Electrocardiogram
   a. Assesses for arrhythmia or MI
   b. If arrhythmia new, will need to be evaluated for possible MI
3. Echocardiogram: assesses for valve disease, cardiac enlargement and chamber function
4. Transesophageal echocardiography (TEE) is performed in patients with a peripheral embolus suspected of originating from a cardiac source. TEE can be used to assess plaque in the ascending aorta as a source of the emboli or determine the presence of a right-to-left shunt through which paradoxical emboli might travel (Eskandari et al., 2012)
5. Complete blood cell count (CBC), platelet count, sedimentation rate, antinuclear antibody (ANA), rheumatoid factor for possible inflammatory or infectious origin, disease-directed laboratories as appropriate
6. Preoperative laboratories for acute ischemia or trauma: CBC, electrolytes, type and crossmatch, consider troponin, creatine kinase, and urine myoglobin if patient has been immobile for a prolonged period of time
7. Hypercoagulable workup: CBC with platelet count, fibrinogen, prothrombin level, partial thromboplastin level, protein C deficiency, protein S deficiency, factor V Leiden mutation, prothrombin gene mutation, antithrombin III deficiency, antiphospholipid antibody/anticardiolipin antibody, and homocysteine level
8. Laboratory evaluation for atherosclerosis: glucose, lipid profile, creatinine and blood urea nitrogen, electrolytes, urinalysis, calcium, phosphorus, possibly homocysteine, high-sensitivity C-reactive protein

B. Noninvasive Vascular Laboratory Studies; perform on both arms for comparison (Gerhard-Herman et al., 2006)

1. Segmental arterial pressures
   a. Pressures taken in the brachial, radial, ulnar, and palmar arch vessels
   b. Pressure in one arm compared to pressure in opposite arm
   c. An abnormally large pressure gradient (>20 mm Hg) between any two segments indicates disease (Eskandari et al., 2012)
   d. Wrist/brachial Index <0.65 begin to be symptomatic
2. Finger pressures
   a. Finger cuff used, with a Doppler probe to measure systolic pressure
   b. An absolute finger pressure <70 mm Hg is considered abnormal (Mowlavi, 2012)
3. Doppler flow studies
   a. Subclavian, axillary, brachial, radial, ulnar, and digital arteries may be examined and analog waveforms recorded at each site
   b. Waveforms will change from triphasic to blunted or monophasic at the level of obstruction
   c. May perform Allen test while obtaining waveforms to document palmar arch status and vessel dominance or evidence of thoracic outlet obstruction respectively (see IV Assessment, palpation)
   d. Duplex scanning will aid in diagnosis of the more proximal vessels.
4. Duplex and color flow scanning
   a. Color flow scanning facilitates more accurate identification and location of vessels as well as visualization of aneurysms, pseudoaneurysms, or arteriovenous malformations
   b. Arterial flow is normally red; venous flow is blue
   c. Absence of color in an artery clearly visualized on B-mode scanning is diagnostic of occlusion; a color shift from red to white identifies stenotic sites with turbulent flow (Eskandari, 2012) (see Fig. 10-1)
   d. Hemodialysis graft flow with Doppler velocity recordings from the proximal anastomosis to the distal and measurements of vein diameter. Assessment of the inflow and outflow vessels and allows anatomic visualization (Eskandari, 2012)

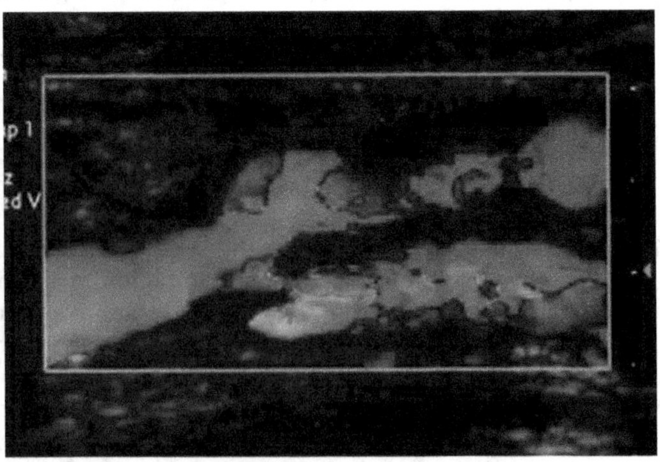

FIGURE 10-1. Arterial duplex.

C. Invasive Tests: Angiography

1. Gold standard for evaluation of upper extremity ischemia, trauma, arteritis, or occlusive disease (Mowlavi, 2012)
   a. Complete arteriography of both upper extremities is necessary to establish the diagnosis and plan an effective treatment
   b. The arteries to the upper extremity must be clearly visualized, beginning with the arch and extending to the digits. Magnification produces detailed studies of the hand (Eskandari et al., 2012)
      1) Plaque, occlusions, emboli, aneurysms, traumatic injuries, arteriovenous malformations, and vasospasm visualized
      2) Arteritis of aortic arch and major vessels shows individual or multiple areas of stenosis with no plaque or ulcerations
2. Additional techniques used to improve visualization of small digital arteries
   a. Hand warming
   b. Use of intra-arterial injection of vasodilators to prevent vasospasm which may occur at time of contrast injection
   c. Primary Raynaud disease (vasospastic hypersensitivity) may be distinguished from secondary Raynaud phenomenon (vasospasm)
   d. Collagen vascular disease: bilateral distal lesions with no findings of atherosclerotic changes; smooth, string-like arteries with or without segmental lesions; collateral circulation has corkscrew appearance
3. Provides the surgeon and interventionist a map with which to plan his intervention, as well as identification of collaterals and distal vessel status
4. Visualization of aortic arch and branches is very important to identify proximal lesions, aneurysms, and plaque
5. May perform maneuvers to evaluate thoracic outlet compression during examination
6. Transfemoral route with use of the Seldinger technique is preferred
7. Allows for the ability to immediately intervene on a lesion using a variety of endovascular techniques—angioplasty, atherectomy, and/or stent

D. Special Procedures (see Chapter 5, Vascular Diagnostic Studies)

1. Chest radiography and cervical spine views reveal a cervical rib or abnormality of the first rib in patients with thoracic outlet syndrome
2. Alternatively, computer tomography angiography (CTA) imaging with three-dimensional reconstruction can be used and is less invasive than angiogram (Eskandari et al., 2012)
3. Magnetic resonance angiography (MRA): gives fully longitudinal and cross-sectional view of the vasculature, much less invasive. MRA may be considered if exposure to contrast dyes or ionizing radiation is of concern; however, it is contraindicated in renal failure persons on dialysis (White et al., 2010)
4. Temporal artery biopsy is the gold standard for diagnosis of temporal and giant cell arteritis

VI. Nonoperative Management of Upper Extremity Arterial Occlusive Disease

A. Medical Management

1. Treatment of vasospasm (see Chapter 17, Raynaud Phenomenon)
   a. Remove external stimulus; avoid cold stimuli

b. Wear gloves, keep extremities warm
c. Warm baths
d. Oral calcium channel blockers
   1) Consider use if symptoms interfere with daily activity, employment, or if digital lesions occur
   2) Minimal effectiveness is reported; therapy is nonspecific
   3) Nifedipine (10 mg PO t.i.d) is used in patients with vasospastic disease of the hand. If this is not tolerated, prazosin at low dose may be tried. A third-line drug with some effectiveness is hydralazine (Eskandari et al., 2012)
   4) Side effects: headache, dizziness, flushing, palpitations, edema, dyspepsia, pruritus
e. Lifestyle changes (Eskandari et al., 2012)
   1) Keep skin from drying or fissuring
   2) Move to warm climate
   3) Avoid severely air conditioned environments
   4) Avoid trauma from work or hobbies

2. Protection from injury
   a. Avoid continued occupational trauma
   b. Caution with athletic injuries; especially hyperabduction
   c. Careful, appropriate insertion of intra-arterial catheters for diagnostic or therapeutic procedures: use of larger vessels whenever possible, femoral artery rather than brachial or axillary, to avoid arterial and nerve injury
   d. Avoid tight casts, prolonged tourniquets, and circumferential dressings
   e. Rehabilitation efforts for illicit drug use
3. Treatment of systemic diseases
   a. Standard medical management of underlying diseases related to atherosclerosis, antihypertensives, lipid lowering agents, diabetes management
   b. Emboli management (see below for additional interventions): long-term oral anticoagulation is recommended in patients with a cardiac source. A normalized ratio (INR) of 2 to 3 is recommended (Eskandari et al., 2012)
      1) Immediate anticoagulation with a parenteral low-molecular-weight heparin or factor Xa inhibitor, such as enoxaparin and others, if no contraindication
      2) Short- and long-term anticoagulation include warfarin or ab oral factor Xa inhibitor (fondaparinux, rivaroxaban, apixaban, or others), if no contraindication
      3) Identify and treat source of emboli
      4) Microemboli to digits: immediate anticoagulation and conservative measures; identify and treat source
   c. Aspirin or clopidogrel as anti-platelet therapy for emboli off the ascending aorta
   d. Regional sympathetic blockade for RSD and causalgia
   e. Steroid therapy for systemic inflammatory diseases such as Takayasu arteritis and giant cell arteritis. Immunosuppression with methotrexate or cyclophosphamide (Cytoxan) may be necessary (Eskandari et al., 2012)
4. Pain management as indicated

B. Interventional Management (European Society of Cardiology [ESC], 2011)

1. Thrombolytic therapy (see Chapter 20, Pulmonary Embolism for thorough discussion)
   a. Role in primary treatment and as adjunct to surgery: restores flow and allows for visualization of underlying lesion
   b. Dissolves a clot at its origin by way of a catheter-directed approach
   c. Serious complications are usually rare
   d. Limited by potential for serious hemorrhage, increased potential for compartment syndrome, and increased possibility of vasospasm
2. Percutaneous angioplasty
   a. Direct dilation of an artery with a catheter-directed balloon
   b. Transfemoral route preferable
   c. Suboptimal results can be improved with the use of an intra-arterial stent
3. Percutaneous atherectomy
   a. Uses laser energy to remove plaque along the intimal arterial wall
   b. Decreases perforation and thermal injury to the treated vessels
   c. Often used with other percutaneous endovascular procedures
   d. More commonly used for lower extremity disease
4. Intravascular stents and stent grafts
   a. Assist in keeping arteries patent after balloon dilation
   b. Longer segments of stenosis can now be treated with stent grafts
   c. Limited studies in upper extremity disease

VII. Operative Management of Upper Extremity Arterial Occlusive Disease

A. Arterial Bypass: traditional for atherosclerotic disease (ESC, 2011)

1. Treatment for significant proximal arterial occlusive lesions and chronic distal lesions
2. Bypass proximal lesions with prosthetic graft; optimal because of approximate size match and proven long-term patency
3. Bypass chronic distal lesions with reversed saphenous vein; proven long-term patency rate
4. Local endarterectomy may be used for focal stenosis
5. Sympathectomy occasionally used as adjunct to bypass when ischemia is severe and small, distal vessels are obstructed
   a. Its role is controversial
   b. Used for patients with underlying connective tissue disease
   c. Provides relief for a limited time, from 6 to 12 months (Eskandari et al., 2012)
6. Aneurysms
   a. Resection with interposition graft
   b. Infected aneurysm or pseudoaneurysm: resection with ligation of proximal and distal vessels without grafting if collateral circulation is adequate
   c. Rarely, extra-anatomic bypass with reversed saphenous vein needed
7. Risks include postoperative hemorrhage, hematoma, graft occlusion, ischemia, phrenic or recurrent nerve injury, brachial plexus or peripheral nerve injury, wound infection, emboli, compartment syndrome, impaired motor

and/or sensory function in the arm or hand, and chronic pain (Eskandari et al., 2012)

B. Thromboembolectomy

1. Operative intervention of choice for acute arterial occlusion secondary to embolic event
2. An arteriotomy is done, followed by removal of the thrombotic debris with a balloon catheter
3. May require systemic heparinization post operatively
4. May alternatively do endarterectomy with patch angioplasty

C. Arterial Resection with Interposition Graft

1. Used for proximal subclavian artery aneurysms or injuries
2. Also indicated for patients with aneurysms in distal arteries of the forearm or hand from occupational trauma

D. Primary Repair of the Artery

1. Used in those patients with laceration trauma or iatrogenic injuries
2. These injuries need prompt repair to prevent fatal hemorrhage
   a. Apply direct pressure to control bleeding
   b. Do not remove penetrating objects or foreign bodies until the patient is stabilized and evaluated
   c. If fatal hemorrhage appears likely, use emergent direct clamping proximal and distal of wound
   d. In operating room, a large vertical incision is needed to allow for proximal and distal control of vessel
   e. Clot should be extracted carefully to prevent fragmentation or embolization
3. Some injuries require vein-patch angioplasty to maintain the diameter of the vessel
4. Some traumatic injuries require extensive debridement prior to repair, such as gunshot wounds and contaminated penetrating injuries

VIII. Nursing Management

A. Alteration in Tissue Perfusion related to upper extremity occlusion as evidenced by diminished or absent upper extremity pulses, upper extremity pain, change in upper extremity color, and delayed digital capillary refill

1. Expected patient outcomes
   a. Patient will maintain upper extremity perfusion
2. Interventions
   a. Keep affected upper extremity in a neutral position; at the level of the heart
   b. Protect arm from further injury; avoid points of pressure for prolonged periods of time
   c. Avoid any circumferential dressings; if casts are necessary, inspect for tightness on a regular basis
   d. Continually assess the forearm for excessive tightness or swelling; this may be a sign of hematoma formation which could precipitate compartment syndrome
   e. Routine circulation, motor, and sensory checks are imperative

3. Evaluation
    a. Monitor circulation, motor function, and sensation to the affected extremity every 2 to 4 hours or as ordered by the provider
    b. Assess pulses and digital capillary refill in affected extremity with each assessment and p.r.n
    c. Monitor vital signs
    d. Observe for any sudden increase in pain or swelling, signs of bleeding, or signs of diminished circulation to the affected extremity

B. Alteration in Comfort, Pain Related to Upper Extremity Occlusive Disease

1. Expected patient outcomes
    a. Patient will be pain free
    b. Patient will be able to use the affected extremity with an acceptable level of pain
2. Interventions
    a. Maintain the affected extremity in a neutral position, in a position of comfort without any areas of pressure
    b. Mild swelling may be relieved by elevation
    c. Analgesia as needed
    d. Activity with upper extremity as tolerated; assist with ADLs as needed
3. Evaluation
    a. Assess pain using a 1 to 10 scale at least every 4 hours and as needed; reassess pain level 30 to 60 minutes after administration of analgesia
    b. Observe and record effectiveness of pain medicine; address provider if pain medicine does not seem to be ablating pain
    c. Notify provider of any sudden increase in pain, swelling, or tightness of affected extremity

C. Alteration in Skin Integrity Related to Surgical Incisions and/or Ischemic Ulcers

1. Expected patient outcomes
    a. Patient will exhibit wound healing without evidence of infection
    b. Patient and significant other will begin to assist with wound care and learn aseptic technique
2. Interventions
    a. Surgical wounds will be covered with a dry sterile dressing for 1 to 2 days postoperatively, or dermabond and no dressing
    b. Ischemic ulcers will need to be cleaned 2 to 4 times daily, gently debrided, and covered with a dressing
    c. Avoid tape to the skin
    d. Traumatic wounds should be kept clean
    e. Gangrenous wounds may need sharp debridement to aid in the healing process
    f. Avoid excessive moisture between the fingers by dressing with light dry dressings
3. Evaluation
    a. Assess for signs of wound closure and healing
    b. Assess for signs of infection, erythema, increased edema, or drainage
    c. Assess patient and significant other's ability to participate in wound care

D. Self-Care Deficit Syndrome related to poorly functioning upper extremity secondary to upper extremity arterial occlusive disease

1. Expected patient outcomes
   a. Patient will be able to participate in self-care
   b. Patient will maintain motor and sensory function of affected upper extremity
2. Interventions
   a. Allow patient to participate as much as possible in self-care activities; allow ample time to complete activities
   b. Occupational and physical therapy consult as soon as possible
   c. Assist patient and family in occupational and physical therapy activities as needed
3. Evaluation
   a. Assess for ability to participate in self-care activities
   b. Assess for sensory or motor impairment in affected extremity
   c. Assess for patient's ability to participate in occupational and physical therapy activities

IX. Patient Teaching

A. Disease Prevention, Health Promotion, and Secondary Prevention

1. Define upper extremity arterial occlusive disease to patient and significant others, explain why it occurred, and discuss patient's specific situation
2. Identify patient's risk factors and plans for modification of risk factors
3. Explain treatment goals
   a. Prevention of further ischemia and occlusive disease
   b. Maintenance of self-care activities, functional status
   c. Avoidance of complications related to therapy
4. Standardized anticoagulation teaching program
   a. Reason why patient will be on warfarin therapy; duration of therapy
   b. Side effects of medication; when to seek medical attention
   c. Importance of routine INR monitoring; with explanation of INR goal
   d. Interactions with other medications and foods
      1) No ASA unless prescribed by provider
      2) No over-the-counter medications unless prescribed by provider
      3) Dietary interactions; discuss foods high in vitamin K; possible dietary consult
   e. Information to patient: pamphlets, books, internet sites, videotape
5. Discuss signs and symptoms that the patient and family will need to look for and explain what to do
   a. Infection; increasing pain, erythema, warmth of the affected extremity: call provider
   b. Incisional dehiscence: call provider
   c. Bleeding:
      1) Major: call 911; go to the emergency department
      2) Minor: call provider
   d. Color change or increasing numbness of affected extremity: call provider

B. Home Care Considerations

1. Activity
   a. Continue occupational and physical therapy exercises as prescribed
   b. Maintain affected extremity in the neutral position
   c. Avoid any strenuous activity; no lifting with affected extremity
2. Diet
   a. Avoid foods high in vitamin K
   b. No alcohol while on narcotic analgesics
   c. No herbal remedies unless prescribed by provider
3. Safety precautions
   a. Avoid constrictive clothing on arm
   b. Protect the affected extremity from injury
   c. If extremity is sensory impaired; do not use any sharp objects, avoid extreme hot or cold
   d. Wear or carry identification that indicates warfarin therapy
   e. Seek immediate attention if a serious head injury is sustained
4. Call provider for
   a. Changes in incision line such as erythema, drainage, wound dehiscence
   b. Changes in the warmth or color of the affected extremity
   c. Changes in medication, diet, or missed medication dose
   d. Any new symptoms such as pain, swelling, or inability to perform self-care activities

CASE STUDY

CC: An 87-year-old female presented to your emergency room by ambulance from her private residence where she was found with a pulseless, cyanotic right arm. The patient is awake and alert.

HPI: Patient states that her right arm suddenly became painful and blue in a matter of a few minutes. She states that she has been doing well at home and denies recent illness. Her medications include warfarin and digoxin.

ROS: History of irregular heartbeat and she takes a blood thinner for this problem. She states that she gets her blood checked regularly, and her doctor adjusts her medicine as needed. The patient states that she has been slightly short of breath for the last few days and she hasn't been eating well. She has no history of myocardial infarction or stroke. According to family, she has been functioning well at home, but has been eating poorly for 2 to 3 weeks.

PE: Pulseless, cyanotic right hand, and pale right arm. The brachial pulse is not palpable, axillary pulse is palpable. There is sluggish capillary refill in the fingers; sensory and motor functions are intact. The patient relays that her hand feels numb. Heart rate is irregular, approximately 95 bpm. EKG shows atrial fibrillation, no signs of ischemia. Otherwise normal female on examination.

Review Questions

1. What pertinent positives in this patient's history and physical examination point to a diagnosis?
   a. History of atrial fibrillation
   b. Patient on warfarin with decreased appetite
   c. Sudden onset of pain and color change
   d. Absence of brachial pulse
   e. All of the above

2. What is the first intervention necessary in the care of this patient?
   a. IV anticoagulation
   b. Preoperative preparation of the patient and family
   c. Doppler studies
   d. BP in both arms

3. What teaching must be done with the patient and family regarding the heparin drip?
   a. Risks and benefits of heparin
   b. When to anticipate the initiation of warfarin therapy
   c. To notify the nurse or provider if any sign of bleeding is noted
   d. All of the above

4. What are the pertinent discharge teaching needs for this patient?
   a. Discussion of the effects and side effects of warfarin therapy
   b. Wound care needs
   c. Discussion of frequency and timing of INR monitoring
   d. Discussion of follow-up appointments with primary care and vascular surgery
   e. All of the above

5. The patient gets home and takes a shower. After her shower, she notices that the incision is bleeding. What should the patient do?
   a. Call 911
   b. Call her family
   c. Go see her primary care provider
   d. Call the vascular surgery office, describe the bleeding, and decide with the surgeon on call based on amount of bleeding

Answers/Rationale

1. e. All of these are pertinent positives in the patient's history and physical examination. They all put this patient at risk for embolization to the upper extremity. Patients with a history of atrial fibrillation, on warfarin with a decreased appetite, have an increased risk of having a sub-therapeutic international normalization ratio and embolizing to the upper extremity or any number of areas in the body. Also, the suddenness of the pain and color change point to an embolic event.

2. b. This patient needs to go to the operating room immediately for an embolectomy. The patient's history is consistent with an embolic event occurring, and an intraoperative angiography can be done if needed. This patient has a successful embolectomy. She returns to the vascular floor after surgery. The orders read to start her on a heparin drip 6 hours after returning to the floor. The heparin drip is initiated as ordered.

3. d. The patient and family need to understand why the patient is on heparin therapy, the therapeutic benefits of heparin, and the necessity of reporting side effects. The patient and family also need to understand that warfarin therapy will be reinitiated very soon after surgery, and that they will get further information about warfarin therapy while in the hospital. The patient progresses through the hospitalization without difficulty. The patient is transitioned to warfarin therapy and the heparin drip is discontinued. The patient is now getting ready to be discharged.

4. e. Patients and their families need to learn about warfarin therapy and be reminded of the blood draws necessary, even if they have had experience with warfarin before. Patients and families need reinforcement of previous teaching and need to build their knowledge base. Wound care and follow-up always need to be reinforced and reiterated at the time of discharge.

5. d. This patient may have only unroofed an incision, or since she is on warfarin, she may have significant bleeding. The vascular provider should be able to give this patient some guidance based on her description of the bleeding. If there is ever any question regarding how much bleeding a patient is experiencing, the patient should be seen in the nearest Emergency Department immediately.

REFERENCES

Andary, M. T., Mahal, B. S., & O'Conner, R. C. (2011). Ischemic monomelic neuropathy. *Emedicine/Medscape.* Retrieved from http://emedicine.medscape.com/article/315915-overview

Arkkila, P. (2006). Thromboangiitis obliterans (Buerger's disease). doi:10.1186/1750-1172-1-14. Retrieved from http://www.ncbi.nlm.nih.gov/pmc/articles/PMC1523324/

Eskandari, M. K. (2012). Upper extremity occlusive disease. *Medscape.* Retrieved from http://reference.medscape.com/article/462289-overview

Eskandari, M. K., Rowe, V. L., & Pearce, W. H. (revised 2012). Upper extremity venous occlusion disease. *Emedicine/Medscape.* Retrieved from http://emedicine.medscape.com/article/462289-overview

Espinoza, L. R. (2009). Buerger's disease: Thromboangiitis obliterans 100 years after the initial description. *The American Journal of the Medical Sciences, 337*(4), 285–286.

European Society of Cardiology (ESC) Task Force on the Diagnosis and Treatment of Peripheral Artery Diseases. (2011). ESC Guidelines on the diagnosis and treatment of peripheral artery diseases. *European Heart Journal, 32,* 2851–2906. doi:10.1093/eurheartj/ehr211. Retrieved from http://eurheartj.oxfordjournals.org/content/32/22/2851.full.pdf

Gerhard-Herman, M., Gardin, J. M., Jaff, M., Mohler, E., Roman, M., Naqvi, T. Z., ... Society of Vascular Medicine and Biology. (2006). Guidelines for noninvasive vascular laboratory testing: A report from the American Society of Echocardiography and the Society of Vascular Medicine and Biology. *Journal of the American Society of Echocardiography, 19,* 955–972. doi:10.1016/j.echo.2006.04.019. Retrieved from http://files.asecho.org/files/VascularGuidelines.pdf

Gradl, G., & Rommel, O. (2007). Early diagnosis in post-traumatic complex regional pain syndrome. *Orthopedics, 30,* 6. Retrieved from http://www.healio.com/orthopedics/journals/ortho/%7Bc7d66bb8-bc77-4af4-a375-30427e779a63%7D/early-diagnosis-in-post-traumatic-complex-regional-pain-syndrome

Higgin, J. P., & McClinton, M. A. (2010). Vascular insufficiency of the upper extremity. *Journal of Hand Surgery, 35,* 1545–1553.

Licht, P. B., Balezantis, T., Wolff, B., Baudier, J. F., & Røder, O. C. (2004). Long-term outcome following thrombembolectomy in the upper extremity. *European Journal of Vascular and Endovascular Surgery, 28*(5), 508–512. Retrieved from http://www.ncbi.nlm.nih.gov/pubmed/15465372

Magishi, K., Izumi, Y., & Shimizu, N. (2010). Short- and long-term outcomes of acute upper extremity arterial thromboembolism. *Annals of Thoracic and Cardiovascular Surgery, 16,* 31–34.

Menard, M. T., & Belkin, M. (2009). Chapter 34: Peripheral aneurysms. In J. W. Hallett, J. L. Mills, J. Earnshaw, J. A. Reekers, & T. Rooke (Eds.), *Comprehensive vascular and endovascular surgery* (2nd ed.). Philadelphia, PA: Elsevier.

Mitchell, R. N. (2010). Chapter 4: Hemodynamic disorders, thromboembolic disease, and shock. In V. Kumar, A. K. Abbas, N. Fausto, & J. C. Aster (Eds.), *Pathologic basis of disease* (8th ed., pp. 111–134). Philadelphia, PA: Saunders-Elsevier.

Mitchell, R. N., & Schoen, F. J. (2010). Chapter 11: Blood vessels. In V. Kumar, A. K. Abbas, N. Fausto, & J. C. Aster (Eds.), *Pathologic basis of disease* (8th ed., pp. 487–528). Philadelphia, PA: Saunders-Elsevier.

Mowlavi, A. (2012). Vascular occlusive syndromes of the upper extremity. *Emedicine/Medscape.* Retrieved from http://emedicine.medscape.com/article/1241088-overview

Nitecki, S., Anekstein, Y., Karram, T., Peer, A., & Bass, A. (2008). Hypothenar hammer syndrome: Apropos of six cases and review of the literature. *Vascular, 16*(5):279–282. Retrieved from http://www.medscape.com/viewarticle/586584

Ramachandran, T. S., & Ramachandran, A. (2012), Temporal/giant cell arteritis. *Emedicine/Medscape.* Retrieved from http://emedicine.medscape.com/article/1147184-overview

Rice, R. D., & Armstrong, P. J. (2009). Brachial artery fibromuscular dysplasia. *Annals of vascular surgery.* Philadelphia, PA: Elsevier. doi:10.1016/j.avsg.2009.05.012

Roberts, J. R., Rossmann, M. G., & Ahmed, M. M. (2011). Takayasu arteritis. *Emedicine/Medscape.* Retrieved from http://emedicine.medscape.com/article/332378-overview

Shepherd, R. F. (2005). Raynaud's syndrome: Vasospastic and occlusive arterial disease involving the distal upper extremity. In R. B. Rutherford (Ed), *Vascular surgery* (6th ed., pp. 1319–1346). Philadelphia, PA: Elsevier Saunders.

Soloway, B. (2013). Peripherally inserted central catheters confer risk for upper-extremity venous thromboembolism. *NEJM Journal Watch,* Reviewing Chopra V et al. Lancet 2013 May 20. Retrieved from http //www.jwatch.org/na31240/2013/06/07/peripherally-inserted-central-catheters-confer-risk-upper

Weinberg, I. (2011). Upper extremity embolism. Vascular medicine evidence-based reviews. Retrieved from http://www.angiologist.com/upper-extremity-embolism/

White, P. W., Gillespie, D. L., Feurstein, I., Aidinian, G., Phinney, S., Cox, M. W.... Fox, C. J. (2010). Sixty-four slice multidetector computed tomographic angiography in the evaluation of vascular trauma. *Journal of Trauma, 68*(1), 96–102.

RELEVANT WEBSITES

http://www.emedicine.com
http://www.svnnet.org
http://www.jvir.org/cgi/content/full/12/1/11
http://www.pvss.org/
http://www.vascularweb.org/Pages/default.aspx
http://www.annalsofvascularsurgery.com/
http://www.vivapvd.com/
http://www.snjourney.com/ClinicalInfo/Systems/PeriphVas.htm

CHAPTER 11

Cerebrovascular Disease

Karen Fitzgerald

OBJECTIVES

1. List three risk factors associated with cerebrovascular disease.
2. Recognize two diagnostic tests to evaluate for cerebrovascular disease.
3. Review two treatments for medical management for the patient with cerebrovascular disease.
4. List three nursing diagnoses for the patient following carotid endarterectomy and patient management.

Introduction/Overview

Carotid artery disease is a major cause of ischemic stroke, the risk of which is directly related to the severity of stenosis and presence of symptoms. Stroke is the third leading cause of death in the United States, with approximately three quarters of a million strokes per year. Stroke is the leading cause of functional impairment, with more than 20% of survivors requiring institutional care and up to one third having a permanent disability (White et al., 2008).

The mortality rate following a stroke ranges from 26% to 52%. According to the most recent American Heart Association statistics, it is estimated that stroke accounts for half of all hospital admissions for acute neurologic disease. In addition, 28% of annual stroke victims are under the age of 65. Although strokes may be caused by a variety of disease entities, atherosclerosis is the most common contributing factor (A to Z Stroke Guide, 2011).

I. Anatomy

A. Carotid Artery (see Fig. 11-1)

1. Anterior blood supply to the brain is provided by the carotid arteries. The right common carotid artery originates from the innominate artery (brachiocephalic trunk), which is the first major branch of the aortic arch.
2. Left common carotid artery originates directly from the arch.
3. Common carotid arteries bifurcate into the internal and external carotid arteries.
4. External carotid arteries lie anterior to the internal carotid artery and gives off numerous branches, which supply the face.

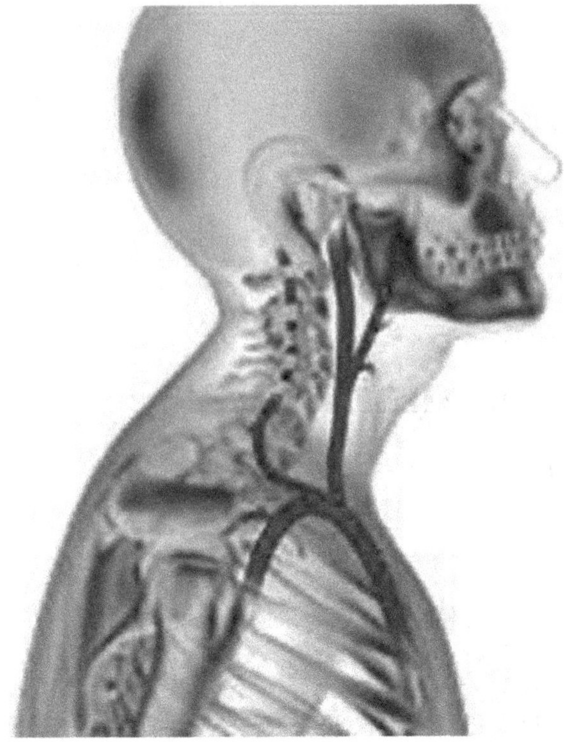

FIGURE 11-1. Carotid, vertebral, and subclavian arteries.

5. Internal carotid artery has no major branch until the ophthalmic artery, which gives rise to the superficial and deep circulation of the eye (Bradley & Pearce, 1999).

B. Vertebral Arteries—Originate from the subclavian arteries bilaterally and provides the posterior circulation.

C. Basilar Artery—Major blood supply to the anterior spinal artery, brain stem, thalamus, cerebellum, and occipital lobe.

D. Circle of Willis—Consists of the four extracranial vessels (two vertebral and two carotid arteries), which join at the base of the skull (Bradley & Pearce, 1999) (see Fig. 11-2).

II. Pathophysiology

A. Atherosclerosis

1. Most common cause of cerebrovascular disease in the United States for individuals 65 years and older (Sullivan & Hertzer, 1996)
2. A diffuse disease characterized by the development of fatty streaks, plaque formation and plaque necrosis, and calcification (Graham & Ford, 1999)
3. Over time, the artery walls thicken, harden, and lose their elasticity, causing a decrease blood flow through the artery and eventually an obstruction of flow (Graham & Ford, 1999)

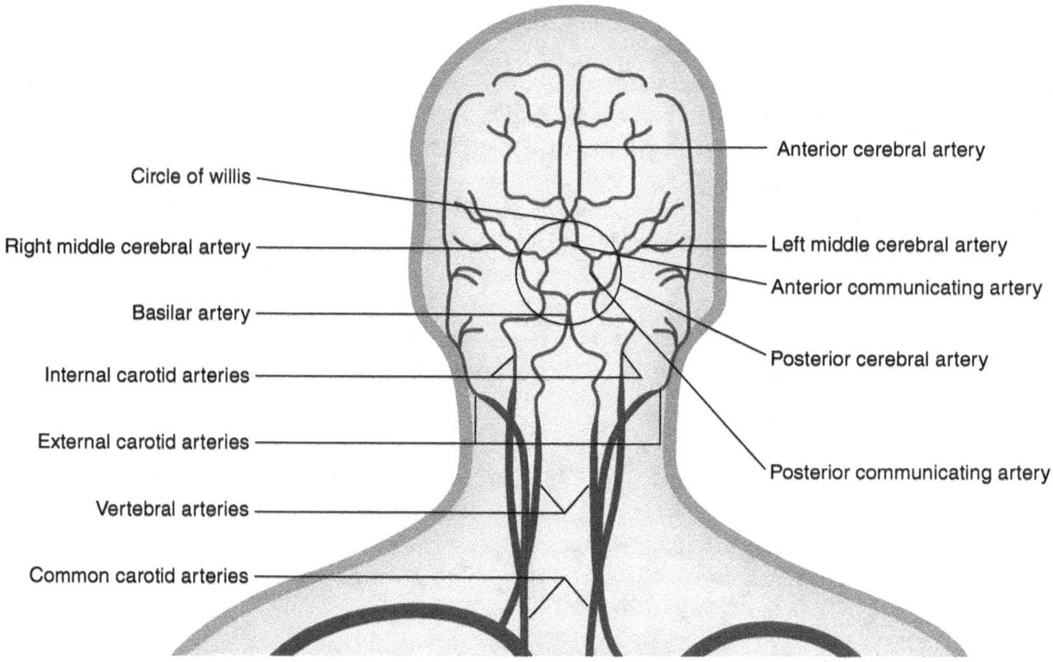

FIGURE 11-2. Carotid and cerebral circulation.

4. The lesions of atherosclerosis accumulate in large- and medium-sized arteries and seem best described by an inflammatory process that comprises a series of highly specific cellular and molecular reactions that lead to the accumulation of atherosclerotic plaque (Oppat & Graham, 2004)
5. Possible causes of inflammation are free radicals formed as by-products of smoking and diabetes, genetic malfunction of healing as might be seen in hyperhomocysteinemia, or infectious agents such as Chlamydia or other yet to be discovered organisms (Oppat & Graham, 2004)
6. The persistent inflammation within the vessel wall results in the accumulation of macrophages and lymphocytes in the vessel wall at the site of a fatty streak (Oppat & Graham, 2004)

B. Asymptomatic Disease

1. A patient with an asymptomatic 50% carotid stenosis has 1% to 2% per year risk of a stroke (Wiebers, Feigin, & Brown, 1997).
2. The risk of stroke is greatest for persons with neurologic symptoms such as transient ischemic attacks (TIAs), but is also increased in patients with asymptomatic lesions. The prevalence of hemodynamically significant carotid stenosis varies with age and other risk factors: population-based studies estimate that 0.5% of persons in their 50s and about 10% of those over 80 years have carotid stenosis greater than 50% (Wiebers et al., 1997).
3. Persons with asymptomatic stenoses are not only at increased risk for cerebrovascular accident, but also early detection can reduce morbidity due to cerebrovascular disease (Wiebers et al., 1997).

C. TIA

1. A TIA is a transient neurological deficit that lasts usually a few minutes. It occurs when the blood supply to part of the brain is briefly interrupted. TIA symptoms, which usually occur suddenly, are similar to those of stroke (Bradley & Pearce, 1999).
2. Symptoms of a TIA disappear within an hour, although they may persist for up to 24 hours (Bradley & Pearce, 1999).
3. Symptoms can include numbness or weakness in the face, arm, or leg, especially on one side of the body; confusion or difficulty in talking or understanding speech; trouble seeing in one or both eyes; and difficulty with walking, dizziness, or loss of balance and coordination (Bradley & Pearce, 1999).

D. Fibromuscular Dysplasia

1. Occurs primarily in White females and involves the larger arteries (renal, iliac, internal carotid arteries).
2. Usually bilateral, characterized by smooth muscle hyperplasia.
3. Internal carotid artery is most often affected, followed by the vertebral arteries (Graham & Ford, 1999).

E. Cervical Irradiation—External irradiation for malignant cervical lesions may damage the entire vessel wall and may accelerate atherosclerosis (Francfort, Smullens, Gallagher, & Fairman, 1989).

F. Carotid Dissection—Blunt trauma, sudden extension of the neck, or even paroxysms of coughing or vomiting may cause intimal tearing with subsequent carotid artery dissection (Spittell & Spittell, 1991).

G. Arteritis—Vasculitis of the giant cell type, often involving the aortic arch and its branches (e.g., Takayasu arteritis) (Bradely & Pearce, 1999).

III. Etiology/Precipitating Factors—Causes of arterial disease are varied. Atherosclerosis is the most common arteriopathy in the United States. A variety of nonatherosclerotic arterial diseases exist. These are less common and often less well defined than is atherosclerotic disease.

IV. Assessment

A. Risk Factors and Primary Prevention

1. A variety of risk factors have been found to influence the atherosclerotic process: age, sex, hereditary, smoking, hypertension, hyperlipidemia, sedentary lifestyle, obesity, diabetes mellitus, and stress (Gotto, 1986)
2. Risk Factor Modification
   a. Smoking cessation
   b. Control of hypertension
   c. Lipid management
   d. Diabetes management
   e. Healthy diet
   f. Regular exercise

B. Patient History—Symptoms vary according to the vessels involved. Timing is also important in the evaluation and classification of symptoms.

1. Subjective findings
   a. TIAs: transient neurologic deficits, which resolve within 24 hours
      1) Slurred or garbled speech or difficulty understanding others
      2) Amaurosis fugax—Ocular TIA: sudden blindness in part of visual field, sometimes as if a gray or black curtain is falling over or crossing visual field
      3) Dizziness, loss of balance, or loss of coordination
      4) Sudden weakness, an abnormal feeling, or paralysis in face, arm or leg, typically on one side of the body
   b. Completed stroke: deficits that persist and are permanent
2. Objective findings
   a. Internal Carotid Artery Stenosis
      1) Deficit whether temporary or permanent affecting one side of the body (hemiparesis, monoparesis, aphasia, dysarthria, monocular blindness). Lesions affect the ipsilateral side of the body.
      2) Ultrasound and/or radiological findings (see V, Pertinent Diagnostic Testing).
   b. Vertebrobasilar insufficiency (VBI)
      1) Atherosclerotic occlusive disease of the vertebral arteries is less common than in carotid system.
      2) Symptoms include dysarthria, global aphasia, diplopia, vertigo, syncope, dizziness, confusion, drop attacks (Bradley & Pearce, 1999).

C. Physical Examination

1. Inspection
   a. Neurological examination: check Cranial nerves (see Table 11-1)
   b. Ophthalmoscopic examination if patient complains of amaurosis fugax to evaluate for retinal emboli (Young, 1996)

TABLE 11-1 Cranial Nerves, Functions, and Impairments

Cranial Nerve	Function	Signs and Symptoms of Impaired Function
Facial (VII)	Movement of facial muscles, taste to anterior two thirds of tongue	Drooping of the corner of the lip on the ipsilateral side and inability to smile symmetrically, loss of taste
Glossopharyngeal (IX)	Tongue movement, taste to posterior third of tongue, palatal and pharyngeal movement	Mild dysphagia, loss of taste
Vagus (X)	Palatal, pharyngeal, and laryngeal movement	Dysphagia and dysphonia; associated with unilateral laryngeal anesthesia and depressed gag reflex
Spinal accessory (XI)	Sternocleidomastoid, trapezius muscle movement	Limitations in neck and shoulder movement in terms of alignment and horizontal motion
Hypoglossal (XII)	Tongue movement	Ipsilateral paresis and atrophy with or without fasciculations in one half of the tongue, dysarthria

2. Palpation
   a. The carotid pulse is palpated in the middle or lower neck between the trachea and the anterior border of the sternocleidomastoid muscle.
   b. Palpate each carotid artery separately.
   c. Check base of the neck and the supraclavicular fossa for pulsatile mass indicating an aneurysm or carotid body tumor (Young, 1996).
3. Auscultation
   a. Listen with bell of stethoscope for bruit.
   b. Carotid bruits are usually loudest in the upper third of the neck in the area of the carotid bifurcation.
   c. A bruit is an audible sound associated with turbulent blood flow created by a change in the diameter of the arterial lumen (Bradley & Pearce, 1999).
   d. Have the patient hold their breath, auscultate the carotid artery from the base of the neck to the angle of the jaw.
   e. If the sound intensifies, it probably originates in the heart or the subclavian artery; a diminished sound usually signifies the bruit originates in the carotid artery (Young, 1996).

D. Considerations Across the Lifespan

1. Young adulthood
   a. Consideration of risk factors, that is, smoking, cholesterol, hypertension, sedentary lifestyle, diet
   b. If risk factors are not controlled there is an increase stroke risk
   c. Fibromuscular dysplasia: most common in young women
2. Elderly
   a. Consideration of risk factors
   b. Age increases one's risk for atherosclerosis therefore increasing one's risk for carotid artery disease
   c. Screening high-risk patients

V. Pertinent Diagnostic Testing

A. Laboratory Testing

1. Complete blood count (CBC) and clotting profile if patient had TIA or stroke to assess for hypercoagulablity
2. Platelet activation is a key step in the development of cerebral ischemia due to atherosclerosis

B. Noninvasive Testing

1. Carotid duplex: uses high-frequency sound waves into the artery which are reflected by moving red blood cells. Identifies blood flow in the arteries
   a. Detects flow disturbances within the vessel (Blackburn & Kennedy, 1999)
   b. High accuracy of the duplex scan; many surgeons are performing surgery based solely upon the duplex scan itself
   c. Is generally the initial test for evaluating carotid stenosis
   d. Used for routine follow-up of the patient to detect recurrent stenosis after carotid endarterectomy (CEA) (Bradley & Pearce, 1999)

2. Magnetic Resonance Angiography (MRA)
    a. Provide anatomic images of blood vessels that can be projected in a format similar to that of conventional angiography and also provide physiologic information
    b. Is increasingly substituted for arteriography because it produces good depiction of blood vessels
    c. The initial test for evaluating the carotids is ultrasound which is a good screening test
    d. Many surgeons will now operate after ultrasound and/or MRA and forego arteriography
3. Computed Tomography (CT) Angiogram
    a. Imaging study utilizing noncontrast and IV contrast to identify specific anatomy of the aortic arch, carotid arteries, and intracerebral arteries
    b. May also be performed to identify those patients whose symptoms are due to tumors, hemangiomas, intracranial vascular disease, or subdural hematomas
    c. Also used to detect stroke and is used postoperatively for any neurologic complication (Bradley & Pearce, 1999)
4. Arteriography: invasive testing
    a. Contrast angiography is an effective method to demonstrate cerebrovascular stenosis (Jensen & Creager, 2003)
    b. Remains the gold standard for diagnosis of carotid and other cerebrovascular stenoses and occlusions (Jensen & Creager, 2003)
    c. In many centers, duplex ultrasonography, often combined with MRA, has replaced the need for most contrast angiograms (Jensen & Creager, 2003)

VI. Medical Management of Carotid Disease

A. Risk Factor Modification

1. Elimination of risk factors such as, smoking, diet, exercise, cholesterol, blood pressure, and diabetes management have a significant impact on the alleviation of symptoms
2. The patient's provider more than likely will recommend one of the following medical treatments prior to intervention such as angioplasty, stent, and/or surgery
3. Serial ultrasounds for progression of disease

B. Antiplatelet Therapy—Platelet activation is a key step in the development of cerebral ischemia due to atherosclerosis, and antiplatelet agents have proven useful therapeutic agents.

1. Aspirin
    a. Indications: prophylaxis for recurrent TIA and stroke due to atherosclerosis
    b. Aspirin in doses of 81 to 325 mg daily, alone or in combination with other agents have shown to have clinical efficacy in large multicenter trials
    c. The mechanism of action of aspirin is to reduce platelet aggregation by inhibiting platelet cyclo-oxygenase and preventing the formation of Thromboxane A2 (Jensen & Creager, 2003)

2. Clopidogrel (Plavix)
   a. Indications: reduction of atherosclerotic events (MI, stroke, and vascular death) in patients with atherosclerosis documented by a recent stroke or MI, or established peripheral artery disease
   b. Is a selective and irreversible inhibitor of ADP-induced platelet aggregation
   c. Normal dose: 75 mg daily (Nunnelee & Fotis, 2004)
3. Ticlopidine (Ticlid) (Discontinued brand in the United States)
   a. Indications: is a thienopyridine, chemically similar to clopidogrel. Not considered as a first-line antiplatelet for stroke prevention because of the side effects and cost. The most severe side effect is neutropenia
   b. Normal dose: 250 mg twice daily (Ticlid® product information, 2013)
4. Prasugrel (Effient)
   a. Indications: a thienopyridine, also chemically similar to clopidogrel that inhibits adenosine diphosphate binding to platelet receptors (a platelet aggregation inhibitor). Thrombocytopenia and bleeding are the most severe side effects; in fact, the bleeding risk is higher than with clopidogrel
   b. Use in caution in patients of 75 years or older secondary to uncertain risk of intracranial bleed and atrial fibrillation
   c. Normal dose: loading dose of 60 mg, then 10 mg daily (Effient® product information, 2013)

C. Anticoagulation

1. Warfarin
   a. Indications: thromboembolic disorders and events (deep vein thrombosis, pulmonary embolism, arterial thrombosis, embolism, arterial or venous graft failures, prosthetic valve, atrial fibrillation, coagulation disorders, cerebrovascular or extracranial carotid artery disease in patients of poor surgical risks; controversial)
   b. Drug of choice in the United States for oral anticoagulation
   c. Normal dose: individualized according to the International Normalized Ratio (INR) (Nunnelee & Fotis, 2004)

D. Interventional Therapies

1. Percutaneous Transluminal Angioplasty (PTA)
   a. Less invasive then surgery
   b. Since 1994, carotid angioplasty with stenting (CAS) has been investigated as an alternative treatment to CEA at multiple centers (Vitek, Roubin, Gishel, Al-Mubarek, & Iyer, 2000)
   c. Generally reserved for nonatherosclerotic lesions such as fibromuscular dysplasia and for patients who have had radiation to the cervical region
2. Carotid artery stenting
   a. Many types of vascular stents with different characteristics, in different stages of clinical use and FDA approval
   b. Patency rate with stenting has been slightly higher compared with angioplasty alone
   c. Candidates include patients with restenosis, previous neck surgery, or radiation on affected side
   d. Patients are put on antiplatelet therapy pre- and postprocedure (Vitek et al., 2000)

VII. Surgical Management

A. CEA—Currently the most frequently performed vascular surgical procedure in the United States. The goal of this surgery is stroke prevention.

1. Overall morbidity and mortality rate is 3% nationally
2. Considered safe for patients with lesions >70%

B. Surgical Procedure

1. CEA (see Fig. 11-3)
   a. Carotid bifurcation is exposed via a vertical incision made parallel to the sternocleidomastoid muscle under general or regional anesthesia (Bradley & Pearce, 1999).
   b. Some surgeons use intraluminal shunting routinely, secondary to comfort level and type of anesthesia, whereas others use it selectively. Other methods of monitoring cerebral perfusion during clamping include electroencephalography (EEG) monitoring (Bradley & Pearce, 1999).
   c. The common carotid artery, internal carotid artery, and the external carotid artery are clamped (Bradley & Pearce, 1999).
   d. A longitudinal arteriotomy is made in the common carotid artery and extended to the internal carotid artery to the end of the plaque (Bradley & Pearce, 1999). Plaque is dissected out down to the media and then removed.

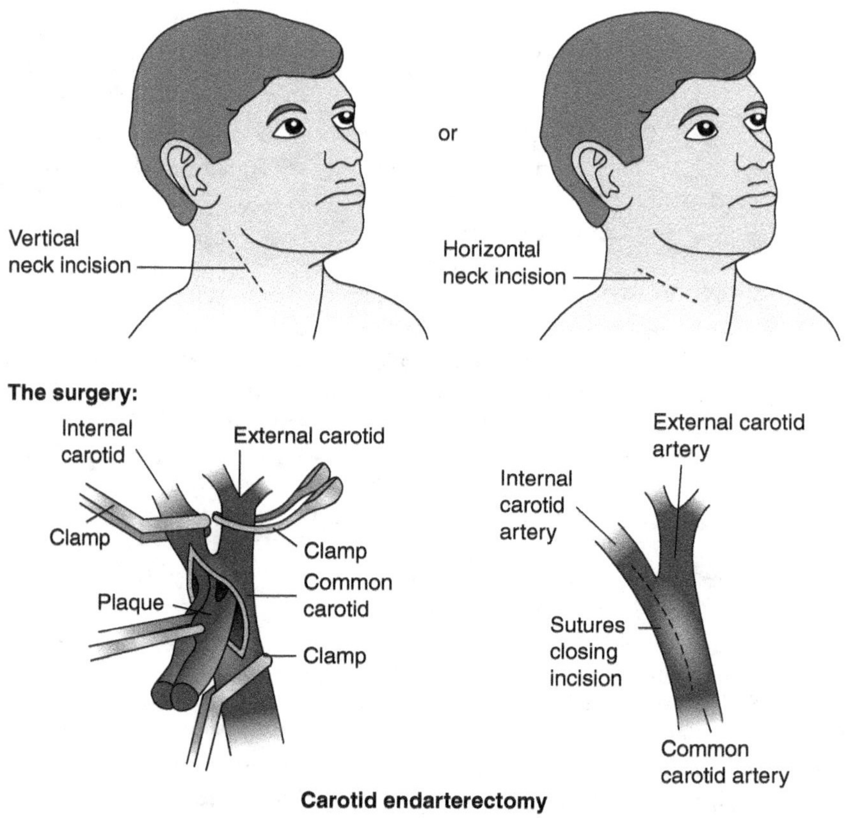

FIGURE 11-3. Carotid endarterectomy.

e. A patch of autogenous vein or prosthetic material may be used if primary closure of the carotid artery will cause narrowing of the artery or when the endarterectomy is being repeated (Bradley & Pearce, 1999).
f. Drain may be inserted subcutaneously (Bradley & Pearce, 1999).

VIII. Research Studies

Research Studies—There are multiple clinical trials to compare and evaluate carotid artery stenting versus CEA.

A. North American Symptomatic Carotid Endarterectomy Trial (NASCET)

1. Reported in 1991, showed the clinical benefit of surgery compared with drug therapy for patients with symptomatic carotid stenoses greater than 70% (Jensen & Creager, 2003)
2. In this trial, patients with carotid artery stenosis of 70% to 99% who had transient hemispheric symptoms, amaurosis fugax, or a nondisabling stroke were randomized to CEA or optimal medical care, including antiplatelet therapy (Jensen & Creager, 2003)
3. The cumulative risk of any ipsilateral stroke at 2 years was 26% in the medical care group and 9% in the surgical group (Jensen & Creager, 2003)
4. This resulted in an absolute risk reduction of 17%
5. CEA was also found to be beneficial when all strokes and deaths were included in the analysis (Jensen & Creager, 2003)

B. Asymptomatic Carotid Artery Study (ACAS)

1. Randomized clinical trial assessing the efficacy of treating asymptomatic carotid stenosis with low-dose aspirin (300 mg/day) alone in comparison to CEA in conjunction with the daily administration of low-dose aspirin (North American Symptomatic Carotid Endarterectomy Trial (NASCET) Steering Committee, 1991)
2. 42,000 patients were screened
3. 1,662 asymptomatic patients were randomized to CEA plus medical therapy ($n = 825$) or medical therapy alone ($n = 834$)
4. The 30-day perioperative stroke or death rate was 2.3%, with an additional 1.2% stroke incidence due to carotid angiography
5. CEA significantly cut the 5-year risk of ipsilateral stroke, perioperative stroke, or death in half (from 11% to 5.1%) (White et al., 2008)

C. Asymptomatic Carotid Stenosis Trial (ACST)

1. Randomized 3,120 asymptomatic patients with >60% carotid artery stenosis by ultrasound
2. There was a 2.8% risk of stroke or death within 30 days for those randomized to CEA
3. The 5-year risk of stroke was reduced significantly for CEA (6.4%) compared with medical therapy (11.8%)
4. At 5 years there was no difference in the rates of all stroke and/or death between medical therapy and CEA (White et al., 2008)

D. Carotid Revascularization Endarterectomy Versus Stent Trial (CREST)

1. It is the largest enrolling randomized clinical trial comparing the efficacy of CAS to CEA.
2. It is the largest trial comparing both symptomatic and asymptomatic patients with carotid artery disease.
3. It has reported on 1,246 patients in the lead-in registry, with a 30-day stroke and death rate of 3.4% for asymptomatic patients (White et al., 2008).

E. Stenting and Angioplasty with Protection in Patients at High Risk for Endarterectomy (SAPPHIRE) trial showed a decrease in perioperative morbidity in high-risk patients undergoing CEA.

1. A multicenter, prospective, randomized trial that enrolled symptomatic (30%) and asymptomatic (70%) patients considered to be at increased risk for surgery.
2. The 30-day ipsilateral major stroke and death rate was 2.6% for CAS and 2.5% for CEA, which compares favorably with both ACAS and ACST results (White et al., 2008).

F. Information on Current Trials—For a list of current stroke clinical trials go to www.strokecenter.org/trials/browse.asp?browse=prevent& condition = 4

IX. Nursing Management/Diagnosis

A. Potential Alteration in Cerebral Tissue Perfusion, Related to Thrombosis of Carotid Artery, Embolization

1. Expected patient outcome: patient will maintain adequate cerebral perfusion; if a deficit occurs it will be recognized promptly.
2. Interventions
   a. Monitor vital signs per unit standards. Close observation of blood pressure is very important
   b. Check for increased blood pressure, decreased heart rate, and Cheyne–Stokes respiration (increased intracranial pressure secondary to hemorrhage)
   c. Decreased blood pressure, increased heart rate, and respirations (due to cerebral ischemia)
   d. Symptomatic bradycardia (due to vagal nerve stimulation)
   e. Neuro checks as per unit standards: cranial nerves II to XII intact
3. Evaluation: patient should have no change from baseline

B. Potential for (Cranial Nerve) Injury, Related to Trauma to Cranial Nerves during Surgery

1. Expected outcome: Patient remains free of cranial nerve deficits; if deficit occurs, patient verbalizes understanding of deficit
2. Intervention
   a. Neuro checks as per unit standards: cranial nerves intact
   b. Be sure to assess patient for presence of a gag reflex; if patient has difficulty swallowing (cranial nerves X or XII), tongue deviation to one side, or biting of tongue when eating

c. Check symmetry of lip movements b.i.d by having patient smile or show teeth (cranial nerve VII)
d. Check speech b.i.d. If patient is hoarse (cranial nerve XII), difficulty attaining high notes (cranial nerve X)
e. Check uvula for symmetry b.i.d
f. Check shoulder alignment b.i.d. Is shoulder sagging noticed (cranial nerve XI)?
g. Check sternocleidomastoid muscle b.i.d (cranial nerve XI). Instruct patient to rotate their head to one side while you provide resistance to head movement

3. Evaluation: patient should have no change from baseline

C. Potential Alteration in Fluid Volume Related to Hemorrhage, Hematoma

1. Expected outcome: patient has maintenance of adequate fluid volume
2. Interventions
   a. Monitor vital signs per unit standards
   b. Monitor dressing and drain (if present) for excessive drainage/output
   c. Check operative site for bruising, excessive swelling
   d. Maintain accurate intake and output
   e. Monitor airway for any compromise related to cervical hematoma
   f. Observe for any signs of tracheal deviation
3. Evaluation: no change from baseline

X. Patient Teaching

A. Disease Prevention/Health Promotion and Secondary Prevention

1. Diet: Low fat, low cholesterol diet unless specified. When appropriate, diet for modification of hyperlipidemia, hypertension, or diabetes should also be reviewed. American Heart Association guidelines specify that a total cholesterol level should be less than 200 mg/dL with low-density lipoprotein (LDL) of less than 130.
2. Smoking: Smoking accelerates atherosclerosis, increases blood pressure, and decreases heart rate. Encourage patient to quit smoking.
3. Hypertension: Patient should resume preoperative antihypertensive medication and emphasize importance of future blood pressure management.

B. Discharge Instructions (may vary from institution to institution)

1. Activity
   a. May go up and down stairs
   b. Move neck normally
   c. No heavy lifting (nothing greater than 10 lbs)
2. Bathing
   a. May shower postoperatively
   b. Clean the incision with mild soap and water
   c. Pat incision dry
3. Wound Care
   a. Staples are generally removed prior to discharge
   b. Patient may have Steri-Strips over incision; these will fall off in 2 to 3 days

   c. Patient may shower, pat incision dry
   d. Inform patient that bruising, discoloration, and swelling are not uncommon and will disappear
   e. Patient may have numbness around the incision, use caution shaving
   f. Men may shave around the incision using an electric razor until swelling resolves
4. What to Report to Provider
   a. Difficulty moving one side of the body
   b. Difficulty speaking
   c. Loss or change in vision
   d. Elevated blood pressure >170/90
   e. Severe headache
   f. Redness, foul smelling drainage from incision
   g. Temperature >101°F
   h. Sudden swelling, erythema of wound or neck

CASE STUDY

MF is a 63-year-old White male who was sitting at his desk at work and had a sudden onset of temporary left eye blindness. He described a "shade being drawn" in front of his eye. The symptom lasted approximately 2 minutes.

He proceeded to the emergency room. After a physical examination a carotid ultrasound was ordered. This showed his right CCA and ECA to be WNL; the ICA had <50% stenosis. The left CCA was WNL, the ECA had 50% stenosis, and the ICA had 70% to 79% stenosis. An MRA was subsequently ordered and confirmed the ultrasounds results.

He has a past medical history of hypertension, hyperlipidemia, and hypothyroidism. Past surgical history of left inguinal hernia repair and appendectomy. Medications: Norvasc 10 mg q.d, Synthroid 25 µg q.d, and Baby aspirin 81 mg q.d. After consultation with a vascular surgeon MF was admitted and the following day had a left CEA. Four hours postoperatively on doing an assessment the RN caring for MF noticed he had difficulty swallowing and that his voice was raspy. His blood pressure was 160/94, pulse 88, and respirations 22. Although he had a dressing on his neck, she noticed his neck to be quite enlarged.

Review Questions

1. What else would you look for?
   a. Observe patient for change in vital signs
   b. Anxiety, restlessness, pallor, cyanosis
   c. Change in level of conscious
   d. Excessive bleeding or swelling at the incisional site
   e. Sudden increase in neck circumference
   f. Check patient's gag reflex and ability to swallow (cranial nerves X or XII)
2. What discharge instructions would you give the patient?

Answers

1. MF had to be taken back to the operating room for an evacuation of a hematoma. He did well postoperatively and was discharged the following day.
2. • Patient may shower 48 hours after surgery, pat incision dry
   • Men may shave

- Contact the doctor's office if the following occur:
  - Difficulty moving one side of the body
  - Difficulty speaking
  - Loss or change of vision
  - Elevated blood pressure >170/90
  - Severe headache
  - Temperature >101°F
  - Sudden swelling, redness along incision

REFERENCES

A to Z Stroke Guide. (2011). Retrieved from http://www.americanheart.org/Heart_and Stroke_A_Z_Guide, accessed June 25, 2011.

Blackburn, D. R., & Kennedy, L. (1999). Noninvasive vascular testing. In V. Fahey (Ed.), *Vascular nursing* (3rd ed., pp. 74–99). Philadelphia, PA: W.B. Saunders.

Bradley, M., & Pearce, W. H. (1999). Extracranial cerebrovascular disease. In V. Fahey (Ed.), *Vascular nursing* (3rd ed., pp. 270–291). Philadelphia, PA: W.B. Saunders.

Effient® (prasugrel) product information. (2013). Retrieved from http://www.effient.com/Pages/index.aspx, accessed August 24, 2013.

Francfort, J. W., Smullens, S. N., Gallagher, J. F., & Fairman, R. M. (1989). Airway compromise after carotid surgery in patients with cervical irradiation. *The Journal of Cardiovascular Surgery, 30*, 877–881.

Gotto, A. M. (1986). Interactions of the major risk factors for coronary heart disease. *American Journal of Medicine, 80*, 48–55.

Graham, L. M., & Ford, M. B. (1999). Arterial disease. In V. Fahey (Ed.), *Vascular nursing* (3rd ed., pp. 2–20). Philadelphia, PA: W.B. Saunders.

Jensen, F. E., & Creager, M. A. (2003). Cerebrovascular disease. In M. A. Creager & E. Braunwald (Ed.), *Vascular disease* (2nd ed., pp. 130–146). Philadelphia, PA: Current Medicine, Inc.

North American Symptomatic Carotid Endarterectomy Trial (NASCET) Steering Committee. (1991). North American symptomatic carotid endarterectomy trial: Methods, patient characteristics and progress. *Stroke, 22*, 711–720. doi: 10.1161/01.STR.22.6.711

Nunnelee, J. D., & Fotis, M. A. (2004). Medications used in vascular patients. In V. Fahey (Ed.), *Vascular nursing* (4th ed., p. 163). Philadelphia, PA: W.B. Saunders.

Oppat, W., & Graham, L. M. (2004). The arterial system. In V. Fahey (Ed.), *Vascular nursing* (4th ed., pp. 10–11). Philadelphia, PA: W.B. Saunders.

Spittell, J. A., & Spittell, P. C. (1991). Dissection of the aorta and other arteries. In J. R. Young, R. A. Graor, J. W. Olin, & J. R. Bartholomew (Eds.), *Peripheral vascular diseases* (pp. 321–329). St Louis, MO: Mosby-Year Book.

Sullivan, E. D., & Herzter, N. R. (1996). Extracranial cerebrovascular arterial disease. In J. R. Young, J. R. Bartholomew, & J. W. Olin, (Eds.), (*Peripheral vascular disease* (2nd ed., pp. 288–304). St. Louis, MO: Mosby-Year Book.

Ticlid® product information. (2013). Retrieved from http://www.medicinenet.com/ticlopidine/article.htm, accessed August 24, 2013.

Vitek, J. J., Roubin, G. S., Gishel, N., Al-Mubarek, N., & Iyer, S. S. (2000). Carotid stenting. *Techniques in Vascular and Interventional Radiology, 3*(2), 75–85.

White, C. J., Beckman, J. A., Cambria, R. P., Comerota, A. J., Gray, W. A., Hobson, R. W., II., & Iyer, S. S. (2008). Atherosclerotic peripheral vascular disease symposium II. Controversies in carotid artery revascularization. *Circulation, 118*, 2852–2859. doi:10.1161/CIRCULATIONAHA.108.191175

Wiebers, D. O., Feigin, V. L., & Brown, R. D. (1997). *Handbook of stroke* (p. 265). New York, NY: Lippincott-Raven Publishers.

Young, J. R. (1996). Physical examination. In J. R. Young, J. R. Bartholomew, & J. W. Olin (Eds.), *Peripheral vascular disease* (2nd ed., pp. 18–32). St. Louis, MO: Mosby-Year Book.

SUGGESTED READING

Kernan, W. N., Ovbiagele, B., Black, H. R., Bravata, D. M., Chimowitz, M. I., Ezekowitz, M. D., ...Wilson, J. A. (2014). Guidelines for the Prevention of Stroke in Patients with Stroke and Transient Ischemic Attack. A Guideline for Healthcare Professionals from the American Heart Association/American Stroke Association. *Stroke*. Published online May 1, 2014. Retrieved from http://Stroke.ahajournals.org/content/early/2014/04/30/STR.0000000000000024, accessed May 13, 2014.

CHAPTER 12

Mesenteric Ischemia

Cynthia Christensen

OBJECTIVES

1. Describe the anatomy and physiology relevant to mesenteric ischemia.
2. List the appropriate diagnostic tests relevant to mesenteric ischemia.
3. Discuss the appropriate medical and surgical interventions relevant to mesenteric ischemia.
4. Identify the nursing implications relevant to mesenteric ischemia.

Introduction/Overview

Mesenteric ischemia ensues when blood flow to the intestines ceases or falls below a critical level, resulting in damage to the bowel ranging from completely reversible functional alterations to total hemorrhagic necrosis. The incidence of mesenteric ischemia accounts for 1 in every 1,000 hospital admissions or 9 Americans in every 100,000 (Assar & Zarins, 2008; Broder, 2007; Herbert & Steele, 2007). Mortality rates for mesenteric ischemia range from 30% to 90% depending on the etiology. This has changed little over the past decades despite advances in medical knowledge and technology (Herbert & Steele, 2007). Poor outcomes of mesenteric ischemia result from the delaying in initiating treatment because of the difficulty in arriving at an accurate diagnosis (Assar & Zarins, 2008; Paral et al., 2007). The natural history of mesenteric ischemia includes three possible results:

1. Establishment of competent collateral circulation that will persist effectively throughout the patient's life or will subsequently break down due to aggravation of the causative factor.
2. Intestinal obstructions without infarction, with blood supply sufficient to sustain life of the gut but not function.
3. Intestinal infarction with the extent of injury varying from a moderate lesion to total necrosis of intestinal tissues (Boley, Brandt, & Sammartano, 1997).

I. Anatomy: Three arteries with a parallel venous system perfuse most of the gastrointestinal tract. These vessels include the celiac axis, the superior mesenteric artery (SMA), and the inferior mesenteric artery (IMA) (see Fig. 12-1).

A. The Celiac Axis

1. Originates from the ventral abdominal aorta at the level of T12 or L1
2. Is only about 1.5 cm long

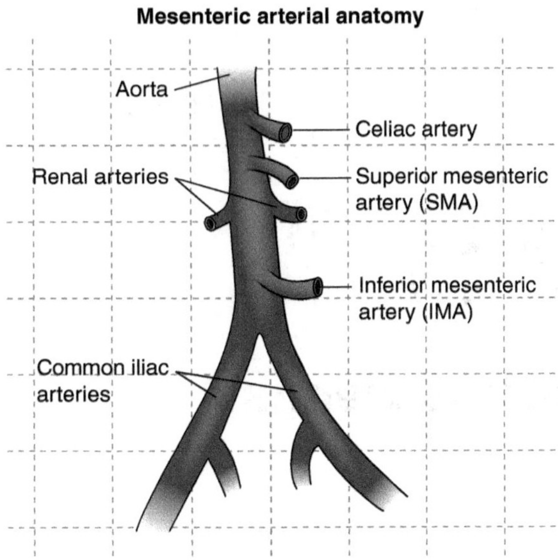

FIGURE 12-1. Mesenteric arterial anatomy.

3. Rapidly divides into the following:
   a. Common hepatic
   b. Left gastric
   c. Splenic arteries
4. The celiac artery provides blood supply to the following:
   a. Liver
   b. Spleen
   c. Pancreas
   d. Gastrointestinal tract from the distal esophagus to the second portion of the duodenum

B. The SMA

1. Exits the aorta anteriorly, about 1 to 2 cm below the celiac axis
2. Is the largest and most important intestinal artery
3. Supplies the following:
   a. Latter portion of the duodenum
   b. Head of pancreas
   c. Jejunum
   d. Ileum
   e. Large bowel proximal to the splenic flexure

C. The IMA

1. Is the smallest of the three intestinal arteries, perfusing only about 10% of the intestine
2. Arises from the aorta about 6 cm distal to the SMA
3. Supplies the left colon and most of the rectum

D. The Venous Anatomy parallels the arterial, eventually draining into the portal system perfusing the liver

1. The superior and inferior mesenteric veins drain the midgut and hindgut

2. The inferior mesenteric vein empties into the splenic vein: these join with the superior mesenteric vein forming the portal vein (Cappell, 1998a; McCutcheon, 2009; Ruotolo & Evans, 1999; Tendler & LaMont, 2011a)

II. Pathophysiology

A. Mesenteric Vessels are uniquely reactive to several intrinsic and extrinsic factors affecting blood flow.

1. Blood flow is increased throughout the visceral vasculature in response to a meal. The SMA undergoes a period of hyperemia 20 to 30 minutes after the ingestion of food. The splenic blood flow can demand 10% to 35% of the total cardiac output during this time.
2. The mucosa uses an autoregulatory mechanism to extract increasing amounts of oxygen to preserve its viability during hypoperfusion or metabolic insult.
3. The mesenteric circulation is under the extrinsic control of the nervous and endocrine systems (Herbert & Steele, 2007; Ruotolo & Evans, 1999; Tendler & LaMont, 2011a).

B. The Results of Vascular Insufficiency are not etiology dependent but are determined by multiple factors. Both ischemic and reperfusion syndromes play a role in tissue breakdown and necrosis.

1. Ischemia attacks the most vulnerable area of the bowel first, the mucosa.
   a. Mucosal sloughing, ulceration, and hemorrhage occur within 3 hours of ischemic insult.
   b. Depending on partial or total occlusion, transmural infarction occurs within 6 hours to several days of ischemic insult.
   c. Once intestinal mucosa begins to slough, the underlying tissue becomes susceptible to the contents of the gut and bacteria begins to flourish, allowing the translocation of bacteria and toxins into the systemic circulation resulting in
      1) Increased capillary permeability
      2) Edema formation
      3) Multiorgan dysfunction or failure
2. Reperfusion leads to the production of oxygen-free radicals, which cause disruption of the cell membrane and mucosal barrier. This release of endotoxins can be associated with:
   a. Disseminated intravascular coagulation
   b. Adult respiratory distress syndrome
   c. Sudden cardiovascular collapse (Hirsch et al., 2006; Ruotolo & Evans, 1999)

III. Etiology/Precipitating Factors. Mesenteric ischemia can be divided into three categories.

A. Acute Mesenteric Ischemia (AMI) occurs when arterial blood and oxygen delivery to the gut is interrupted by the following:

1. Arterial embolism or thrombosis
   a. Atherosclerosis
   b. Advanced age

c. Low cardiac output states
d. Severe cardiac valvular disease
e. Intra-abdominal malignancy
f. Dysrhythmias
g. Atrial fibrillation
h. Myocardial infarction (Assar & Zarins, 2008; Broder, 2007; Levy, 2007; Tendler & LaMont, 2011a)

2. Mechanical occlusion
   a. Trauma
   b. Adhesive bands
   c. Presence of diagnostic devices within the vessels (Mansour, 1999; Vincente & Kazmers, 1999)
3. Nonocclusive mesenteric ischemia (NOMI) in response to systemic hypoperfusion
   a. Congestive heart failure
   b. Sepsis
   c. Renal failure
   d. Hypoperfusion
   e. Hemorrhagic shock
   f. Hypovolemia
   g. Cardiac surgery
   h. Medications
      1) Digitalis
      2) Ergotamines
      3) Cocaine
      4) Norepinephrine
      5) Diuretics
      6) Alpha-adrenergic agonists
      7) Arginine-vasopressin & angiotensin (Assar & Zarins, 2008; Broder, 2007; Herbert & Steele, 2007; Hirsch et al., 2006; Levy, 2007; Tendler & LaMont, 2011a)

B. Mesenteric Venous Thrombosis (MVT) is the least common cause of AMI. MVT may be primary or idiopathic, or secondary due to one or more other disorders (Assar & Zarins, 2008) such as:

1. Intra-abdominal trauma
2. Sepsis
3. Portal hypertension
4. Hypercoagulable states
   a. Protein C deficiency
   b. Protein S deficiency
   c. Factor V Leiden mutation
   d. Antithrombin III deficiency
   e. Anticardiolipin antibodies
   f. These may be associated with oral contraceptive use
5. Previous abdominal operation
6. Intra-abdominal malignancy
7. Sickle cell disease
8. Smoking
9. Homocysteinemia
10. Immobilization
11. Use of steroids

12. Irritable bowel syndrome
13. Cirrhosis
14. Myeloproliferative syndromes
15. Polycythemia vera
16. Antiphospholipid syndrome
17. Nocturnal paroxysmal hemoglobinuria (Herbert & Steele, 2007; Hugon, deClercq, & Landen, 2007; Levy, 2007; McCutcheon, 2009; Tendler & LaMont, 2011a)

C. Chronic Mesenteric Ischemia (CMI)

C. Chronic Mesenteric Ischemia (CMI) occurs in the presence of advanced atherosclerosis with insufficient splenic blood flow during periods of increased intestinal demand. Factors associated with this include the following:

1. Atherosclerosis
2. Radiation therapy
3. Celiac compression syndrome
4. Vasculitides
   a. Polyarteritis nodosa
   b. Takayasu disease
5. Fibromuscular dysplasia
6. Peripheral vascular disease with
   a. Advanced age
   b. Hypertension
   c. Smoking
7. Median arcuate ligament (MAL) syndrome (Gupta, Horan, Turaga, Miller, & Pipinos, 2010; Herbert & Steele, 2007; Kougias, El Sayed, Zhou, & Lin, 2007; Levy, 2007; Tendler & LaMont, 2011b)

IV. Assessment

A. Risk Factors and Primary Prevention

1. Risk factors
   a. Cardiac arrhythmias
   b. Advanced age
   c. Low cardiac output states
   d. Generalized atherosclerosis
   e. Hypercoagulable states
   f. Severe valvular cardiac disease
   g. Recent myocardial infarction
   h. Intra-abdominal malignancy (Hirsch et al., 2006; McCutcheon, 2009; Tendler & LaMont, 2011a)
2. Primary prevention includes eliminating or controlling those risk factors associated with vascular disease:
   a. Hypertension
   b. Smoking
   c. Hyperlipidemia
   d. Diabetes (Nunnelee, 1999)

B. Patient History

1. Subjective findings
   a. AMI

1) Rapid onset of peri-umbilical pain out of proportion to examination is the hallmark sign
2) Nausea and vomiting
3) Forceful bowel evacuation
4) Mental status change
5) Feculent odor to breath (Assar & Zarins, 2008; Broder, 2007; Hirsch et al., 2006; Levy, 2007; Tendler & LaMont, 2011a)

b. NOMI
1) Abdominal pain absent in up to 25% of patients
2) Pain varies in character, intensity, and location (Assar & Zarins, 2008; Tendler & LaMont, 2011a)

c. MVT
1) Depends on size of thrombus, size of vessel involved, depth of bowel wall ischemia
2) Diffuse, nonlocalized, moderately severe, constant, colicky type pain disproportionate to examination is the hallmark sign
3) Diarrhea
4) Gastrointestinal bleeding
5) Nausea/vomiting
6) Chills
7) Esophageal variceal hemorrhage
8) Mild abdominal pain evolving over 7 to 10 days
9) May be asymptomatic (Hugon et al., 2007; Levy, 2007; McCutcheon, 2009; Safieddine, Mamazza, Common, & Prabhudesai, 2007)

d. CMI
1) Pain described as "abdominal angina" occurs within 30 minutes of eating, increases in severity, and slowly resolves after 1 to 3 hours
2) Pain may be acute episodes of dull, crampy pain within 1 hour of eating
3) Pain may vary in intensity and radiate to back
4) Diarrhea
5) Nausea/vomiting
6) Constipation
7) Food fear related to pain
8) Early satiety
9) May be asymptomatic (Dupee, 2011; Gupta et al., 2010; Herbert & Steele, 2007; Kougias et al., 2007; Levy, 2007; Tendler & LaMont, 2011b)

2. Objective findings
a. Cachectic appearance
b. Leukocytosis
c. Hypotension
d. Acidosis
e. Pyrexia
f. Increased serum amylase
g. Increased lactate level
h. Hypovolemia
i. Cardiac arrhythmia
j. Weight loss (Broder, 2007; Dupee, 2011; Gupta et al., 2010; Herbert & Steele, 2007; Kougias et al., 2007; Levy, 2007; McCutcheon, 2009; Tendler & LaMont, 2011a, 2011b)

C. Physical Examination

1. Inspection
   a. Overall appearance of being uncomfortable
   b. Fecal occult blood
   c. Abdominal distension
2. Palpation
   a. Abdominal pain
      1) See subjective finding for description
      2) Abdomen soft, nontender with CMI
   b. Abdominal rigidity
   c. Rebound abdominal tenderness
   d. Guarding (except with arterial embolism)
3. Percussion for distension and ascites
4. Auscultation
   a. Abdominal or epigastric bruit for CMI
   b. Bowel sounds may be absent in AMI
   c. Presence of dysrhythmia in NOMI (Assar & Zarins, 2008; Broder, 2007; Herbert & Steele, 2007; Hugon et al., 2007; Levy, 2007; McCutcheon, 2009; Safieddine et al., 2007; Tendler & LaMont, 2011a, 2011b)

D. Considerations Across the Life Span

1. Younger patients develop ischemia but usually have an underlying disease or condition that predisposes them to an abnormality in splanchnic blood flow such as
   a. Collagen vascular disease
   b. Vasculitis
   c. Hypercoagulable states
   d. Vasoactive medication
   e. Cocaine use
   f. Extrinsic compression of the celiac artery
2. Elderly—Mesenteric ischemia is described as a disease of the elderly with most occurring within the sixth or seventh decade of life (Assar & Zarins, 2008; Broder, 2007; Herbert & Steele, 2007; Levy, 2007; Tendler & LaMont, 2011a)

V. Pertinent Diagnostic Testing.

Most diagnostic tests are performed to evaluate other more common causes of abdominal pain and to help rule out other causes.

A. Laboratory Tests (complete chemistry and hematology profiles) to assess for the following:

1. Leukocytosis
2. Hypercoagulable states
3. Shift to immature leukocytes in differential
4. Metabolic acidosis
5. Hyperamylasemia
6. Hemoconcentration
7. Elevated serum lactase
8. Elevated serum phosphate

9. Elevated serum alkaline phosphatase
10. Azotemia

B. Experimental Laboratory Tests Include:

1. Alpha-glutathione s-transferase (Alpha-GST)
2. Intestinal fatty acid–binding protein (I-FABP)
3. Cobalt–albumin binding assay (CABA)
4. Ischemia-modified albumin, a sensitive marker of myocardial ischemia, skeletal muscle ischemia, PE, and stroke; can be used as a diagnostic marker. May have a place in early diagnosis of acute mesenteric embolism (Assar & Zarins, 2008; Broder, 2007; Gunduz et al., 2008; Hugon et al., 2007; McCutcheon, 2009; Tendler & LaMont, 2011a)

C. Noninvasive Tests Include:

1. Endoscopy
   a. Little value in diagnosing CMI
   b. Often needed to exclude other causes of abdominal pain
   c. Contraindicated in SMV with acute symptoms (Cappell, 1998a; McCutcheon, 2009)
2. Sonogram of gallbladder: to exclude gallbladder disease as a source of abdominal pain (Nunnelee, 1999)
3. Intravenous pyelogram: to exclude renal stones as a source of abdominal pain (Nunnelee, 1999)
4. Echocardiography:
   a. Used to identify whether the source of embolization is cardiac in origin
   b. Useful in postoperative management, especially if anticoagulation is considered (Mansour, 1999)
5. Barium enema/swallow
   a. Upper gastrointestinal series may demonstrate nonspecific findings as follows:
      1) Malabsorption of contrast segmentation, flocculation, and dilution
      2) Bowel dilatation and hypoperistalsis
      3) Mural thickening
   b. The most common finding of barium enema is thumbprinting:
      1) Caused by submucosal edema and hemorrhage
      2) Appears as multiple, round, smooth, soft tissue densities projecting into the air-filled colonic lumen
   c. Thumbprinting can also occur with the following:
      1) Inflammatory bowel disease
      2) Pseudomembranous colitis
      3) Amebic colitis
      4) Intramural hemorrhage from Henoch–Schönlein purpura or anticoagulation therapy
   d. Acute findings of barium enema may resemble findings of the following:
      1) Diverticulitis
      2) Colon cancer
      3) Ulcerative, infectious, or Crohn colitis
   e. Contraindicated when
      1) There is suspected SMV
      2) Intraluminal barium contraindicated as it interferes with visualization during angiography (Cappell, 1998b; McCutcheon, 2009; Tendler & LaMont, 2011a)

6. Colonoscopy is required when gastrointestinal bleeding occurs
   a. It is preferred over sigmoidoscopy because about 50% of ischemic colonic lesions are proximal to the sigmoid colon.
   b. The entire colon is visualized.
   c. It is highly important in diagnosing ischemic colitis.
   d. It is usually nondiagnostic for CMI (Cappell, 1998b).
7. Plain abdominal roentgenograms:
   a. A standard diagnostic tool to evaluate acute abdominal pain
   b. Most common findings include the following:
      1) Adynamic ileus
      2) Associated distention, air–fluid levels, and fixed, dilated loops of bowel
      3) Thumbprinting or thickening of bowel loops
   c. May see calcification of mesenteric vessels in CMI
   d. After infarction the following may be seen:
      1) Pneumatosis intestinalis: the presence of thin-walled, gas-filled cysts in the intestines
      2) Gas in portal vein
      3) Both are signs of poor prognosis
   e. A negative radiographic finding in the setting of acute, severe abdominal pain may be the earliest indicator of an ischemic event (Assar & Zarins, 2008; McCutcheon, 2009; Ruotolo & Evans, 1999; Tendler & LaMont, 2011a, 2011b)
8. CT scan: superior to plain films for imaging specific signs of mesenteric ischemia
   a. Bowel wall thickening is the most common finding.
   b. Relatively specific findings of mesenteric ischemia include the following:
      1) Abnormal gas in the bowel wall of portal system
      2) Acute embolic infarction of the spleen
      3) Thrombi in the mesenteric vessels
      4) Absence of bowel wall enhancement
      5) Intestinal pneumatosis
   c. Gold standard for diagnosing MVT demonstrating
      1) Defect in filling or occlusion of SMV
      2) Mesenteric congestion
      3) Wall thickening in the small bowel
      4) Establishes 90% of diagnoses except in cases of early thrombosis in small vessels
      5) Magnetic Resonance Angiography (MRA) may be highly sensitive to MVT but CT preferred due to cost and availability (Hirsch et al., 2006; Levy, 2007; McCutcheon, 2009; Tendler & LaMont, 2011a)
9. Doppler ultrasonography
   a. A sensitive and specific screening examination for CMI
   b. Useful as an alternative to arteriography in evaluating celiac and mesenteric stenosis, 96% accuracy for >70% stenosis
   c. May show dilated SMV and presence of collaterals in chronic occlusion with MVT
   d. Accuracy of the test requires considerable training and expertise for the ultrasonographer
   e. Accuracy may be limited by the following:
      1) Respiratory motion
      2) Intraperitoneal gas
      3) Previous laparotomy

4) Obesity
5) Air-filled loops of distended bowel (Herbert & Steele, 2007; Kougias et al., 2007; McCutcheon, 2009; Tendler & LaMont, 2011a, 2011b)

D. Invasive Tests: Angiography is the gold standard for acute arterial ischemia with digital subtraction angiography the most accurate to determine degree of stenosis

1. Anteroposterior and lateral views are essential for complete arteriographic evaluation to
   a. Visualize the collateral arcades
   b. Visualize origins of major visceral vessels
   c. Exclude other causes of mesenteric ischemia such as MAL syndrome also known as celiac compression syndrome
   d. Absence of collateralization is suggestive of an acute process
2. Four reliable arteriographic criteria for the diagnosis of mesenteric vasospasm include
   a. Narrowing of the origins of multiple branches of the SMA
   b. Alternate dilatation and narrowing of the intestinal branches, the "string of sausages" sign
   c. Spasm of the mesenteric arcades
   d. Impaired filling of the intramural vessels
3. In MVT, angiography may reveal
   a. Reflux of contrast material backs into the aorta due to extremely slow flow and heightened outflow resistance
   b. Characteristic sign is a prolonged arterial phase with accumulation of contrast and thickened bowel walls
   c. Extravasation of contrast material into the bowel lumen may indicate active bleeding
   d. Definitive diagnosis of MVT is made during the venous phase by
      1) Filling the defect within the portal vein
      2) In extensive thrombosis there is an absence of the entire venous phase (Assar & Zarins, 2008; Bassiouny, 1997; Herbert & Steele, 2007; Kougias et al., 2007; McCutcheon, 2009; McKinsey & Gewertz, 1997; Moawad et al., 1997; Tendler & LaMont, 2011a)

E. Special Procedures

1. Tonometry has been proposed as a useful screening tool for abdominal pain in suspected CMI.
   a. Two measurements may identify CMI:
      1) A drop in the intramural pH of the jejunum after introduction of a test meal, along with the onset of abdominal pain
      2) Increased gastric PCo_2 during exercise
2. Endoscopic visible light spectroscopy
   a. Abnormally low mucosal oxygen saturations are measured in the proximal small bowel of patients with CMI
   b. Measures mucosal capillary hemoglobin oxygen saturation, a direct measure of the adequacy of mucosal perfusion
   c. Currently limited to point measurements rather than assessing entire endoscopic field (Friedland, Benaron, Coogan, Sze, & Soetikno, 2007; Herbert & Steele, 2007; Kolkman, Groeneveld, Van der Berg, Rauwerda, & Meuwissen, 1999; Moawad & Gewertz, 1997; Tendler & LaMont, 2011b)

3. Fluorescein-assisted laparoscopy (FAL)
   a. The luminescence markedly differentiates the perfused, viable tissue from ischemic tissues.
      1) Perfused segments are highlighted with the bright yellow-green dye
      2) Ischemic areas remain dark
   b. Used to assess early stage acute bowel ischemia and second look 24 to 48 hours after surgery
   c. May be laparoscopically which is associated with less postoperative morbidity (Paral et al., 2007)

VI. Medical Management

A. Therapy Depends on

1. Cause
2. Disease severity
3. Timing of presentation
4. Presence of comorbidity (Cappell, 1998b)

B. Patients are treated with medical therapy unless they present with physical signs or laboratory evidence of peritonitis that requires surgery (Cappell, 1998b; Tendler & LaMont, 2011a)

C. Initial Management Includes:

1. Conditions that decrease mesenteric perfusion are treated
   a. Volume resuscitation for hypovolemia
   b. Cardiac function optimized
   c. Medications that cause mesenteric vasoconstriction are discontinued or avoided
2. Correction of acidosis if possible
3. Administration of appropriate antibiotics
4. Anticoagulation with heparin is initiated to prevent further thrombus propagation
5. Hyperalimentation is initiated for
   a. Malnourishment
   b. Profuse diarrhea
   c. Prolonged clinical course
6. A Foley catheter and peripheral arterial line are placed to monitor intravascular volume and hemodynamic status
7. Nasogastric tube is placed to decrease chances of aspiration and for gastric decompression
8. Narcotics are not initially given because they can blunt the signs of peritonitis
9. Cathartics are contraindicated because they can cause colonic perforation
10. In patients with NOMI, vasodilators such as papaverine may be administered (Assar & Zarins, 2008; Cappell, 1998b; Herbert & Steele, 2007; Mansour, 1999; McKinsey & Gewertz, 1997; Tendler & LaMont, 2011a)

TABLE 12-1 Occurrence, Treatments, Recurrence, and Prevention of Mesenteric Ischemia

Type of Ischemia	Occurrence	Treatment	Recurrence and Prevention
AMI	Embolic 30–50% of cases	Embolic–traditional treatment is laparotomy with embolectomy and resection as needed along with second look laparotomy in 24–48 hrs. Catheter-directed thrombolysis or PTA has been used. Endoscopic remains controversial but is an alternative for patients with increased operative risk without peritoneal signs or those with contaminated peritoneal cavity and lack of autogenous conduit for bypass	Long-term prevention of embolic events with anticoagulants
	Thrombotic 15–30%, highest mortality at 90%	Thrombotic observation while on anticoagulation in patients. With no peritoneal signs and angiographic evidence of collateral flow. Surgical repair with bypass before resection and evaluate bowel viability	Use of antiplatelet agents
NOMI	20–30% of cases <0.01% of population. Most lethal form of acute ischemia second to vasospasm that may persist even after correction of initial event. Mortality 70% due to difficulty in diagnosis and reversing ischemia	Primary treatment includes reversal of underlying cause and use of papaverine through angiocatheter. If no peritoneal signs a second angio in 24 hrs is done to verify resolution. A laparotomy is done for any signs of bowel infarction	Careful monitoring of at-risk patients for hypoperfusion and vasoconstriction that may lead to NOMI
MVT	5–15% of cases. Mortality is 20–50%	Work up for hypercoagulable condition. If asymptomatic no treatment or anticoagulation ranging from 3 mos to lifetime dependent on cause. Venous thrombolysis with streptokinase, urokinase, or tissue plasminogen activator is considered experimental. If bowel infarction, perforation, or peritonitis is present, surgery with thrombectomy and/or bowel resection with second look laparotomy if damage is extensive	Recurrence rate is 32–71% with most occurring 30 d after presentation. Prevention includes anticoagulation, ambulation, and compression
CMI	<5% of all ischemia. Women > men. Surgical mortality of 4.5–15%; endo mortality of 2–5%	Open surgery has been the gold standard but PTA with stenting surpassed surgery by 2005 due to the decrease in hospital length of stay, in-hospital mortality (4% endo vs. 15% open), and decrease in bowel resections. Need to examine bowel after revascularization to determine resolution of ischemia and bowel involvement with second look laparotomy if needed	Initial success of 88–100% with patency rates at 1 yr down to 70–80%

Assar & Zarins (2008), Dupee (2011), Gupta, Horan, Turaga, Miller, & Pipinos (2010), Herbert & Steele (2007), Hugon, deClercq, & Landen (2007), Kougias, El Sayed, Zhou, & Lin (2007) Levy (2007), McCutcheon (2009), Oderich (2010), Safieddine, Mamazza, Common, & Prabhudesai (2007), Schermerhorn, Giles, Hamdan, Wyers, & Pomposelli (2009) and Tendler & LaMont (2011a).

D. **Thrombolytic Therapy** has been reported to be successful for acute mesenteric embolus or thrombus

1. Thrombolytic therapy should be limited to patients with onset of abdominal pain within 8 hours without signs of peritoneal irritation
2. If there are no signs of lysis within 4 hours, or if the patient develops peritoneal signs, the thrombolytic infusion should be discontinued and surgical exploration emergently performed (Cappell, 1998b; McKinsey & Gewertz, 1997; Tendler & LaMont, 2011a)

E. **Percutaneous Transluminal Angioplasty (PTA)** is an option when vessel stenosis is found to be the cause of ischemia

1. PTA has advantages over surgical interventions
   a. Avoids general anesthesia
   b. Avoids laparotomy
   c. Reduces cost
2. Clinical success rates range from 85% to 96%, comparable to surgical success rates
3. Unsatisfactory results after PTA indicate the need for stenting to improve long-term results
   a. Residual stenosis >30% or >15 mm Hg pressure gradient across a lesion
   b. High-grade eccentric stenosis
   c. Chronic occlusion
   d. Presence of dissection
4. Restenosis rates for PTA are approximately 30% (Kougias et al., 2007; Oderich, 2010)
5. Occurrence, treatments, recurrence, and prevention (see Table 12-1)

VII. Surgical Management

A. **Surgical Exploration** is required if the patient develops signs of necrosis or continued bowel ischemia

1. Signs of bowel ischemia or necrosis include
   a. Rebound tenderness
   b. Guarding
   c. Absent bowel sounds (Broder, 2007; Herbert & Steele, 2007; Tendler & LaMont, 2011a)

B. **If the Cause of Mesenteric Ischemia** is an embolus/thrombus, an embolectomy or thrombectomy may be performed

1. The occluded mesenteric artery is identified and an arteriotomy is made
   a. A balloon-tipped embolectomy catheter is inserted retrograde and the embolus/thrombus is extracted
2. The arteriotomy is closed and the vessel is palpated for the presence of a pulse (Tendler & LaMont, 2011a)

C. **Resection** is performed with or without a second look procedure if the bowel is determined to be nonviable

1. Nonviable bowel is
   a. Dull gray or black in color
   b. Edematous
   c. Distended
   d. Lacks peristaltic activity and Doppler flow along the antimesenteric border
2. Intestinal continuity is restored after resection if the intestinal margins are unequivocally viable
3. If marginally viable segments remain, a second look procedure should be performed in 12 to 24 hours to reassess tissue viability, regardless of clinical improvement in the immediate postoperative period
4. If viability is questionable, the most conservative approach is to avoid primary anastomosis and bring the ends out as stomas. This allows
   a. Frequent assessment of bowel viability
   b. Aids in determining the time of another operation (Assar & Zarins, 2008; Bassiouny, 1997; Mansour, 1999)

D. **Mesenteric Artery Reimplantation** is performed by transecting the mesenteric artery distal to the occlusion and anastomosing the distal segment directly to the aorta. Reimplantation is not widely accepted due to

1. Technical difficulty
2. Frequent requirement of short-segment grafts (Cappell, 1998b)

E. **Aortomesenteric** bypass from the aorta to beyond the mesenteric obstruction is the most commonly performed procedure (see Fig. 12-2).

1. Bypass graft
   a. Antegrade from the supraceliac aorta
   b. Retrograde from the infrarenal aorta
2. Bypass materials
   a. Dacron
   b. Polytetrafluoroethylene (PTFE)
   c. Autogenous saphenous vein grafts
3. Bypass grafts have a long-term success rate of 89% to 94% (Assar & Zarins, 2008; Herbert & Steele, 2007)

F. **Mesenteric Endarterectomy** is an alternative to bypass, especially when no suitable vein is available and there is a contraindication to using a prosthetic graft

1. An arteriotomy is made in the occluded vessel and plaque is removed under direct vision
2. Transaortic endarterectomy is contraindicated in patients with severe cardiopulmonary disease due to
   a. Extensive dissection and surgical exposure
   b. Prolonged intraoperative time
   c. Technical difficulty requiring great expertise
3. There are related risks of renal and lower extremity ischemia due to
   a. Suprarenal aortic clamping
   b. Emboli of atheromatous debris
4. Mesenteric endarterectomy has a long-term success rate of 80% to 90% (Cappell, 1998b; Mansour, 1999)

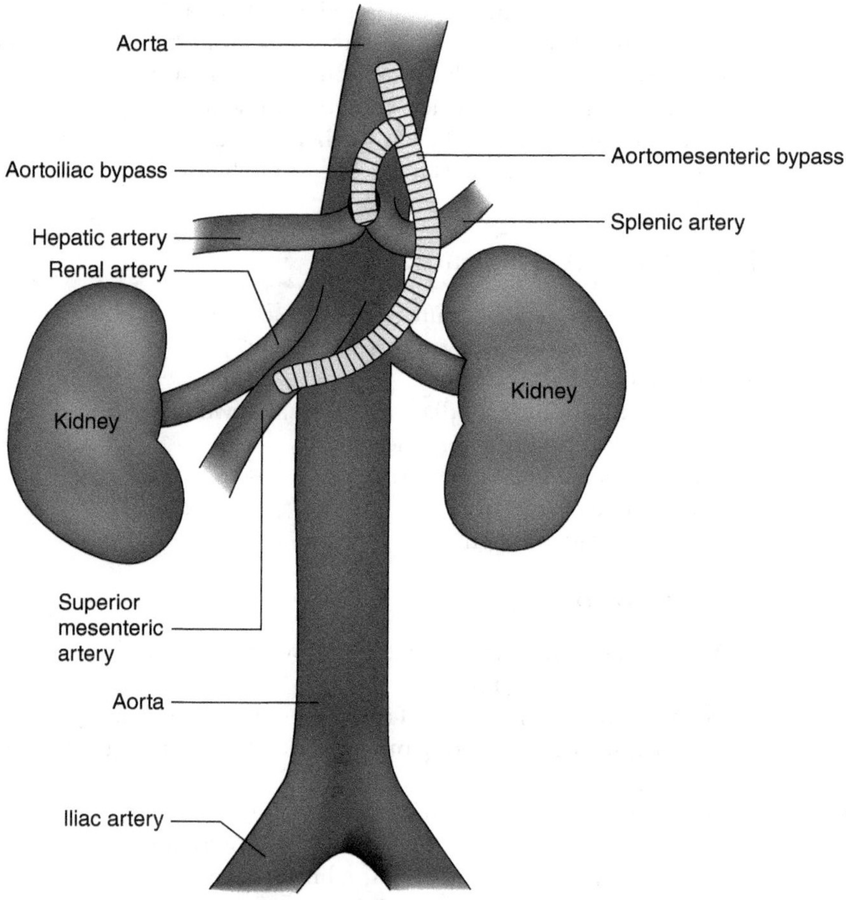

FIGURE 12-2. Aortomesenteric bypass.

G. Regardless of which Surgical Option is utilized, upon restoration of blood flow the mesenteric vessels and bowel should be reassessed for persistent ischemia. This can be accomplished as follows:

1. Palpating the entire length of the mesenteric artery
2. Using various techniques
   a. Continuous-wave Doppler
   b. Pulse oximetry
   c. Fluorescein injection and inspection with Wood lamp (Assar & Zarins, 2008; Bassiouny, 1997; Herbert & Steele, 2007; Mansour, 1999; McKinsey & Gewertz, 1997)

VIII. Nursing Management

A. Nursing Diagnoses Include:

1. Potential for temperature loss related to a cold operating room environment and intra-abdominal tissue exposure
2. Potential for hypotension related to administration of vasodilators (Bassiouny, 1997)

3. Potential fluid volume deficit related to ischemia changes
4. Alteration in bowel function, diarrhea related to mesenteric ischemia
5. Alteration in comfort related to ischemia and treatment
6. Alteration in tissue perfusion related to mesenteric ischemia
7. Potential for infection related to ischemia and possible incision
8. Alteration in nutritional status related to ischemia and postprandial pain (Ekers, 1994)

B. Expected Outcomes are:

1. Will maintain a temperature of at least 36°C
2. Will remain normotensive (Bassiouny, 1997)
3. Restore fluid balance
4. No complications from diarrhea, normal bowel function
5. Pain will be controlled or relieved
6. Attain improved tissue perfusion
7. Remain free of infection
8. Maintain or gain weight

C. Interventions

1. To maintain temperature use the following:
   a. Warm operating room
   b. Warm blankets on patient upon entering the operating room
   c. Warming devices during procedure such as Bair Huggers or radiant heat lamps
   d. Warm irrigation and prep sets
   e. Keep head covered during procedure, if possible
   f. Cover exposed tissue with warm linen (Bassiouny, 1997; Carpenito, 1999)
2. Monitor BP and pulse hourly while using vasodilators. Stop medication, infuse saline, and report to physician if hypotension occurs (Bassiouny, 1997).
3. To restore fluid balance use the following:
   a. Maintain a patent intravenous line
   b. Monitor intake and output accurately
   c. Weigh daily
   d. Monitor levels of serum electrolytes, blood urea nitrogen, urine and serum osmolality, creatinine, hematocrit, and hemoglobin
   e. Consider additional fluid loss associated with vomiting, diarrhea, fever, tubes, and drains (Carpenito, 1999; Ekers, 1994; Gordon & Christensen, 2011)
4. To avoid complications of diarrhea and to normalize bowel function
   a. Provide meticulous skin care
   b. Monitor fluid and electrolytes
   c. Provide nutritional support
   d. Reduce diarrhea as follows:
      1) Discontinue solids
      2) Ingest clear liquids
      3) Avoid milk, fat, high-fiber foods
      4) Gradually add solids and semisolids into the diet
   e. Observe for the following:
      1) Fever
      2) Tachycardia
      3) Lethargy

        4) Leukocytosis
        5) Decreased serum protein
        6) Anxiety
        7) Prostration (Doenges, Moorhouse, & Geissler, 2000; Ekers, 1994)

5. Reduce pain
    a. Reduce lack of knowledge through the following:
        1) Explain causes of pain, if known
        2) Relate how long pain will last, if known
        3) Explain diagnostic tests and procedures
    b. Provide opportunities for rest during the day and uninterrupted sleep at night
    c. Use noninvasive pain relief through the following:
        1) Distraction
        2) Relaxation
        3) Cutaneous stimulation
    d. Provide optimal pain relief with prescribed analgesics
    e. Return in 30 minutes to assess effectiveness of analgesics
    f. Assist with coping mechanisms (Carpenito, 1999; Ekers, 1994; Leary, 2011)
6. Assess tissue perfusion
    a. Investigate changes in level of conscience, dizziness, and headaches
    b. Monitor cardiac rate and rhythm
    c. Assess skin for the following:
        1) Coolness
        2) Pallor
        3) Diaphoresis
        4) Delayed capillary refill
        5) Weak, thready pulses
    d. Note urine output and specific gravity
    e. Hemoccult all stools
    f. Administer vasodilators as ordered
    g. Monitor pulse oximetry and give oxygen as needed (Doenges et al., 2000; Ekers, 1994; Gordon & Christensen, 2011)
7. Reduce potential for infection
    a. Identify individuals at risk for nosocomial infections
    b. Reduce entry of organisms into individuals by the following:
        1) Meticulous handwashing
        2) Aseptic technique
    c. Reduce individual's susceptibility to infection by the following:
        1) Encourage and maintain caloric and protein intake
        2) Monitor overuse of antimicrobial therapy
        3) Administer prescribed antimicrobial therapy within 15 minutes of scheduled time
        4) Minimize length of hospital stay (Carpenito, 1999)
8. Maintain nutritional status
    a. Determine daily caloric requirements, consult dietary as needed
    b. Weigh daily
    c. Explain importance of adequate nutrition
    d. Teach person to use spices to improve taste and aroma of food
    e. Offer favorite foods when able
    f. Plan care so unpleasant, painful procedures are not performed before meals

g. Provide a pleasant, relaxed atmosphere for eating
h. Control pain
i. Maintain good oral hygiene
j. Offer frequent small feedings (Carpenito, 1999; Ekers, 1994)

D. Evaluation of Interventions

1. Temperature maintained with no vasospasms or increase in ischemia
2. BP will be ±20 mm Hg of their normal BP (Bassiouny, 1997)
3. There will be greater than 30 cc/hr of urine output and good skin turgor
4. Skin will remain intact, normal electrolytes maintained
5. Report of pain ≤3 on a 0-to-10 pain scale
6. Stools hemoccult negative, denies postprandial pain
7. No signs or symptoms of infection
8. Weight is maintained or increased if necessary (Ekers, 1994)

IX. Patient Teaching

A. Disease Prevention should be encouraged through lifestyle changes by including

1. Smoking cessation
2. Low-fat diet
3. Use of regular exercise (Gordon & Christensen, 2011; Nunnelee, 1999)

B. Patients should also be taught the signs and symptoms of mesenteric artery reocclusion, especially when medical intervention is used (Cappell, 1998a)

C. Home Care Consideration Includes:

1. Wound care
2. Maintenance/increase of nutritional status (Nunnelee, 1999)

CASE STUDY

A 62-year-old White female presents to the ER at 5:00 p.m. with complaints of nausea, vomiting, and intense diarrhea. Today she began having severe abdominal pain after breakfast at 7:00 a.m., which she describes as the worst pain she has ever had. Her past medical history includes congestive heart failure and dysrhythmia. Her medications include digitalis and furosemide.

Review Questions

1. What symptoms would you expect to see on physical examination?
2. What medication(s) would you expect to be discontinued and why?
3. Severe, sudden abdominal pain out of proportion to physical findings is the cardinal symptom of AMI. What other subjective findings would you expect to find?
4. What would your initial management of the patient include?
5. If initial management efforts provide no symptomatic relief, what other management options would you choose or not choose?

Answers/Rationale

1. Symptoms would include abdominal distension, absent bowel sounds, direct abdominal tenderness, fecal occult blood, abdominal rigidity, and rebound abdominal tenderness (Assar & Zarins, 2008; Broder, 2007; Herbert & Steele, 2007; Hugon et al., 2007; Levy, 2007; McCutcheon, 2009; Safieddine et al., 2007; Tendler & LaMont, 2011a, 2011b).
2. Discontinue both digitalis and furosemide. Digitalis can cause vasoconstriction and furosemide can lead to dehydration and hypovolemia. Both of these conditions could exacerbate AMI (Assar & Zarins, 2008; Bassiouny, 1997; Herbert & Steele, 2007; Tendler & LaMont, 2011a).
3. Findings would include diarrhea, nausea, vomiting, mental status change, and feculent odor to breath (Assar & Zarins, 2008; Broder, 2007; Hirsch et al., 2006; Levy, 2007; Tendler & LaMont, 2011a).
4. Management would include: (1) Conditions that decrease mesenteric perfusion are treated; (2) Correction of acidosis if possible; (3) Administration of appropriate antibiotics; (4) Anticoagulation with heparin is initiated to prevent further thrombus propagation; (5) Hyperalimentation is initiated for malnourishment, profuse diarrhea, and prolonged clinical course; (6) A Foley catheter and peripheral arterial line are placed to monitor intravascular volume and hemodynamic status; (7) Nasogastric tube is placed to decrease chances of aspiration and for gastric decompression; (8) Narcotics are not initially given because they can blunt the signs of peritonitis; (9) Cathartics are contraindicated because they can cause colonic perforation (Assar & Zarins, 2008; Cappell, 1998b; Herbert & Steele, 2007; Mansour, 1999; McKinsey & Gewertz, 1997; Tendler & LaMont, 2011a).
5. Thrombolytic therapy would not be an option because her onset of pain exceeds 8 hours. Endovascular treatments are considered controversial but may be an option if she was found to be a high surgical risk without peritoneal signs. An embolectomy or thrombectomy may be done. Observation with anticoagulation if thrombus is the source; however most cases of thrombosis involve a stenosis requiring revascularization with bowel resection as needed (Assar & Zarins, 2008; Kougias et al., 2007; Tendler & LaMont, 2011a).

REFERENCES

Assar, A. N., & Zarins, C. K. (2008). Acute mesenteric ischaemia: Facts and perspectives. *British Journal of Hospital Medicine, 69*(12), 686–691.

Bassiouny, H. S. (1997). Nonocclusive mesenteric ischemia. *Surgical Clinics of North America, 77*(2), 319–326.

Boley, S. J., Brandt, L. J., & Sammartano, R. J. (1997). History of mesenteric ischemia. The evolution of a diagnosis and management. *Surgical Clinics of North America, 77*(2), 275–288.

Broder, J. (2007). Abdominal vascular emergencies: A unified approach. *Emergency Medicine, 39*, 20–30.

Cappell, M. S. (1998a). Intestinal (mesenteric) vasculopathy I. *Gastroenterology Clinics of North America, 27*(4), 783–825.

Cappell, M. S. (1998b). Intestinal (mesenteric) vasculopathy II. *Gastroenterology Clinics of North America, 27*(4), 827–860.

Carpenito, L. J. (1999). *Handbook of nursing diagnosis.* Philadelphia, PA: Lippincott.

Doenges, M. E., Moorhouse, M. F., & Geissler, A. C. (2000). *Nursing care plans, guidelines for individualizing patient care.* Philadelphia, PA: F.A. Davis Company.

Dupee, R. M. (2011). Acute intestinal ischemia in the elderly. Retrieved from http://www.annalsoflongtermcare.com/article/8428, accessed April 11, 2011.

Ekers, M. A. (1994). Mesenteric ischemia. In V. A. Fahey (Ed.), *Vascular nursing* (pp. 391–401). Philadelphia, PA: W.B. Saunders Company.

Friedland, S., Benaron, D., Coogan, S., Sze, D. Y., & Soetikno, R. (2007). Diagnosis of chronic mesenteric ischemia by visible light spectroscopy during endoscopy. *Gastrointestinal Endoscopy, 65*(2), 294–300.

Gordon, P., & Christensen, C. R. (2011). Cardiac and vascular disorders, peripheral vascular disease. In M. S. Baird & S. Bethel (Eds.), *Manual of critical care nursing: Nursing interventions and collaborative management* (6th ed., pp. 546–565). St. Louis, MO: Elsevier, Mosby.

Gunduz, A., Turedi, S., Mentese, A., Karahan, S. C., Hos, G., That, O., ... Topbas, M. (2008). Ischemia-modified albumin in the diagnosis of acute mesenteric ischemia: A preliminary study. *American Journal of Emergency Medicine, 26*, 202–205.

Gupta, P. K., Horan, S. M., Turoga, K. K., Miller, W. J., & Pipinos, I. I. (2010). Chronic mesenteric ischemia: Endovascular versus open revascularization. *Journal of Endovascular Therapy, 15*, 540–549.

Herbert, G. S., & Steele, S. R. (2007). Acute and chronic mesenteric ischemia. *Surgical Clinics of North America, 87*, 1115–1134.

Hirsch, A. T., Haskal, Z. J., Hertzer, N. R., Bakal, C. W., Creager, M. A., Halperin, J. L., . . . White, R. A. (2006). ACC/AHA 2005 Practice guidelines for the management of patients with peripheral arterial disease (lower extremity, renal, mesenteric, and abdominal aortic): A collaborative report from the American Association for Vascular Surgery/Society for Vascular Surgery, Society for Cardiovascular Angiography and Interventions, Society for Vascular Medicine and Biology, Society of Interventional Radiology, and the ACC/AHA Task Force on Practice Guidelines. *Circulation, 113*, e463–e465.

Hugon, S., deClercq, P., & Landen, S. (2007). Acute mesenteric vein thrombosis. *Annals of Emergency Medicine, 50*(5), 623–624.

Kolkman, J. J., Groeneveld, A. B. J., Van der Berg, F. G., Rauwerda, J. A., & Meuwissen, S. G. M. (1999). Increased gastric PCO_2 during exercise is indicative of gastric ischaemia: A tonometric study. *Gut, 44*(2), 163–167.

Kougias, P., El Sayed, H. F., Zhou, W., & Lin, P. H. (2007). Management of chronic mesenteric ischemia. The role of endovascular therapy. *Journal of Endovascular Therapy, 14*, 395–405.

Leary, L. L. (2011). General concepts in caring for the critically ill; Pain. In M. S. Baird & S. Bethel (Eds.), *Manual of critical care nursing: Nursing interventions and collaborative management* (6th ed., pp. 135–149). St. Louis, MO: Elsevier, Mosby.

Levy, A. D. (2007). Mesenteric ischemia. *Radiologic Clinics of North America, 45*, 593–599.

Mansour, M. A. (1999). Management of acute mesenteric ischemia. *Archives of Surgery, 134*(3), 328–331.

McCutcheon, T. (2009). Superior mesenteric vein thrombosis after bowel resection in patients with inflammatory bowel disease. *Gastroenterology Nursing, 32*(2), 85–91.

McKinsey, J. F., & Gewertz, B. L. (1997). Acute mesenteric ischemia. *Surgical Clinics of North America, 77*(2), 307–318.

Moawad, J., & Gewertz, B. L. (1997). Chronic mesenteric ischemia, clinical presentation and diagnosis. *Surgical Clinics of North America, 77*(2), 357–369.

Moawad, J., McKinsey, J. F., Wyble, C. W., Bassiouny, H. S., Schwartz, L. B., & Gewertz, B. L. (1997). Current results of surgical therapy for chronic mesenteric ischemia. *Archives of Surgery, 132*(6), 613–618.

Nunnelee, J. D. (1999). Chronic mesenteric ischemia: Role of the nurse practitioner in diagnosis and management. *Clinical Excellence for Nurse Practitioners, 3*(4), 205–209.

Oderich, G. S. (2010). How do we decide when to stent and when to cut for mesenteric ischemia? *Journal of Endovascular Therapy, 17*, 550–553.

Paral, J., Ferko, A., Plodr, M., Raupach, J., Hadzi-Nikolov, D., Dolezal, D., & Chovanec, V. (2007). Laparoscopic diagnostics of acute bowel ischemia using ultraviolet light and fluorescein dye: An experimental study. *Surgical Laparoscopy, Endoscopy & Percutaneous Techniques, 17*(4), 291–295.

Ruotolo, R. A., & Evans, S. R. T. (1999). Mesenteric ischemia in the elderly. *Clinics in Geriatric Medicine, 15*(3), 527–557.

Safieddine, N., Mamazza, J., Common, A., & Prabhudesai, V. (2007). Splenic and superior mesenteric artery thrombolytic infusion therapy for acute portal and mesenteric vein thrombosis. *Canadian Journal of Surgery, 50*(1), 68–69.

Schermerhorn, M. L., Giles, K. A., Hamdan, A. D., Wyers, M. C., & Pomposelli, F. B. (2009). Mesenteric revascularization: Management and outcomes in the United States 1988–2006. *Journal of Vascular Surgery, 50*(2), 341–348.

Tendler, D. A., & LaMont, J. T. (2011a). Acute mesenteric ischemia. Retrieved from http://www.uptodate.com/contents/acute-mesenteric-ischemia?view=print, accessed April 11, 2011.

Tendler, D. A., & LaMont, J. T. (2011b). Chronic mesenteric ischemia. Retrieved from http://www.uptodate.com/contents/chronic-mesenteric-ischemia?view=print, accessed April 11, 2011.

Vincente, D. C., & Kazmers, A. (1999). Acute mesenteric ischemia. *Current Opinion in Cardiology, 14*(5), 453–458.

RELEVANT WEBSITES

http://www.emedicine.com/emerg/topic311.htm
http://www.vascularweb.org/vascularhealth/Pages/mesenteric-ischemia.aspx
http://www.mayoclinic.com/health-information/
http://www.nlm.nih.gov/medlineplus/ency/article/001156.htm
http://my.clevelandclinic.org/heart/disorders/vascular/visceralischemiasyndrome.aspx

CHAPTER 13

Aneurysmal Disease

Victoria R. Latessa
Anne Aquila

OBJECTIVES

1. Describe the anatomy and physiology relevant to aortic aneurysms and aneurysmal disease.
2. List appropriate diagnostic tests relevant to the diagnosis of aneurysmal disease.
3. Discuss the appropriate medical and surgical interventions relevant to aneurysmal disease.
4. Identify the nursing implications relevant to aneurysmal disease.

Introduction/Overview

The Ad hoc Committee of the Society for Vascular Surgery and International Society for Cardiovascular Surgery defines an aneurysm as a permanent localized dilation of an artery; an increase in diameter of greater than 50% or 1.5 times its normal diameter, normal diameter being determined by age, sex, and blood pressure (Johnston et al., 1991). Abdominal aortic aneurysm (AAA) is present in more than 5% of older men who have smoked. Aortic aneurysms constitute the 14th leading cause of death in the United States and the 10th leading cause of death in older men, who are the principal victims (Lederle, 2009).

Statistical data show that there is a 1% per year rupture rate for AAAs with a maximal diameter of less than 5.5 cm. The 1-year incidence of probable rupture for aneurysms between 5.5 and 5.9 cm was 9.4%, and there was a 10.2% rupture rate for aneurysms of 6 to 6.9 cm. Aneurysms greater than 7 cm had a 6-month rupture rate of 32.5%. These data indicate that due to the low incidence of rupture, physicians can recommend close observation of AAAs less than 5.5 cm. Aneurysms between 5.5 and 6.9 cm should be repaired promptly and those greater than 7 cm in diameter require urgent repair (Pappas, 2002). These are general recommendations that do not take into account the threshold for rupture in women that may be closer to 5 cm as opposed to men at 6 cm (Hannawa, Elias, & Upchurch, 2009).

A ruptured AAA is a catastrophic event. Overall, mortality of AAA rupture is 71% to 77% which includes all out-of-hospital and in-hospital deaths as compared to 2% to 6% for elective open surgical repair (Fillinger, 2010).

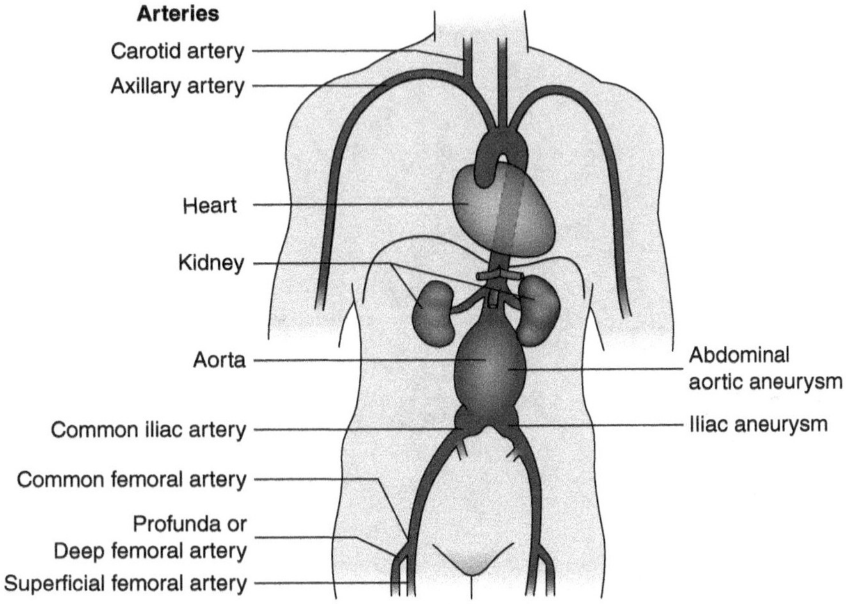

FIGURE 13-1. Aneurysms of some of the abdominal arteries.

I. Aortic Anatomy and Aneurysm Location (see Fig. 13-1)

A. Aorta Begins at the Aortic Valve, ascends in the anterior mediastinum, arches posteriorly, descends in the posterior mediastinum, and traverses the retroperitoneum to end at the bifurcation into the common iliac arteries (Matsumura, 2004).

B. It is Posteriorly Situated in the chest and abdomen and is considered a posterior mediastinal and retroperitoneal structure once past the aortic arch.

C. The First Branches of the aorta are the left and right coronary arteries that feed the myocardium.

D. The Arch Vessels include the innominate artery that branches into the right subclavian and right common carotid arteries and the left common carotid artery and left subclavian artery.

E. The Descending Aorta gives off intercostal branches, some of which (usually in the T9 to L1 area) anastomose with the critical artery of Adamkiewicz, which feeds the spinal cord.

F. Abdominal Branches of the aorta include the celiac artery, the superior mesenteric artery (SMA), renal arteries, and the inferior mesenteric artery (IMA).

G. At the Level of the Umbilicus, the aorta divides into the common iliac arteries.

H. In the Pelvis, the common iliac arteries bifurcate into the external and internal iliac arteries.

I. The External Iliac Artery continues under the inguinal ligament and becomes the common femoral artery.

J. Adult's Aorta normally measures approximately 2 cm (3/4") in diameter at the celiac axis level, narrowing as it nears the aortic bifurcation.

K. Twelve Percent of aneurysms occur in the thoracoabdominal aorta.

1. Involves the segment of the aorta where the celiac axis, SMA, and renal arteries arise
2. Extent of aortic involvement for thoracoabdominal aortic aneurysms based upon Crawford Classification (see Fig. 13-2)
   a. Type I: proximal descending thoracic aorta (DTA) to upper abdominal aorta
   b. Type II: proximal TA to below renal arteries
   c. Type III: distal DTA and abdominal aorta
   d. Type IV: suprarenal and infrarenal

L. Eighty Percent of Aneurysms Occur in the Infrarenal Abdominal Aorta (Lederle, 2009; O'Connor, 2013).

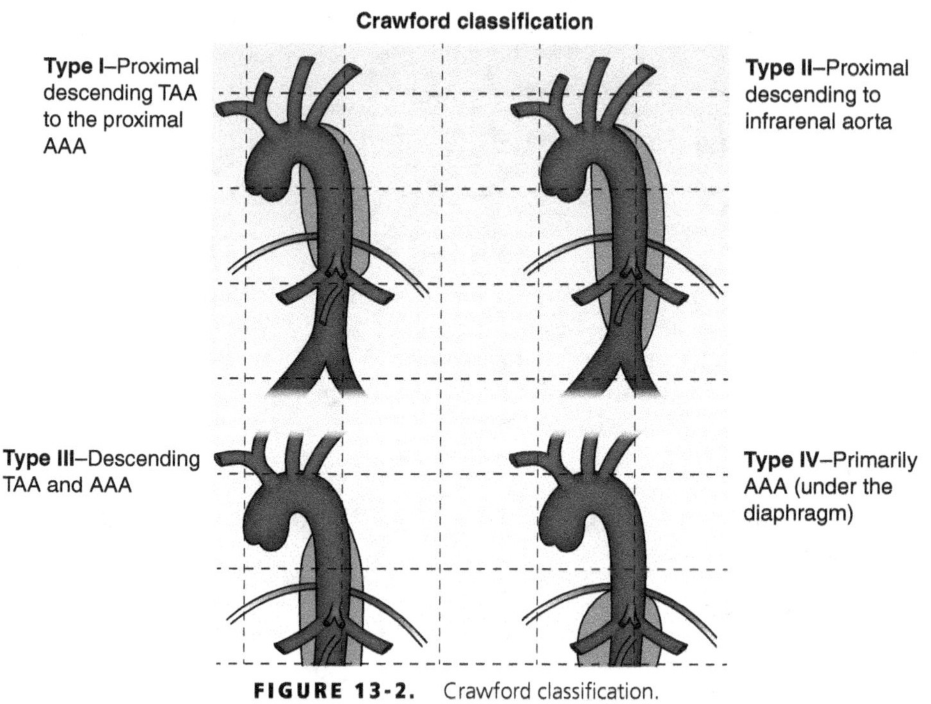

FIGURE 13-2. Crawford classification.

II. Pathophysiology

A. Arteriosclerosis/Atherosclerosis: Plays a role in the development of most aneurysms (Cohen, 1990; Lawrence & Rigbirg, 2010; Lovell & Harris, 1991).

1. Traditional views held that most aneurysms were caused by degenerative atherosclerotic disease.
2. Atherosclerotic lesions weaken arterial wall rendering it brittle and susceptible to thinning.

B. Genetic Predisposition to Aneurysm Development

1. Clinical observations and biochemical data suggest that atherosclerosis/arteriosclerosis may not be the unique pathogenic factor of aneurysmal disease.
2. Some studies suggest that genetic predisposition is isolated to a single dominant gene with low penetrance that increases with age (Majumder, Jean, Ferrell, Webster, & Steed, 1991).
3. There may be a genetic predisposition to their development—alteration in systemic connective tissue metabolism (Anderson, 1994; Cohen, 1990, Curci, Baxter, & Thompson, 2005; Greenberg, Messina, & Thompson, 2000; Reilly & Tilson, 1989; Tilson, 1990).
4. Data over the past 20 years have revealed:
   a. Presence of matrix metalloproteins (MMPs), a family of enzymes involved in breaking down elastin and collagen (Curci, Lee, & Thompson, 2001)
   b. Chronic increase in aortic elastin breakdown brings about weakening of the wall and aneurysm dilation
   c. Current theories suggest a spectrum of inflammation with all AAA (Lawrence & Rigbirg, 2010)
   d. Cigarette smoking has major effect on enzyme activity—increasing serum elastase activity
   e. Definite familial tendency; 15% to 25% of patients undergoing AAA repair have a first-degree relative with clinically apparent AAA (Curci et al., 2005; Lawrence & Rigbirg, 2010)

C. Aneurysmal Growth

1. Aneurysm thought to grow according to law of Laplace: tension = pressure × radius ($T = P \times r$). With increasing pressure on the aortic wall or increase in wall radius, the wall tension becomes close to that of the tensile strength of collagen, resulting in rupture with any local wall weakness (Cohen, 1990).
2. Size of an aneurysm is the most important risk factor that determines risk of rupture, pressure (Goldstone, 2002; U.S. Preventive Services Task Force, 2005).
3. Sudden rupture of AAA accounts for approximately 15,000 deaths in the United States (Goldstone, 2002).

III. Etiology or Precipitating Factors (Cronenwett, Krupski, & Rutherford, 2000)

A. Degenerative

1. Atherosclerosis
2. Medial necrosis

3. Fibrodysplasia
4. Pregnancy related
5. Site of graft anastomosis

B. Inflammatory

1. Arteritis
2. Bacterial/fungal/viral infections

C. Mechanical

1. Traumatic
2. Poststenotic
3. Anastomotic
4. Prosthetic

D. Congenital

1. Born with abnormal dilations of arteries
2. Marfan syndrome
3. Ehlers–Danlos syndrome

IV. Assessment

A. Risk Factors

1. Gender
    a. Males three to six times more likely to have AAA than females
    b. Occurs in of every 20 elderly men (Lederle, 2003)
    c. Males have a 40% higher likelihood of presenting with ruptured aneurysm and are older than females for intact and ruptured AAA (Fillinger, 2010)
    d. Women more likely to fare worse, whether open repair of EVAR, elective surgery, or repair with rupture (Hannawa et al., 2009; Schermerhorn & Giles, 2010)
2. Age
    a. Prevalence of AAA increases with age
    b. Highest percent of patients with AAA between 70 and 80 years of age (Schermerhorn & Giles, 2010)
    c. Ninety-five percent of patients dying with rupture AAA are older than 65 years (Singh, Bonaa, Jacobsen, Bjork, & Solberg, 2001)
3. Smoking
    a. Smokers three to five times more likely than nonsmokers
    b. Length of time smoking more important than amount
    c. By-products of smoking are destructive to aortic wall (Lederle, 2003)
4. Hypertension
    a. Accelerates the degeneration of the aortic wall
    b. Higher intra-aortic pressure increases risk of rupture
5. Family history
    a. AAA not an inherited disorder
    b. Evidence of familial clustering
    c. Risk of AAA for brother of patient treated for AAA is increased fourfold (Powell, 2003)

6. Aneurysm elsewhere
    a. Patient with unilateral popliteal artery aneurysm has 8% chance of having AAA
    b. Patient with bilateral popliteal artery aneurysms has 30% chance of AAA
    c. Patient with AAA has 12% chance of thoracic aortic aneurysm (Goldstone, 2002)
7. Known history of connective tissue disease
    a. Ehlers–Danlos
    b. Marfan
8. Primary prevention
    a. No biochemical markers available to detect early changes in matrix of aortic wall
    b. Screen those at high risk for developing AAA with ultrasound (U.S. Preventive Services Task Force, 2005)
        1) One time screening for all males 60 to 75 years old who have ever smoked or 55 years old for those with family history of AAA
        2) Ultrasound screening for women 65 years and older who have smoked or have positive family history of AAA (Chaikof et al., 2009)
        3) Screen men 60 to 85 years of age or older who are either the sibling or offspring of patients with AAA (Hirsch et al., 2006)

B. Patient History

1. Subjective findings
    a. Asymptomatic
        1) Usually found incidentally during evaluation for chronic back pain or kidney stones
        2) Rarely symptomatic unless there is rapid expansion or rupture (Cronenwett et al., 2000; Lederle, 2009; Winterstein & Baxter, 2000).
        3) Can have diffuse mid-abdominal pain caused by compression of adjacent structures
        4) AAA rupture may have back, flank, or groin pain and tenderness
        5) Gastrointestinal (GI) dysfunction, urinary dysfunction, syncope, hypotension, and shock (Lederle, 2009)
    b. Past health history—Broad in scope but focused on vascular risk factors such as hypertension, angina, myocardial infarction, peripheral artery disease, transient ischemic attack, DM, dyslipidemias, chronic obstructive pulmonary disease (COPD)
    c. Family history
        1) Vascular, heart disease, hypertension
        2) Aneurysmal disease
    d. Social history—Cigarette smoking; a history of heavy tobacco use or family history of AAA should heighten awareness in older persons particularly men (Lederle, 2009)
    e. Medication history—All current therapeutic drugs
2. Objective findings on physical examination
    a. Inspection
        1) Pulsatile abdomen
        2) Mottling, cyanosis may be present with rupture
        3) "Blue toes" may be evident with distal embolization (Fahey, 2004)

b. Palpation
    1) Widened aortic pulsation or pulsatile abdominal mass at or above the umbilicus usually at least 5 cm to be reliably identified except in a very thin person
    2) Has only moderate overall sensitivity for detecting AAA but appears to be highly sensitive for diagnosis of AAA large enough to warrant elective intervention in patients who do not have a large girth (Fink et al., 2000)
    3) Check for associated femoral and popliteal aneurysms

3. Auscultation—Abdominal bruit rarely present

V. Considerations Across the Life Span

A. Aging

1. Estimated incidence: 3% to 5% of elderly population >65 years of age (about one million people) have aneurysmal disease (Ohki, 2002)
2. Frequency of aneurysms increases steadily in men older than 55 years, reaching a peak of 5.9% at 80 to 85 years (Goldstone, 2002)
3. Astute physical examination needed in this population to identify aneurysms, follow individuals, and intervene when necessary
4. Continuous and diligent assessment of risk factors
5. Screening at risk populations (U.S. Preventive Services Task Force, 2005)

VI. Pertinent Diagnostic Testing

A. Laboratory Tests: Complete blood count, platelet count, prothrombin time, partial prothrombin time, fibrinogen, electrolytes, blood urea nitrogen, creatinine, liver profile, urinalysis

B. Noninvasive Testing

1. Chest roentgenograms (CXR)
    a. Anteroposterior (AP) and lateral x-rays
    b. May be able to demonstrate aneurysm if there is sufficient calcium in the wall of the aneurysm sac (Lovell & Harris, 1991)
    c. Advantages—With thoracic aneurysm, may be mediastinal widening; if leaking or rupture may have pleural effusion or pleural hematoma
    d. Disadvantages—CXR is nondiagnostic, requires additional diagnostic studies
2. Abdominal ultrasonography (Barkin & Rosen, 2004; Nowygrod, 2001; Vogelzang, 2004)
    a. Based on Doppler ultrasound principles—abdomen is scanned using a transducer utilizing low frequency such as 3 MHz
    b. Sound waves are reflected and refracted by the structures beneath the transducer and are detected by the same transducer that is sending the signals
    c. Returning sound waves are then converted to images and displayed on a monitor
    d. Advantages
        1) Provides noninvasive quantitative determination of severity of disease; gives estimate of size: length, width, AP diameter

2) Suitable for screening, diagnosis, and follow-up evaluation
3) Highly accurate (95%) with experienced technologist
4) Relatively inexpensive compared to invasive testing, without risks of complications

e. Disadvantages
1) Bowel gas may cause an inadequate study, so overnight fasting is usually successful in obtaining images
2) Resolution impaired by body habitus
3) Technician dependent

3. Computed tomography (CT) scan (Vogelzang, 2004)
a. Produces axial slices of the body, so that anatomy is depicted in cross-section
b. Patient placed supine in circular open gantry with x-ray tube and multiple x-ray detectors
c. Tube moves around body while emitting x-rays confined to narrow slice varying from 2 to 10 mm. Rays pass through body and are detected on opposite side by detectors
d. Advantages
1) More accurate in estimating size than ultrasonography
2) Demonstrates the relationship of the aneurysm to renal arteries and involvement of the iliac arteries
3) Helpful in identifying suprarenal extension of the aneurysm
4) Better at identifying extravasated blood and confirming the suspicion of a contained rupture

e. Disadvantages
1) Use of ionizing radiation
2) Use of intravenous contrast for best results (nephrotoxicity or allergic reaction)
3) Expensive equipment requiring experienced technical support staff and a radiologist who is familiar with interpretation of results
4) Patient must be able to lie flat in gantry without moving and intermittently hold breath for optimal imaging

4. Magnetic resonance angiography (MRA) (Vogelzang, 2004)
a. Images formed by placing patient in a magnetic field strong enough to cause a small fraction of atomic nuclei to orient with magnetic field
b. A radio frequency pulse wiggles the nuclei so that they emit signal. Through the collection of signals from hundreds of pulses, an image is created
c. Advantages
1) No ionizing radiation is used
2) Images are multiplanar (three-dimensional)
3) No arterial catheter

d. Disadvantages
1) If claustrophobia, patient will not tolerate
2) Careful screening for metals within body because of powerful magnet: avoid patients with pacemakers, implanted defibrillators, metal implants in eyes, cochlear implants
3) For patients with intracavitary metal such as staples or stents, images will reflect scatter effect from metal and may be difficult to interpret
4) User and equipment dependent for quality images

5) Gadolinium must be used with extreme caution in patients with renal insufficiency or renal failure due to increased incidence of nephrogenic systemic fibrosis (Diego, 2010)
6) Not suitable for unstable patient (O'Connor, 2013)

C. Invasive Testing

1. Arteriography (Vogelzang, 2004) (Gold Standard in outlining the vascular tree and patency of vessels)
   a. Radiographic images of various segments of the arterial circulation via catheter-based injection of contrast media to outline vessel lumen
   b. Transfemoral approach is the most widely used, safest, and most effective route of arteriography
   c. Virtually all arteriography procedures are performed using the Seldinger technique, which involves a needle puncture of the artery followed by placement of a wire through the needle into the lumen of the vessel
   d. Over this wire a catheter may be safely placed within the vessel, with the wire acting as a "guide" to the catheter
   e. The wire is then withdrawn and the catheter can be directed to a specific location and an injection made with iodine contrast agent
      1) Total contrast does not usually exceed 350 mL
      2) Heparinized flush solution constantly infused to prevent thrombosis
   f. Advantages
      1) Useful in delineating anatomy of renal arteries and mesenteric circulation
      2) Helpful in evaluating patency and involvement of iliac arteries and distal runoff below the aorta, as sites of stenosis or occlusion are identified by partial filling defect or complete lack of filling of vessel with contrast medium
   g. Disadvantages
      1) Invasive, arterial contrast dye injection required which may limit or prevent testing
      2) Potential for arterial injury, distal embolization, or vessel occlusion from catheter
      3) May require overnight hospital stay
   h. Not routinely required unless reason to suspect complicating features such as associated renovascular hypertension or suspected additional aneurysms (femoral, popliteal)

VII. Medical Management (Nonoperative)

A. No known Evidence-Based medical treatment at present time other than optimal treatment of risk factors: hypertension, hyperlipidemia, diabetes, and smoking cessation (Chaikof et al., 2009)

B. Standard of Care is Surgical Repair to Prevent Rupture

C. Research Underway

1. Develop biochemical markers that would indicate changes in the composition and matrix of abdominal wall

2. High-resolution CT scans may be able to detect progressive loss of elasticity in aorta that might warrant closer observation

D. Research in Pharmacology (Cronenwett et al., 2000; Curciet al., 2001)

1. Beta blockers (propranolol): hemodynamic properties and biochemical effects on matrix proteins (Baxter, Terrin, & Dalman, 2008)
   a. Sustained control of elevated BP
   b. Blocks circulating tissue plasminogen activator and may decrease expansion by reducing plasminogen-mediated MMP activation
2. Indomethacin
   a. Inhibition of aneurysm formation by lowering MMP-9 levels
3. MMP inhibitors such as doxycycline and roxithromycin
   a. Inhibit a number of MMPs that stimulate the production and release of MMPs from medial smooth muscle cells (Fillinger, 2010)
   b. Decrease inflammatory cell infiltrate thereby reducing expansion of small AAAs (Takagi, Masafumi, & Umemoto, 2010)
   c. Need larger clinical trials
4. Statins
   a. Reduce atherogenic lipoproteins, inhibit inflammation and protease inhibition in arterial wall (Buth, 2008)
   b. Reduction of C-reactive protein levels that may be relevant to the pathogenesis of AAA disease (Baxter et al., 2008)

VIII. Surgical Management (Operative)

A. Risk of Rupture

1. Natural history of AAA is enlargement and rupture
2. As a rule, the greater the size of the aneurysm, the more likely it is to rupture
3. Growth rate is 0.2 to 0.4 cm/yr and depends on aneurysm size, diastolic blood pressure, and COPD (Goldstone, 2002)
4. Information regarding growth rate and rupture risk is useful in balancing the risk of associated disease and its progression against the risk of aneurysm rupture as it increases in size
5. Aneurysms are repaired to avoid rupture

B. Indications for Surgery (Pappas, 2002)

1. Size >5.5 cm
2. Symptomatic: symptoms believed to come from aneurysm and pressure on adjacent structures
3. Rapid enlargement
4. Distal emboli: thrombotic material and atheromatous debris that line almost all AAAs may come loose and carry emboli distally to lower extremities
5. GI hemorrhage: stretching of duodenum over the enlarging aneurysm may bring about partial intestinal obstruction, or if erosion occurs, upper GI bleeding
6. Rupture

C. Preoperative Evaluation

1. Identification of preoperative risk factors as they may influence intraoperative and postoperative periods
   a. Smoking
   b. Angiographically significant coronary artery disease
   c. Coronary artery disease
      1) Angina
      2) Myocardial infarction
      3) Coronary artery bypass grafting
   d. Hypertension
   e. Peripheral vascular disease
   f. Lung dysfunction
   g. Congestive heart failure
   h. Renal dysfunction
   i. Cerebrovascular disease
   j. Diabetes mellitus
2. Selective testing based upon patient status
   a. Stress testing to identify underlying heart disease; if abnormal proceed with cardiac catheterization
   b. Echocardiography to assess valvular function; valvular incompetence is a relative contraindication to cross-clamping of proximal aorta unless shunt or bypass technique is used
   c. Carotid duplex scan to determine significant carotid stenosis
   d. Pulmonary function testing to determine significant pulmonary disease; optimization may be needed prior to surgery
   e. Ankle–brachial index to assess for lower-extremity disease

D. Types of Repair

1. Open aneurysmectomy (see Fig. 13-3)
   a. First report of successful surgical resection and graft replacement of an infrarenal AAA in 1952

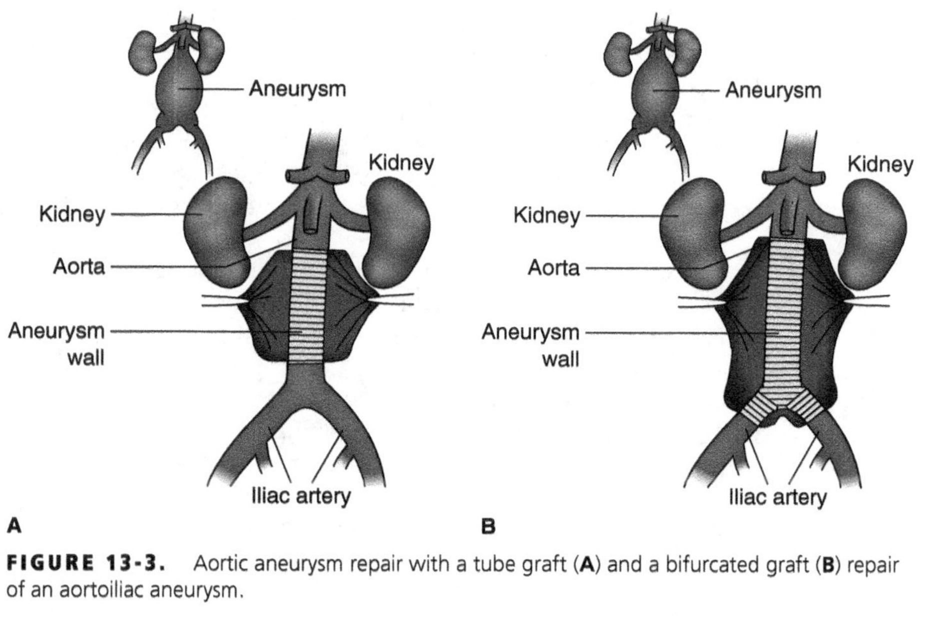

FIGURE 13-3. Aortic aneurysm repair with a tube graft (**A**) and a bifurcated graft (**B**) repair of an aortoiliac aneurysm.

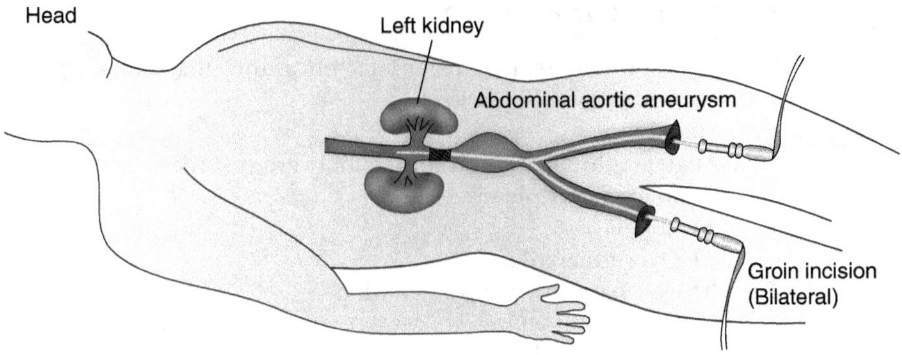

FIGURE 13-4. Endovascular repair of an aortic aneurysm.

   b. Approaches to aneurysm—transperitoneally or retroperitoneally
      1) Retroperitoneal approach may be performed for patients with lung dysfunction to avoid midline incision or those patients with a hostile abdomen
      2) Technically and physiologically advantageous for all types of aortic repair (Darling, Paty, & Saltzberg, 2010)
   c. Control of aneurysm is achieved as neck and iliac arteries are dissected out
   d. Aorta and appropriate distal vessels are clamped
      1) Clamping stops blood flow to extremities
      2) Workload of heart increases as there is an increase in resistance the heart must beat against
   e. Aneurysm is opened along its full length, laminated thrombus that lines vessel wall is removed, and any bleeding lumbar arteries are oversewn from within the aneurysm
   f. Graft is placed
      1) Knitted Dacron preclotted
      2) Tube graft for aortic involvement
      3) Bifurcated graft for extension into iliac arteries
   g. Graft is sewn in place distally and proximally
   h. Old aneurysm wall often closed over new graft as cover to reinforce and isolate it from abdominal contents
   i. Incision is closed
2. Endovascular stent graft (EVSG) repair (see Fig. 13-4)
   a. Accounts for more than one half of all AAA repairs performed in the United States (Paraskevas, Bessias, Giannoukas, & Mikhailidis, 2010)
   b. Intraluminal repair of aneurysm via remote access site under fluoroscopic guidance
   c. First endovascular repair of AAA using transfemoral insertion of prosthetic graft reported by Juan Parodi of Buenos Aires in 1991
   d. Types of grafts: tube, bifurcated, aorto-uni-iliac; type used based upon anatomy (see Fig. 13-5)
   e. Candidates for consideration of EVSG anatomy dependent
   f. Anatomic considerations for graft placement
      1) Diameter of iliac or femoral artery must be large enough to accommodate device
      2) Tortuosity may limit access and prohibit navigation of device
      3) Calcification may prohibit navigation of device and predispose to arterial injury or rupture

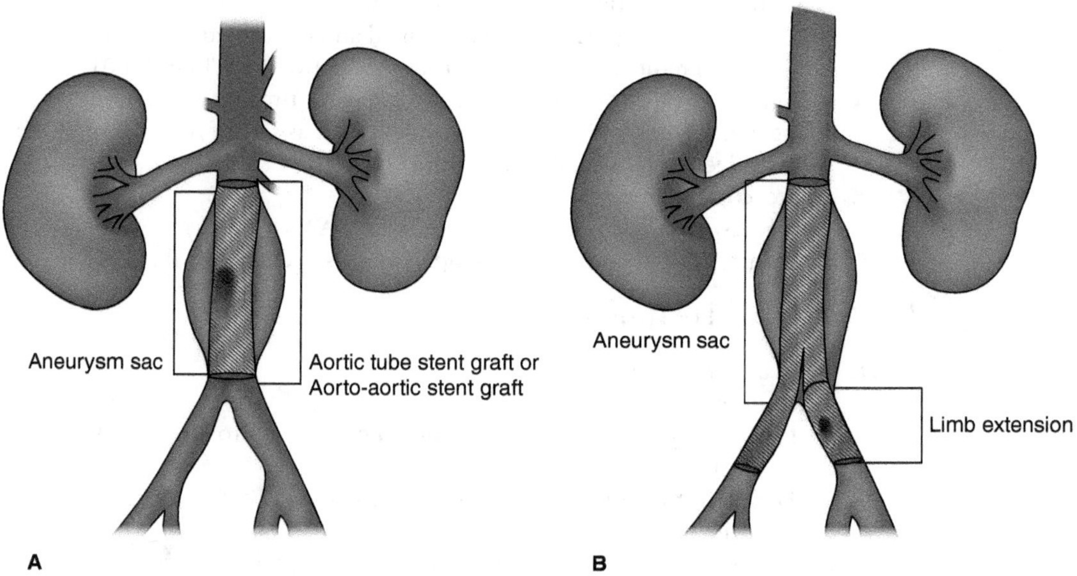

FIGURE 13-5. Endovascular stent graft placement as a tube graft (**A**) and with limb extension to create a bifurcated graft (**B**).

4) Proximal neck: that area of normal aorta above the aneurysm and below the renal arteries in which the graft must attach to the aortic wall to provide an adequate seal
5) Distal neck: the area of normal aorta below the aneurysm in the aorta or in the iliac artery that will be the distal landing zone of the graft (Green, 2002)

g. Preoperative screening.
   1) Same as for open procedure
   2) Ankle–brachial indices documented
   3) CT scan of abdomen and pelvis with 3-mm cuts used to determine the diameter of the aorta and iliac arteries so that the device can be sized to fit snug against aortic wall (GRAFT DIAMETER)
   4) CTA with three-dimensional reconstruction or angiogram with marker catheter: may be used to determine the length of the endovascular graft (GRAFT LENGTH)
   5) Type of imaging used depends on surgeon and imaging availability (Van der Laan, Milner, & Blankensteijn, 2002)

h. Procedure
   1) Performed in operating room or interventional radiology with C-arm
   2) Epidural, spinal, or general anesthesia
   3) Mark distal pulses
   4) Cutdown to iliac or common femoral artery
   5) Placement of protective sheath through which all instrumentation takes place
   6) Patient is heparinized
   7) Advancement of guidewire into abdominal aorta, navigation of endovascular device over the guidewire into proper position above

and below the aneurysm excluding it from the general circulation, may use multiple injections of contrast
        8) Once proper positioning is obtained and confirmed, heparin reversed, sheath removed, and arteriotomy closed (May & White, 2000)
    i. Follow-up is lifelong with imaging at specific time intervals monitoring graft for migration and endoleak as well as size of AAA (Clair, 2010; Eastridge, Rodriguez, & Matusmura, 2004)
3. Laparoscopic aneurysmectomy
    a. Very few laparoscopic surgeries done for AAA
    b. Requires vascular and laparoscopic expertise (Olinde et al., 2010)

E. Results of Treatment

1. Open aneurysmectomy
    a. Mortality rate
        1) For infrarenal AAA, aortic reconstruction is approximately 5% (Pappas, 2002)
        2) Emergency surgery for rupture approximately 45%
        3) Patients in shock, 80%
    b. Improvement in mortality rates for elective repair is related to
        1) Better preoperative assessment of concomitant coronary artery disease
        2) Better operative technique
        3) Better graft material
        4) Autotransfusion intraoperatively
        5) More sophisticated intraoperative monitoring and fluid/drug management
    c. Advantages
        1) Low mortality rate 2% to 6% (Forsdahl, Singh, Solberg, & Jacobson, 2009)
        2) Long-term, regular follow-up of graft not necessary
        3) Durable procedure, usually lasts a lifetime
    d. Disadvantages
        1) Overall morbidity rate is 32.4% (Pappas, 2002)
        2) Cardiac and pulmonary status must be acceptable for general anesthesia and anticipated recovery
        3) Large abdominal or left flank incision
        4) Longer length of hospital stay
        5) Recovery time 4 to 6 weeks
2. EVSG repair
    a. Mortality rates
        1) 1% to 2% (Pappas, 2002)
        2) Early complications include damage to iliac or femoral artery, graft limb thrombosis, branch artery occlusion, distal embolization
        3) Late complications: stent migration or endoleak (Clair, 2010)
    b. Advantages
        1) Regional anesthesia with conscious sedation alternative to general anesthesia
        2) One/two groin incisions instead of abdominal incision
        3) Can be used in conjunction with supraceliac balloon to control bleeding in event of ruptured aneurysm (Clair, 2010)
        4) Hospitalization 24 to 72 hours
        5) Recuperation 7 to 10 days

c. Disadvantages
   1) Anatomy dependent
   2) Requires long-term follow-up due to potential for complications including endoleak, graft migration, continued expansion of the aneurysm
d. Endoleak
   1) Complication unique to EVSG repair of aneurysm
   2) Definition: persistence of blood flow around the endograft within the aneurysm sac (May & White, 2000)
   3) Classification of endoleaks (Clair, 2010)
      a) Type I: persistent flow of blood into the aneurysm sac develops due to inadequate seal at proximal or distal ends of graft. Treatment: proximal or distal extension, embolization, secondary endograft, convert to open
      b) Type II: persistent blood flow into the aneurysm sac due to retrograde blood flow from lumbar arteries, the IMA, or other collateral vessels. Treatment: observation, most resolve without intervention. For those that do not resolve, coil embolization or laparoscopic clipping of vessel
      c) Type III: arises at the midgraft region because of leakage through a defect within the graft or at the junction between pieces. Treatment: secondary endograft
      d) Type IV: seen on completion angiography or subsequent contrast studies as any minor blush of contrast that is presumed to emanate from blood diffusion across the pores of a highly porous graft fabric. Treatment: usually subside in 30 days (Deitch & Yano, 2000)
      e) Type V: endotension; persistent growth of aneurysm sac without demonstrable endoleak; can lead to open repair

IX. Nursing Diagnosis Following AAA Repair (extent to which each system is affected will depend to a certain extent upon the type of procedure performed)

A. Alteration in Ventilation related to anesthesia, surgical incision, decreased functional residual capacity, pain

1. Expected outcome: experience adequate respiratory function
2. Nursing interventions
   a. Assess rate, depth, effort of breathing
   b. Institute lung expansion maneuvers as appropriate
      1) Activity/positioning
      2) Incentive spirometry with deep breathing and coughing
      3) Chest physiotherapy when indicated
      4) Respiratory treatments when indicated
   c. Oxygen therapy
   d. Monitoring of pulse oximetry
   e. Monitoring of ABGs
3. Evaluation of nursing care
   a. Respiratory status assessed frequently with documentation and reporting of alterations

   b. Lung expansion maneuvers are taught, instituted, and patient performance evaluated and importance reinforced

B. Potential for Cardiac Instability related to stress of aortic surgery, pre-existing coronary artery disease, aortic cross-clamping (open repair), hypokalemia. During EVSG hypotension may be induced to ease deployment of the graft or may be caused by venous dilatation with regional anesthesia (Ouriel & Green, 1999)

1. Expected outcome: maintenance of optimal cardiovascular function
2. Nursing interventions
   a. Serial EKGs when indicated
   b. Monitoring serum potassium levels
   c. Cardiac enzymes when indicated
   d. Assess for chest pain, dyspnea, diaphoresis, nausea, vomiting
   e. Monitoring of vital signs and hemodynamic parameters
3. Evaluation of nursing care
   a. Cardiovascular status is assessed frequently with documentation and reporting of alterations

C. Potential for Renal Failure related to decreased cardiac output, hypotension, declamping shock (unusual event now during open repair), and renal artery injury, occlusion, or embolism. EVSG repair necessitates significant contrast during the procedure that can result in renal insufficiency or failure

1. Expected outcome: experience adequate kidney function
2. Nursing interventions
   a. Accurate intake/output
   b. Daily weights as ordered
   c. Monitoring of urine specific gravity
   d. Monitoring of urine electrolytes and osmolality when indicated
   e. Monitoring of BUN, creatinine, and serum potassium; compare with baseline
   f. Fluids/diuretics when indicated
   g. Fluid restriction, acid–base balance, and electrolyte management when indicated
3. Evaluation of nursing care
   a. Kidney function assessed frequently with documentation and reporting of alterations

D. Potential Fluid Volume Deficit related to hemorrhage or hematoma, third spacing of fluids

1. Expected outcome: maintenance of adequate vascular fluid volume
2. Nursing interventions
   a. Monitoring of vital signs and hemodynamic parameters
   b. Monitoring of change in mental status and level of consciousness
   c. Examination of skin for color and temperature
   d. Examination of back/scrotum for ecchymosis
   e. Inspection of nasogastric tube (NGT) aspirate, replace NGT output as ordered
   f. Monitor dressings for excessive drainage

g. Monitor incisions for hematoma formation
h. Accurate intake/output
i. Volume replacement (crystalloid/colloid)
j. Attention to laboratory values including hemoglobin, hematocrit, and coagulation studies
3. Evaluation of nursing care
a. Fluid volume status assessed frequently with documentation and reporting of alterations

E. **Potential Alteration in Peripheral Tissue Perfusion** related to presence of arterial occlusive disease, graft thrombosis, distal embolization

1. Expected outcome: maintenance of adequate lower-extremity tissue perfusion
2. Nursing interventions
a. Monitor lower extremities at specified intervals noting color, temperature, pulses, motor and sensory function
b. Provide patient with pressure-reducing devices as appropriate
c. Avoid raising knee gatch and placing pillows under the knees
3. Evaluation of nursing care
a. Lower-extremity tissue perfusion will be assessed frequently with documentation and reporting of alterations

F. **Potential Alteration in Skin Integrity** related to decreased circulation, altered nutritional status, presence of infection, multiple surgical procedures

1. Expected outcome: maintenance of adequate skin integrity
2. Nursing interventions
a. Monitor lower extremities at specified intervals noting color, temperature, pulses, motor and sensory function, and any areas of skin breakdown
b. Provide patient with pressure-reducing devices as appropriate
c. Separate toes that press on each other with lamb's wool or dry gauze
d. Remove pressure on the toes from bed linen as appropriate
e. Encourage a diet high in protein and vitamins for wound healing
f. Involve dietitian as needed to assist with diet education
3. Evaluation of nursing care
a. Lower-extremity skin integrity will be assessed frequently with documentation and treatment of alterations

G. **Alteration in GI Function** related to anesthesia, bowel manipulation during surgery (open repair), ileus with spinal or epidural anesthesia (EVSG repair), pain medication, decrease in activity

1. Expected outcome: maintenance of adequate GI function
2. Nursing interventions
a. Assess for return of bowel sounds/flatus
b. Monitor for any abdominal distension, bloody diarrhea, or severe abdominal pain (could indicate bowel ischemia)
c. Monitor and record NGT output with attention to patency
d. Out of bed with progressive ambulation
e. Assess need for some type of laxative postoperatively

3. Evaluation of nursing care
   a. GI status assessed frequently with documentation and reporting of alterations

H. Potential Alteration in Tissue Perfusion to the Bowel related to division of IMA in surgery, embolization of mesenteric arteries, decreased perfusion during aortic cross-clamping

1. Expected outcome: maintenance of adequate perfusion to the bowel
2. Nursing interventions
   a. Monitor for any abdominal distension, bloody or nonbloody diarrhea, or severe abdominal pain that could indicate bowel ischemia
   b. Monitor for any sudden elevation in white blood cell count or fever
   c. If bowel ischemia is suspected, prepare patient for bedside sigmoidoscopy to determine extent of bowel injury
   d. For any symptoms indicative of mild bowel ischemia resulting in superficial (mucosal) bowel injury
      1) Maintain NGT
      2) Ensure adequate hydration
      3) Initiate antibiotic therapy
   e. For more severe injury
      1) Treat as a surgical emergency
      2) Plan for exploratory surgery with resection without a primary anastomosis
      3) Initiate antibiotic therapy
      4) Patient may require second look operation as indicated
3. Evaluation of nursing care
   a. Bowel ischemia will be assessed for, identified promptly should it occur, and be promptly treated

I. Alteration in Comfort related to surgical incision/procedure and variety of tubes, drains, lines, and monitors

1. Expected outcome: pain will be appropriately assessed and managed
2. Nursing interventions
   a. Assess pain noting location, intensity, quality, aggravating/alleviating factors, effect on mood and functioning
   b. Determine with patient an acceptable pain level
   c. Institute appropriate pain management strategies
      1) Pharmacologic modalities
      2) Nonpharmacologic modalities
   d. Reassess patient at specified intervals to determine the appropriateness and effectiveness of pain management strategies instituted
3. Evaluation of nursing care
   a. Pain is assessed at specified intervals with appropriate interventions and follow-up of patient provided

J. Potential for Endoleak related to incomplete seal at the proximal or distal ends of the graft; retrograde blood flow from patent lumbar arteries, the IMA, or other collateral vessels; ineffective seal between graft joints or graft porosity

1. Expected outcome: patient will remain free from endoleak

2. Nursing interventions
   a. Review timing and importance of follow-up examinations and diagnostic tests to monitor the integrity and placement of the graft
   b. Physical examination to palpate aneurysm noting tenderness or pulsations
   c. Monitor lower extremities noting pulses for evidence of embolization or graft limb thrombosis
   d. Plain films of the abdomen: PA, lateral, right/left obliques to monitor for fracture of struts that support graft (would predispose to endoleak)
   e. CT scan of the abdomen and pelvis with intravenous contrast to check for extravasation of dye into aneurysm sac or increase in size of the aneurysm
   f. Review warning signs of AAA leak, expansion, or rupture (asymptomatic, new onset of abdominal or chest pain, severe or unusual abdominal or chest pain, sudden weakness, syncope, collapse)
3. Evaluation of nursing care
   a. Endoleak will be assessed for, identified promptly should it occur, and be promptly treated, if indicated. Follow up 1 to 2 weeks postoperative, 6 months, 12 months, and annually thereafter for life (Eastridge et al., 2004)

X. Patient Teaching

A. Preoperative

1. Knowledge deficit regarding disease process and treatment indications
   a. Explain treatment options using diagrams and written instructions when appropriate
   b. Review and discuss pre-and postoperative routines including preoperative testing, hospital and posthospital recovery
   c. Encourage patient to ask questions, and provide support and encouragement

B. Postoperative (review the following with the patient)

1. Activity
   a. Ambulate as tolerated and increase activity gradually
   b. Expect to feel a little weaker and more tired at home; this is normal and it may take 4 to 6 weeks to return to baseline
   c. Pace activities and stop any activity when you begin to feel tired
   d. Climbing stairs is acceptable in moderation
   e. Going outdoors is acceptable
   f. No heavy lifting (more than 5 lbs) until first follow-up visit
2. Bathing
   a. Bathing or showering is usually allowed by the fifth day following, but this will vary depending on surgeon's preference
   b. Cleanse incision with soap and water; pat dry
3. Driving: Do not drive a car until you have permission from your surgeon
4. Wound care
   a. No special wound care is needed unless otherwise indicated
   b. Observe wound for signs of redness, swelling, or drainage

5. Avoiding injury/foot care
   a. Inspect feet every day
   b. Do not go barefoot
   c. Shoes and socks protect your feet. Wear shoes that fit well and provide good support
   d. Break in a new pair of shoes slowly by wearing them for 30 minutes the first day, then an hour longer on the following days. Always inspect feet for any signs of redness or blisters
   e. Change socks daily and avoid tight socks and panty hose
   f. Protect limbs from excessive heat or cold to prevent against injury
   g. Wash feet daily with mild soap and water (no longer than 10 minutes), rinse well and dry completely, especially between your toes
   h. Have a foot doctor (podiatrist) care for corns, calluses, or ingrown nails
   i. Moisturizing lotions may be used, but avoid perfumed preparations because of drying effects
6. Diet
   a. A decrease in appetite is normal after surgery, as are changes in bowel habits. Appetite will slowly return to normal
   b. Proper nutrition is needed (protein, vitamin C) for wound healing
7. Medications: medication management: purpose, dosage, side effects
8. Fever
   a. Monitor temperature after EVSG repair of AAA
   b. Small percentage of patients with EVSG repair will develop postimplantation syndrome characterized by low-grade fever that lasts from 2 to 10 days
   c. Treatment is symptomatic, acetaminophen or ibuprofen for comfort
   d. Call health care provider for temperature greater than 101°F, shaking chills, shortness of breath, or any difficulty breathing
9. Follow up with health care provider/surgeon
   a. Emphasize need for patient to maintain contact with health care provider
      1) Patients undergoing open repair will follow up with surgeon 7 to 10 days with physical examination, inspection of wounds, and palpation of pulses.
      2) EVSG patients will require follow-up in 7 to 10 days postoperatively with physical examination, inspection of wounds, and palpation of pulses. One week to 1 month postoperative will need an ultrasound or CT scan of abdomen to check for endoleak. Examination will be repeated at 6 months postoperative and every 6 to 12 months thereafter to check the status of the graft and the size of the aneurysm sac.
   b. Significant number of patients with AAA will have or develop thoracic aneurysm, so continued follow-up and monitoring is important
   c. Be alert to the following in the immediate postoperative period
      1) Redness/swelling around the incision, increase or change in wound drainage, increase in wound pain, or warmth at the incision site
      2) Fever greater than 100°F
      3) Unusual or severe increase in pain in lower back or legs
      4) Sudden weight gain or swelling of legs/feet

    5) Skin breakdown of legs/feet
    6) Tingling/coldness/discoloration of legs/feet
10. Risk factor modification
    a. Smoking cessation
    b. Monitor cardiac status
    c. Target HgbA1c for control of diabetes
    d. Lipid management
    e. Hypertension control
    f. Stress reduction
    g. Regular exercise
    h. Weight control as needed

CASE STUDY

AL is a 68-year-old female who presented to her primary care physician for her annual physical examination. She felt well and had no complaints other that arthritic pain in both knees relieved by acetaminophen and occasional heartburn relieved by antacids. She denied abdominal pain, back pain, or symptoms of intermittent claudication. She had no history of chest pain, angina, or MI. Her weight was stable, appetite was good, and she was physically active in many volunteer activities.

Her past health history was significant for mild hypertension treated with Atacand HC 32/12.5 (candesartan cilexetil, hydrochlorothiazide). She also was found to have hyperlipidemia 2 years ago and was prescribed atorvastatin which she took intermittently. This patient was a reformed smoker, having quit 16 years ago. She previously had smoked one pack of cigarettes a day for 30 years.

Her past surgical history included a hysterectomy for dysfunctional uterine bleeding at age 50, and a cholecystectomy at age 62 for acute cholecystitis.

Her family health history revealed that her father died at age 70 of a probable MI. Her mother died suddenly at age 67, cause of death unknown, and a maternal aunt died of a ruptured AAA. The patient has one daughter and two sons ranging in ages from 45 to 52 years old, all in good health.

The physical examination by her primary care physician was found to be normal, excluding a pulsatile mass in her abdomen at the level of the umbilicus. She subsequently had an ultrasound of the abdominal aorta that disclosed a 5.8-cm AAA. She was referred to a vascular surgeon for consultation. The surgeon recommended repair of her aneurysm.

Review Questions

1. List four factors that may have contributed to aneurysm formation in this patient.
2. Discuss the treatment options for this patient including advantages and disadvantages of each possible option.
3. AL has an open repair of her AAA. On the first postoperative day she develops unusually severe abdominal pain. Her abdomen becomes distended and she passes a small amount of bloody stool. What is the most likely cause of these symptoms?
4. Let us say that while AL could have undergone an open repair, she opted for an EVSG repair of her AAA. Her postoperative course was unremarkable and she was discharged from the hospital on her second postoperative day. She was scheduled for follow-up in 10 days but calls you on her third postoperative day complaining of fever, malaise, and vague backache

that has remained since her surgery. As the telephone triage nurse, what do you advise her to do?

5. AL is concerned that her children may develop an aneurysm. Are her concerns valid and if so, why?
6. What is the most common complication of endovascular repair of an AAA? What are the symptoms of endoleak?

Answers

1. (A) Age; (B) Smoking history; (C) Hypertension; (D) Family health history
2. Most surgeons agree that repair of an AAA that is 5.8 cm in greatest diameter is indicated especially in a female where the threshold for rupture is lower than in males. At this point, the risk of morbidity and mortality with surgery are less than the morbidity and mortality of no treatment. Her two options are continued medical observation or surgical repair.
   a. The nonoperative option is that of observation. AL can be followed with serial ultrasound examinations to monitor growth pattern or until symptoms occur. This can be dangerous, as most aneurysms are asymptomatic until rupture, so observation until symptomatic is not a reliable indicator for repair. Aneurysms can be unpredictable, even small ones can rupture.
   b. The second option is open surgical repair. AL is in reasonably good health. If her cardiac and pulmonary status are relatively normal and she is an acceptable candidate for general anesthesia, this type of repair would offer her a lifetime repair with little follow-up.
   c. The third option is endovascular repair if the patient is anatomically suited. This method was previously reserved for high-risk patients who were not candidates for open surgery and were therefore denied treatment. This method avoids laparotomy, cross-clamping of the aorta, and the blood loss associated with open repair. Preparation for open repair and endovascular repair are similar—both methods require the patient be optimized preoperatively. EVSG repair can be done under general, spinal, or epidural anesthesia. It is a good alternative for those patients who cannot tolerate general anesthesia or might have a prolonged recovery such as those with COPD. It might also be a good choice for those with a hostile abdomen where open repair would be very complicated and risky.

   Considering AL's history and her reported good health, an acceptable physical examination, normal laboratory studies, EKG, CXR, and stress test, as well as her active lifestyle, the recommendation was for conventional (open) repair.
3. Ischemic colitis is the most likely cause of these symptoms and occurs as a result of interruption of blood flow to the bowel mainly via the IMA. The injury can be superficial and limited to the mucosa which is self-limiting. It can, however, involve the full thickness of the bowel which would require resection of the involved part of the intestine to prevent contamination of the graft.
4. After careful attempts to rule out all other common causes of postoperative fever (pulmonary, urinary, vascular, deep vein thrombosis or wound), one could conclude she has postimplantation syndrome. Since her back pain had been present in the immediate postoperative period while hospitalized and has not increased in intensity, it would be safe to treat her symptomatically with acetaminophen or nonsteroidal anti-inflammatory medication. If, however, her pain is increasing, she should be seen and examined with plans for immediate CT scan with intravenous contrast to make sure that her repair is not compromised or that there is no injury to other vessels.
5. Yes, this patient has valid concerns. Her family health history is indeed strong, with her aunt and possibly her mother having aortic aneurysms. Therefore the chance of her children developing an aortic aneurysm is much higher than that of the general population. Her children should be advised to have screening ultrasounds of the abdomen starting at age 50 and every

3 to 5 years thereafter. The patient herself is also at risk for developing an aneurysm elsewhere. She should have a CT scan of the chest every 5 years to monitor for thoracic aneurysm as well as palpation of distal pulses noting widening of popliteal pulsation that may indicate a popliteal aneurysm.

6. The most common complication is an endoleak. This occurs in approximately 10% of patients undergoing this procedure. Endoleak refers to continued perfusion of the aneurysm sac. The treatment of the endoleak depends on the type of leak, whether it is related to the device itself, the positioning of the device, and back flow from other vessels such as the hypogastric arteries or patent lumbar arteries that continue to perfuse the aneurysm sac. Endoleaks are almost always asymptomatic and found on postoperative imaging. It is therefore essential that patients understand the necessity of lifelong follow-up with appropriate imaging.

REFERENCES

Anderson, L. A. (1994). An update on the cause of abdominal aortic aneurysms. *Journal of Vascular Nursing, 12*(4), 95–100.

Barkin, A. Z., & Rosen, C. L. (2004). Ultrasound detection of abdominal aortic aneurysm. *Emergency Medical Clinics of North America, 22*, 675–682.

Baxter, T. M., Terrin, M. C., & Dalman, R. L. (2008). Medical management of abdominal aortic aneurysms. *Circulation, 117*, 1883–1889.

Buth, J. (2008). *Should patient receive statins before EVAR; after EVAR; what dosage is best.* Presented at the Veith symposium, New York.

Chaikof, E. L., Brewster, D. C., Dalman, R. L., Makaroun, M. S., Illig, K. A., Sicard, G. A., . . . Veith, F. J. (2009). SVS practice guidelines for care of patients with abdominal aortic aneurysm: Executive summary. *Journal of Vascular Surgery, 50*, 880–896.

Clair, D. (2010). Management of ischemic complications following endovascular graft repair. In M. D. Morasch, W. H. Pearce, & J. S. Yao (Eds.), *Modern trends in vascular surgery: The aorta and its body branches* (pp. 333–345). Shelton, CT: People's Medical Publishing House-USA.

Cohen, J. R. (1990). Current concepts for the pathogenesis of abdominal aortic aneurysms. *Perspectives in Vascular Surgery, 3*(2), 103–111.

Cronenwett, J. L., Krupski, W. C., & Rutherford, R. B. (2000). Abdominal aortic and iliac aneurysms. In R. B. Rutherford (Ed.), *Vascular surgery* (5th ed., pp. 1246–1274). Philadelphia, PA: W. B. Saunders.

Curci, J. A., Baxter, B. T., & Thompson, R. W. (2005). Arterial aneurysms: Etiological considerations. In R. B. Rutherford (Ed.), *Vascular surgery* (6th ed., pp. 475–492). Philadelphia, PA: W.B. Saunders.

Curci, J. A., Lee, J. K., & Thompson, R. W. (2001). Pathogenesis of abdominal aortic aneurysm. In C. B. Ernst & J. C. Stanley (Eds.), *Current therapy in vascular surgery* (4th ed., pp. 199–206). St Louis, MO: Mosby.

Darling, R. C., Paty, P. S., & Saltzberg, S. (2010). The retroperitoneal approach for abdominal aortic surgery. In M. D. Morasch, W. H. Pearce, & J. S. T. Yao (Eds.), *Modern trends in vascular surgery: Surgery of the aorta and its body branches* (pp. 33–41). Shelton, CT: People's Medical Publishing House-USA.

Deitch, J. S., & Yano, O. J. (2000). Description and classification of endoleaks. In M. L. Marin & L. H. Hollier (Eds.), *Endovascular grafting: Advanced treatment for vascular disease.* Armonk, NY: Futura.

Diego, R. M. (2010). Nephrogenic systemic fibrosis and gadolinium-enhanced magnetic resonance imaging: Does a U.S. Food and Drug Administration influence practice patterns in CKD? *American Journal of Kidney Diseases, 56*(3), 427–430.

Eastridge, D., Rodriguez, H., & Matusmura, J. S. (2004). In V. Fahey (Ed.), *Vascular nursing* (4th ed., pp. 237–249). Philadelphia, PA: W. B. Saunders.

Fahey, V. (2004). Clinical assessment of the vascular system. In V. Fahey (Ed.), *Vascular nursing* (4th ed., pp. 49–71). St. Louis, MO: Saunders.

Fillinger, M. F. (2010). Abdominal aortic aneurysms: Evaluation and decision making. In J. L. Cronenwett & K. W. Johnston (Eds.), *Rutherford's vascular surgery* (7th ed., pp. 1928–1948). Philadelphia, PA: Saunders Elsevier.

Fink, H. A., Lederele, F. A., Roth, C. S., Bowles, C. A., Nelson, D. B., & Haas, M. A. (2000). The accuracy of physical examination to detect abdominal aortic aneurysm. *Archives of Internal Medicine, 160*, 833–836.

Forsdahl, F. H., Singh, K., Solberg, S., & Jacobson, B. K. 2009). Risk factors for abdominal aortic aneurysm-a 7 year prospective study: The Tromso Study, 1994–2001. *Circulation, 199*, 2202–2208.

Goldstone, J. (2002). Aneurysms of the aorta and iliac arteries. In W. S. Moore (Ed.), *Vascular surgery: A comprehensive review* (6th ed., pp. 457–480). Philadelphia, PA: W. B. Saunders.

Green, R. (2002). Patient selection for endovascular AAA repair. *Endovascular Today*, 31–33.

Greenberg, R. K., Messina, L. M., & Thompson, R. W. (2000). Symposium: Open and endovascular repairs for abdominal aortic aneurysms. K. C. Kent (Moderator). *Contemporary Surgery, 56*(5), 298–301, 305–306, 308–309.

Hannawa, K. K., Elias, J. L., & Upchurch, G. R. (2009). Gender differences in abdominal aortic aneurysms. *Vascular, 17*(Suppl. 1), S30–S39. Supplement to International Society for Vascular Surgery.

Hirsch, A. T., Haskal, Z. J., Hertzer, N. R., Bakal, C. W., Creager, M. A., Halperin, J. L., . . . Riegel, B. (2006). ACC/AHA 2005 Practice Guidelines for the management of patients with peripheral arterial disease (lower extremity, renal, mesenteric, and abdominal aortic): A collaborative report from the American Association for Vascular Surgery/Society for Vascular Surgery, Society for Cardiovascular Angiography and Interventions, Society for Vascular Medicine and Biology, Society of Interventional Radiology, and the ACC/AHA Task Force on Practice Guidelines. *Circulation, 113*(11), e463–e654.

Johnston, K. W., Rutherford, R. B., Tilson, M. D., Shah, D. M., Hollier, L. H., & Stanley, J. C. (1991). Suggested standards for reporting on arterial aneurysms. *Journal of Vascular Surgery, 13*(3), 452–458.

Lawrence, P. F., & Rigbirg, D. (2010). Arterial aneurysms: General considerations. In J. L. Cronenwett & K. W. Johnston (Eds.), *Rutherford's vascular surgery* (7th ed., pp. 1920–1927). Philadelphia, PA: Saunders Elsevier.

Lederle, F. A. (2003). Ultrasonographic screening for abdominal aortic aneurysms. *Annals of Internal Medicine, 139*(6), 516–521.

Lederle, F. A. (2009). In the clinic: Abdominal aortic aneurysms. *Annals of Internal Medicine, 150*(9), ITC5–1–15.

Lovell, M. B., & Harris, K. A. (1991). Abdominal aortic aneurysms. *Journal of Vascular Nursing, 9*(1), 2–6.

Majumder, P. P., Jean, L. S., Ferrell, R. E., Webster, M. W., & Steed, D. L. (1991). On the inheritance of abdominal aortic aneurysm. *American Journal of Human Genetics, 48*(1), 164–170.

Matsumura, J. S. (2004). Surgery of the aorta. In V. Fahey (Ed.), *Vascular nursing* (4th ed., pp. 215–236). Philadelphia, PA: W.B. Saunders Company.

May, J., & White, G. H. (2000). Endovascular treatment of aortic aneurysms. In R. B. Rutherford (Ed.), *Vascular surgery* (5th ed., pp. 1281–1291), Philadelphia, PA: W. B. Saunders.

Nowygrod, R. (2001). Ultrasound and comprehensive tomography in evaluation of abdominal aortic aneurysm. In C. B. Ernst & J. C. Stanley (Eds.), *Current therapy in vascular surgery* (pp. 221–224). St. Louis, MO: Mosby.

O'Connor, R. E. (2013). *Abdominal aortic aneurysm rupture.* Retrieved from http://emedicine.medscape.com/article/756735-overview, accessed August 17, 2013.

Ohki, T. (2002). Endovascular treatment of AAAs: A failed experiment or a technology in evolution. *Endovascular Today, 1*(2), 5.

Olinde, A. J., Dion, Y.-M., Sam, A. D., II., McNeil, J. W., Herbert, S. A., & Fruscha, J. D. (2010). Totally laparoscopic aorta surgery: The North American experience. In M. D. Morasch, W. H. Pearce, & J. S. T. Yao (Eds.), *Surgery of the aorta and its body branches, modern trends in vascular surgery* (pp. 197–206). Shelton, CT: People's Medical Publishing House.

Ouriel, K., & Green, R. M. (1999). Arterial disease. In S. I. Schwartz (Ed.), *Principles of surgery* (7th ed.). New York, NY: McGraw Hill.

Pappas, P. J. (2002). Open surgical repair: Some AAA patients simply fare better with surgery. *Endovascular Today, 1*(2), 58–60.

Paraskevas, K. I., Bessias, N., Giannoukas, A. D., & Mikhailidis, D. P. (2010). Endovascular abdominal aortic aneurysm repair (EVAR) procedures: Counterbalancing the benefits with the costs. *Vascular & Endovascular Surgery, 44*(4), 319–320. doi:10.1177/1538574410362119

Powell, J. T. (2003). Familial clustering of abdominal aortic aneurysms. *British Journal of Surgery, 90*(1), 173–174.

Reilly, J. M., & Tilson, M. D. (1989). Incidence and etiology of abdominal aortic aneurysms. *Surgical Clinics of North America, 69*, 705–711.

Schermerhorn, M. L., & Giles, K. A. (2010). Population-based comparison of open and EVAR. In M. D. Morasch, W. H. Pearce., & J. S. T. Yao (Eds.), *Surgery of the aorta and its body branches* (pp. 159–172). Shelton, CT: People's Medical Publishing House-USA.

Singh, K., Bonaa, K. H., Jacobsen, L., Bjork, L., & Solberg, S. (2001). Prevalence of and risk factors for AAA in population based study: The tromso study. *American Journal of Epidemiology, 154*(3), 236–244.

Takagi, H., Masafumi, M., & Umemoto, T. (2010). Antibiotics for preventing progression of abdominal aortic aneurysms: A meta-analysis of randomized trials. *Vascular & Endovascular Surgery, 44*(7), 613–614.

Tilson, M. D. (1990). Atherosclerosis and aneurysm disease. *Journal of Vascular Surgery, 12*, 372–374.

U.S. Preventative Services Task Force for Abdominal Aortic Aneurysm. (2005). *Recommendation statement.* AHRQ Publication No. 05-0569-A. Retrieved from www.uspreventiveservicestaskforce.org/uspstf05/aaascr/aaa./htm

Van der Laan, M., Milner, R., & Blankensteijn, J. D. (2002, November/December). Preprocedural imaging. *Endovascular Today*, pp. 34–39.

Vogelzang, R. L. (2004). Percutaneous vascular intervention and imaging techniques. In V. Fahey (Ed.), *Vascular nursing* (4th ed., pp. 97–125). Philadelphia, PA: W. B. Saunders Company.

Winterstein, B. A., & Baxter, B. T. (2000). Diseases of the aorta and its branches. In J. A. Norton, R. R. Bollinger, A. E. Chang, S. F. Lowry, S. J. Mulville, H. I. Pass, & R. W. Thompson (Eds.), *Surgery: Basic science and clinical evidence* (pp. 1051–1066). New York, NY: Springer.

SUGGESTED READINGS

Assar, A. N., & Zarins, C. K. (2009). Ruptured abdominal aortic aneurysm; a surgical emergency with many clinical manifestations. *Postgraduate Medical Journal, 85*(1003), 268–273.

Natalin, R. A., Prince, M. R., Grossman, M. E., Silvers, D., & Landman, J. (2010). Contemporary applications and limitations of magnetic resonance imaging and contrast materials. *Journal of Urology, 183*(1), 27–33.

Schwarze, M. L., Shen, Y., Hemmerick, J., & Dale, W. (2009). Age related trends in utilization and outcomes of open and endovascular repair for abdominal aortic aneurysm in the United States, 2001–2006. *Journal Vascular Surgery, 50*(4),722–729e2. doi:10.1016/j.jvs.2009.05.010

Veith, F. (2010, January). Veith reports EVAR is superior to open repair for ruptured aneurysms. *Vascular News, 45*, p. 1.

RELEVANT WEBSITES

Agency for Healthcare Research and Quality, Public Health Service, U.S. Department of Health and Human Services, National Guideline Clearinghouse: http://www.ahrq.gov and http://www.guidelines.gov

American Heart Association: http://www.americanheart.org

National Heart, Lung and Blood Institute: http://www.nhlbi.nih.gov

Society for Vascular Surgery: http://www.vascularweb.org

Society for Vascular Nursing: http://www.svnnet.org

Society of Vascular Technology: http://www.svtnet.org

U.S. Preventive Services Task Force: Screening for Abdominal Aortic Aneurysm: http://www.uspreventiveservicestaskforce.org/uspst05/aaa.scr/aaars.htm

CHAPTER 14

Renovascular Disease and Ischemic Nephropathy

L. Beth Sossoman

First Edition Authors: *Maria Henderson-Everhardus and J. Hal. Van Bockel*

OBJECTIVES

1. Identify the components of a comprehensive physical examination (including clinical clues for proceeding to diagnostic testing) for people with renovascular hypertension.
2. Perform a comprehensive renovascular health assessment.
3. List the appropriate diagnostic tests relevant to renovascular hypertension.
4. Discuss the appropriate medical, radiological, and surgical interventions relevant to renovascular hypertension.
5. Identify the nursing implications of renovascular hypertension.

Introduction

Renovascular disease (RVD) encompasses atherosclerotic, fibromuscular, and inflammatory diseases. RVD can lead to renovascular hypertension (RVH) which causes reduced kidney perfusion and renal ischemia (Fenves & Ram, 2006). Hypertension affects an estimated 78 million American adults (Go et al., 2013). It is estimated that RVH accounts for 5% of all cases of hypertension. This accounts for upward of 4 million people (Hartman & Kawashima, 2009). Renal artery stenosis (RAS) may be a cause of RVH. RAS has been found to be associated with atherosclerosis in other vascular beds (i.e., carotids and peripheral vessels) and is associated with adverse coronary events (Hirsch et al., 2006). RAS is caused by narrowing of the artery resulting predominately from either atherosclerosis or fibromuscular dysplasia (FMD). Diminished perfusion to the kidney results in increased renin secretion and production of angiotensin II. This results in systemic vasoconstriction and retention of salt and water. If RAS leads to renal impairment, the long-term outcome is poor (Hirsch et al., 2006).

The etiology of renal vascular disease may affect one or more vessels in one or both of the kidneys. The most common cause of RVH is atherosclerosis, which is seen in 90% of cases (Plouin & Bax, 2010). This is primarily seen in people over 50 years of age, especially men, smokers, with a history of treatment-resistant hypertension, and atherosclerosis in other blood vessels (Colyer, Eltahawy, & Cooper, 2011). RVH caused by fibrodysplastic RAS occurs primarily in children, young adults, and in women of childbearing age (Colyer et al., 2011).

The natural history of RVH differs by the cause of RAS. Arteriosclerotic RAS (ARAS) is characterized by intimal thickening, subintimal lipid deposition, progressive narrowing, and finally occlusion of the arterial lumen. Atherosclerotic lesions usually occur at the ostium of the renal artery or in the proximal one third of the vessel. ARAS is progressive and is manifested with high-grade lesions (between 50% and 70% depending on the measurement methodology) and systemic hypertension (usually defined as a systolic pressure >160 mm Hg). Renal insufficiency/failure is associated with atherosclerotic RAS when coupled with an abnormal baseline creatinine and bilateral stenosis (Dworkin & Cooper, 2009). ARAS is also associated with increased mortality and morbidity, usually from cardiovascular disease (Edwards, Craven, Burke, Dean, & Hansen, 2005; Hirsch et al., 2006). Manifestations on echocardiogram are left ventricular hypertrophy and diastolic dysfunction (Chrysochou & Kalra, 2010).

FMD is classified into three categories: intimal fibroplasia, medial fibroplasia, and perimedial dysplasia. Medial fibroplasia is the predominant type making up 85% of cases and is characterized by the typical "string of pearls" on angiographic studies (Hirsch et al., 2006). Other arteries can be affected including the carotid, vertebral, iliac, and mesenteric arteries (Coffman, Falk, Molitoris, Nelson, & Schrier, 2013). FMD may also be familial in 10% of cases. Complications, which result from the dysplastic process, include renal artery aneurysms, stenosis, dissections, and thrombosis (Colyer et al., 2011).

Either type of RAS can lead to a reduction of renal parenchymal blood flow sufficient to provoke sustained renin production, which may result in hypertension (RVH). If only one kidney is affected, the renin–angiotensin–aldosterone system is activated, causing renin-dependent hypertension (Hirsch et al., 2006). If both kidneys are affected or only a solitary kidney is present, renin production is inhibited and hypertension becomes more fluid dependent, which results in cardiac failure from fluid overload (Chrysochou & Kalra, 2010). Having bilateral RAS is associated with a higher mortality rate (Rocha-Singh et al., 2008). In both types of RAS, renal impairment and ischemic nephropathy, defined as a decrease in glomerular filtration rate (GFR) may result (Elliott, 2008). Intervention with either surgery or catheter-based technology may or may not improve one's hypertension, serum creatinine, or GFR.

I. Anatomy (see Fig. 14-1)

A. The Kidneys are located in the retroperitoneal space (posterior to the abdominal organs) on either side of the aorta and vena cava.

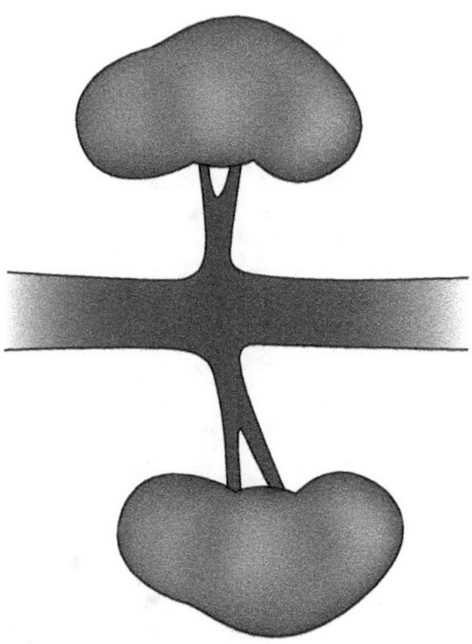

FIGURE 14-1. Normal renal vasculature and kidneys.

B. The Adult Kidney is 115 to 117 g in weight, 9 to 11 cm long, 5 to 7 cm wide, and 2 to 3.5 cm thick.

C. The Right Kidney is 1 to 2 cm lower than the left kidney because of the liver (Jarvis, 2012).

D. Kidney Size Varies by Sex and Age.

1. Adult women have slightly smaller kidneys than adult men.
2. Infants and young children have proportionately smaller kidneys than adults.

E. The Blood Supply of the kidneys arises from the abdominal aorta.

F. The Renal Artery enters the kidney at the renal hilus.

G. Duplicate or Multiple Arteries are frequently found.

H. The Main Renal Artery bifurcates into several segmental branches, which progressively branch within the kidney into the lobar, arcuate, and interlobular arteries.

I. Interlobular Arteries are located in the outer zone of the kidney (cortical layer) and give rise to the afferent arterioles, which supply the glomerulus and the nephrons.

J. The Renal Vein is paired with the renal artery and is connected to the inferior vena cava.

II. Pathophysiology (see Fig. 14-2)

A. RAS (from atherosclerotic occlusive disease)

1. ARAS usually occurs at the ostium and proximal one third of the main renal artery, as well as the nearby aorta (Colyer et al., 2011).

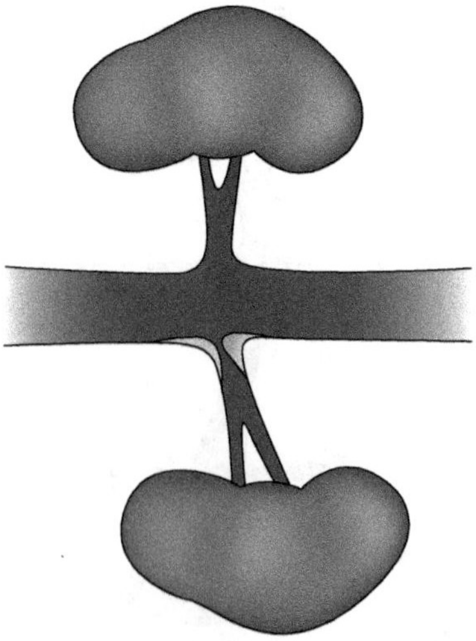

FIGURE 14-2. Unilateral renal artery ostial stenosis.

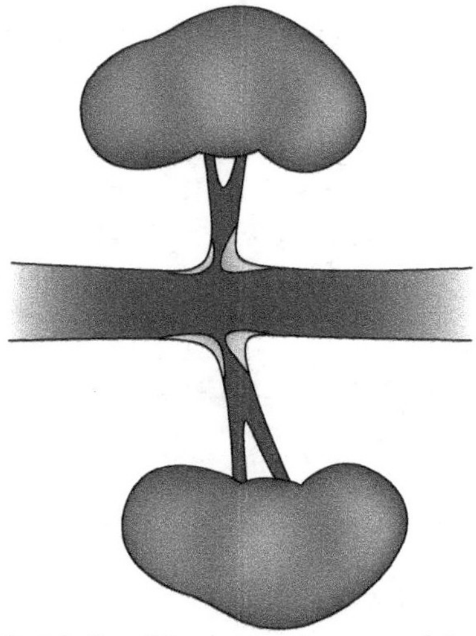

FIGURE 14-3. Bilateral renal artery ostial stenosis.

2. Changes from arteriosclerosis lead to intimal thickening and subintimal lipid deposition, which gradually narrows and eventually occludes the arterial lumen.
3. Stenosis or occlusion can be unilateral or bilateral (see Figs. 14-3 and 14-4).
4. As the renal artery narrows, the kidney becomes ischemic, atrophied, fibrotic, and ultimately, shrinks.
5. Decreased pressure in the arterioles stimulates the juxtaglomerular apparatus to increase renin secretion, leading to RVH (Hallett, Mills, Earnshaw, & Reekers, 2004).
6. With stenosis or occlusion of the renal artery, the kidney ultimately suffers ischemia or infarction.

B. FMD

1. FMD is commonly found in the middle and distal two thirds of renal arteries (Hirsch et al., 2006).
2. FMD causes defects in the medial portion of the artery (Plouin & Bax, 2010).

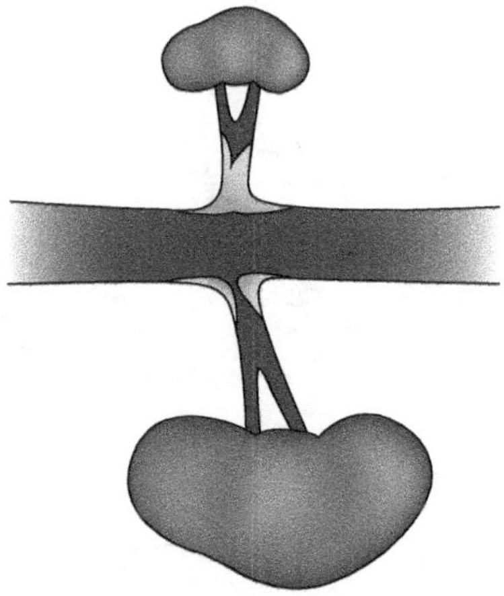

FIGURE 14-4. Unilateral renal artery ostial stenosis and contralateral occlusion with a shrunken kidney.

3. It rarely causes intimal hyperplasia or adventitial fibroplasia (Plouin & Bax, 2010).
4. FMD commonly impacts small and mid-sized arteries. Most commonly affected arteries are renal (60% to 75% of cases) and cerebral (25% to 30% of cases) (Coffman et al., 2013).
5. FMD rarely results in renal artery occlusion or ischemic nephropathy.
6. FMD can lead to development of saccular aneurysms, microaneurysms, and stenosis.

C. Renovascular Hypertension (see Fig. 14-5) (Hallett et al., 2004; Munden, 2007)

1. Blood pressure is controlled by the renin–angiotensin–aldosterone mechanism.
2. RVH occurs when the renin–angiotensin system is activated secondary to RAS.

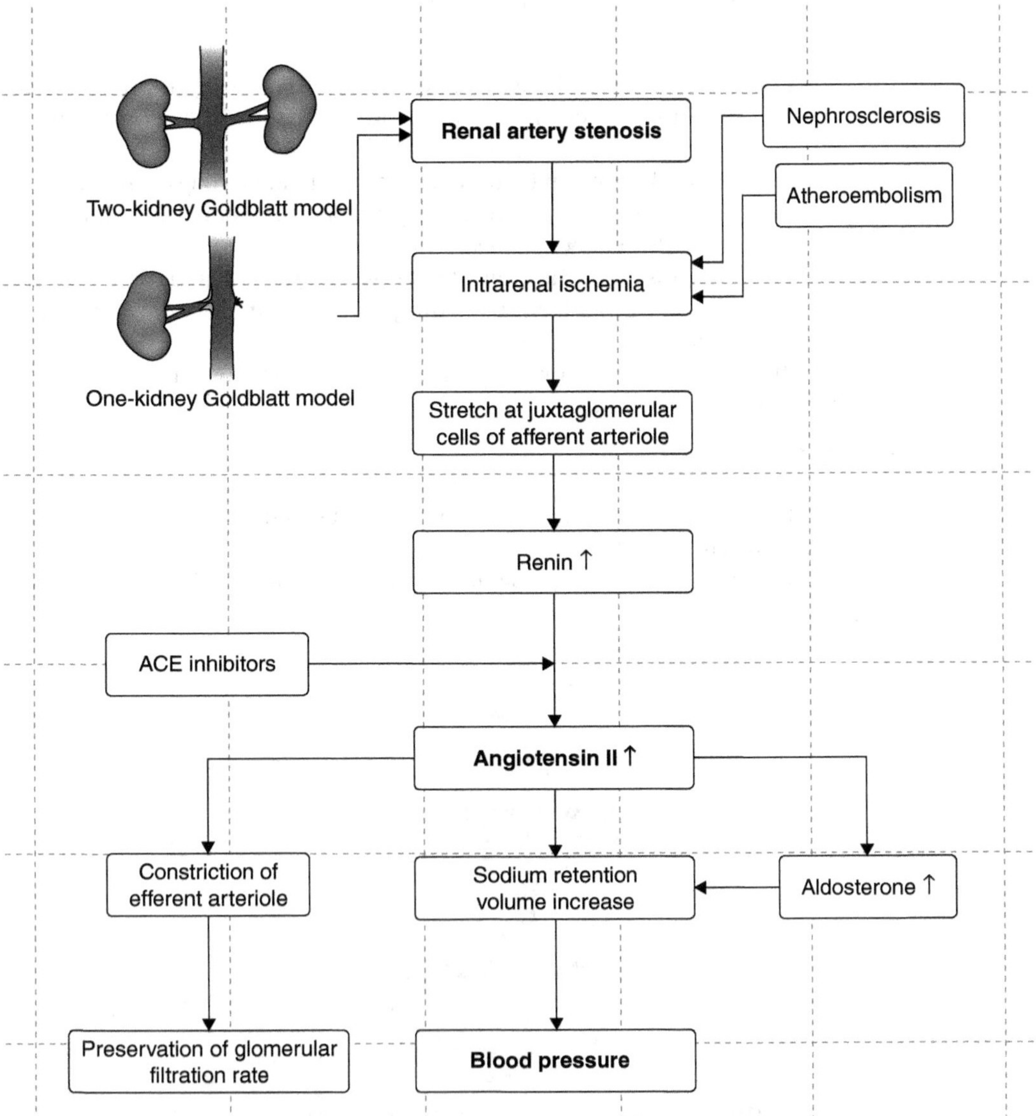

FIGURE 14-5. Pathophysiologic algorithm of renovascular hypertension.

3. When blood pressure within the kidneys falls, the kidneys release renin into the bloodstream.
4. Renin and angiotensinogen, in the liver, combine to form angiotensin I.
5. Angiotensin I is converted to angiotensin II in the lungs.
6. Angiotensin II causes vasoconstriction, increased peripheral resistance, and elevated blood pressure.
7. Angiotensin II has direct renal actions causing reabsorption of sodium and water.
8. Angiotensin II stimulates the adrenal gland to release aldosterone.
9. Aldosterone causes the kidneys to retain sodium and water.
10. Sodium in the kidney causes retention of water.
11. Extra fluid retention expands the volume of blood in the body, leading to increased blood pressure.

III. Etiology

A. Arteriosclerosis

1. Arteriosclerosis is the cause of RVH in approximately 90% of cases (Hirsch et al., 2006).
2. In arteriosclerosis, intimal thickening and subintimal lipid deposition leads to artery occlusion. The disease process is progressive.
3. Arteriosclerosis and the resulting stenosis or occlusion increases the risk of renal failure.

B. FMD

1. It is the second most common cause of RVH. It is seen in 10% of cases (Coyler et al., 2011).
2. FMD is not an inflammatory or atherosclerotic process (Hirsch et al., 2006)

C. Other Causes (Coyler et al., 2011; Plouin & Bax, 2010)

1. Takayasu arteritis: form of systemic vasculitis. Found most commonly in China, Japan, and India
2. Renal artery aneurysms: seen in saccular forms at the bifurcation of the renal artery
3. Embolism: either spontaneous or occurring during vascular procedures
4. Renal artery occlusion during endovascular procedures for aortic aneurysm repair (EVAR) (Coffman et al., 2013)
5. Aortic dissection
6. Polyarteritis nodosa: a form of vasculitis causing aneurysms
7. Arteriovenous fistula
8. RAS after transplantation

IV. Complications

A. Of Atherosclerosis

1. Hypertension, including refractory hypertension (Plouin & Bax, 2010)
2. Renal dysfunction (Plouin & Bax, 2010). Most common cause of end-stage renal disease in individuals over the age of 60 on renal replacement therapy (Hallett et al., 2004)
3. Renal atrophy or injury (Hirsch et al., 2006)
4. Pulmonary edema (Plouin & Bax, 2010)

B. Of FMD (Plouin & Bax, 2010)

1. Renal artery dissection
2. Acute renal infarction
3. Rarely causes renal function impairment

V. Assessment

A. Risk Factors

1. Race: more prevalent in Caucasians than African Americans
2. Age
   a. 15 to 30 years of age (FMD)
   b. 55 years of age (arteriosclerotic disease)
3. Arteriosclerotic disease of the heart and/or peripheral blood vessels (Chrysochou & Kalra, 2010)
4. Smoking (current or previous history)
5. Hypertension (Hirsch et al., 2006)
   a. Onset before age 30
   b. Onset of severe hypertension after age 55
   c. Accelerated hypertension (sudden/persistent worsening of previously controlled hypertension)
   d. Resistant hypertension (on full dose of three antihypertensive agents including a diuretic and not achieving target blood pressure)
   e. Malignant hypertension (hypertension with end-organ system damage)

B. Patient History (McLaughlin, Jardine, & Moss, 2000)

1. RVH resulting from FMD
   a. Subjective findings
      1) Asymptomatic
      2) Usually discovered by physical examination with elevation of blood pressure
   b. Objective findings
      1) History of etiologic factors
      2) Bilateral retinopathy (grade III or IV) on fundoscopic examination
      3) Aortic-renal bruit usually heard midline or toward flank
      4) Elevated bilateral arm blood pressure with diastolic hypertension >110 mm Hg
      5) Higher nocturnal blood pressures (Coffman et al., 2013)
2. RVH resulting from arteriosclerotic disease
   a. Subjective findings
      1) Fatigue
      2) Visual changes
      3) Headache
      4) Pain from coronary artery disease, peripheral artery disease, and ischemia
      5) Peripheral edema
      6) Inability to regulate blood pressure with medications
      7) Pulmonary edema and wheezing (rare, but can occur)
   b. Objective findings
      1) History of etiologic factors
      2) Bilateral retinopathy (grade III or IV) on fundoscopic examination

3) Aortic-renal bruit
4) Flank pain present with severe kidney ischemia
5) Decreased peripheral pulses with CAD and PAD
6) Bilateral arm blood pressure readings elevated, systolic >160 mm Hg
7) Higher nocturnal blood pressures (Coffman et al., 2013)

C. Physical Examination

1. Inspection
   a. Venous distention or peripheral swelling
   b. On fundoscopic examination, arteriolar narrowing, arteriovenous nicking, hemorrhage, exudates, or papilledema (grade III or IV)
   c. Peripheral edema
2. Palpation
   a. Decreased or absent aortic and peripheral pulses (indicative of peripheral artery disease)
   b. Jugular venous distention and central venous pressure elevation
   c. Peripheral edema
   d. Percussion
   e. Flank tenderness over kidneys
   f. Pulmonary edema
3. Auscultation
   a. Bruits in aorta, carotid, renal, and femoral arteries
   b. Changes in bilateral arm blood pressures with change in position (sitting, lying, and standing)
   c. Elevated blood pressure
   d. Abnormal breath sounds resulting from pulmonary edema

VI. Considerations Across the Life Span

A. Children and Young Adults

1. Suspect RVH in children and young adults presenting with sudden onset severe hypertension.
2. Take blood pressure at every visit to monitor for any sudden elevations in blood pressure.
3. Evaluate flank pain, if present
   a. Flank pain is most often the result of an infection, but in some cases may be due to renal ischemia.
   b. Renal artery disease should be ruled out if RVH is suspected.
4. Clinical clues for a high level of suspicion for RVH
   a. Age <25 years at onset of hypertension
   b. Sudden onset of hypertension in the absence of family history of hypertension
   c. Onset of moderate to severe hypertension (defined as BP >160/100) develops into malignant hypertension
   d. Headaches
   e. Resistance to standard pharmacological management

B. Women of Childbearing Age

1. Have a higher risk of developing fibrodysplastic RAS than atherosclerotic RAS

2. Suspect RVH in cases of abrupt onset hypertension or treatment-resistant hypertension
3. Clinical clues same as for children and young adults

C. Adult/Elderly

1. People >50 years are more likely to have arteriosclerotic disease
2. Monitor blood pressure and renal function regularly, in anyone with CAD, PAD, or renal disease
3. Clinical clues for a high level of suspicion for RVH (Harvin et al., 2012)
   a. Abdominal bruit
   b. Malignant or accelerated hypertension
   c. Significant (diastolic pressure >110 mm Hg) in a young adult (<35 years old)
   d. New onset after the age of 50 (or age 55, depending on the source)
   e. Sudden development or worsening of hypertension
   f. Refractory hypertension
   g. Deterioration of GFR in response to ACE inhibitors or angiotensin receptor blocking agents
   h. Generalized arteriosclerosis in other major organs
   i. Atrophy of one kidney or discrepancy of more than 1.5 cm between the kidneys (Hirsch et al., 2006)
   j. Unexplained pulmonary edema (Hirsch et al., 2006)

VII. Diagnostic Testing

A. General Information

1. ACC/AHA (Hirsch et al., 2006) recommends one of the following for detection of RAS: duplex ultrasonography, computerized tomographic angiography (CTA, in patients with normal renal function), and MRA.
2. If there is a high level of clinical suspicion and the noninvasive tests are inconclusive, then invasive catheter angiography is indicated (Hirsch et al., 2006).
3. The index of suspicion for RVH is based on clinical clues, as outlined above.
4. Calculations of sensitivity, specificity, and accuracy are usually based on a gold standard comparison like angiography with standard definitions. However, there is no clear definition of significant RAS. Based on the study, the definition of significant RAS can be based on the degree of stenosis (ranging from 50% to 75%) or improvement in blood pressure post intervention (Harvin et al., 2012).

B. Anatomical Studies for RVD

1. Renal duplex ultrasound (Hallett et al., 2004)
   a. Description
      1) First-line screening test
      2) Direct visualization of the renal arteries (B-mode) and hemodynamic blood flow measurements (Doppler) to evaluate renal artery blood flow, parenchymal blood flow, and kidney size
   b. Interpretation of findings
      1) Normal kidney length: 9 to 11 cm
      2) Size difference between kidneys <1.5 cm

3) Criteria that correlates with >60% stenosis (Harvin et al., 2012; Hirsch et al., 2006)
 a) Direct peak velocity >180 to 200 cm/sec (higher velocity correlates with a greater pressure differential across the stenosis)
 b) Renal to aortic velocity ratio (RAR) >3.5 is indicative of stenosis >60%
 c) Rise time >0.07 seconds
 d) Difference in renal or segmental resistive index >0.15

c. Advantages
 1) Poses no nephrotoxic risk
 2) Noninvasive test that visualizes the kidney, renal arteries, perfusion through the kidney
 3) May be able to determine bilateral or unilateral stenosis at the origin of the renal artery
 4) Requires fasting before testing
 5) Can also use bowel prep, like a colonoscopy to improve visualization by reducing colonic contents (Elliott, 2008)
 6) Medications do not affect the outcome of the study

d. Disadvantages
 1) Technique is operator dependent
 2) Even with overnight fasting, the renal arteries are difficult to image because of abdominal artifacts such as obesity, bowel gas, and anatomical location
 3) Does not reliably identify renal artery, branch, or polar renal artery disease
 4) Can overlook small accessory arteries

e. Sensitivity/specificity (Harvin et al., 2012)
 1) Varies by published report
 2) 85% to 90% sensitive; however, some investigators have reported sensitivity of 0% (that correlated with a >60% stenosis) as listed above
 3) 95% specific

2. CTA (Hirsch et al., 2006)
 a. Description
  1) Used to evaluate soft tissue and blood flow by taking multiple computerized x-ray photos of the kidney (with the addition of a contrast agent, blood flow can be evaluated).
  2) Spiral images are obtained with rotation of the x-rays to reconstruct three-dimensional images (requires iodinated contrast).
  3) Densities of various tissues are visualized to determine if stenosis or aneurysms are present.
 b. Interpretation of findings (normal)
  1) Blood flow is normal throughout the aorta, renal arteries, and renal branches.
  2) Vessel lumen size is normal without obstructions or aneurysms present.
 c. Advantages
  1) Correlates very well with digital subtraction angiography (DSA)
  2) Can visualize the kidney in multiple planes and determine any ostial lesions or multiple accessory vessels
  3) Visualization of renal tumors and cysts, ureteral obstructions, calculi, and abnormalities

4) Can use in patients with metal stents and can assess for in-stent restenosis

d. Disadvantages
 1) Allergic reactions or acute renal toxicity resulting from contrast agent
 2) High cost
 3) Contraindicated in patients with claustrophobia

e. Sensitivity/Specificity
 1) 59% to 96% sensitive
 2) 82% to 99% specific

3. Magnetic resonance imaging/angiography (MRA) (Hirsch et al., 2006)
 a. Description
  1) Radiofrequency signals are passed through a magnetic field and behavior of hydrogen atoms in the field is recorded
  2) Gadolinium, a contrast agent with low nephrotoxicity, is used to detail the structures and blood flow of the aorta and renal arteries
   a) Agent has to be used with caution in patients with stage III or IV chronic kidney disease; can cause nephrogenic systemic fibrosis (Coyler et al., 2011)
   b) Blood flow and vessel lumens are visualized
 b. Interpretation of findings (normal)
  1) Blood flow is normal throughout the aorta, renal arteries, and renal branches
  2) Vessel lumen size is normal without obstructions or aneurysms present
 c. Advantages
  1) Good visualization of ostial, proximal, and distal renal lesions that are atherosclerotic
  2) No need for nephrotoxic contrast
 d. Disadvantages
  1) Preparation and time of procedure
  2) High cost
  3) Contraindicated for patients with metal implants
  4) Contraindicated in patients with claustrophobia
  5) Limited availability
 e. Sensitivity/specificity
  1) 90% to 100% sensitive
  2) 76% to 94% specific
  3) Reduced accuracy in small branch or distal renal arteries
  4) Tendency to overestimate moderate stenosis (40% to 69%)

4. Angiography, intra-arterial DSA, intravascular Doppler ultrasound (IVUS) (Hallett et al., 2004)
 a. Description
  1) Renal arteriography, can be combined with intra-arterial pressure measurements and IVUS
  2) Provides accurate identification and location of soft tissue organs and blood vessels and size and contour of lumens
  3) Ultrasound is sound waves which detect the speed of blood cells, determining the flow of blood and noting any turbulence or obstruction
 b. Interpretation of findings
  1) Normal
   a) Kidneys are 9 to 11 cm in length
   b) Origin of the aorta and renal arteries are patent without calcification, aneurysm, or obstruction

c) Blood flow within the artery is regular without turbulence noted in the lumen
2) Abnormal
a) Unilateral or bilateral stenosis at the origin of the renal artery (atherosclerosis) or in the main renal artery or its extrarenal or intrarenal branches
b) May include (micro)aneurysms or dissections
c. Advantages
1) Balloon dilatation or stenting can occur in the same setting
2) Can be done in the same setting as a coronary/peripheral arteriography
d. Disadvantages
1) Allergic reactions or acute renal toxicity resulting from contrast agent
2) Dehydration makes patients more susceptible to contrast-induced renal failure, especially in patients with impaired renal function and patients with diabetic nephropathy
3) Contrast-induced renal failure
4) Atheroembolization resulting from catheter manipulations
5) Pseudoaneurysm, hemorrhage, and hematoma may result from femoral puncture

C. Functional Studies for RVD (performed when the patient exhibits hypertension and has unilateral RVD)

1. Currently, there is not a test that can conclusively establish the functional significance of a lesion or predict the response to revascularization
2. Renal venous renin (Harvin et al., 2012; Hirsch et al., 2006)
a. Description
1) Helps to identify functionally significant lesions (Zarins & Gewertz, 2005)
2) Not indicated as an initial screening test
b. Interpretation of findings
1) In patients with unilateral RAS, the ischemic kidney secretes increased renin and the contralateral kidney has relative suppression of renin release
2) With bilateral RAS, the renal vein with the higher renin level has the greatest degree of stenosis (there may be no lateralization of renin levels due to both kidneys being hyper-reninemic)
3) A 1.5:1 renal vein/renin ratio for the involved versus uninvolved kidney can be considered positive for renovascular lesion
c. Advantages—Has been used to select patients for arteriography
d. Disadvantages
1) High rate of false-negative and false-positive results
2) Operator sensitive as it relates to specimen collection
3) Patient hydration is key to accurate results
e. Sensitivity/specificity (Harvin et al., 2012)
1) 72% to 92% sensitive
2) 29% to 42% specific
3. Captopril-augmented nuclear renography (Hartman & Kawashima, 2009)
a. Description (Hirsch et al., 2006)
1) ACC/AHA does not recommend this for initial diagnosis
2) This is a functional assessment of renal perfusion and function
3) Baseline plasma renin level is drawn

4) An ACE inhibitor, captopril, is given in a single oral dose
5) Plasma renin assays are repeated at 60 minutes
6) Blood pressure measurements are repeated at 15-minute intervals of a total of 60 minutes
7) Scintigraphic images and time–activity curves are measured after the injection to evaluate the degree of renal update before and after administration of captopril

b. Interpretation of findings
1) When the renin–angiotensin–aldosterone system is blocked, blood pressure falls
2) Normal finding shows a rapid uptake, followed by excretion of the contrast agent. Fifty percent of the contrast should be excreted in 10 minutes
3) Abnormal findings show delayed uptake and excretion, indicating RAS

c. Advantages
1) Only used in persons with unilateral stenosis when RVH is predominantly the result of inhibition of the renin–angiotensin–aldosterone system
2) Best identifies patients who will likely have improvement in blood pressure after revascularization
3) May be helpful in borderline lesions

d. Disadvantages
1) Not reliable if renal insufficiency and intrinsic parenchymal disease present
2) Not valid for patients with elevated creatinine levels (>2.0 mg/dL)
3) If stenosis is bilateral, ACE inhibitors are effective because there is not enough fluid to affect the renin–angiotensin–aldosterone system

e. Sensitivity/specificity
1) 81% sensitive
2) 59% specific (see Fig. 14-6)

D. Laboratory Tests

1. Blood urea nitrogen (BUN)
   a. Description—Provides indirect and rough measure of renal function and GFR, if normal liver function exists
   b. Interpretation of findings
      1) Normal (Dunning & Fischbach, 2011)
         a) Children: 5 to 18 mg/dL or 1.8 to 6.4 mmol/L
         b) Adults: 7 to 18 mg/dL or 3.6 to 7.1 mmol/L (SI units)
         c) Elderly: 8 to 20 mg/dL or 2.9 to 7.5 mmol/L
      2) Abnormal—Increased BUN, indicating a drop in GFR
   c. Advantages—Used to establish baseline values for evaluating abnormal function
   d. Disadvantages
      1) Accurate only if liver function normal
      2) Changes in protein intake and hydration may affect BUN levels
2. Serum creatinine
   a. Description
      1) Used to estimate clearance of creatinine, which is excreted entirely by the kidneys

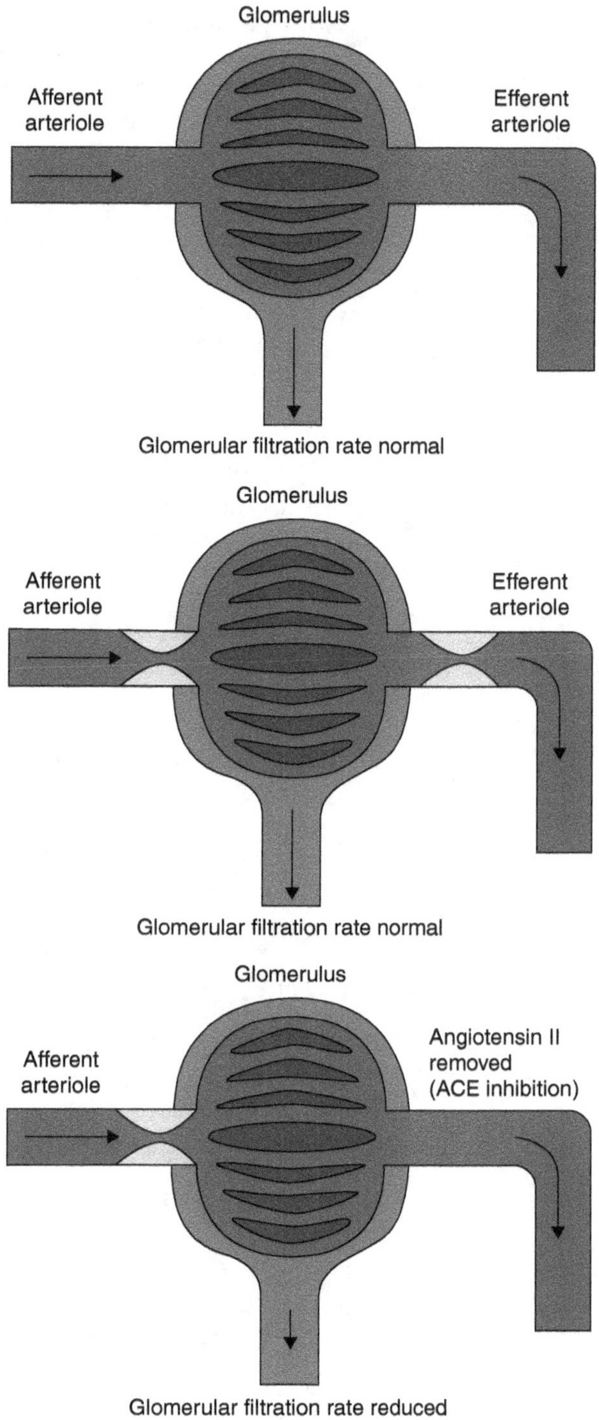

FIGURE 14-6. Glomerular function (**top**). There is a normal supply of blood without any pressure-reducing stenosis or occlusion in the efferent arteriole resulting in a normal perfusion pressure and a normal glomerular filtration. No compensation of the efferent arteriole is required to maintain the perfusion pressure (**middle**). Diagram of glomerulus in the presence of a renal artery stenosis (afferent arteriole). This results in a reduced perfusion pressure, which might result in a reduced filtration rate. However, autoregulation resulting in vasoconstriction of the efferent arteriole by angiotensin II results in maintaining the perfusion pressure. This results in a normal glomerular filtration (**bottom**). The same as in the middle figure. However, high blood pressure is treated by an angiotensin-converting enzyme inhibitor. This results in prevention of the vasoconstrictive effect of angiotensin II on the efferent arteriole. As a result, vasoconstriction of the efferent arteriole is released resulting in a reduction of the perfusion pressure and, consequently, in a reduced glomerular filtration rate. This is usually clinically observed (in particular in the presence of a monokidney) as an increase of the serum creatinine level, reduced perfusion pressure on a renal scan, or a decrease in the volume of the urine production.

2) Excretion is directly proportional to renal excretory function
3) May be elevated in atherosclerotic RAS (Colyer et al., 2011)
4) Rarely elevated in FMD (Plouin & Bax, 2010)
5) GFR (Dunning & Fischbach, 2011)—The National Kidney Disease Education Program (NKDEP) recommends that clinical laboratories report an estimated GFR when reporting a serum creatinine

b. Interpretation of findings
   1) Normal (Dunning & Fischbach, 2011)
      a) Children: 0.3 to 0.7 mg/dL
      b) Adults: 0.8 to 1.2 mg/dL
      c) Elderly: values may be slightly lower because of decreased muscle mass
   2) Abnormal
      a) Doubling of creatinine, which suggests a 50% reduction in the GFR
      b) Elevation of creatinine, which suggests a chronic disease process

c. Advantages—Quick procedure that provides baseline and surveillance monitoring of kidney function

d. Disadvantages
   1) Results are influenced by technique and by endogenous and exogenous substances
   2) Results are also influenced by age, sex, body weight, muscle mass, diet, and drugs
   3) Creatinine levels must be interpreted in conjunction with BUN levels
   4) A high protein (meat) diet may cause elevation in creatinine
   5) Drugs (aminoglycosides, cimetidine, heavy metal chemotherapeutic agents, and cephalosporins) increase creatinine levels

3. Creatinine clearance
   a. Description—Used to measure GFR of the kidneys as determined through a series of blood tests and a 24-hour urine collection
   b. Interpretation of findings
      1) The amount of blood present for filtration depends on the ability of glomeruli to act as a filter
      2) Filtration is decreased in renal artery atherosclerosis or obstruction
      3) When one kidney becomes diseased, the opposite kidney, if functioning normally, can compensate by increasing its GFR; therefore, creatinine clearance will be normal if one kidney has compensated for a stenotic or absent kidney
      4) Normal (Dunning & Fischbach, 2011)
         a) Males: 94 to 140 mL/min/1.73 m^2 or 0.91 to 1.35 mL/s/m^2
         b) Females: 72 to 110 mL/min/1.73 m^2 or 0.69 to 1.06 mL/s/m^2
         c) Elderly: values decrease 6.5 mL/min/decade of life after age 20 with decline in GFR
   c. Advantages
      1) Daily production of creatinine depends on muscle mass, which fluctuates very little
      2) Creatinine is directly proportional to GFR
   d. Disadvantages
      1) The amount of filtrate made in the kidney depends on the amount of blood to be filtered and the ability of the glomeruli to filter the blood
      2) Unilateral disease may not cause a decrease in creatinine clearance because the normal kidney will compensate
      3) Ingestion of large amounts of protein (meat) will increase creatinine levels
      4) Requires 24-hour collection of urine

4. Urine specific gravity (Dunning & Fischbach, 2011)
   a. Description—Is used to assess the ability of the kidney to concentrate urine. A comparison is made with distilled water, which has a specific gravity of 1.000

b. Interpretation of findings
   1) Normal: 1.005 to 1.030 (usually 1.010 and 1.025). Specific gravity varies inversely with the amount of urine excreted (i.e., decreased urine output, increased specific gravity)
   2) Abnormal
      a) Concentrated urine: >1.025
      b) Dilute urine: 1.001 to 1.010
c. Advantages
   1) In early renal disease, clinician will see increased volume and decreased specific gravity
   2) In hypertension, clinician will see normal volume and decreased specific gravity
d. Disadvantages—Results are altered by multiple medications (including diuretics and antibiotics), proteinuria, and temperature of the sample

5. Urine protein
   a. Description—Assess the severity of renal disease and to assess for nephrotic syndrome
   b. Interpretation of findings (Dunning & Fischbach, 2011)—Normal: 24-hour urine: 10 to 140 mg/24 hours
   c. Advantages
      1) Occurs in renal disease with glomerular damage
      2) Can be elevated in vascular disease, like hypertension
   d. Disadvantages—Requires 24-hour collection of urine
6. Lipid profile (Dworkin & Cooper, 2009)
   a. Description
      1) Used to profile lipoproteins in the blood that transport cholesterol, triglycerides, and other insoluble fats within the body
      2) High levels of high density lipoprotein (HDL) are associated with a lower risk of atherosclerosis and occlusive disease
      3) High levels of low density lipoprotein (LDL) and very low density lipoprotein (VLDL) are associated with a higher risk of atherosclerosis and occlusive disease
   b. Interpretation of findings (Dunning & Fischbach, 2011)
      1) Normal
         a) Total cholesterol: 140 to 199 mg/dL
         b) Triglyceride: <150 mg/dL
         c) HDL: 35 to 65 mg/dL (men); 35 to 80 mg/dL (women)
         d) LDL: 60 to 130 mg/dL
         e) VLDL: 25% to 50% of total triglyceride levels
      2) Abnormal—Elevation of atherosclerotic etiology
   c. Advantages—Establish baseline and sequential follow-up measurements of lipid profile
   d. Disadvantages—Not specific for RAS

VIII. Medical Management

A. Description

1. The goal is to control all atherosclerotic risk factors
2. Maximal medical therapy may be equal to PTRA with or without stenting (Kumbhani et al., 2011)

B. Smoking/Use of Tobacco Products

1. Tobacco use is known to damage vascular endothelium, promote intravascular coagulation, and accelerate progression of atherosclerosis
2. Strategies include tobacco cessation, nicotine replacement therapy, pharmacological agents, and behavioral support

C. Blood Pressure Management

1. Exercise/increased physical activity
2. Diet management/low salt diet
3. Antihypertensive medications
   a. ACE inhibitors
      1) Used as first-line therapy in cases of unilateral RAS. Reduced BP in 86% to 92% of patients with RVH
      2) Reduces incidence of proteinuria
      3) Because they inhibit renal perfusion, can be used diagnostically to distinguish between unilateral and bilateral disease
         a) In presence of unilateral disease, will cause blood pressure to fall
         b) In presence of bilateral disease, will cause creatinine levels to rise
      4) BUN/creatinine should be assessed at baseline and within 1 week of the initiation of therapy. A rise in serum creatinine (as much as 25% above baseline) with ACE inhibitors and angiotensin receptor blockers (ARBs) is not a reason to withhold treatment unless hyperkalemia develops (Chrysochou & Kalra, 2010)
   b. ARBs
      1) Used as first-line therapy, if allergic to ACE inhibitors
      2) Reduce incidence of proteinuria
      3) Both ACE inhibitors and ARBs have demonstrated favorable effects on the progression of diabetic and nondiabetic renal disease
   c. Beta blockers
      1) ACC/AHA guideline recommendation for patients with RAS (Hirsch et al., 2006)
      2) Reduce heart rate. Beta-1 agonists. Negative inotrope. Reduces renin
   d. Calcium channel blockers
      1) ACC/AHA guideline recommendation for patients with unilateral RAS (Hirsch et al., 2006)
      2) Decreases heart rate by prolonging the refractory period. Reduces blood pressure through vasodilation
   e. Diuretics
      1) Mechanism: agents reduce sodium reabsorption in the nephron promoting diuresis
      2) Reduction in glomerular hydrostatic pressure can reduce GFR. Clinician needs to monitor (Chrysochou & Kalra, 2010)

D. Control of Dyslipidemia

1. Exercise
2. Diet management
3. Drug management
   a. Statins
      1) Reduces total and LDL cholesterol
      2) Lower overall cardiovascular mortality and morbidity

3) May reduce progression of renal stenosis (Chrysochou & Kalra, 2010)
4) Niacin—Raises HDL levels

E. Antiplatelet Agent for Atherosclerotic Disease

1. Should be considered if there is associated cardiac or vascular disease (Hallet et al., 2004)
2. Aspirin is recommended
3. Dual antiplatelet therapy is not required unless there are other indications (i.e., coronary stent)

F. Monitor for Worsening Renal Function

G. Monitor for End-Organ disease of hypertension including angina, CHF, and cerebrovascular ischemia (Rocha-Singh et al., 2008)

IX. Catheter-Based/Surgical Management

A. Renal Revascularizaion Therapy is Controversial

B. The ACC/AHA guidelines' only class I indication is for individuals with atherosclerotic RAS with recurrent heart failure or sudden, unexplained pulmonary edema

C. Rocha-Singh et al. (2008) suggested a grading scale for RAS and clinical outcomes. This grading scale may guide the need for renal revascularization with a focus on intervention in grade III individuals

1. Grade I: RAS is present, but there are no clinical manifestations (normal blood pressure with normal renal function)
2. Grade II: RAS is present, but patients have hypertension that is controlled medically and normal renal function
3. Grade III: RAS is present, and patients have evidence of abnormal renal function, medically refractory hypertension, or volume overload

D. Revascularization for renal disease shows a trend toward catheter-based intervention and a more limited use of surgical renal revascularization

E. Preprocedure/Preoperative Management

1. Preoperative explanation of the procedure
   a. Discussion of the procedure's risks and benefits to obtain informed consent
   b. Importance of preoperative pulmonary toilet and proper nutrition
   c. Discussion of preoperative testing and clearance
   d. Discussion of the catheter-based procedure and postprocedural recovery
   e. Discussion of the operative procedure and postoperative stages of recovery

F. Angioplasty with or without Stenting (PTRA)

1. Indications
   a. Generally, open repair provides superior results, but angioplasty is less invasive

b. As a result, angioplasty is often preferred as the first intervention (Hirsch et al., 2006)
c. In fibrodysplastic lesions, PTRA without stent is recommended (Hallett et al., 2004)
d. Addition of an expandable stent to PTRA is indicated in ostial atherosclerotic lesions (Hirsch et al., 2006)
e. Procedure—The vessel is dilated by a balloon-tipped catheter, which stretches the vessel wall and portions of the media, resulting in dilation of the vessel wall

2. Results
   a. PTRA of fibromusclar dysplastic stenosis
      1) Satisfactory patency is achieved
      2) In terms of blood pressure response, 46% cure hypertension (Trinquart, Mounier-Vehier, Sapoval, Gagnon, & Plouin, 2010)
      3) 10-year patency of 87% in young adults (Hallett et al., 2004)
      4) Hypertension cure rates 67% to 80% in children treated with PTRA (Trinquart et al., 2010)
   b. PTRA of ostial atherosclerotic lesions
      1) Patency of >80% is achieved, but repeat angioplasty is often required. Restenosis occurs in approximately 48% of cases (Hirsch et al., 2006)
      2) Improvement in blood pressure is common. Cure is rare (Hirsch et al., 2006)
   c. PTRA with stenting
      1) Meta-analysis showed procedural success of 96%, with procedural mortality <1% and restenosis rate of 16% at 12 months (Hirsch et al., 2006)
      2) Stenting may reduce complications due to local dissection, prevent elastic recoil, and nearly eliminate pressure gradients (Elliott, 2008)
      3) Demonstrate improvement/stabilization of renal function (Hirsch et al., 2006)
      4) Some clinicians have reported that the results are no better than those achieved by optimal medical therapy (Kumbhani et al., 2011)
3. Complications
   a. Bleeding
   b. Atheroembolization
      1) Can be caused during an intervention due to disruption of the atherosclerotic plaque
      2) Suspected if worsening renal function or peripheral evidence of embolization (i.e., blue toes, livedo reticularis)
      3) Can impair renal function, ESRD and death (Rocha-Singh et al., 2008)
   c. Renal artery restenosis
      1) Cause is neointimal hyperplasia in response to arterial injury
      2) Can occur within the stents, gaps between stents, or as new focal stenosis outside of the stents
      3) Incidence is between 17% and 22% within the first 12 months post intervention (Rocha-Singh et al., 2008)
      4) Treatment includes additional stents or balloon angioplasty

G. Surgical Revascularization

1. Indications: for both fibrodysplastic and atherosclerotic lesions
2. In patients with ostial atherosclerosis with renal insufficiency, surgical repair is superior (Hallet et al., 2004)
3. Has similar morbidity and mortality when compared to PTRA with stenting in atherosclerotic lesions (Balzer et al., 2009)
4. Bypass grafts have a long-term patency of 90% or greater (Zarins & Gewetz, 2005)
5. In patients with nonatherosclerotic renal disease (i.e., FMD or Takayasu arteritis) surgery demonstrated longer 5- and 10-year patency rates than PTRA (Ham, Kumar, Wang, Rowe, & Weaver, 2010)
6. Hypertension improved in 90% of patients with FMD or Takayasu arteritis (Ham et al., 2010)
7. Conduits include the use of autogenous saphenous vein, autogenous hypogastric artery (in children), and prosthetic bypasses
8. Mortality is approximately 5% and morbidity is 30%, related to secondary atherosclerosis and risk factors (Zarins & Gewetz, 2005)
9. Complications following surgery include myocardial infarction, arrhythmias, stroke, pneumonia, and worsening renal function (Hallet et al., 2004)
10. Aortorenal bypass (see Fig. 14-7) (Hallet et al., 2004; Zarins & Gewertz, 2005)
    a. Indication: atherosclerotic RAS
    b. Most common open surgical procedure (Hirsch et al., 2006)
    c. Procedure
        1) Xiphoid-to-pubis abdominal incision
        2) Preferred conduit is a reversed saphenous vein
        3) Anastomosis between the renal artery and graft is performed first
        4) Aortic anastomosis is then performed
11. Renal artery thromboendarterectomy (Hallet et al., 2004; Zarins & Gewertz, 2005)
    a. Indication: atherosclerotic RAS
    b. Procedure
        1) Xiphoid-to-pubis abdominal incision
        2) A transverse aortotomy is made and the renal artery is opened

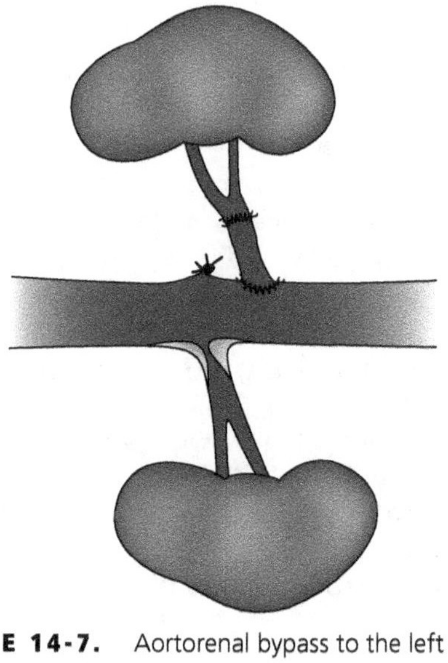

FIGURE 14-7. Aortorenal bypass to the left kidney.

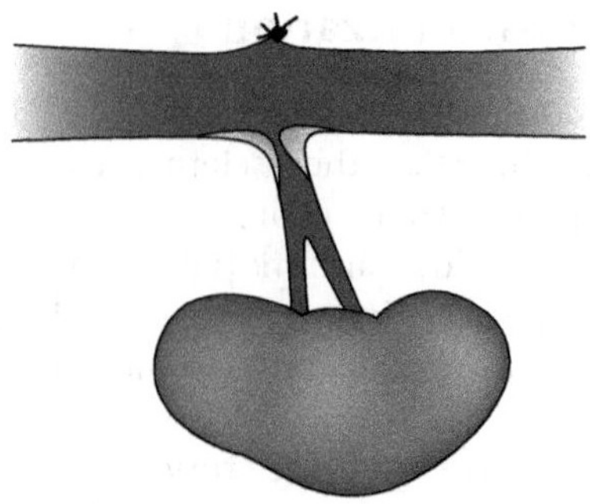

FIGURE 14-8. Nephrectomy of the left kidney.

3) Incision must extend beyond the stenosis
4) The arteriosclerosis and the media are excised
5) The renal artery is closed usually with a Dacron patch to ensure that the artery is widely patent

c. Renal artery reimplantation (Hallet et al., 2004)—When the artery has redundancy, reimplantation at a slightly lower level may be required

12. Autotransplantation and ex vivo reconstruction for treatment of fibrodysplastic branch lesions (Hallet et al., 2004)
    a. Indication: FMD, renal aneurysm, or stenosis involving the renal artery branches
    b. Procedure
        1) The kidney is removed from the body and preserved by hypothermic perfusion as done for renal transplantation
        2) Then the renal artery and branches are reconstructed outside the body
        3) A saphenous vein or internal iliac artery is used as a new conduit for the renal artery
        4) The kidney is implanted back into the patient's body
13. Nephrectomy (Hallet et al., 2004)
    a. Surgical removal of the kidney (see Fig. 14-8)
    b. Rarely performed because of the improvements in medical, interventional, and surgical management
    c. Indication
        1) Nonfunctioning kidney (<10% of function)
        2) After renal infarction, in which the kidney usually has shrunken to <6 to 7 cm in length
    d. Procedure
        1) The kidney is excised via lumbotomy
        2) The artery, vein, and ureter are ligated

X. Recent Randomized Controlled Trials (RCTs)

A. **STAR Trial** (Stenting in Renal Dysfunction Caused by Atherosclerotic Renal Artery): 140 patients were studied. No benefit was found with stenting plus medical therapy versus medical therapy only on prevention of loss of kidney function. Stenting resulted in a total of three deaths (two procedural deaths and one death later due to infected hematoma) (Bax et al., 2009).

B. **ASTRAL Trial** (Angioplasty and Stent for Renal Artery Lesions): Trial that compared endovascular revascularization plus medical therapy versus standard medical therapy in patients with atherosclerotic RVD. Eight hundred and six patients were studied over a mean of 33.5 months and there was no added benefit with revascularization in renal function, blood pressure control, renal/CV events, and mortality (Wheatley et al., 2009).

1. Inclusion criteria limited to asymptomatic, which may have resulted in bias. Symptomatic patients that may have seen more benefit.
2. Blood pressure control was improved in both limbs of the study, but was not clinically significant.
3. The study demonstrated that surgical and endovascular treatment was equivocal with reduced mortality/morbidity in the endovascular treatment group. There were higher patency rates at 2 years in the surgical treatment group (Wheatley et al., 2009).

C. **CORAL** (Cardiovascular Outcomes in Renal Atherosclerotic Lesions) trial is an NIH sponsored trial that randomized 1,080 hypertensive patients (SBP >155 mm Hg) with severe atherosclerotic renal artery lesions (>60% diameter stenosis) to optimal medical management with or without renal stenting. Enrollment ended in January 2010. Study data is not available at this time. This study will help clarify the role of stenting in ARAS lesions (Cooper et al., 2006)

D. **DRASTIC** (Dutch Renal Artery Stenosis Intervention Cooperative) was an early study comparing medical management versus intervention (at the time PTRA, before the era of stents). Outcome at 3 months showed an advantage in the PTRA in terms of blood pressure control (van Jaarsveld et al., 2000)

XI. Nursing Management

A. Risk for Ineffective Renal Perfusion

1. Definition per NANDA (Herdman, 2012): "At risk for a decrease in blood circulation to the kidney that may compromise health"
2. Risk factors: RAS
3. Expected outcomes
   a. Patient will exhibit normal renal function
   b. Patient will exhibit systolic blood pressure <140 mm Hg and diastolic blood pressure <90 mm Hg
4. Nursing interventions
   a. Monitor and document intake and output to ensure kidney function is adequate
   b. Monitor urine specific gravity, serum electrolytes, BUN, and creatinine. Rising levels may indicate decreased kidney function
   c. Monitor and record blood pressure to ensure that there is not a sudden increase in blood pressure
   d. Monitor and record urinary output to ensure that there is not a sudden decrease in urine output
   e. Monitor vital signs, hemoglobin, hematocrit to detect signs of hemorrhage or shock after intervention/surgery

5. Evaluation of nursing care
   a. Patient maintains adequate fluid and electrolyte balance and hemodynamic stability
   b. Patient's vital signs remain within set limits
   c. Patient maintains adequate urine output
   d. Patient identifies his/her risk factors that impact renal perfusion, long term

B. Acute Pain

1. Definition per NANDA (Herdman, 2012): "Sudden or slow onset of any intensity from mild to severe with an anticipated or predictable end and a duration <6 months"
2. Defining characteristics
   a. Coded report (e.g., use of pain scale)
   b. Reports pain
   c. Observed evidence of pain
   d. Positioning to avoid pain
3. Related factors—Injury agents: physical
4. Expected outcomes
   a. Patient will identify specific characteristics of pain
   b. Patient will express reduction of pain level within a reasonable time after taking prescribed medication
   c. Patient will identify alternative strategies to reduce pain other than pharmacological agents
5. Nursing interventions
   a. Assess physical symptoms
   b. Administer physical measures of massage, rest/activity, and pharmacological agents
   c. Discuss possible association of exacerbation of pain
   d. Provide positive encouragement of progression toward reaching goals
6. Evaluation of nursing care
   a. Patient is able to discuss characteristics of postinterventional/postoperative pain and methods that improve/alleviate pain
   b. Patient acknowledges that acute pain is reduced with pharmacological agents and alternative strategies

C. Risk for Imbalanced Fluid Volume

1. Definition per NANDA (Herdman, 2012): "At risk for an increase or decrease in intravascular/interstitial and/or intracellular fluid that may compromise health. The result may be body fluid loss or gain"
2. Risk factors
   a. Abdominal surgery, if applicable
   b. Compromised regulatory mechanisms associated with RAS
3. Expected outcomes
   a. Blood pressure will remain between 90 and 140 mm Hg systolic
   b. BUN, creatinine, sodium, and potassium levels will be within normal levels
   c. Urine output will return to normal
4. Nursing interventions
   a. Monitor blood pressure, pulse rate, cardiac rhythm, temperature, and breath sounds at least every 4 hours, while the patient is in the hospital

b. Carefully monitor intake, output, and urine specific gravity at least every 4 hours. Intake greater than output and elevated specific gravity may indicate fluid retention or volume overload
c. Monitor BUN, creatinine, electrolytes, hemoglobin, and hematocrit
   1) BUN and creatinine indicates renal function
   2) Electrolytes, hemoglobin, and hematocrit help indicate fluid status
d. Weigh patient daily before breakfast to check for signs of fluid retention
e. Physical examination includes assessment of degree of peripheral edema at baseline and at least every 12 hours

5. Evaluation of nursing care
   a. Blood pressure remains within established limits
   b. Urine specific gravity remains within established limits
   c. Hemoglobin, hematocrit, and electrolytes remain within established limits
   d. No weight gain
   e. Reduction in peripheral edema

D. Risk for Bleeding

1. Definition per NANDA (Herdman, 2012): "At risk for a decrease in blood volume that may compromise health"
2. Risk factors: treatment-related side effect of angioplasty with or without stenting or surgery
3. Expected outcomes
   a. Patient will maintain hemodynamic stability
   b. Patient will not experience bleeding
4. Nursing interventions
   a. Monitor blood pressure, pulse rate, and cardiac rhythm, at least every 4 hours, while the patient is in the hospital
   b. Monitor vital signs, hemoglobin, hematocrit to detect signs of hemorrhage or shock after intervention/surgery
   c. Monitor surgical incisions for signs of bleeding
   d. Monitor puncture sites for signs of overt bleeding or hematoma
   e. Monitor for signs of retroperitoneal bleeding
5. Evaluation of nursing care
   a. Hemoglobin and hematocrit remain within established limits
   b. Patient maintains hemodynamic stability
   c. Patient's vital signs remain within set limits

E. Ineffective Breathing Pattern

1. Definition per NANDA (Herdman, 2012): "Inspiration and/or expiration that does not provide adequate ventilation"
2. Defining characteristics. Alterations in depth of breathing
3. Related factors
   a. Anesthesia
   b. Pulmonary edema
   c. Surgical incision
   d. Pain
   e. Decreased functional residual capacity
4. Expected outcomes
   a. Patient will achieve comfort without depressing respirations
   b. Patient will demonstrate correct use of incentive spirometer and/or Acapella device

c. Auscultation of lungs will reveal no adventitious breath sounds
d. Patient will state importance of pulmonary toilet (taking deep breaths, use of devices)
e. Patient will report ability to breathe comfortably

5. Nursing interventions
   a. Assess for pain and reduced respiratory effort and ventilation during postoperative period
   b. Give pain medication to allow maximal chest expansion
   c. Assist patient with incisional splinting and use of incentive spirometer/ Acapella device to ensure proper use and help prevent atelectasis
   d. Teach relaxation techniques to help reduce anxiety
6. Evaluation of nursing care
   a. Patient's respiratory rate improves, and patient expresses feelings that pain is manageable
   b. Breath sounds remain clear
   c. Patient reports breathing comfortably and being able to move without any shortness of breath and minimal incisional discomfort

XII. Patient Education

A. When Looking for Reputable information sites for patient/family education, the following sites are recommended

1. National Institute of Diabetes and Digestive and Kidney Diseases (NIH Publication No. 07-6020, May 2007)
2. AHRQ's *Renal Artery Stenosis Treatments: A guide for consumers* (AHRQ Publication No. 07-EHC004-2 A, June 2007)
3. Society for Vascular Surgery—Vascular Web (www.vascularweb.org)
4. Society for Vascular Nursing—www.svnnet.org

B. Disease Prevention/Health Promotion (secondary prevention)

1. Lifestyle modifications to improve health, promote circulation, and decrease weight through smoking cessation, change in diet, and change in exercise program
2. Importance of frequent physical examinations to monitor blood pressure
3. Importance of frequent physical examinations to monitor patency of renal arteries, kidney function, and other vascular functions
4. Use and side effects of antihypertensive, antiplatelet, and dyslipidemia medications
5. Evaluation of medication effectiveness
6. Identification of early signs of RAS and renal failure

C. Diagnostic Phase

1. Knowledge of preparation and completion of blood and urine testing
2. Knowledge of specific renal testing (noninvasive and invasive)

D. Acute Phase (interventions, repair, reconstruction, nephrectomy)

1. Knowledge deficit regarding disease process and treatment indications
2. Knowledge of activity levels during postoperative, recovery, and discharge phases

3. Knowledge of importance of rest during postoperative phase to promote healing
4. Knowledge of restrictions on bathing during immediate postoperative period
5. Knowledge of maintaining a clean and dry incision
6. Knowledge of need to report any increase in temperature, any wound drainage, increasing wound pain, or change in the appearance of the wound
7. Knowledge of maintaining a healthy high-protein diet and adequate vitamin intake to promote healing
8. Knowledge of indication and side effects of medications, including pain medications
9. Knowledge of signs and symptoms of renal failure, surgical complications, and decreased circulation resulting from progression of arteriosclerotic disease
10. Knowledge of home care and follow-up health checkups to evaluate renal function and overall health status

E. Home Care Considerations

1. Availability of health care resources for support with recovery
2. Importance of medication compliance and knowledge of contraindications for herbal supplements
3. Compliance with lifestyle changes, including smoking cessation, medication regimen, heart/vascular healthy diet, and changes in exercise habits
4. Monitoring blood pressure at home, with parameters that are preferred and when to call the health care provider
5. Family support (physical, psychological, social, and economic)
6. Importance of preserving kidney function and decreasing risk of loss of renal function

CASE STUDIES

CASE STUDY 1 (RVH RESULTING FROM FMD)

A 30-year-old female presents with the new onset of severe hypertension with systolic blood pressures 180 to 200, heart rates in the 60 to 65 range, and frequent headaches. No focal neurologic changes. Her medical history reveals no clues to the etiology. Social history reveals that she currently smokes one half pack of cigarettes per day. Negative for alcohol or illicit drug use. Family history is negative for hypertension or cardiovascular disease. She was admitted to the hospital for management of her hypertension and expedite her diagnostic workup.

Current Medications

1. Multivitamin (One a Day® Women) one tablet daily
2. Loestrin 24 Fe one tablet daily

Laboratory data: WBC, 7,200/μL; Hgb, 12.3 gm/dL; HCT, 36.8%; Platelets, 225,000/μL; BUN, 24 mg/dL; Creatinine, 1.30 mg/dL; Potassium, 4.9 mmol/L. Urine studies were normal. Urine creatinine, 93.5 mg/dL; Urine protein, 3.4 mg/dL; Random urine sodium, 58 mmol/L.

Diagnostics: She underwent a CT scan of the brain which was negative for any acute or chronic changes. She underwent a CT angiogram of the chest, abdomen, and pelvis. CTA of the chest was normal. Abdominal aorta was of normal caliber and was without disease. She was noted to have 80% left RAS and 40% right RAS.

Physical examination: Vital signs: Height, 5′3″; Weight, 125 lbs; BP right arm, 180/65; BP left arm, 188/68; Heart rate, 65 and regular. General: Pleasant, well-developed African American female in no acute distress. HEENT: Head atraumatic, normocephalic. Extraocular movements intact. Sclerae nonicteric. Oropharynx clear. Neck: Supple, no JVD. 2+ carotids. Chest: Lungs clear anteriorly and posteriorly. Cardiac: S1, S2, no murmurs, rubs, or gallops. Abdomen: No bruits appreciated. Extremities: No peripheral edema, skin intact, feet warm to the touch. 2+ dorsalis pedis and posterior tibial arteries. Neuro: Alert and oriented × 3.

Impression and Plan

1. RVD with severe left RAS and mild right RAS
2. Malignant hypertension
3. Chronic headaches secondary to #2
4. Renal insufficiency secondary to #1

She was admitted to the hospital for IV hydration and IV management of her malignant hypertension. After completion of her CTA and appropriate hydration, she underwent bilateral selective renal angiography. Angiogram confirmed an 80% proximal left RAS with a string of pearls–like appearance and 40% proximal lesion in the right RAS. A diagnosis of FMD was made. She underwent angioplasty of the left renal artery with minimal residual, good flow, and no complications. She was discharged home on oral antihypertensive medications. Patient education included how to monitor her blood pressure at home. She is advised to stop her oral contraceptives that can contribute to her hypertension until her blood pressure is under better control. She is to follow-up with her Primary Care Provider to discuss alternatives to oral contraceptives. Team discussed the need for smoking cessation and its impact on her overall cardiovascular health.

CASE STUDY 2 (RVH RESULTING FROM ATHEROSCLEROSIS)

A 73-year-old man presents for routine follow-up at the vascular medicine clinic. He has a history of diffuse vascular disease. He had a right carotid endarterectomy in June 2012, bilateral renal artery stenting in September 2011, and left fem-popliteal bypass in March 2011. Medical history includes hypertension and dyslipidemia.

He denies any neurologic changes. Blood pressure at home is up per the patient's report. His primary care physician recently added amlodipine 5 mg daily. His BP log shows a range of 160 to 190/80 to 96 over the past 2 weeks. He denies claudication symptoms or peripheral edema. He does not smoke. He is compliant with his medications (listed below).

Current Medications

1. Amlodipine 5 mg daily	6. Losartan 50 mg b.i.d.
2. Aspirin 81 mg daily	7. Lovastatin 40 mg daily
3. Caltrate 600 + Vitamin D daily	8. Metoprolol 25 mg b.i.d.
4. Clopidogrel 75 mg daily	9. Omega-3 fatty acids 1 tablet daily
5. Hydrochlorothiazide 12.5 mg daily	

Laboratory data: WBC, 7,700/μL; Hgb: 13.3 gm/dL; HCT, 38.5%; Platelets, 232,000/μL; BUN, 22 mg/dL; Creatinine, 0.68 mg/dL; Potassium, 3.6 mmol/L. Urine creatinine, 367.1 mg/dL; Urine protein, 18.2 mg/dL.

Diagnostics: In the vascular laboratory, he underwent a bilateral duplex scan which shows normal kidney size bilaterally with recurrent RAS bilaterally with peak systolic velocity of 320 to 350 cm/sec. Bilateral carotid duplex scan shows right internal carotid stenosis of 10% to 39%, left 40% to 69% with peak systolic velocity of 303 cm/sec.

Physical examination: Vital signs: Height, 5′7″; Weight, 188 lbs; BP right arm, 168/94; BP left arm, 170/88; Heart rate, 74 and regular. General: Pleasant, well-developed White male in no acute distress. HEENT: Head atraumatic, normocephalic. Extraocular movements intact. Sclerae nonicteric. Oropharynx clear. Neck: Supple, no JVD. 2+ carotids. Left carotid bruit noted. Well-healed carotid endarterectomy on right. Chest: Lungs clear anteriorly and posteriorly. Cardiac: S1, S2, no murmurs, rubs, or gallops. Abdomen: No bruits appreciated. Extremities: No peripheral edema, skin intact, feet warm to the touch. 2+ dorsalis pedis and posterior tibial arteries. Well-healed left femoral vascularization scar.

Impression and Plan

1. Carotid occlusive disease, status post right carotid revascularization, widely patent on ultrasound. The patient has moderate disease on the left, stable from last examination, asymptomatic. The patient will follow up in 6 months with bilateral carotid duplex scan. He will call for any acute neurological changes.
2. Peripheral artery disease with history of previous left surgical revascularization. Continue aspirin, clopidogrel, and statin. Exercise regimen encouraged. He will have lower extremity arterial studies at his next follow-up.
3. Renal vascular disease with a history of bilateral renal artery interventions including stenting, RVH. The patient has recurrent elevated blood pressure (at home and in office). Duplex scan shows severe RAS. Continue medical management for treatment of hypertension. Continue aspirin, clopidogrel, and statin. He is to be scheduled for angiogram and possible intervention.

He was admitted to the hospital for bilateral selective renal angiography with bilateral cutting balloon angioplasty. Procedure was successful. He had minimal in-stent residual stenosis. He had no postprocedural complication and was discharged the following day on medications, as outlined above. He is to continue to monitor his blood pressure at home. He is to return to the vascular medicine clinic in 2 weeks to evaluate changes to his antihypertensive medication.

REFERENCES

Balzer, K. M., Pfeiffer, T., Rossbach, S., Voiculescu, A., Mödder, U., Godehardt, E., & Sandmann, W. (2009). Prospective randomized trial of operative vs. interventional treatment for renal artery ostial occlusive disease (RAOOD). *Journal of Vascular Surgery, 49*(3), 667–675.

Bax, L., Woittiez, A. J., Kouwenberg, H. J., Mali, W. P., Buskens, E., Beek, F. J., ... Beutler, J. J. (2009). Stent placement in patients with atherosclerotic renal artery stenosis and impaired renal function: A randomized trial. *Annals of Internal Medicine, 150*, 840–848.

Chrysochou, C., & Kalra, P. A. (2010). Atherosclerotic renovascular disease and the heart. *Journal of Renal Care, 36*(Suppl. 1), 146–153.

Coffman, T. M., Falk, R. J., Molitoris, B. A., Neilson, E. G., & Schrier, R. W. (2013). *Schrier's diseases of the kidney* (9th ed., Vol. 1.) Philadelphia, PA: Wolters Kluwer.

Colyer, W. R., Eltahawy, E., & Cooper, C. J. (2011). Renal artery stenosis: Optimizing diagnosis and treatment. *Progress in Cardiovascular Diseases, 54*(1), 29–35.

Cooper, C. J., Murphy, T. P., Matsumoto, A., Steffes, M., Cohen, D. J., Jaff, M., ... Dworkin, L. (2006). Stent revascularization for the prevention of cardiovascular and renal events among patients with renal artery stenosis and systolic hypertension: Rationale and design of the CORAL trial. *American Heart Journal, 152*, 59–66.

Dunning, M. B., & Fischbach, F. (2011). *Nurses' quick reference to common laboratory & diagnostic tests* (5th ed.) Philadelphia, PA: Lippincott, Williams, & Wilkins.

Dworkin, L. D., & Cooper, C. J. (2009). Renal artery stenosis. *New England Journal of Medicine, 361*(20), 1972–1978.

Edwards, M. S., Craven, T. E., Burke, G. L., Dean, R. H., & Hansen, R. J. (2005). Renovascular disease and the risk of adverse coronary events in the elderly: A prospective, population study. *Archives of Internal Medicine, 165*(2), 207–213.

Elliott, W. J. (2008). Renovascular hypertension: An update. *The Journal of Clinical Hypertension, 10*(7), 522–533.

Fenves, A. Z., & Ram, C. V. (2006). Renovascular hypertension: Clinical concepts. *Minerva Medica, 97*(4), 313–324.

Go, A. S., Mozaffarian, D., Roger, V. L., Benjamin, E. J., Berry, J. D., Borden, W. B., ... American Heart Association Statistics Committee and Stroke Statistics Subcommittee. (2013). Heart disease and stroke statistics—2013 update: A report from the American Heart Association. *Circulation:* published online before print December 12, 2012, doi:10.1161/CIR.0b013e31828124ad

Hallet, J. W., Jr., Mills, J. L., Earnshaw, J. J., & Reekers, J. A. (Eds). (2004). *Comprehensive vascular and endovascular surgery.* Edinburgh: Mosby.

Ham, S. W., Kumar, S. R., Wang, B. R., Rowe, V. L., & Weaver, F. A. (2010). Late outcomes of endovascular and open revascularization for nonatherosclerotic renal artery disease. *Archives of Surgery, 145*(9), 832–839.

Hartman, R. P., & Kawashima, A. (2009). Radiologic evaluation of suspected renovascular hypertension. *American Family Physician, 80*(3), 273–279.

Harvin, H. J., Casalino, D. D., Remer, E. M., Bishoff, J. T., Coursey, C. A., Dighe, M., ... Vikram, R. (2012). Expert panel on urologic imaging. ACR Appropriateness Criteria® renovascular hypertension. Reston (VA). *American College of Radiology (ACR).* Retrieved from http://www.acr.org/~/media/ACR/Documents/AppCriteria/Diagnostic/RenovascularHypertension.pdf, accessed August 17, 2013.

Herdman, T. H. (Ed). (2012). *NANDA International nursing diagnoses definition and classification 2012–2014.* Oxford: Wiley-Blackwell.

Hirsch, A. T., Haskal, Z. J., Hertzer, N. R., Bakal, C. W., Creager, M. A., Halperin, J. L., ... White, R. A. (2006). ACC/AHA 2005 Practice guidelines for the management of patients with peripheral arterial disease (lower extremity, renal, mesenteric, and abdominal aortic): A collaborative report from the American Association for Vascular Surgery/Society for Vascular Surgery, Society for Cardiovascular Angiography and Interventions, Society for Vascular Medicine and Biology, Society of Interventional Radiology, and the American College of Cardiology/American Heart Association (ACC/AHA) Task Force on Practice Guidelines, *Circulation, 113*(11), e463–e654.

Jarvis, C. (2012). *Physical examination and health assessment* (6th ed.). St. Louis, MO: Elsevier, Saunders.

Kumbhani, D. J., Bavry, A. A., Harvey, J. E., de Souza, R., Scarpioni, R., Bhatt, D. L., & Kapadia, S. R. (2011). Clinical outcomes after percutaneous revascularization versus medical management in patients with significant renal artery stenosis: A meta-analysis of randomized controlled trials. *American Heart Journal, 161*(3), 622–630.

McLaughlin, K., Jardine, A. G., & Moss, J. G. (2000). ABC of arterial and venous disease. Renal artery stenosis. *British Medical Journal, 320,* 1124–1127.

Munden, L. (Ed). (2007). *Professional guide to pathophysiology* (2nd ed.). Philadelphia, PA: Lippincott Williams & Wilkins.

Plouin, P. F., & Bax, L. (2010). Diagnosis and treatment of renal artery stenosis. *Nature Reviews Nephrology, 6*(3), 151–159.

Rocha-Singh, K. J., Eisenhauer, A. C., Textor, S. C., Copper, C. J., Tan, W. A., Matsumoto, A. H., & Rosenfield, K. (2008). Atherosclerotic peripheral vascular disease symposium II: Intervention for renal artery disease. *Circulation, 118*(25), 2873–2878.

Trinquart, L., Mounier-Vehier, C., Sapoval, M., Gagnon, N., & Plouin, P. F. (2010). Efficacy of revascularization for renal artery stenosis caused by fibromuscular dysplasia: A systematic review and meta-analysis. *Hypertension, 56*(3), 525–532.

Van Jaarsveld, B. C., Krijnen, P., Pieterman, H., Derkx, F. H. M., Deinum, J., Postma, C. T., . . . Schalekamp, M. (2000). The effect of balloon angioplasty on hypertension in atherosclerotic renal artery stenosis. *New England Journal of Medicine, 342,* 1007–1017.

Wheatley, K., Ives, N., Gray, R., Kalra, P. A., Moss, J. G., Baigent, C., ... Scoble, J. (2009). Revascularization versus medical therapy for renal-artery stenosis. *New England Journal of Medicine, 361,* 1953–1962.

Zarins, C. K., & Gewertz, B. L. (2005). *Atlas of vascular surgery* (2nd ed.). Philadelphia, PA: Elsevier.

SUGGESTED READINGS

Alhadad, A., Mattiasson, I., Ivancev, K., Gottsäter, A., & Lindblad, B. (2005). Revascularisation of renal artery stenosis caused by fibromuscular dysplasia: Effects on blood pressure during 7-year follow-up are influenced by duration of hypertension and branch artery stenosis. *Journal of Human Hypertension, 19,* 761–767.

ASTRAL Investigators. (2009). Revascularization versus medical therapy for renal-artery stenosis. *New England Journal of Medicine, 361,* 1953–1962.

Baumgartner, I., & Lerman, L. O. (2011). Renovascular hypertension: Screening and modern management. *European Heart Journal, 32*(13), 1590–1598.

Cheung, C. M., Patel, A., Shaheen, N., Cain, S., Eddington, H., Hegarty, J., ... Kalra, P. A. (2007). The effects of statins on the progress of atherosclerotic renovascular disease. *Nephron Clinical Practice, 107*(2), c35–c42.

Corriere, M. A., Edwards, M. S., Pearce, J. D., Andrews, J. S., Geary, R. L., & Hansen, K. J. (2009). Restenosis after renal artery angioplasty and stenting: Incidence and risk factors. *Journal of Vascular Surgery, 50*(4), 813–819.

Fischbach, F., & Dunning, M. B., III., (2009). *A manual of laboratory and diagnostic tests* (8th ed.). Philadelphia, PA: Wolters Kluwer Health.

Goto, A., & Kawauchi, N. (2001). Captopril-augmented renal scan. *New England Journal of Medicine, 344*, 430.

Kalra, P. A., Guo, H., Kausz, A. T., Gilbertson, D. T., Liu, J., Chen, S. C., … Foley, R. N. (2005). Atherosclerotic renovascular disease in United States patients aged 67 years or older: Risk factors, revascularization, and prognosis. *Kidney International, 68*, 293–301.

Kumar, S. K., MacGinley, R., Mantha, M., Mount, P., Roberts, M., & Mangos, G. (2010). Natural history and progression of atherosclerotic renal vascular stenosis. *Nephrology, 15*, S204–S209.

Lao, D., Paraher, P. S., Cho, K. C., & Yeghiazarians, Y. (2011). Atherosclerotic renal artery stenosis – diagnosis and treatment. *Mayo Clinic Proceedings, 86*(7), 649–657.

Martin, L. G., Rundback, J. H., Wallace, M. J., Cardella, J. F., Angle, J. F., Kundu, S., … Wojak, J. C. (2010). Quality improvement guidelines for angiography, angioplasty, and stent placement for the diagnosis and treatment of renal artery stenosis in adults. *Journal of Vascular and Interventional Radiology, 21*, 421–430.

Mehta, A. N., & Fenves, A. (2010). Current opinions in renovascular hypertension. *Hypertension, 56*(3), 525–536.

Modrall, J. G., Rosero, E. B., Smith, S. T., Arko, F. R., III., Valentine, R. J., Clagett, G. P., & Timaran, C. H. (2008). Operative mortality for renal artery bypass in the Unites States: Results from the National Inpatient Sample. *Journal of Vascular Surgery, 48*, 317–322.

Olin, J. W., Allie, D. E., Belkin, M., Bonow, R. O., Casey, D. E., Jr., Creager, M. A., … Zheng, Z. (2010). ACCF/AHA/ACR/SCAI/SIR/SVM/ SVN/SVS 2010 Performance measures for adults with peripheral artery disease: A report of the American College of Cardiology Foundation/American Heart Association Task Force on Performances Measures, the American College of Radiology, the Society for Cardiac Angiography and Interventions, the Society for Interventional Radiology, the Society for Vascular Medicine, the Society for Vascular Nursing, and the Society for Vascular Surgery (Writing Committee to Develop Clinical Performance Measures for Peripheral Artery Disease) developed in collaboration with the American Association of Cardiovascular and Pulmonary Rehabilitation; the American Diabetes Association; the Society for Atherosclerosis Imaging and Prevention; the Society for Cardiovascular Magnetic Resonance; the Society of Cardiovascular Computed Tomography; and the PAD Coalition Endorsed by the American Academy of Podiatric Practice Management. *Journal of the American College of Cardiology, 56*, 2147–2181.

Rooke, T. W., Hirsch, A. T., Misra, S., Sidawy, A. N., Beckman, J. A., Findeiss, L. K., … Zierler, R. E. (2011). 2011 ACCF/AHA focused update of the guideline for the management of patients with peripheral artery disease (updating the 2005 guideline); A report of the American College of Cardiology Foundation/American Heart Association Task Force on Practice Guidelines. *Journal of the American College of Cardiology, 58*, 2020–2045.

Shuman, L. S. (2008). Diagnostic imaging and endovascular treatment of renovascular hypertension. *The Journal of Lancaster General Hospital, 3*(3), 98–101.

Vasbinder, G. B., Nelemans, P. J., Kessels, A. G., Kroon, A. A., Maki, J. H., Leiner, T., … van Engleshoven, J. M. (2004). Accuracy of computed tomographic angiography and magnetic resonance angiography for diagnosing renal artery stenosis. *Annals of Internal Medicine, 141*(9), 674–682.

Zierler, R. E., Bergelin, R. O., Polissar, N. L., Beach, K. W., Caps, M. T., Cantwell-Gab, K., … Strandness, D. E., Jr. (1998). Carotid and lower extremity arterial disease in patients with renal artery atherosclerosis. *Archives of Internal Medicine, 158*(7), 761–767.

WEBSITES

Agency for Healthcare Research and Quality (AHRQ). (2007). *Renal artery stenosis treatments: A guide for consumers,* Pub #: 07-EHC004-2 A. Houston TX: Eisenberg Center. (Also available at www.ahrq.gov)

CORAL (Cardiovascular Outcomes in Renal Atherosclerotic Lesions) trial (website http://www.coralclinicaltrial.org)

National Kidney Foundation (2002). K/DOQI guidelines on hypertension and antihypertensive agents in chronic kidney disease. Accessed on 1/3/2013. (http://www.kidney.org/professionals/kdoqi/guidelines_bp/guide_4.htm)

National Kidney and Urologic Diseases Information Clearinghouse. (2007). *Renal artery stenosis.* Washington, DC: U.S. Department of Health and Human Services. Pub #: 07-602. (Also available at www.kidney.niddk.nih.gov)

Society for Vascular Surgery. (2009). *Renovascular conditions.* Chicago: Society for Vascular Surgery (Also available at www.vascularweb.org)

CHAPTER 15

Vascular Access

Ellen Malone

First Edition Author: *Jeanne Doyle*

OBJECTIVES

1. Identify three indications for long-term vascular access.
2. Name three common anatomical locations to obtain vascular access.
3. Differentiate between catheter, autogenous, and synthetic graft access.
4. Identify three potential complications of long-term vascular access.

Introduction and Overview

Vascular access is a term used to describe techniques designed to provide readily obtainable and dependable long-term/chronic access to the venous system for treatment interventions, such as hemodialysis, or the delivery of chemotherapy or nutritional supplementation. In most cases, vascular access devices provide a simple and relatively painless means of drawing blood or administering treatment. The most common types of vascular access are surgically created fistulae between an artery and vein (AV fistulae), and implantable (tunneled or non-tunneled) intravenous catheters or port devices. This chapter provides an overview of these approaches.

I. Vascular Access for Advanced Chronic Kidney Disease

A. Incidence and Significance

1. Chronic kidney disease (CKD) affects as many as 26 million people in the United States (13% of the population).
2. The incidence is significantly increased in those older than age 65.
3. More than 480,000 people with kidney failure are receiving hemodialysis requiring permanent, "durable" long-term access.
4. In addition to surgically created fistulae, an estimated 2.75 million vascular access devices are placed per year.

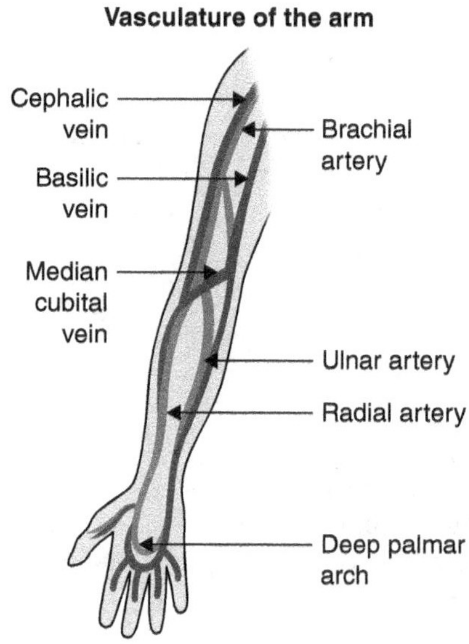

FIGURE 15-1. Vasculature of the arm.

II. Surgical Vascular Access for End-Stage Renal Disease

(Note: Theoretically, an AV fistula can be surgically created anywhere in the body where an artery and vein of suitable size are available. Considerations such as patient comfort, accessibility, and ease of use for dialysis are important. Thus, the upper extremity is the most commonly used site.)

A. Anatomy (see Fig. 15-1)

1. Upper extremity arteries
   a. Radial: located on lateral side of wrist, communicates with palmer arch
   b. Ulnar: located on the medial side of wrist, also communicated with palmer arch
   c. Brachial: located in antecubital area extending into the upper arm, joins proximally with (axillary artery which becomes the) subclavian artery
2. Upper extremity veins
   a. Cephalic: located on lateral side of arm, courses from wrist to upper arm—joins the axillary vein in the upper arm, superficial in forearm so it is frequently visualized on physical examination
   b. Basilic: located on medial side of arm, courses from wrist to upper arm—becomes the axillary vein at upper arm. It lies deeper in the tissue making it hard to visualize on physical examination

B. Assessment

1. Determination of dominant arm, (nondominant arm used if feasible)
2. Risk factors for poor vein quality in upper extremities include history of frequent or prolonged intravenous catheter including central lines and peripherally inserted central catheters (PICC), history of IV drug use, vein or arterial harvest, prior surgery or trauma to upper extremity, (primary prevention avoid trauma to or venipuncture of the arm vessels)
3. Palpation of radial, ulnar, and brachial arterial pulses

4. Allen test
   a. Determines the ability of the ulnar artery to perfuse the hand via the palmer arch
   b. Pressure is applied over the ulnar and the radial artery simultaneously resulting in pallor of the hand
   c. Release of pressure over the ulnar artery will result in return of color due to rapid reperfusion of the hand if blood supply through the ulnar system is adequate and the palmar arch is intact

C. Diagnostic Testing

1. Blood pressure in both arms
2. Doppler systolic pressures of wrist arteries
3. Ultrasound vein mapping determines caliber of vessels and suitability for use
4. Doppler ultrasound arterial velocities to evaluate for stenosis
5. Venogram if there is a concern regarding vein quality or central venous stenosis

D. Surgical Management

1. Access to the vascular system for hemodialysis is most often achieved by surgical creation of an autogenous arteriovenous fistula
2. Fistulae should be created using the distal-most vessels in the upper extremity (e.g., the radial-cephalic fistula) to preserve more proximal vessels for future fistula formation (see Fig. 15-2)
3. More proximal surgical fistulae can be created using the brachial artery and cephalic or basilic veins in the upper arm
4. In the most extreme cases, vein can be harvested from the lower extremity for interposition fistula or a fistula can be created in the lower extremities
5. When suitable autogenous vein is not available, synthetic graft materials (i.e., PTFE, Dacron) may be used to create a "bridge" fistula between the artery and vein. Long-term patency rates with synthetic interposition grafts are inferior to autogenous fistulae

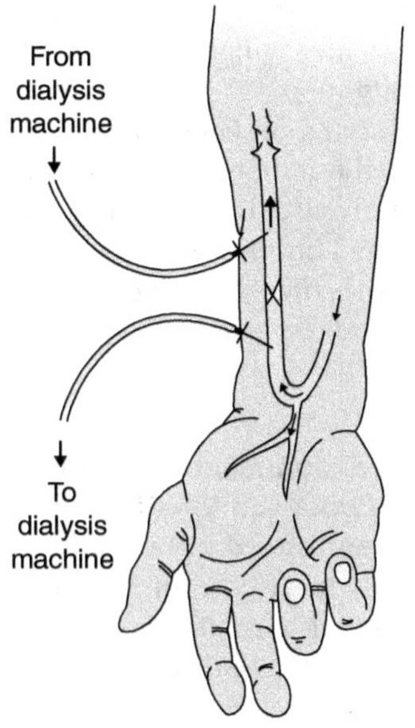

FIGURE 15-2. Brescia–Cimino (radial-cephalic) fistula.

E. Postsurgical Nursing Management

1. Acute postoperative care
   a. Potential for acute thrombosis of fistula (often secondary to technical factors such as lack of adequate venous run-off)
      1) Palpate/auscultate fistula for thrill/bruit
      2) Report diminished or absence of thrill/bruit to surgeon
      3) Maintain adequate blood pressure and fluid status
   b. Potential for infection
      1) Inspect surgical incision for signs/symptoms of infection or abscess
      2) Report any fevers, increased pain, swelling or drainage
   c. Potential for hemorrhage
      1) Inspect surgical incision for development of hematoma or excessive bleeding
   d. Potential for postoperative edema (anticipated because of changes in local hemodynamics and soft tissue injury)
      1) Elevate arm with pillow or splint
      2) Monitor for improvement of edema with time
      3) Report persistent/worsening edema to surgeon (may be indicative of venous thrombosis or central venous stenosis)
2. Long-term care
   a. Potential for late thrombosis (related to repeated trauma to outflow vein by needle punctures leading to fibrosis)
      1) Palpate/auscultate for presence of thrill/bruit
      2) Report absence to surgeon
      3) Increase flow rate on hemodialysis
   b. Potential for hemodynamic complications
      1) Congestive heart failure related to increased venous return, resulting in compensatory increase in cardiac output and workload
      2) "Steal syndrome" shunting of blood from the artery to the vein away from the palmar arch may result in pain in the hand on exertion
      3) Pseudoaneurysm formation from repeated venipunctures that fail to seal
      4) Distal venous hypertension/chronic edema (may worsen as fistula matures and valvular incompetence develops) characterized by edema, blue discoloration, and pigmentation of overlying skin
      5) Aneurysm formation—may require surgical repair
      6) Neuropathy/carpal tunnel syndrome
3. Preoperative patient teaching considerations
   a. Psychological: effect of disease on perception of health and well-being
   b. Psychosocial: impact on daily activities, time commitment for treatment, transportation to dialysis, and so forth
   c. Physical: formation and care of fistula
   d. Dialysis procedure
   e. Nutritional counseling
4. Postoperative patient teaching considerations
   a. Check for palpable thrill several times daily (report absence)
   b. Report any signs/symptoms of infection
   c. Avoid constrictive or circumferential dressing
   d. No blood pressure cuffs or devices on operative arm
   e. Avoid tight sleeves, wristwatch, or bracelets on operative arm
   f. Avoid carrying heavy objects with operative arm
   g. Encourage hand grip exercises several times a day post operation

III. Percutaneous Catheter Access to the Venous System

A. Seldinger Technique: advancing a catheter over a guidewire, into a central vein

1. First reported for use in emergency fluid volume resuscitation and central venous pressure measurement. Led to the first use of central venous access for nutritional support (total parenteral nutrition)
2. The development of large-bore silicone catheters (e.g., Hickman, Broviac) has vastly improved the lives of patients requiring long-term parenteral therapy for nutrition, antibiotics for resistant infections, and chemotherapy
3. Further technical advancements have resulted in multiple-lumen catheters, allowing for infusion as well as outflow (e.g., blood sampling)

B. Central Venous Anatomy (see Fig. 15-3)

1. Subclavian vein
2. Internal jugular vein
3. Femoral vein (rarely used)

C. Insertion Technique

1. Neck and chest are prepped with cleansing solution and draped using sterile conditions
2. Patient is placed in slight Trendelenburg position
3. Local anesthesia is infused over the vessel being cannulated
4. Fluoroscopic guidance or ultrasound is optimal

Note: Catheters may be inserted via a surgical cut-down technique in patients with bleeding dyscrasias or in whom "blind" puncture might carry an increased risk.

D. Types of Catheters

1. Central venous tunneled catheters/ports (see Figs. 15-4 and 15-5)
   a. First introduced by Broviac and colleagues in 1973
   b. Composed of silicone with a Dacron polyester cuff that anchors the catheter in a subcutaneous tunnel
   c. Newest catheters have an additional antimicrobial-impregnated cuff creating a physical barrier to bacteria
   d. Available in single, double, or triple lumens

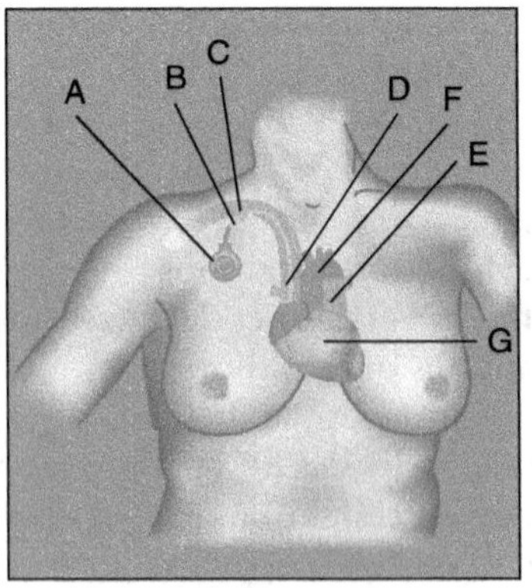

Central venous anatomy
A Port
B Catheter (tubing)
C Subclavian vein
D Superior vena cava
E Pulmonary vein
F Aorta
G Heart

FIGURE 15-3. Central venous anatomy.

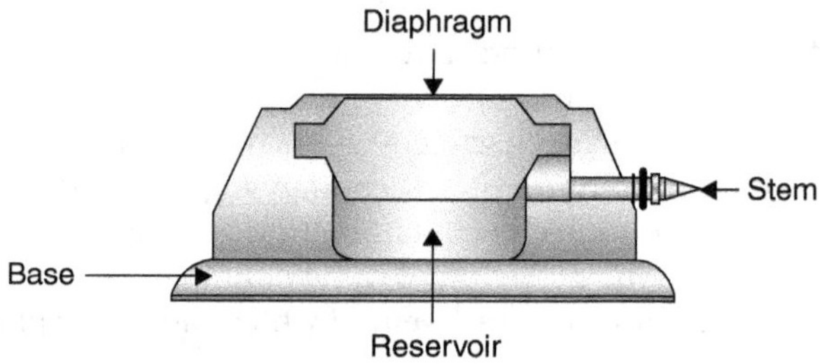

FIGURE 15-4. Subcutaneous hub of central venous port.

   e. Advantages
      1) Lower risk of infection
      2) "Discreet" cosmetic placement
      3) Multiple lumens allow for dual therapy (e.g., chemotherapy/total parenteral nutrition [TPN]) or blood sampling
   f. Disadvantages
      1) Daily dressing changes
      2) Daily heparin flush required
      3) Cost of maintenance supplies
2. PICC inserted from antecubital or axillary vein into central venous system
   a. Advantages
      1) Inexpensive placement: does not require surgery/OR cost
      2) Ease of removal
   b. Disadvantages
      1) Daily care requirements: sterile cleansing of insertion site with dressing change
      2) Need for occlusive dressings
      3) Increased risk of infection
3. Hemodialysis catheters
   a. Nontunneled: temporary, used in acute care settings. Not for long-term use
   b. Tunneled dialysis catheters (TDC)
   c. Strict protocol for dressing changes and access of catheters usually performed by hemodialysis staff
   d. Catheters are used for hemodialysis only

E. Complications of Central Venous Catheters

1. Acute complications from needle or catheter injury
   a. Pneumothorax (most common with subclavian catheter insertion)
   b. Hemothorax

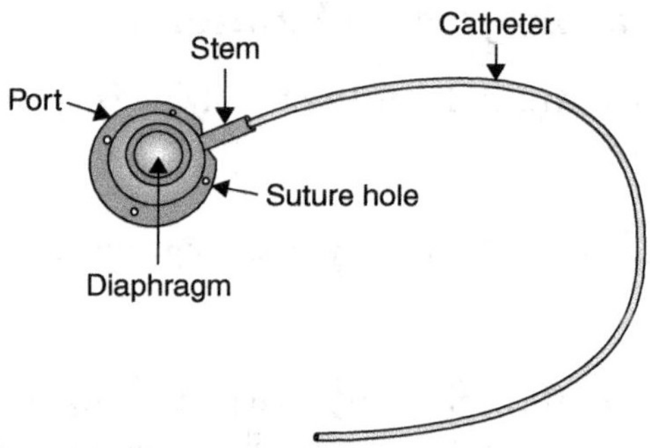

FIGURE 15-5. Implantable central venous port/catheter.

c. Air embolism
d. Cardiac perforation/tamponade

2. Late complications
    a. Catheter-related bacteremia—increase prevalence in patients who are immunocompromised secondary to primary disease or therapy; most common source of contamination is the skin
    b. Thrombotic occlusion of catheter lumen
    c. Thrombosis of "host" vein in which catheter is placed—risk of pulmonary embolism
    d. Stenosis of vein

IV. Nursing Diagnosis/Outcomes

A. **Potential for Infection** related to venous cannulation/patient will not develop catheter-related sepsis

1. Use meticulous sterile techniques (cleansing, antibiotic ointment, and dry sterile dressing) over catheter insertion site daily
2. Inspect site during dressing changes for signs of infection
3. Ascertain symptoms of infection from patient (e.g., fever)

B. **Potential for Luminal/Venous Thrombosis** related to long-term cannulation/patient will not develop thrombotic complications related to venous catheter

1. Flush catheter with saline or heparin solution as ordered
2. Report difficulty with infusion through and/or withdrawal from catheter
3. Assess surrounding area (e.g., neck, upper extremity) for evidence of edema, discoloration, or venous distention, which may suggest venous occlusion, and report to surgeon

C. **Alteration in Body Image** related to external catheter/patient will experience minimal negative impact on body image

1. Instruct patient on ways to "minimize" presence of catheter (e.g., wearing long-sleeved clothing)
2. Advise patient regarding personal hygiene while avoiding contamination of catheter insertion site

V. Patient Teaching Considerations

A. **Instruct Patient/Family** on daily care requirements for catheter insertion site

B. **Instruct Patient/Family** regarding catheter flushing technique and frequency

C. **Instruct Patient/Family** to report any signs/symptoms of local or systemic infection to surgeon/family physician immediately

CASE STUDY

Mr. S., a 72-year-old insulin-dependent diabetic man with end-stage renal disease, visited his nephrologists with symptoms of increased lethargy, mental "cloudiness," and decreased urine output. Serum chemistry revealed a creatinine of 5.4 mg/dL, which had been 4.6 mg/dL at last assessment several months previously. Arrangements were made to admit Mr. S. to hospital for surgical creation of an arteriovenous (AV) fistula, anticipating need for hemodialysis in the near future. He is also scheduled for insertion of a central venous catheter, should the need for dialysis become emergent.

Review Questions

1. The preferred anatomic location for creation of an AV fistula is:
   a. femoral artery to femoral vein
   b. innominate artery to subclavian vein
   c. radial artery to cephalic vein
   d. iliac artery to inferior vena cava
2. Considerations before surgical creation of an AV fistula include:
   a. allowing time for the fistula to "mature"
   b. use of vessels in nondominant extremity
   c. ease of access to fistula for intervention
   d. all of the above
3. The most common complication of an AV fistula is:
   a. infection
   b. hemorrhage
   c. thrombosis
   d. pseudoaneurysm formation
4. Postoperative nursing management of Mr. S. would include:
   1. incisional care using sterile technique
   2. assessment of a bruit and thrill over the fistula
   3. assessment of signs and symptoms of infection
   4. frequent blood pressure assessment in the operative arm
   a. 2, 3, and 4
   b. 1, 3, and 4
   c. 1, 2, and 4
   d. 1, 2, and 3
5. Chronic central venous catheters are most commonly used for:
   1. chemotherapy
   2. hemodialysis
   3. total parenteral nutrition
   4. plasmapheresis
   a. 1 and 3
   b. 2 and 3
   c. 1 and 4
   d. 2 and 4

Answers/Rationale

1. c. The radial artery to cephalic vein (Brescia–Cimino) AV fistula remains the preferred surgical procedure because it is distal-most in the extremity (allowing for use of more proximal vessels should complications arise), has the best long-term patency rates, and has a low incidence of infection.

2. d. All options are important considerations for the surgeon before creating an AV fistula. Fistulae typically take 4 to 6 weeks to "mature," should be most convenient for the patient (nondominant arm), and should allow for ease of access for hemodialysis.
3. c. Although all listed are potential complications, thrombosis is the most common. It can occur early, secondary to technical inadequacy, or late (after 3 months) related to repeated needle trauma leading to fibrosis and stenosis of the outflow vein.
4. d. Blood pressure should not be taken in the operative arm. In addition, restrictive clothing, carrying heavy objects, venipuncture proximal to the fistula, and so forth should be avoided in the operative arm.
5. a. Chronic central venous catheters are most commonly used for chemotherapy and total parenteral nutrition. Use of a central venous catheter for hemodialysis would be an interim intervention only, as chronic use is associated with serious complications of infection, thrombosis, and inadequate filtration. Hemofiltration is synonymous with hemodialysis.

SUGGESTED READINGS

Coresh, J., Selvin, E., Stevens, L. A., Manzi, J., Kusek, J. W., Eggers, P., ... Levey, A. S. (2007). Prevalence of chronic kidney disease in the United States. *Journal of the American Medical Association, 298*(17), 2038–2047.

Fitzgerald, J. T., Schanzer, A., Chin, A. I, McVicar, J. P, Perez, R. V, & Troppman, C. (2004). Outcomes of upper arm arteriovenous fistulas for maintenance hemodialysis access. *Archives of Surgery, 139,* 201–208.

Gillies, D., O'Riordan, E., Carr, D., O'Brien, I., Frost, J., & Gunning, R. (2003). Central venous catheter dressings: A systematic review. *Journal of Advanced Nursing, 44,* 623–632.

Goldstein, L. J., & Gupta, S. (2003). Use of the radial artery for hemodialysis access. *Archives of Surgery, 138,* 1130–1134.

Jacobsen, J. (1999). Vascular access surgery. In V. A. Fahey (Ed.), *Vascular nursing* (3rd ed., pp. 390–415). Philadelphia: Saunders.

Klerk, C. P., Smorenburg, S. M., & Büller, H. R. (2003). Thrombosis prophylaxis in patient populations with a central venous catheter: A systematic review. *Archives of Internal Medicine, 163,* 1913–1921.

Padberg, F. T., Jr., Calligaro, K. D., & Sidawy, A. N. (2008). Complications of arteriovenous hemodialysis access: Recognition and management. *Journal of Vascular Surgery, 48,* 55S–80S.

Rayner, H. C., Pisoni, R. L., Gillespie, B. W., Goodkin, D. A., Akiba, T., Akizawa, T., . . . Port, F. K. (2003). Creation, cannulation and survival of arteriovenous fistulae: Data from the Dialysis Outcomes and Practice Patterns Study. *Kidney International, 63,* 323–330.

Sidawy, A. N., Spergel, L. M., Besarab, A., Allon, M., Jennings, W. C., Padberg, F. T., Jr., . . . Ascher, E. (2008). The Society for Vascular Surgery: Clinical practice guidelines for the surgical placement and maintenance of arteriovenous hemodialysis access. *Journal of Vascular Surgery, 48*(5 Suppl.), 2S–25S.

RELEVANT WEBSITES

PROFESSIONAL

http://clinicalcenter.nih.gov/index.html
Home page of the National Institute of Health Clinical Center, request Vascular Access Device

www.vascularaccesssociety.com
Home page of the Vascular Access Society

www.rsna.org/
Home page of the Radiological Society of North America

CONSUMER

www niddk.nih.gov
Website of the National Institute of Diabetes and Digestive and Kidney Diseases

www.esrdnetworks.org
Website of the End-Stage Renal Disease Networks. Includes link to "Caring for Your Vascular Access". Details related to the Fistula First program of the National Vascular Access Improvement Initiative

www.ikidney.com
Website "bringing the worldwide kidney disease community together." Sponsored by an educational grant from Watson Pharma, Inc.

CHAPTER 16

Buerger Disease (Thromboangiitis Obliterans)

Rita C. Clark

OBJECTIVES

1. Define the pathophysiology of Buerger disease.
2. Identify three diagnostic criteria for Buerger disease.
3. Identify the major risk factor for development of Buerger disease.
4. List five criteria which must be ruled out for a diagnosis of Buerger disease.
5. Discuss medical and surgical treatment options, considerations, and limitations.
6. List three nursing diagnoses relevant to care of the patient with Buerger disease.

Introduction/Overview

Buerger disease or Thromboangiitis Obliterans (TAO) is a "nonatherosclerotic segmental inflammatory disease that most commonly affects the small- and medium-sized arteries, veins, and nerves of the arms and legs" (Olin, 2000). The cause is unknown but it is widely accepted that tobacco use in some form is critical to the onset and progression of Buerger disease (Mills, 2003).

In 1879 von Winter, of the University Clinic in Vienna, published his autopsy findings of a patient with a 12-year history of leg ischemia culminating in "spontaneous gangrene" and limb loss (Mills, 2003). Twenty-nine years later, Leo Buerger, from Mount Sinai Hospital in New York, described detailed pathologic findings of the disease process in 11 amputated limbs of males with ongoing limb ischemia commencing between the ages of 20 and 40 years. Buerger coined the term TAO to describe the clinical and pathologic characteristics of this disease process, which has since taken on the eponym Buerger disease (Mills, 2003).

I. Incidence

A. **The True Incidence Worldwide** is unknown due to the lack of epidemiologic studies in many countries and inconsistencies in diagnosis.

B. North American incidence estimated at 8 to11.6/100,000/yr (Cooper et al., 2004). Olin (2000) reported annual incidence in the United States to be 12.6/100,000. Prevalence in North American incidence has declined in last 30 years (Olin & Shih, 2006). More prevalent in the Mediterranean, the Middle East, and Asia (Olin & Shih, 2006).

C. Erroneously, Dr. Buerger thought the disease was primarily limited to the Jewish population, but that observation was found to be reflective of his patient population at Mount Sinai Hospital. Authors have quoted an extraordinary high incidence (80%) of Buerger disease among Israeli Jews of Ashkenazi ancestry with peripheral vascular disease (Małecki, Zdrojowy, & Adamiec, 2009; Olin, 2000). In response to Małecki et al., 2009, Adar (2010) claims the incidence among Ashkenazi Jews has been erroneously quoted from the original 1965 article printed in the American Journal of Medicine. In the original source document 80% (63 of 80) was the percent of Ashkenazi Jews studied in Israel for that paper. This preponderance of Ashkenazi Jews was not reflective of incidence or prevalence, but rather imperfect sampling and the inclination of affluent Ashkenazi Jews to participate in scientific studies during the 60s.

D. Strong Association exists between the disease and tobacco use. Type of tobacco used affects prevalence. Cigarette smoking carries the greatest risk. Cigars, chewing tobacco, snuff, and marijuana have also been implicated (Olin & Shih, 2006). Higher prevalence in India among smokers of bidis, homemade cigarettes made of raw tobacco (Olin, 2000). Prevalence higher among Indonesians smoking homegrown Kawung cigarettes (Mills, 2003).

II. Epidemiology

A. Generally presents in young adults before the age of 40 to 45 years (Olin, 2000). Median age at onset of 34 years (Mills, 2003).

B. Historically, more men than women. In early reports women constituted only 1% to 2%; but over the years there has been a relative increase among women, paralleling the increase of tobacco use among young women (Joyce, 1996). Joyce (1996) and Olin (2000) reported increased incidence among women from 11% in 1971 to 23% in 1990.

C. In a Series of 112 Patients evaluated at the Cleveland Clinic between 1970 and 1987, the mean age at diagnosis was 42 (range 20 to 75) with a presence among women of 23% (Olin & Lie, 1992).

D. Mills (2003) cited a men to women ratio of 7.5:1 (13%) compared with a previously documented ratio of 9:1 (11%) in past series, as cited by Olin and Lie in 1992

E. **In a Mayo Clinic Review** of 111 Buerger patients, the mean age was 33.6 ± 8.4 years; and the percentage of female patients was 40.5%, which had increased from 1976 to 2000 (Cooper et al., 2004).

III. Clinical Features

A. **Most Commonly Affects** the small- and medium-sized arteries and veins in the arms, hands, legs, and feet.

B. **Reports of the Disease** affecting cerebral, coronary, pulmonary, renal, mesenteric, aorta, and iliac arteries exist (Olin, 2000). Hoppe, Lu, Thistlewaite, Yi & Mahmud (2002) published a case report of a 39-year-old female with affected left and right internal mammary arteries (IMAs) and the associated implications for coronary artery bypass; hence, coronary angiography to include IMAs in Buerger patients pre CABG is recommended.

C. **Typically Presents as Ischemia** of the distal small arteries and veins of the digits, hands, and feet, manifested by rest pain, ulceration, or gangrene (Mills, 2003; Olin, 2000).

D. **Claudication** of the instep of the foot rather than typical calf claudication is also a frequent complaint (Mill, 2003).

E. **Calf Claudication** may be present as the disease progresses more proximally.

F. **Superficial Thrombophlebitis** (38%), Raynaud disease (44%), an abnormal Allen test (63%), and nonspecific sensory findings (69%) are frequent signs and symptoms of the disease (Olin & Lie, 1992).

G. **Affects** any or all of the limbs. Isolated lower-extremity involvement in 50% of patients; isolated upper-extremity involvement in 10%; and both upper- and lower-extremity involvement in 30% to 40% of patients (Mills, 2003).

H. **Ischemia of Upper Extremity** clinically evident in 40% to 50% of patients. Disease detected in 63% by Allen test, and 91% with arteriography of the hand and forearm (Puéchal & Fiessinger, 2007).

I. **Rheumatic Manifestations:** Joint manifestations occur in 12.5% of patients in the preocclusive phase. Recurrent episodes of arthritis with local signs of inflammation. Duration of symptoms 2 to 14 days. Nonerosive arthritis. Wrists and knees most frequently involved. Joint problems precede diagnosis of Buerger by about 10 years. Arthritis disappears with appearance of ischemic signs (Puéchal & Fiessinger, 2007).

IV. Pathophysiology

A. Type of Vasculitis.

Nonatherosclerotic segmental inflammatory disease of small- and medium-sized arteries, veins, and nerves of arms and legs (Hooten, Burns, & Hays, 1998; Olin, 2000)

B. Segments of Involved Vessels

interspersed between segments of normal vessels

C. Three Phases of the Disease (Joyce, 1996)

1. Acute phase lesions
   a. Essential for histological diagnosis
   b. Artery or vein is swollen
   c. Acutely inflamed superficial vein is excellent biopsy source
   d. Arterial biopsy jeopardizes blood flow
   e. Observations are limited due to contraindications of arterial biopsy
   f. Inflammatory cell infiltration throughout adventitia and media
   g. Lumen is occluded by a highly cellular, unique thrombus with characteristic microabscesses
   h. Lymphocytes exceed neutrophils
   i. Occasional giant cells and eosinophils present
2. Subacute lesions
   a. Recanalization of lumen begins
   b. Cellularity of vessel wall and thrombus lessens
   c. Microabscesses disappear
3. Late lesions
   a. Organized and recanalized thrombus in fibrotic, small vessels. In all three phases, the normal architecture of vessel wall, including the internal elastic membrane, remains intact, and no necrosis is seen. These findings distinguish Buerger disease from atherosclerosis and other vasculitides that have disruption of the internal elastic membrane (Joyce, 1996)

V. Etiology/Precipitating Factors:

Definitive etiology of Buerger disease is unknown, although there is a strong association with exposure to tobacco.

A. Tobacco Use

1. Clear correlation between active tobacco use and disease onset and progression
2. Smoking cessation brings remission
3. Recurrence linked to resumption of tobacco use
4. Persistent tobacco use related to increased frequency of amputation
5. Most reports document the use of 20 to 40 cigarettes daily (Joyce, 1996)
6. Exacerbation noted in patients smoking only 4 to 8 cigarettes a few days a week (Joyce, 1996)
7. Disease has been reported with other forms of tobacco: cigar, pipe, chewing tobacco and snuff, and marijuana (Joyce, 1996; Olin, 2000; Olin & Shih, 2006)
8. Effect of passive smoke unknown

B. Autoimmune Pathogenesis

1. Increased cellular sensitivity to types I and III collagen (Hoppe et al., 2002; Mills, 2003; Szuba & Cooke, 1998; Tanaka, 1998)
2. Cellular and humoral sensitivity to tobacco glycoproteins (Hooten et al., 1998)
3. Elevated antiendothelial cell antibodies (Mills, 2003)
4. Impaired endothelium-dependent vasorelaxation in peripheral vasculature (Olin & Shih, 2006; Piazza & Creager, 2010)
5. Deposition of immunoglobulins and complement factors along the internal elastic lamina (Mills, 2003)
6. Intima infiltration of human leukocyte antigen (HLA)—DR antigen-bearing macrophages and dendritic cells (Mills, 2003)

C. Genetic

1. Increased HLA-AP9 and HLA-B5 haplotypes (Tanaka, 1998)
2. MICA gene polymorphism (Tanaka, 1998)

D. Possible Etiologic link between Buerger disease and periodontal disease and oral bacterial infections. DNA of oral bacteria found in 13 of 14 patient samples of occluded arteries of patients with Buerger disease; all 14 had moderate to severe periodontitis; and none of the control patient arterial samples were positive (Iwai et al., 2005)

VI. Assessment: Risk Factors and Primary/Prevention

A. Diagnostic Criteria (Mills, 2003)

Major criteria

1. Onset of distal extremity ischemic symptoms before 45 years of age
2. Tobacco abuse
3. Exclusion of proximal embolic source, trauma and local lesions, autoimmune disease, hypercoagulable state, atherosclerosis, diabetes, hyperlipidemia, hypertension, and renal failure
4. Undiseased arteries proximal to the popliteal or distal brachial level
5. Objective documentation of distal occlusive disease by means of histopathology, segmental arterial Doppler studies, four-limb plethysmography, and four-limb invasive contrast arteriography. Advances in computed tomography angiography (CTA) and magnetic resonance angiography (MRA) show promise for imaging distal arteries but may not be sufficient for detection of small-artery pathology (Piazza & Creager, 2010)

Minor criteria

1. Migratory superficial phlebitis
2. Raynaud disease present in >40% of patients with Buerger disease and may be asymmetrical (Piazza & Creager, 2010)
3. Upper limb involvement
4. Instep claudication

B. Patient History

1. Subjective findings
   a. Arch or forefoot claudication
   b. Development of ulcers or gangrene of tips of digits
   c. Rest pain of distal extremities, toes, foot, fingers, hand
   d. Skin color changes, distal cyanosis
   e. Intermittent claudication of hand or forearm
   f. Paresthesia: numbness, tingling, aching in extremity
   g. Coldness of extremity
2. Objective findings
   a. Skin: coldness to touch, dependent rubor, elevation pallor, ulcerations or gangrene
   b. Diminished or absent distal pulses
   c. Abnormal Allen test
   d. Delayed venous filling time
   e. Superficial phlebitis (phlebitis migrans)
   f. Raynaud disease
   g. Tobacco use
   h. Neurologic examination to assess for peripheral nerve involvement

C. Physical Examination

1. Inspection of skin
   a. Color of extremities, fingers, toes
   b. Dependent rubor, elevation pallor
   c. Capillary refill time (normal ≤ 3 seconds)
   d. Size and symmetry of extremities: muscle atrophy, edema
   e. Trophic changes: hair loss, shiny taut skin, thickened nails, tapering of toes or fingers, skin breakdown, ulceration, or gangrene
   f. Thrombophlebitis: swollen, erythematous, painful veins
2. Palpation
   a. Complete pulse examination, upper and lower extremities
   b. Allen test to determine arterial patency of the palmar arch
   c. Skin temperature
   d. Palpate for cord along phlebitic veins and increased skin temperature
3. Auscultation
   a. Bruits over carotid, abdominal vessels and femoral sites for stenosis
   b. Continuous wave Doppler assessment of nonpalpable pulses (posterior tibial, dorsalis pedis, radial, ulnar)
   c. Ankle–brachial indices (ABI)
   d. Wrist pressures

D. Considerations Across the Life Span

1. Generally presents in young adults before the age of 40 to 45 years (Olin, 2000)
2. Life expectancy approximates that of the general population at 5 (97%) and 10 (94%) years (Mills, 2003). However, Cooper et al. (2004) found lower long-term (>10 years after diagnosis) survival rates among TAO cohort compared to matched US population. Fifteen of 111 (13.5%) patients died in median of 14.8 years after diagnosis, at average age of 52.2 years

VII. Pertinent Diagnostic Testing

A. Laboratory Tests (Mills, 2003; Olin & Lie, 1992; Szuba & Cooke, 1998)

There are no serologic tests for diagnosing Buerger disease, and most results are within normal ranges; however, erythrocyte sedimentation rate (ESR), fibrinogen, and platelet count may be elevated in the presence of active ulcer or necrosis. Hematocrit, RBC rigidity, and blood viscosity may be elevated in Buerger disease compared to atherosclerosis. Presence of anticardiolipin antibodies and prothrombin gene mutation 20210 is associated with increased risk of disease. Lupus anticoagulant and anticardiolipin antibodies may be present but could also indicate an isolated thrombophilia (Piazza & Creager, 2010).

1. Exclude hypercoagulable states
   a. Protein C and S levels
   b. Prothrombin time (PT) and partial thromboplastin time (PTT)
   c. Complete blood count (CBC)
   d. Antithrombin III
   e. Antiphospholipid antibody
   f. Activated protein C
   g. Homocysteine
   h. Factor V Leiden
   i. Prothrombin G20210A
   j. Lupus anticoagulant
   k. Anticardiolipin antibody
2. Exclude autoimmune disorders and vasculitis, such as CREST syndrome, scleroderma, rheumatoid arthritis, systemic lupus erythematous, and antiphospholipid antibody syndrome (Olin, 2000)
   a. Antinuclear antibody level
   b. ESR
   c. Rheumatoid factor
   d. C-reactive protein
   e. VDRL antigen
   f. Hepatitis serology
   g. Serum complement levels
   h. Cryoglobulins
   i. Anticentromere antibody
   j. Anti-DNA
   k. Anti-SCL-70

B. Noninvasive Tests

1. Vascular laboratory studies
   a. Segmental arterial pressures
   b. Pulse volume recordings
   c. ABI
   d. Transcutaneous oximetry ($TcPO_2$)
   e. Digital temperatures and pressures
   f. Finger photoplethysmography
   g. Laser Doppler
2. Transthoracic echocardiography to rule out cardiac source of emboli
3. Ultrasound to rule out aortic, iliac, femoral, popliteal aneurysm source of emboli

4. CTA or MRA to exclude proximal source of emboli and to define anatomy and extent of disease

C. Invasive Tests

1. Arteriography (Joyce, 1996; Mills, 2003)
   a. Diagnostic versus supportive
   b. Essential findings are multiple, bilateral focal segments of stenosis or occlusion with normal intervening and proximal vessels. Stenosis may be a few millimeters or several centimeters long
   c. Identifies involvement of radial, ulnar, palmar, popliteal, tibial, and pedal arteries
   d. Pattern of occlusive disease parallels the distribution and clinical severity of the disease
   e. Occlusions abrupt or tapering
   f. Generous collaterals, "tree-root," spiderlike, or corkscrew
   g. Arterial calcification and atheroma absent
   h. Arteriographic abnormalities may be seen in limbs not yet clinically involved
   i. Identifies other arterial abnormalities: aneurysms, atherosclerosis, vasculitides
   j. Identifies those patients amenable to bypass surgery
2. Transesophageal echocardiography to rule out proximal source of emboli

VIII. Medical Management (Joyce, 1996; Małecki et al., 2009; Mills, 2003; Olin, 2000; Olin & Lie, 1992; Olin & Shih, 2006; Piazza & Creager, 2010; Puéchal & Fiessinger, 2007)

A. Abstinence from all forms of tobacco is the cornerstone of therapy

1. "Except for discontinuation of tobacco use, there is no other definitive therapy" (Puéchal & Fiessinger, 2007). Critical for therapeutic success. Favorably affects the prognosis of disease at any stage
2. Follow urinary nicotine and cotinine levels for questionable active smoking
3. Consider inpatient nicotine dependence treatment
4. Avoid nicotine replacement therapy as it may contribute to disease activity
5. Use bupropion and varenicline for pharmacotherapy
6. Secondhand smoke exposure may perpetuate disease process

B. Improve Arterial Flow to the Limb

1. Avoid vasoconstriction
2. Encourage vasodilation
3. Use of vasodilating agents: calcium channel blocker, α-blockers, and sildenafil; efficacy not proven (Piazza & Creager, 2010)
4. Antiplatelet drugs, heparinization, thrombolysis of anecdotal success
5. Epidural spinal cord stimulation to improve regional perfusion (Małecki et al., 2009; Olin & Shih, 2006)
6. Intermittent pneumatic compression (IPC)
7. Prostacyclin derivatives: alprostadil alfadex (Prostaglandin E_1) or iloprost (prostacyclin analog). Iloprost more effective than placebo and aspirin for wound healing, relief of rest pain, and reduction in need for amputation.

Intravenous iloprost more effective than oral iloprost. Within 28 days of treatment 35% of iloprost group had healed ulcerations versus 13% in the aspirin group. Rest pain was relieved in 63% of iloprost patients versus 28% in aspirin group. Response rate at 6 months was 88% for iloprost group versus 21% for aspirin group. Iloprost more effective than lumbar sympathectomy (Małecki et al. 2009; Piazza & Creager, 2010; Puéchal & Fiessinger, 2007). More studies are needed to support efficacy.

8. Gene therapy: intramuscular injection of vascular endothelial growth factor (VEGF) increases limb perfusion and collateral vessel development, improves clinical symptoms, and promotes ulcer healing (Olin & Shih, 2006; Szuba & Cooke, 1998)
9. Intramuscular transplantation of autologous bone marrow mononuclear cells (BM-MNC), including progenitor cells, into ischemic limbs, promotes ulcer healing, increases collateral vessel development and decreases pain (Miyamoto et al., 2006; Motukuru, Suresh, Vivekanand, Raj, & Girija, 2008; Puéchal & Fiessinger, 2007; Saito et al., 2007). Long-term safety and efficacy is promising. Idei et al. (2011) showed 4-year amputation free survival post BM-MNC transplantation to be 95% in Buerger disease patients with critical limb ischemia (CLI) and 48% in peripheral artery disease (PAD) patients with CLI compared to 6% and 0% in control patients with Buerger disease and PAD, respectively. Four-year overall survival post BM-MNC transplantation was 100% in Buerger patients and 76% in PAD patients, compared to 100% and 67% in control Buerger and PAD patients, respectively. Matoba et al. (2008) showed the safety and efficacy of intramuscular transplantation of BM-MNC was not inferior to conventional revascularization therapies. Primary outcomes of death and amputation-free survival were better in Buerger patients with 3-year overall survival of 100% in the Buerger cohort and 80% in the PAD cohort, and amputation-free survival was 91% and 60%, respectively. Significant secondary outcomes included improvements in leg pain, ulcer healing, and pain-free walking distance. Change in ABIs and $TcPO_2$ values were not significant. In contrast, Miyamoto et al. (2006) found long-term adverse events in four of eight Buerger patients. Sudden death occurred in a 30 year old at 20 months post transplantation and three developed worsening or recurrence of ischemic symptoms.
10. Autologous whole bone marrow stem cell transplantation by fenestration of tibial bone in affected leg effective in inducing therapeutic angiogenesis, improving ischemic symptoms, and promoting ulcer healing and collateral vessel development (Kim, Kim et al., 2006; Puéchal & Fiessinger, 2007)
11. Stem cell therapy using umbilical cord blood-derived multipotent cells helpful in relieving pain, healing necrotic lesions, and promoting angiogenesis (Kim, Han et al., 2006; Puéchal & Fiessinger, 2007)
12. Feasibility, safety, and efficacy of gene therapy and cell therapy have been established; hence, these are promising new strategies for treatment of CLI. Large-scale, randomized control trials are needed to confirm the effects of gene therapy and cell therapy alone and in combination with one another on clinical symptoms and cardiovascular outcomes (Idei et al., 2011).

C. Treat Concomitant Infection and Cellulitis

1. Antibiotics
2. Drainage and debridement
3. Circulator boot therapy

D. Treat Thrombophlebitis

1. Nonsteroidal anti-inflammatory agents

E. Wound Healing

1. Debridement
2. Appropriate wound agents and dressings
3. IPC

F. Control Pain

1. Narcotic analgesic
2. Prolonged epidural analgesic

IX. Surgical Management (Joyce, 1996; Mills, 2003; Olin & Lie, 1992; Shigehiko, 1995)

A. Amputation of Digit(s) or Limb(s)

1. Unremitting rest pain and/or pain associated with ischemic ulcerations
2. Infection
3. Unsalvageable digit(s) or limb(s) with ulcerations or demarcated gangrene
4. Potential consequence: 85% of Buerger patients who underwent major amputation lost their jobs (Piazza & Creager, 2010)

B. Sympathectomy

1. Removes vasoconstrictor tone in the distal part of the limb
2. Relieves vasomotor symptoms of coolness and mild pain
3. Ischemic ulcers failing to heal
4. Efficacy not proven
5. Ischemia rarely worsens after sympathectomy
6. Performed on about 20% of patients
7. Chemical or surgical
8. Lumbar or thoracic, open versus laparoscopy or thoracoscopy

C. Surgical Revascularization

1. Generally precluded by extensive distal disease
2. Less than 10% of patients have suitable distal target arteries
3. Graft patency rates inferior to bypasses in diabetics and nondiabetics with atherosclerosis
4. Graft patency rates nearly 50% lower in Buerger patients who continue to smoke (Piazza & Creager, 2010)
5. Poor vein quality for conduit because of previous phlebitis

D. Omental Transfer (Olin, 2000)

1. Use for rest pain, nonhealing ischemic ulcers
2. Increases skin temperatures
3. Decreases rest pain
4. Promotes ulcer healing

X. Nursing Management

A. Nursing Diagnoses (Ackley & Ladwig, 2004; Carpenito-Moyet, 2004)

1. Ineffective tissue perfusion related to arterial insufficiency
2. Impaired tissue integrity related to altered circulation
3. Risk for impaired skin integrity related to altered circulation
4. Risk for peripheral neurovascular dysfunction related to vascular obstruction
5. Ineffective health maintenance related to tobacco use
6. Disturbed body image related to disease manifestations and/or amputation
7. Impaired physical mobility related to tissue loss, pain, amputation
8. Pain related to arterial insufficiency, tissue loss, amputation

B. Expected Patient Outcomes

1. Demonstrate adequate tissue perfusion. Verbalize knowledge of treatment regimen. Identify lifestyle changes needed to increase tissue perfusion.
2. Report sensory and pain changes at site of tissue impairment. Verbalize understanding of plan of care to heal tissue and prevent injury. Identify measures to heal and protect the tissue. Attain wound healing with increase in granulation tissue and decrease in wound size.
3. Verbalize understanding of personal risk factors related to impairment of skin integrity.
4. Maintain circulation, sensation, and movement of extremity. Explain signs of neurovascular compromise.
5. Eliminate use of all tobacco products. Demonstrate understanding of short-term and long-term health effects of tobacco use. Describe benefits of abstinence from tobacco use. Verbalize desire to eliminate tobacco use and commitment to personal health. Identify strategies to assist in tobacco cessation.
6. State or demonstrate acceptance of affected and/or lost body parts. State or demonstrate an ability to adjust to lifestyle change.
7. Increase physical activity. Set mutually defined goals and meet those goals. Verbalize feelings of accomplishment. Demonstrate use of adaptive equipment and other aids.
8. Rate intensity of pain using a pain scale. Determine comfort and function goals. Describe pharmacologic and nonpharmacologic pain relief plan. Function at an acceptable activity level with minimal interference from pain and medication side effects

C. Interventions

1. Assessments: pulses, skin color and temperature; capillary refill; skin texture and presence of hair, ulcers, or gangrene; edema; and pain. Do not elevate legs above heart level. Keep extremities warm.
2. Assessment and monitoring of tissue integrity and wound. Initiate and maintain appropriate wound care and dressing changes. Assess nutritional status.
3. Monitor skin condition and skin-care practices. Identify areas at risk and potential causative factors/agents. Prevent pressure over areas at risk. Assess nutritional status.

4. Perform neurovascular assessment using six Ps: pain, pulselessness, pallor/poikilothermia, paresthesia, paralysis, and pressure. Monitor for evidence of compartment syndrome.
5. Discuss risks of smoking; relevance to disease process, and rewards and benefits of cessation. Promote understanding of tobacco use behaviors. Explore strategies for cessation and minimizing weight gain. Discuss withdrawal symptoms and management of symptoms.
6. Acknowledge denial, anger, or depression as normal feelings when adapting to body and lifestyle changes. Encourage patient to make own decisions and to participate in plan of care.
7. Assess mobility skills and limitations. Assess for and treat pain prior to activities. Obtain assistive devices as needed for activity. Increase independence with activities of daily living (ADL) and discourage helplessness.
8. Assess pain level using pain-rating scale. Explore need for pain medication and class of analgesia needed for pain relief. Reassess pain after administration of analgesic and treat unrelieved pain. Explore nonpharmacologic measures for pain control. Explain to the patient the pain management plan that has been ordered.

D. Evaluation

1. Patient implements and adheres to treatment regimen
2. Wound shows signs of healing
3. Patient describes measures to prevent trauma to limb and further tissue loss
4. Patient is able to describe altered sensation and motor function in the limb
5. Patient successfully refrains from all tobacco products
6. Patient verbalizes feelings regarding loss of body part and the associated impact on lifestyle
7. Patient has increased physical activity and exhibits independence with ADL
8. Patient is able to control pain with acceptable types and amounts of medications and to maintain acceptable activity level with minimal interference from pain and medication side effects

XI. Patient Teaching

A. Disease Prevention/Health Promotion/Secondary Prevention

1. Educate, counsel patient repeatedly regarding the importance of discontinuing use of all tobacco products and exposure to tobacco smoke
   a. No cigarettes, cigars, or pipe tobacco
   b. No smokeless tobacco
   c. No nicotine replacement products
   d. Avoid passive smoke
2. Tobacco cessation strongly associated with disease progression and amputation rate
3. Patients without gangrene at the time of tobacco cessation usually do not require amputation—94% avoided amputations, whereas 43% of persistent smokers went on to one or more amputations (Olin, 2000)
4. Intermittent claudication, rest pain, ischemic ulceration, thrombophlebitis are most common among patients who continue to smoke (Hooten et al., 1998)

5. Inpatient treatment for tobacco abuse if necessary
6. Avoid illicit drug use and ergotamine
   a. Marijuana may have similar effects as tobacco
   b. Cocaine may induce vasospasm and acute arterial thrombosis (Marder & Mellinghoff, 2000)
   c. Ergotamine tartrate may induce vasospasm (Oppat & Graham, 2004)

B. Home Care Considerations

1. Avoid all tobacco products and passive smoke.
2. Maintain a healthy diet and appropriate caloric intake.
3. Lower-extremity protection.
   a. Avoid thermal, mechanical, and chemical trauma.
   b. Wear proper-fitting shoes made of soft, flexible leather.
   c. Avoid walking barefoot.
   d. Wash feet and clean between toes with mild soap and warm water, dry thoroughly, and inspect daily.
   e. Use clean cotton or wool socks, unmended and without seams.
   f. Avoid constricting socks, stockings, and clothing.
   g. Keep feet dry and warm. Hypoallergenic, nonmedicated talcum powder may be used lightly twice daily, avoiding nonintact skin. Rooke boot may be used for warmth.
   h. Sparingly apply a lubricating cream to intact skin but not between toes. Avoid perfumed creams.
   i. Use lamb's wool or gauze pads between toes to prevent pressure.
   j. Exercise meticulous nail care with podiatry assistance.
   k. Avoid heating pads, heat lamps, hot water bottles, and cold packs.
   l. Do not use cream hair removers, adhesive corn patches, or any harsh chemicals.
   m. Avoid use of tape and adhesive bandages on skin.
4. Upper-extremity protection
   a. Avoid vasospastic stimuli. Keep hands warm: wear gloves, mittens, cotton batting, or use warm water baths.
   b. Cleanse with mild soap and warm water.
   c. Sparingly apply lubricating cream to intact skin.
   d. Exercise meticulous nail care.
   e. Avoid heating pads, heat lamps, hot water bottles, and cold packs.
   f. Avoid irritants, such as cleaning solutions and other chemicals.
   g. Avoid use of tape and adhesive bandages on skin.
   h. Avoid constricting clothing and jewelry.
5. Wound care
   a. Apply wound care agents and dressings as instructed.
   b. Inspect wounds daily.
   c. Notify health care provider of development of new ulcerations or gangrene.
   d. Notify health care provider of worsening of wound; unusual color, amount, or odor of drainage; increase in inflammation, redness, tenderness, or pain.
   e. Do not soak the affected areas.
6. Activity
   a. Discuss activity restrictions with health care provider.
   b. Remain as active as possible and exercise regularly.

7. Postamputation rehabilitation
   a. Attend physical therapy and perform exercises at home as directed.
   b. Employ residual limb care as directed to control shrinkage, prevent edema, prevent trauma, and reduce wound pain.
   c. Use ace wraps, shrinkers, rigid removable dressing, as instructed.
   d. Identify functional outcomes and goals that correspond to maximal level of independence, lifestyle, and quality of life.
   e. Treat depression.
   f. Prosthesis fitting and gait-training when appropriate
   g. Determine ability to drive a vehicle, modifications needed to do so, and any required driving license validation.
   h. Application for handicap parking permit, as necessary, dependent on level and location of amputation.
   i. Phantom limb pain management.

CASE STUDY

Chief complaint: Six-month history of nonhealing left great toe ulceration. Bilateral upper-extremity coolness, discoloration, burning, and tingling paresthesia to all fingers upon cold exposure.

History of present illness: CB was a single White male high school senior referred to our vascular center at age 18 with 6-month history of nonhealing left great toe ulceration following an accidental glass injury to the toe. An episode of infection had been treated with antibiotics, and he had been using Epsom salt soaks to the ulcerative toe. He reported activity restrictions in gym class because of the ulceration and development of bilateral foot pain with exercise, which was relieved after a 5-minute rest. He reported awakening with nocturnal pain in the ulcerative toe, which was relieved by dangling the leg over the side of the bed.

He also had complaints of progressive bilateral upper-extremity coolness, purplish discoloration, burning and tingling paresthesia of all fingers upon cold exposure. Symptoms typically resolved with rewarming after 15 minutes. No prior or current tissue loss was evident on either side. Symptoms were not present during the warmer summer months. Two years previous to presentation, his symptoms had been limited to the right index finger.

Medical and surgical history: none other than the above

Social history: Significant for cigarette smoking of up to seven cigarettes per day for previous 2 years. Quit 5 weeks prior to presentation. His initiation of smoking predated the onset of right index finger symptoms. No alcohol consumption.

Family history: Noncontributory

Medications: Nifedipine, pentoxifylline, meperidine, enoxaparin, aspirin, and vitamin E. Recently completed a course of amoxicillin clavulanate. Previously on prazosin, but discontinued due to dizziness.

Allergies: NKDA

Examination

Heart: Regular, rate with normal S1 and S2 without S3, S4, or murmur.

Vessels: Diminished right radial pulse; normal left radial pulse; absent ulnar pulses bilaterally; normal brachial pulses bilaterally; normal carotid pulses bilaterally without bruits; normal femoral pulses; diminished right popliteal pulse; absent left popliteal; absent dorsalis pedis; and posterior tibial pulses bilaterally. Right foot had reduced biphasic Doppler signals. Left foot had monophasic Doppler signals. No abdominal bruits audible.

Lower extremities: Large, distal left great toe ulceration with eschar and fibrinous debris with associated tenderness to touch. Small superficial ulceration with erythematous base on the bottom of the left fifth toe, which had been debrided by his local physician a few days prior to presentation. Rubor of the toes bilaterally and elevation pallor of the left foot within 30 seconds.

Upper extremities: Digits of both hands were notably cooler than the corresponding wrist and arm. Bilateral Allen test was indeterminate.

Laboratory Studies

Outside Studies 1 Month Prior to Referral

Sedimentation rate normal; antinuclear antibody negative; Factor V Leiden negative; anticardiolipin antibodies negative; protein S and C levels normal; lupus anticoagulant negative; antithrombin III activity normal; homocysteine level normal; total, HDL, and LDL cholesterol levels normal.

Bilateral upper- and lower-extremity arteriography was notable for major arterial occlusions at the wrist and ankle levels; multiple arterial occlusions and stenoses involving the palmar region and the digital arteries of the hands; arterial occlusion within the radial and ulnar arteries and tibial arteries; 8 cm left proximal popliteal segmental occlusion; and right deep femoral artery occlusion. Angiographic findings were consistent with a diagnosis of Buerger disease. Proximal arterial segments of the aorta, renal arteries, superior mesenteric artery, and brachiocephalic arteries were noted to be normal. There was a slight narrowing at the origin of the celiac of indeterminate etiology.

Echocardiogram was noted to be negative for intracardiac thrombus.

Additional Studies upon Presentation

Lipoprotein (a) normal, cryoglobulin (S) negative; cryofibrinogen (P) negative; total complement normal; rheumatoid factor normal; antinuclear antibody negative; extractable nuclear antigen antibody screen normal; IgM phospholipid antibody negative; IgG phospholipid antibody negative; and sensitive thyrotropin normal. Serum protein electrophoresis was notable for polyclonal gammopathy.

Lower-extremity vascular laboratory studies revealed bilateral arterial occlusive disease of moderate severity in the infrapopliteal segments and severe multilevel disease on the left side. Posterior tibial and anterior tibial Doppler signals were biphasic on the right and monophasic on the left. The highest resting ABIs were 0.66 on the right and 0.48 on the left. $TcPO_2$ values were mildly reduced at the distal right forefoot site with absolute values of 74 (RPI 0.85) and 68 mm Hg (RPI 0.78) in supine position, worsening to 67 (RPI 0.77) and 60 mm Hg (RPI 0.69) with elevation. Oximetries were severely reduced at both left forefoot sites with absolute values of 19 and 5 mm Hg (RPI 0.22 and 0.06, respectively) in supine position, worsening to 0 and 0 with elevation.

Upper-extremity vascular laboratory studies revealed arterial occlusive disease involving the right radial and ulnar arteries and the left radial and possibly the ulnar arteries. The digital pressures were markedly reduced compared to brachial pressures. Triphasic Doppler signals were present at all arterial sites in the arms, hands, and digits. The digital temperatures were noted to be 4°C to 8°C cooler than the corresponding wrist temperatures. No vasospastic processes were evident.

A vascular medicine specialist completed his medical evaluation. Vascular surgery consultation was obtained. Surgical revascularization deferred at that time due to suboptimal revascularization potential and the potential for improved wound healing following smoking cessation. Aggressive local wound care, with discontinuation of foot soaks, and a 5-day course of circulator boot therapy with cefazolin ensued, followed by home therapy with IPC 6 to 8 hours per day and local wound care with a Curasol/Iodosorb mixture to the ulceration. He was instructed in the importance of proper foot care and footwear.

He returned for wound care follow-up and local wound debridement over the next few months, with noted improvement in ulcer healing and 100% epithelization of the base. Three months later, his local physician reported worsening of the ulceration following discontinuation of IPC by the patient and resumption of smoking. He returned to the wound care clinic 1 month later, having quit smoking 4 weeks prior to his return. His ulceration was definitely worse, with a dense eschar, evidence of exposed bone, and increased cyanosis of and pain in the left great toe. Bone destruction and osteomyelitis were not evident on radiograph. Repeat vascular laboratory studies revealed worsening of left foot ischemia with a decrease in ABI and $TcPO_2$ values when compared to studies 6 months previously. Orthopedic consultation ensued for consideration of amputation. Considering the probability of a nonhealing great toe amputation site and infection, IPC was reinstituted in addition to local wound therapy with the Curasol/Iodosorb mixture.

He returned 1 month later with complaints of unrelenting rest pain in the toe unresponsive to increasing dosages of narcotic medications. Despite continued use of the arterial flow pump, local wound care, and continued smoking cessation his ulceration had worsened; and in fact, he had developed an additional ulcer on the dorsum of the toe. Repeat arteriography was recommended to ascertain the feasibility of percutaneous intervention versus surgical revascularization. Patient returned home and thereafter was lost to follow-up at our institution until 34 months later.

Shortly after his return home from our institution 34 months prior to his return, he underwent surgical revascularization with a left femoropopliteal bypass and left great toe amputation, accompanied by good initial success and near complete healing of his wounds during a period of tobacco cessation. Within 6 months of those procedures, he had resumed smoking; and the graft thrombosed culminating in a below-the-knee amputation.

During the intervening years his numerous attempts with permanent smoking cessation had been unsuccessful, despite psychiatric therapy and progression of Buerger disease with limb loss and threatened limb loss. Within the year preceding his return, he had developed persistent atraumatic ulcerations of the right first and left fifth digits of the hands. There was physical evidence of past tissue loss in multiple upper-extremity digits.

A couple of weeks preceding his return, he developed acute ischemia, rest pain, and threatening tissue loss of the right foot requiring hospitalization. At that time, he had been off cigarettes for about 4 weeks. Per report he had absent posterior tibial and dorsalis pedis Doppler signals; and angiography demonstrated right deep femoral, popliteal, and tibial artery occlusions. Repeat studies at our clinic confirmed absence of Doppler signals in the right foot and severe ischemia from the infrapopliteal level downward, as evidenced by critically reduced $TcPO_2$ values. The left below-knee amputation stump was also noted to have a severely reduced $TcPO_2$ value in the supine position, with improvement when dependent.

Medical management options discussed included a trial of circulator boot therapy, IPC, or referral to other centers for hyperbaric oxygen treatment, or participation in a clinical trial utilizing vascular growth factor. His pharmacologic regimen had been maximized previously with the use of a calcium channel blocker, platelet inhibitor, hemorheologic agent (blood viscosity modifier, i.e., pentoxifylline), and an anticoagulant.

During the course of his evaluation, he exhibited inappropriate behavior manifested by loud, profane, and abusive language, aggressive actions, and threatening statements directed toward the physicians and other personnel. At that point, intervention by security and the administrative staff was mandated, resulting in cancellation of a vascular surgery consultation. By way of phone the following day, his mother reported additional escalation of his verbally abusive behavior. He was, therefore, referred to the emergency room for an emergency neurology and psychiatric evaluation. He was found to be neurologically intact. Psychiatric evaluation was consistent with an ongoing major depressive disorder related to medical issues with recent insomnia, anhedonia, feelings of excessive guilt, and passive suicidal thoughts. Previous use of Zoloft and Wellbutrin were noted, and a decision was made to resume Wellbutrin. Hospitalization was deemed unnecessary at that time, and he was advised to seek additional psychiatric care in his local area.

Upon his return to the wound care clinic 2 weeks later, he was noted to have progression of his ulcerations and development of "kissing" ulcers between all toes without evidence of any granulation tissue. Dependent rubor, cyanosis, pitting edema, and extensive tenderness in the foot were evident. He complained of ongoing, unrelenting rest pain despite use of a fentanyl patch and hydrocodone for breakthrough pain.

In light of a severely reduced $TcPO_2$ value below the knee, he would likely need an above-knee amputation. In lieu of amputation, he was admitted to the hospital for reversal of his Coumadin anticoagulation and to be covered transiently with intravenous heparin in preparation for repeat arteriography and thrombolytic therapy in an attempt to lyse any recent thrombus contributing to the acute event 3 weeks previously. Lytic therapy with alteplase into the thrombosed popliteal and peroneal arteries and attempted angioplasty of the popliteal artery were ultimately unsuccessful. The distal popliteal and all tibial arteries and all plantar branches were noted to be occluded, precluding any revascularization options. He was dismissed home with home health care assistance for continuation of IPC to the upper and right lower extremities, local wound care, and antibiotic therapy. Arrangements were made for him to proceed with a right lower-extremity amputation by his local vascular surgeon 3 days later.

Review Questions

1. Buerger disease most commonly affects
   a. Medium- to large-sized arteries in the thorax, abdomen, and pelvis
   b. Carotid and cerebral arteries
   c. Small- to medium-sized arteries and veins in the upper and lower extremities

2. While a definitive etiology of Buerger disease is unknown, possible causes or precipitating factors include
   a. Autoimmune process
   b. Tobacco use
   c. Genetic disorder
   d. All of the above

3. Buerger disease most commonly presents in
   a. Men before age 40 to 45
   b. Men after age 50
   c. Women before age 40 to 45
   d. Women after age 50

4. The best diagnostic test(s) to support the clinical diagnosis of Buerger disease is
   a. Biopsy of an acutely inflamed artery or vein
   b. Four-limb arteriography
   c. CTA or MRA
   d. ABIs, segmental pressures, transcutaneous oximetry, digital pressures, and temperatures
   e. Doppler ultrasound
   f. a and b
   g. a, b, and c
   h. All of the above

5. Primary treatment of Buerger disease is
   a. Arterial bypass
   b. Cessation of all tobacco products
   c. Sympathectomy
   d. Omental transfer
   e. Amputation

6. Manifestations of Buerger disease include
   a. Superficial thrombophlebitis
   b. Rest pain of distal extremity
   c. Atypical claudication of pedal arch, forefoot, hand, or forearm
   d. Ulcers or gangrene of tips of digits
   e. All of the above

7. Promising gene and cell therapy promoting angiogenesis and ulcer healing for patients with Buerger disease include
   a. Intramuscular injection of vascular endothelial growth factor (VEGF)
   b. Fenestration of the tibia for autologous whole bone marrow stem cell transplantation
   c. Stem-cell therapy using umbilical cord blood-derived multipotent cells
   d. Intramuscular transplantation of autologous bone marrow mononuclear cells
   e. All of the above
   f. None of the above

Answers/Rationale

1. c. The small- to medium-sized vessels of the arms, hands, legs, and feet are the most frequently affected, although there have been reports of the disease affecting other arteries.

2. d. In addition to a strong association with tobacco use, there may be autoimmune and genetic processes contributing to disease onset.

3. a. The disease generally presents before age 40 to 45 years. Historically, men have been afflicted more frequently, but this situation appears to be changing as tobacco use among women increases.

4. f. While all of these tests may be obtained during the investigation, a biopsy of an affected artery or vein in the acute phase and/or arteriography is diagnostic/supportive of the disease. A biopsy may be contraindicated as blood flow to an already-ischemic limb may be further jeopardized. Arteriography is usually attainable, revealing distinctive arterial abnormalities to support the diagnosis or to rule out other causes of ischemia. CTA and MRA may be used to rule out other causes of ischemia but may not be sufficient for imaging of distal arteries and detection of the small artery pathology seen in Buerger disease. This will likely change with improvements in CTA and MRA technology.

5. b. Discontinued use of all tobacco products is essential for disease remission and limb salvage. Avoidance of passive smoke is advised, although exposure to passive smoke has not been proven to affect disease onset or progression. Amputation of digits or limb may be necessary for control of unremitting rest pain, infection, or ulceration/gangrene. Arterial bypass, sympathectomy, and omental transfer are applicable to a minority of Buerger patients.

6. e. All of the above

7. e. All of the above. Feasibility, safety, and efficacy of gene and cell therapy have been established, but further study with large-scale, randomized control trials are needed to confirm effects of gene and cell therapy alone and in combination with one another.

REFERENCES

Ackley, B. J., & Ladwig, G. B. (Eds.). (2004). *Nursing diagnosis handbook: A guide to planning care* (6th ed.). St. Louis, MO: Mosby.

Adar, R. (2010). Epidemiology of TAO—Correction of an error. *Atherosclerosis, 211*, 24. doi:10.1016/j.atherosclerosis.2010.01.027

Carpenito-Moyet, L. J. (2004). *Nursing diagnosis; application to clinical practice* (10th ed., pp. 377–379). Philadelphia, PA: Lippincott Williams & Wilkins.

Cooper, L. T., Tse, T. S., Mikhail, M. A., McBane, R. D., Stanson, A. W., & Ballman, K. V. (2004). Long-term survival and amputation risk in thromboangiitis obliterans (Buerger's disease). *Journal of the American College of Cardiology, 44*, 2410–2411. doi:10.1016/j.jacc.2004.09.029

Hooten, W. M., Burns, H. K., & Hays, J. T. (1998). Inpatient treatment of severe nicotine dependence in a patient with thromboangiitis obliterans (Buerger's disease). *Mayo Clinic Proceedings, 73*, 529–532. doi:10.4065/73.6.529

Hoppe, B., Lu, J. T., Thistlewaite, P., Yi, E. S., & Mahmud, E. (2002). Beyond peripheral arteries in Buerger's disease: Angiographic considerations in thromboangiitis obliterans. *Catheterization and Cardiovascular Interventions, 57*, 363–366. doi:10.1002/ccd.10330

Idei, N., Soga, J., Hata, T., Fujii, Y., Fujimura, N., Mikami, S., ... Higashi, Y. (2011). Autologous bone-marrow mononuclear cell transplantation reduces long-term major amputation risk in patients with critical limb ischemia: A comparison of atherosclerotic peripheral arterial disease and Buerger disease. *Circulation: Cardiovascular Interventions, 4*, 15–25. doi:10.1161/CIRCINTERVENTIONS.110.955724

Iwai, T., Inoue, Y., Umeda, M., Huang, Y., Kurihara, N., Koike, M., & Ishikawa, I. (2005). Oral bacteria in the occluded arteries of patients with Buerger's disease. *Journal of Vascular Surgery, 42*, 107–115. doi:10.1016/j.jvs.2005.03.016

Joyce, J. W. (1996). Thromboangiitis obliterans (Buerger's disease). In J. R. Young, J. W. Olin, & J. R. Bartholomew. (Eds.), *Peripheral vascular diseases* (2nd ed., pp. 371–379). St. Louis, MO: Mosby.

Kim, D. I., Kim, M. J., Joh, J. H., Shin, S. W., Do, Y.S., Moon, J. Y., . . . Shim, J.-S. (2006). Angiogenesis facilitated by autologous whole bone marrow stem cell transplantation for Buerger's disease. *Stem Cells, 24*, 1194–1200. doi:10.1634/stemcells.2005-0349

Kim, S. W., Han, H., Chae, G. T., Lee, S.-H., Bo, S., Yoon, J. H., ... Kang, K.-S. (2006). Successful stem cell therapy using umbilical cord blood-derived mulitpotent stem cells for Buerger's disease and ischemic limb disease animal model. *Stem Cells, 24*, 1620–1626. doi:10.1634/stemcells.2005-0365

Małecki, R., Zdrojowy, K., & Adamiec, R. (2009). Thromboangiitis obliterans in the 21st century: A new face of disease. *Atherosclerosis, 206*, 328–334. doi:10.1016/j.atherosclerosis.2009.01.042

Marder, V. J., & Mellinghoff, I. K. (2000). Cocaine and Buerger's disease: Is there a pathogenetic association? *Archives of Internal Medicine, 160*, 2057–2060.

Matoba, S., Tatsumi, T., Murohara, T., Imaizumi, T., Katsuda, Y., Ito, M., . . . Matsubara, H. (2008). Long-term clinical outcomes after intramuscular implantation of bone marrow mononuclear cells (Therapeutic Angiogenesis by Cell Transplantation [TACT] trial) in patients with chronic limb ischemia. *American Heart Journal, 156*, 1010–1018. doi:10.1016/j.ahj.2008.06.025

Mills, J. L. (2003). Buerger's disease in the 21st century: Diagnosis, clinical features, and therapy. *Seminars in Vascular Surgery, 16*, 179–189.

Miyamoto, K., Nishigami, K., Nagaya, N., Akutsu, K., Chiku, M., Kamei, M., . . . Takeshita, S. (2006). Unblinded pilot study of autologous transplantation of bone marrow mononuclear cells in patients with thromboangiitis obliterans. *Circulation, 114*, 2679–2684. doi:10.1161/CIRCULATIONAHA.106.644203

Motukuru, V., Suresh, K. R., Vivekanand, V., Raj, S., & Girija, K. R. (2008). Therapeutic angiogenesis in Buerger's disease (thromboangiitis obliterans) patients with critical limb ischemia by autologous transplantation of bone marrow mononuclear cells. *Journal of Vascular Surgery, 48*, 53S–60S. doi:10.1016/j.jvs.2008.09.005

Olin, J. W. (2000). Current concepts: Thromboangiitis obliterans (Buerger's disease). *New England Journal of Medicine, 343*, 864–869.

Olin, J. W., & Lie, J. T. (1992). Thromboangiitis obliterans (Buerger's disease). In J. P. Cooke & E. D. Frohlich (Eds.), *Current management of hypertensive and vascular diseases* (pp. 265–271). Philadelphia, PA: Decker.

Olin, J. W., & Shih, A. (2006). Thromboangiitis obliterans (Buerger's disease). *Current Opinion in Rheumatology, 18*, 18–24.

Oppat, W., & Graham, L. M. (2004). The arterial system. In V. A. Fahey (Ed.), *Vascular nursing* (4th ed., p. 14). St. Louis, MO: Saunders.

Piazza, G., & Creager, M. A. (2010). Thromboangiitis obliterans. *Circulation, 121*, 1858–1861. doi:10.1161/CIRCULATIONAHA.110.942383

Puéchal, X., & Fiessinger, J. N. (2007). Thromboangiitis obliterans or Buerger's disease: Challenges for the rheumatologist. *Rheumatology, 46*, 192–199. doi:10.1093/rheumatology/kel388

Saito, Y., Sasaki, K.-I., Katsuda, Y., Murohara, T., Takeshita, Y., Okazaki, T., … Imaizumi, T. (2007). Effect of autologous bone-marrow cell transplantation on ischemic ulcer in patients with Buerger's disease. *Circulation Journal, 71*, 1187–1192. doi:10.1253/circj.71.1187

Shigehiko, S. (1995). Buerger's disease (thromboangiitis obliterans). In R. B. Rutherford (Ed.), *Vascular surgery* (4th ed., Vol. 1, pp. 235–245). Philadelphia, PA: Saunders.

Szuba, A., & Cooke, J. P. (1998). Thromboangiitis obliterans: An update on Buerger's disease. *Western Journal of Medicine, 168*, 255–260. PMCID: PMC1304949.

Tanaka, K. (1998). Pathology and pathogenesis of Buerger's disease. *International Journal of Cardiology, 66*(Suppl. 1), S237–S242.

CHAPTER 17

Raynaud Phenomenon

Patricia A. Lewis

First Edition Authors: *Patricia A. Lewis and Sue Monaro*

OBJECTIVES

1. Distinguish between primary and secondary Raynaud phenomenon.
2. Identify physical examination findings consistent with Raynaud phenomenon.
3. List medical treatment options for Raynaud phenomenon.
4. Discuss key elements in nursing management of patients with Raynaud phenomenon.

Introduction

In 1862, Maurice Raynaud noticed that some people developed transient digital ischemia when exposed to cold. He attributed this response to an overreaction of the central nervous system (Bakst, Merola, Franks, & Sanchez, 2008; Wigley, 2002). Raynaud phenomenon is now defined as a vasospastic disorder resulting in intermittent digital or body part ischemia. The other vasospastic disorders include acrocyanosis (continuous cyanosis of hands or feet aggravated by cold), pernio or chilblains (pruritic burning lesions affecting skin exposed to cold), and livedo reticularis (semipermanent bluish discoloration of hands and legs that worsens with cold exposure). Attacks of Raynaud's are characterized by well-demarcated, sudden pale or cyanotic changes of digits, ears, nose, or, rarely, other body parts such as the nipple (Barclay, 2004) or penis (Kropman, 2004) in response to cold or emotional stress. The affected body part often becomes bright red as rewarming and reactive hyperemia occur, resulting in the classic sequential white, blue, then red color changes. However, not all affected individuals will demonstrate this triphasic color sequence; many will have only pallor or cyanosis (Creager & Dzau, 2005).

Primary Raynaud's occurs without other associated diseases or causes and is also known as Raynaud disease or syndrome. Secondary Raynaud phenomenon has similar symptoms with an associated vasospastic or immunologic disease process (e.g., scleroderma) as the cause of the disorder. The distinction between primary and secondary Raynaud phenomenon is not always clear (Anders, Sigi, & Schattenkirchner, 2001), but generally the vasospasm of primary Raynaud's is less severe, totally reversible, and does not result in permanent ischemic changes, such as ulceration. However, a small quality of life study on the psychosocial effects of primary Raynaud disease showed a reduction is quality of life and increased anxiety compared to age-matched controls (DeAngelis, Slaffi, & Grassi, 2008). Because secondary Raynaud's is associated with underlying connective tissue disease, particularly scleroderma, permanent skin changes with ulceration may occur. Studies suggest that between 10% and 30% of patients who have primary disease will eventually be diagnosed with a systemic connective tissue disorder over a period of as long as 20 years (Hodges, 1995), thus making the transition to secondary Raynaud phenomenon (Kahaleh, 2004; Wigley, 2002). Although approximately 15% of patients who have primary disease will improve spontaneously (Craeger & Dzau, 2005), health care providers should be cautious about assuming that primary Raynaud's remains a relatively benign problem over the course of an individual's lifetime.

Although true incidence of Raynaud's is unknown because a standardized definition and testing are lacking and mild cases are underreported, surveys estimate that between 4% and 30% of the general population have symptoms of the phenomenon (Coffman, 1996; Klippel, Crofford, Stone, & Weyand, 2001). More than 50% of patients with symptoms have primary Raynaud's (Creager & Dzau, 2005). A familial tendency toward the disease has been identified, and females are affected in a ratio of 4:1 over males, with the usual age of onset between the second and fourth decades (Coffman, 1996). One study documented 15% prevalence in children aged 12 to 15 years; prevalence was higher in girls (18%), increased with age, and had no association with psychosocial factors (Jones et al., 2003). Prevalence, as well as frequency and severity of attacks, varies depending on natural environment (increased in a cold, damp climate or in winter) and occupation (especially use of vibrating heavy equipment, such as a jackhammer). "Evidently, any disease, persistent vasoconstrictor stimulus, or constant trauma that causes damage to blood vessels or tissue may lead to one of the vasospastic syndromes, perhaps by the common mechanism of ischemia" (Coffman, 1996).

I. Anatomy (Refer to Chapter 3, Anatomy and Physiology of the Vascular System, for a complete anatomic description.)

A. Upper Extremity Digits are More Often Affected (Wigley, 2002).

1. Radial and ulnar arteries are the major suppliers of hand circulation.
   a. Multiple intercommunications occur at palmar level.
   b. One dorsal and two palmar arches (superficial and deep) provide a variety of inflow pathways to digits (see Fig. 17-1).
   c. Superficial palmar arch is usually the dominant arterial circulation to fingers, supplying common digital arteries that branch into proper digital arteries on either side of fingers.
   d. Distal circulation of the hand is much more variable than proximal, larger vessels of upper extremities.
2. In addition to capillary circulation, human digits contain multiple arteriovenous anastomoses, connecting arterial and venous circulation directly (Coffman, 1996).
   a. These bypass the capillary bed.
   b. Shunts allow a large blood flow to pass through digits in a warm environment and close when exposed to cold, thus allowing the body to regulate core temperature.
   c. They are under control of the sympathetic nervous system by means of alpha receptors.
   d. During body cooling, arteriovenous shunts constrict and close, but capillary and nutritional blood flow is normally maintained unless vasospastic disease is present.
3. Attack usually begins in a single digit.
4. Attack spreads to other digits symmetrically in both hands.

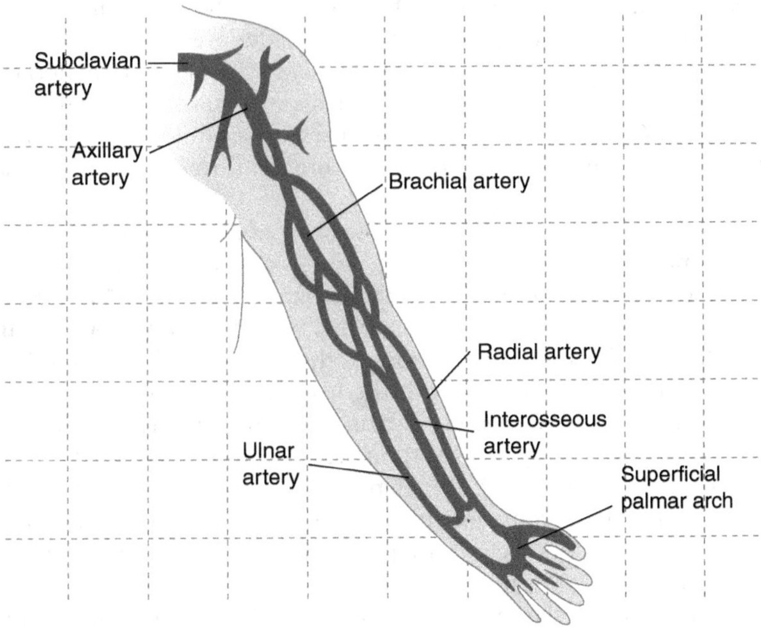

FIGURE 17-1. Anatomy of the major arteries of the upper extremity.

5. Index, middle, and ring fingers are most frequently affected; thumb is usually not involved.

B. Toes are Commonly Involved, but Patients are Less Likely to Complain of Symptoms.

C. Other Affected Sites

1. Ears, nose, face, knees
2. Nipples of breastfeeding mothers (Barclay, 2004)
   a. Involves painful breastfeeding with symptoms brought on by cold exposure.
   b. Nipple blanching is followed by cyanosis and/or erythema.
   c. Symptoms may also be present during pregnancy.
   d. Attack is treatable (refer to Medical Management); does not result in permanent damage.
3. Penis (Kropman, 2004)

II. Pathology and Pathophysiology

A. Primary Raynaud Disease

1. Pathology
   a. Mild (early) diseased limited data; no tissue abnormalities noted (Coffman, 1996).
   b. Severe diseased intimal hyperplasia, narrowing or total occlusion of digital arteries, thrombi, possible cellular or basement membrane changes; conflicting reports of abnormalities in digital arteries seen on arteriograms: some show stenoses/occlusions; others are normal (Coffman, 1996).

2. Pathophysiology
   a. Normal physiology: digital flow depends on pressure gradient across vessel, and resistance is determined by blood viscosity and vessel radius.
      1) Blood flow in vascular bed is regulated by central nervous system via sympathetic system; hypothalamus controls arteriovenous anastomoses to regulate body temperature; emotional response is also related to hypothalamus activity.
      2) Messages from cerebral cortex are passed to vasomotor centers in medulla to stimulate either pressor or depressor activity.
      3) Baroreceptors, chemoreceptors, and somatic afferent nerves also affect activity of vasomotor center. Messages are sent from medulla to sympathetic ganglia and then to sympathetic nerves.
      4) Sympathetic activity regulates vessel smooth muscle tone and vessel wall thickness, changing the radius.
      5) Increased sympathetic stimulation (stress) or cold causes secretion of norepinephrine, which stimulates alpha-adrenoreceptors and leads to vasoconstriction, with closure of arteriovenous shunts as already described.
      6) Serotonin receptors are also present in hand, which have similar activity but are independent of alpha receptors. Stimulation of serotonin receptors causes vasoconstriction.
   b. Abnormal/pathophysiology: primary Raynaud's is associated with an extreme alpha-2 response to cold exposure, but cause is unknown.
      1) Three physiology alterations are identified
         a) Sympathetic nervous system
         b) Adrenoreceptor number and function
         c) Naturally occurring vasoactive peptides
      2) Triggers (cold and stress) induce an abnormally forceful contraction of arterial wall smooth muscle.
      3) Total finger and capillary flow is decreased in patients with primary Raynaud's in both warm and cool environments (Coffman, 1996).
      4) Patients who have primary Raynaud's have lower brachial and finger systolic blood pressure and fingertip perfusion pressure than normal subjects, but not all individuals who have low systolic pressure have vasospastic attacks.
      5) Increased number of peripheral alpha-receptors augments vasoconstriction; at the same time, decrease in beta and calcitonin receptors limits normal vasodilatation capacity (Hodges, 1995).
      6) Hard red blood cells, increased plasma viscosity, and decreased fibrinolysis contribute to increased vascular resistance and sluggish microcirculatory blood flow (Hodges, 1995).
      7) Endothelin, a potent vasoconstrictor, is elevated, whereas endothelium-derived relaxation factor (EDRF), a vasodilator, is decreased (Hodges, 1995).
      8) Central nervous system pathology is suggested by decreased baseline microvascular flow and increased systemic levels of norepinephrine (Hodges, 1995).
      9) The "local fault" theory was proposed by Sir Thomas Lewis, 1930: abnormality exists at digital artery level; local cooling produces ischemic attacks in a single finger, even with a sympathetic block (Wigley, 2002).

10) Raynaud's "sympathetic overactivity" theory posits an exaggerated response of digital blood flow to body position and stress as well as to cold, implicating more of a sympathetic reaction than a local reaction. This theory is supported by positive response of some patients to the use of alpha-adrenergic blockers or sympathectomy. However, sympathectomy does not consistently provide relief, and sympathetic overactivity should alter blood and urine catecholamines, but these changes have not been demonstrated (Coffman, 1996).

11) Theory of generalized functional abnormality of vascular smooth muscle rests on close correlation of primary Raynaud symptoms to other vasospastic disorders, especially migraine headache, as well as to pulmonary, renal, and macular capillary vasospasm (Coffman, 1996).

B. Secondary Raynaud Phenomenon

1. Decreased blood flow and blood pressure in digits are due to atherosclerotic, vinyl chloride, or connective tissue diseases.
   a. Underlying disease disrupts normal mechanisms of vessel reactivity.
   b. Example: scleroderma involves intimal fibrosis and endothelial dysfunction; endothelial cell damage is associated with increased platelet adhesion, decreased storage of von Willebrand factor, and decreased adenosine uptake. Cold- or stress-induced vasospasm similar to Raynaud response is also documented in other circulatory beds (gastrointestinal, coronary, placental, and genitourinary) in these patients.
   c. Reperfusion injury follows ischemia, leading to altered smooth muscle receptor expression and vascular function (Wigley, 2002).
2. Hyperviscosity related to blood abnormalities (e.g., cryoglobulinemia) also leads to reduced flow state.
3. Persistent vasoconstriction is secondary to drug therapy or sympathetic nerve damage related to thoracic outlet syndrome (refer to Chapter 18, Thoracic Outlet Syndrome).
4. Vibration injury: degeneration of sensory vibration receptors produces reflex vasoconstriction by means of alpha-receptor activity; centrally mediated sympathetic hyperactivity is also increased with vibration (Hodges, 1995).
5. End-stage renal disease: Raynaud phenomenon related to endothelial dysfunction, rather than AV shunt steal syndrome, is responsible for symptoms in hemodialysis patients (Czupryniak et al., 2005).

C. Triphasic Color Change (white to blue to red) Episode.

Cold exposure/emotional stress

↓

Vasospasm of palmar and digital arteries/arterioles

↓

Cessation of capillary perfusion

↓

Pallor

↓

Reflexive dilatation of capillaries and venules from regional hypoxia and byproducts of anaerobic metabolism

↓

Slight relaxation of arterial spasm

↓

Blood flow into dilated capillary bed
↓
Desaturation
↓
Cyanosis
↓
Increased amounts of blood entering dilated capillaries
↓
Rubor
↓
Relaxation of arterial spasm
↓
Return of normal blood flow
↓
Capillary perfusion

III. Causation and Precipitating Factors

A. Primary Raynaud Disease

1. Causation is idiopathic and possibly genetic. Genome-wide screen among families with disease has tentatively identified five genetic loci on X chromosome and chromosomes 6, 7, 9, and 17 (Wigley, 2002).
2. Precipitating factors include cold exposure and increased stress.

B. Secondary Raynaud Phenomenon (see Table 17-1)

1. Most common causes are drugs and connective tissue disorders.
2. Other causes include atherosclerosis, trauma, increased blood viscosity, compression of nerves/blood vessels, vasculitis.
3. Strong association with autoimmune disorders: most of these conditions have element of distal upper-extremity small artery obstruction.
4. Drugs
   a. Beta-adrenergic antagonists, both nonselective and cardioselective
      1) Affect males and females; all ages affected equally
      2) No relationship to dose
      3) Incidence: 4% to 40% of patients using these drugs (Coffman, 1996)
      4) Substitution with alpha-adrenergic blockers does not always alleviate symptoms.
      5) Exact mechanism of effect unknown; may be due to unopposed alpha-adrenergic vasoconstriction, reduced blood pressure and cardiac output with reflexive vasoconstriction, or central cardiovascular vasoconstriction effect.
   b. Ergot derivatives
      1) Produce intense vasospasm by stimulation of alpha-adrenoceptors.
      2) Ergot intoxication leads to proliferation of endothelium, thrombosis, hyaline degeneration, and fibrosis of the vascular wall.
      3) Vasospasm occurs with ingestion of more than 10 mg/week.
      4) Females are affected more than males.
      5) Incidence of toxicity is 0.01%.
      6) Large and small vessels are involved: digital, carotid, axillary, renal, coronary, ophthalmic, and splanchnic circulation.

TABLE 17-1 Conditions Associated with Secondary Raynaud Phenomenon

Connective Tissue Disorders/Collagen Vascular Disease	
Scleroderma	Spinal cord tumors
Systemic lupus erythematosus	Syringomyelia
Sjögren syndrome	Stroke
Rheumatoid arthritis	Poliomyelitis
Dermatomyositis	Carpal tunnel syndrome
Polyarteritis nodosa	Reflex sympathetic dystrophy
Mixed connective tissue disease	Trauma
Hematologic disorders/blood dyscrasia	Vibration injury; hypothenar hammer (hammer hand) syndrome
Polycythemia vera; thrombocythemia	Frostbite
Cold agglutinins	Electric shock
Cryoglobulinemia; cryofibrinogenemia	Upper extremity trauma
Myeloproliferative disorders	Drug-induced conditions
Dysproteinemia and hyperviscosity syndromes	Ergot derivatives
Waldenstrom macroglobulinemia	Methysergide
Hemoglobinopathies	Beta-adrenergic receptor blockers (e.g., metoprolol)
Arterial occlusive disease	Chemotherapy—bleomycin, vinblastine, cisplatin
Atherosclerosis of extremities	Caffeine—excess intake
Acute arterial occlusion	Drug-induced vasculitis
Thromboangiitis obliterans	Other conditions associated with vasospasm
Thoracic outlet syndrome; crutch pressure	Carcinoid syndrome
Inflammatory arterial disease (e.g., Takayasu's)	Pheochromocytoma
Arteriovenous fistula	Polyvinyl chloride disease
Pulmonary hypertension	Hypothyroidism
Neurologic disorders	Paraneoplastic conditions
Migraine headache	Hepatitis
Intervertebral disc disease	

Adapted from Hodges, H. (1995). Raynaud's disease: Pathophysiology, diagnosis, and treatment. *Journal of the American Academy of Nurse Practitioners*, *7*(4), 159–164.

7) Symptoms include painful, cold, discolored extremities or intermittent claudication; occasional intense burning pain in extremities (known as St. Anthony's fire). Large vessel pulses may be palpable; gangrene may occur.
8) Arteriographic findings: uniform smooth tapering of large- and medium-sized vessels that disappears at forearm or calf level.
9) Treatment: if patient does not have a limb-threatening condition, bed rest with heparinization for 3 days to allow for resolution of spasm. For severe cases: intra-arterial or intravenous nitroprusside with or without oral nifedipine.

c. Chemotherapeutics: vinblastine and bleomycin
   1) 2.6% to 37% of patients may develop Raynaud's (Coffman, 1996) with this combination.
   2) Symptoms usually appear after 10 months of therapy.
   3) It is unknown which drug is the causative agent.
   4) Vinblastine causes nephrotoxicity; bleomycin causes skin toxicity.
   5) Arteriographic findings: diffuse narrowing of digital arteries or multiple small vessel occlusions
   6) Attacks may continue even after drugs are discontinued.

d. ADHD medications: methylphenidate and dextroamphetamine—case studies have suggested an association with Raynaud symptoms (Syed & Moore, 2008).
e. Other drugs associated with Raynaud's include bromocriptine, clonidine, imipramine, amphetamine, cyclosporine; withdrawal from nitroglycerine products. Inconclusive data regarding oral contraceptives (Coffman, 1996).

5. Connective tissue disease
   a. Scleroderma/systemic sclerosis: Raynaud's is the earliest and most common symptom (Kahaleh, 2004).
      1) Initial complaint of 50% of patients with scleroderma (Coffman, 1996)
      2) 90% of scleroderma patients have Raynaud's (Klippel et al., 2001)
      3) CREST syndrome (limited systemic sclerosis): **C**alcifications in subcutaneous tissue, **R**aynaud's, **E**sophageal motility abnormalities, **S**kin thickening or tightness, **T**elangiectasias
      4) Other associated symptoms: sclerodactyly (loss of digital pads on fingertips), digital ulcerations, ischemic demarcation leading to amputation
      5) Scleroderma is associated with vascular occlusion caused by fibrosis of intima, platelet activation, stimulation of clotting cascade, and fibrin deposition (see section on Pathophysiology). Walls of small arteries are thickened and trapped in fibrous tissue.
      6) "(There is) strong evidence for "systemic" Raynaud phenomenon, a generalized vasospastic disorder involving vasculopathy of the terminal arterial circulation of the lungs, kidneys, and heart" (Klippel et al., 2001).
      7) Cause of scleroderma and associated Raynaud's is unknown.
   b. Systemic lupus erythematosus (SLE)
      1) 10% to 44% of patients have Raynaud's symptoms.
      2) Affects women in third to fourth decade; Blacks more than Whites.
      3) Other signs and symptoms: photosensitive rash in butterfly distribution on face, arthralgias or arthritis, seizures, alopecia, pericarditis, nephritis, anemia, leukopenia, thrombocytopenia
      4) Pathology: generalized vasculitis affecting both arterioles and venules; fibrinoid necrosis of blood vessels
      5) Cause unknown: believed to be autoimmune, but some drugs can induce similar clinical presentation, such as procainamide, isoniazid, hydralazine.
   c. Rheumatoid arthritis
      1) Focal ischemic lesion and microinfarction
      2) Arteriographic findings: occlusion of one or more digital arteries
   d. Sjögren syndrome
      1) Raynaud's associated with symptoms of dry eyes and mouth with enlargement of salivary or lacrimal glands
      2) Usually associated with rheumatoid arthritis or SLE
6. Trauma and occupational vasospasm
   a. Also known as "vibration-induced white fingers"
   b. Equipment: pneumatic hammers, chain saws, riveting machines, pounding machines, brush saws
   c. Occupations: construction and demolition workers, typists, telephone operators, pianists, meat cutters, sewing machine operators

d. Incidence: 30% to 84% of workers using vibratory tools develop symptoms after 6,000 to 7,000 hours of work (Coffman, 1996).
e. Symptoms: blanching and numbness of fingers; pain and cyanosis rare; feet usually spared; attacks may also be brought on by cold exposure. Attacks lessen with avoidance of equipment use, but sensitivity to cold persists.
f. Pathology: usually normal but may show medial muscular hypertrophy or subintimal fibrosis of digital arteries (Coffman, 1996)

7. Hypothenar hammer syndrome
   a. Use of palm of hand as a hammer or during karate exercise, bowling, or pushing a walker may cause ulnar artery occlusion.
   b. Patient develops Raynaud symptoms in only one hand.
      1) Pallor or cyanosis with numbness on exposure to cold
      2) No reactive hyperemia
   c. 1.7% of patients with Raynaud's symptoms; usually affects men in third to fourth decade; calluses over palm suggest diagnosis (Coffman, 1996)
   d. Radial and ulnar pulses are usually palpable, normal
   e. Allen test: color restored with release of radial artery (refer to Chapter 10, Upper Extremity Arterial Occlusive Disease for complete description)
   f. Arteriographic findings: ulnar artery thrombosed, irregular, or aneurismal at level of hamate bone; possible multiple digital artery occlusions caused by emboli
8. Carpal tunnel syndrome
   a. Numbness, burning, tingling of first three fingers of hand; worse at night; pain may radiate to elbow or shoulder; symptoms usually bilateral
   b. Raynaud's symptoms may precede other symptoms by 6 to 12 months.
   c. Weakness and atrophy of muscles on thenar eminence with sensory complaints below the wrist
   d. Symptoms related to compression of median nerve by swelling, inflammation, or infiltration of tissue of the transverse ligament that crosses the ventral surface of wrist
   e. Common occupational disease: affects keyboard operators or others who overuse wrist, hand.
9. Thoracic outlet syndrome (refer to Chapter 18, Thoracic Outlet Syndrome)
   a. 38.6% of patients who have hyperabduction and 5.3% of those who have other causes of thoracic outlet syndrome have Raynaud's symptoms (Coffman, 1996).
   b. Attacks may affect one or both hands.
   c. Attacks are caused by either compression of nerves in thoracic outlet or by distal emboli from thrombi in subclavian artery.
10. Blood dyscrasias (See Table 17-1)
    a. Raynaud's symptoms develop as a result of clumping of red blood cells in small arteries and arterioles.
    b. Cryoglobulinemia: patients develop purpura of legs, joint pain, leg ulcers, renal failure; twice as common in females, with symptoms starting in third to fourth decade; may be secondary to infections, autoimmune or connective tissue disease, lymphoproliferative disease, or liver disease.
    c. Cold agglutinins: antibodies of -IgM type; Raynaud's symptoms with or without pallor or cyanosis of entire hand. Affects men aged 30 to 90 years; need not be accompanied by underlying disease but may be associated with viral infection or lymphoma (Coffman, 1996).

11. Atherosclerosis of upper extremities
    a. Atherosclerosis of extremities: frequent cause of Raynaud symptoms in men older than 50 years (refer to Chapter 10, Upper Extremity Arterial Occlusive Disease).
    b. Arteriosclerosis obliterans: attacks of pallor and cyanosis occur in one or two toes with no reactive hyperemia; only one leg involved; pulses absent and patient has history of intermittent claudication.
    c. Thromboangiitis obliterans (Buerger disease): Raynaud's symptoms in as many as 57%; lower extremities usually affected but upper extremities affected in as many as 70% (Coffman, 1996) (refer to Chapter 16, Buerger Disease).
    d. Acute arterial occlusion: Raynaud's symptoms may follow acute occlusion of proximal large- or medium-sized vessels but should not be confused with embolization to smaller digital vessels, which involves only one or two digits and may lead to ischemic changes.
    e. Inflammatory arterial disease/vasculitis: any of the many vasculitides may be associated with Raynaud's symptoms owing to immune complexes that can induce inflammatory reactions in small arteries.
    f. Arteriovenous fistula: more than 50% of patients with fistulas have Raynaud's symptoms; peripheral coolness and trophic skin changes may develop; in addition to reduced blood flow to digits, other factors are probably involved, because the unaffected hand also develops symptoms with exposure to cold (Coffman, 1996).
12. Other conditions associated with secondary Raynaud's
    a. Polyvinyl chloride disease
        1) Occurs in workers who clean autoclaves
        2) Results in multisystem disease resembling scleroderma: thickening of skin on hands and arms, nodule formation, thinning of bones, thrombocytopenia, hepatic and pulmonary dysfunction, angiosarcoma of liver
        3) Arteriographic findings: stenoses or occlusions of digital arteries
    b. Hypothyroidism
        1) Incidence may be as high as 24% (Coffman, 1996)
        2) Vasoconstriction may be due to decreased production of body heat
    c. Primary pulmonary hypertension
        1) Incidence of Raynaud's is 10% to 30% (Coffman, 1996)
        2) Marked intimal thickening of pulmonary arterioles while skin and muscle biopsies are normal; no evidence of systemic disease
        3) It is theorized that neurohumoral changes affecting both pulmonary and digital circulations cause vasospasm that could lead to permanent damage to small vessels (Creager & Dzau, 2005)
    d. Heavy metal: Raynaud's symptoms have been associated with toxicity from lead, arsenic, thallium, and mercury.
    e. Neoplasms
        1) Raynaud phenomenon or digital ischemia has been associated with stomach, kidney, colon, ovarian, breast, cervical, and lung cancers and leukemia.
        2) No extrinsic compression from tumor needed for symptoms; no consistent identifiable causative relationship.
        3) Raynaud's symptoms preceded diagnosis of tumor in 63 of 180 patients by an average of 9 years (Coffman, 1996).
    f. Drug-induced: ADHD medications and renal clearance.

IV. Assessment

A. Assess for Risk Factors

1. Primary Raynaud disease: family history. As mentioned earlier, this idiopathic condition may have a genetic link; despite longstanding evidence for familial patterns, further longitudinal studies are needed (Kahaleh, 2004; Wigley, 2002).
2. Secondary Raynaud phenomenon
   a. Risk associated with cause
   b. Drugs: use of ergot derivatives, methysergide, excessive caffeine, beta blockers, ADHD medications, hemotherapeutics as listed
   c. Connective tissue disorders
      1) "One of the most difficult clinical challenges faced when evaluating patients with Raynaud phenomenon is the assessment of risk for transition to connective tissue disease" (Kahaleh, 2004).
      2) 10% to 30% conversion from primary Raynaud disease to secondary Raynaud phenomenon occurs over 20 years (Hodges, 1995).
   d. Trauma (see causes listed earlier)
      1) Occupational hazards: use of vibratory tools, jackhammers, or chain saws; use of electrical wires; chronic exposure to cold; professional sports injuries; injuries from strenuous use of upper extremities in certain professions (e.g., commercial fishermen, lumberjacks, masons, farmers, meat cutters)
      2) Frostbite
      3) Recreational injuries from sports such as bowling, baseball, karate
      4) Any limb trauma resulting in reflex sympathetic dystrophy, thoracic outlet syndrome, or carpal tunnel syndrome; use of hand as a hammer
   e. Risk factors associated with atherosclerosis
      1) Smoking
      2) Hypertension
      3) Hyperlipidemia
      4) Advancing age
      5) Male gender
      6) Family history, including aneurysmal disease
      7) Medical history of coronary artery disease, stroke, renal failure, diabetes mellitus
   f. Medical conditions as listed earlier
   g. Risks associated with other occupations: typists, pianists, sewing machine operators, workers who clean autoclaves (vinyl chloride exposure), workers who are exposed to heavy metal

B. Patient History

1. Subjective
   a. Triphasic color changes of digits with exposure to cold or stressful situations.
      1) Classic symptoms may or may not be present.
      2) Onset is sudden with sharp demarcation of color changes; pallor/ischemic changes last 15 to 20 minutes.
      3) Patient reports sensitivity to cold: avoids shopping in frozen food section of store or air conditioning; winter activities worsen complaints.

4) Involvement is usually bilateral and symmetric but may be unilateral, depending on cause.
5) General body chill may provoke attack.
6) Upper extremity complaints include tips of fingers distal to metacarpophalangeal joint and thumb.
7) Initially, only one or two digits are involved; condition progresses to other digits over time. Index, middle, and ring finger are most frequently involved (Wigley, 2002).
8) Fewer than 50% also have attacks in toes (Coffman, 1996).
9) Other areas of involvement include nose, ears, lips, face, chest, and nipples during breastfeeding.

b. Symptoms of low blood flow: sensation of pins and needles, numbness, clumsiness of hands, finger aching
c. Age at onset: primary disease symptoms reported in younger years; secondary phenomenon usually reported in third decade and later.
d. Trophic skin changes: thickening of skin, pitting scars, chronic paronychia, fissuring of fingers, ulcerations, digital gangrene
e. Symptoms of associated disorders as listed earlier: thorough review of systems required.
  1) Constitutional: fatigue, fevers, night sweats, weight changes
  2) Skin: changes as listed earlier; rashes, telangiectasias, jaundice, hyper- or hypopigmentation
  3) HEENT (Head, Ears, Eyes, Nose Throat): headache, vision change, dry eyes or mouth, oral ulcers
  4) Respiratory: cough, exertional dyspnea, wheezing, frequent infections
  5) Cardiovascular: chest pain/pressure, palpitations, limb swelling, claudication, rest pain
  6) Gastrointestinal: appetite, dysphagia, abdominal pain, change in color or caliber of stools
  7) Genitourinary: painful breastfeeding, vaginal dryness, erectile dysfunction, frequency, miscarriage
  8) Musculoskeletal: painful, swollen joints; limitation of range of motion; muscular atrophy, especially of thenar eminence
  9) Endocrine: intolerance to heat/cold, excessive thirst, urinary frequency
  10) Hematologic: easy bruisability, petechiae, history of blood clots
  11) Neurologic: numbness, tremor, seizure activity, symptoms of stroke, bilateral or unilateral weakness, changes in sensation
  12) Psychiatric: anxiety, depression, panic attack, psychosis

2. Objective
  a. Primary disease: physical examination is normal except for cool digits.
    1) Triphasic color changes may be observed with cold exposure, nervousness, or startle reaction; completely reversed with rewarming.
    2) Radial, ulnar, dorsalis pedis, posterior tibial pulses are palpable.
    3) Livedo reticularis: mottling of skin of arms and legs during cold response; reversible with rewarming
  b. Secondary phenomenon: wide variety of findings depend on causative agent.
    1) Temperature and color changes as previously described
    2) Trophic skin changes: skin thickening, fissuring, digital ulcerations or gangrene

3) Other signs of connective tissue disease: digital skin binding, dry eyes and mouth with or without oral ulcers, inflammatory joint changes, skin rash, alopecia, sclerodactyly, telangiectasia, xerostomia
4) Signs of atherosclerosis: hairlessness, decreased pulses
5) Evidence or history of trauma
6) Presence of dialysis fistula
7) Positive Allen test (assessment of palmar arch patency) or Adson maneuver (assessment of thoracic outlet)

3. Medical history, including medical or surgical conditions and medication use to identify secondary causes as listed
4. Social history, including occupation, tobacco and drug use, diet and caffeine consumption, recreational activities
5. Family history
   a. Raynaud disease
   b. Connective tissue disease
   c. Atherosclerosis
   d. Blood dyscrasias
   e. Endocrine disorders: thyroid disease, diabetes mellitus

C. Physical Examination

1. Inspection
   a. Primary disease: normal skin condition with visible color changes (as described) with exposure to cold or stressful situation.
   b. Secondary phenomenon: trophic skin changes with fissures, ulcerations, gangrene; evidence of trauma; presence of fistula; swelling; muscle atrophy of thenar eminence; arthritic or inflammatory joint changes; punctate lesions on fingertips associated with cyanosis indicating microemboli; other signs of systemic disease as previously listed.
2. Palpation
   a. Primary disease: normal skin turgor and texture; bilateral cool hands/feet; normal palpable proximal and distal pulses of upper and lower extremities
   b. Secondary phenomenon: variable depending on cause; pulses may be diminished or absent; aneurysmal changes of native vessels or hemodialysis fistula (palpable thrill should be present); skin or joint nodules or calcifications may be present
   c. Perform Allen test to assess patency of palmar arch: Radial and ulnar arteries are compressed while patient clenches fist to evacuate blood from hand. When hand is opened, the palm appears pale and mottled. In a patient with normally patent palmar arch, release of either the radial or ulnar artery results in prompt reactive hyperemia of the entire palm, with disappearance of pallor and mottling. In the presence of radial artery occlusion, releasing radial artery compression while maintaining occlusion of the ulnar artery results in continued pallor and mottling. Release of the ulnar artery compression restores hand perfusion. With ulnar artery occlusion, color returns to the hand only after release of the radial artery (Bruni, 2004)
   d. Perform Adson maneuver to assess for subclavian artery compression at thoracic outlet: With patient sitting erect, palpate radial pulse as patient deeply inhales and turns head strongly to the affected side. If subclavian artery is compressed by this maneuver, radial pulse will weaken or

disappear and return as patient resumes original position facing forward (Bruni, 2004)

e. All pulses, including abdominal aorta, should be palpated to assess for presence of other vascular conditions

3. Percussion of chest and abdomen assesses for pulmonary consolidation or hepatic/splenic enlargement
4. Auscultation
   a. Primary disease: no bruits will be heard at any level.
   b. Secondary phenomenon: assess for presence of bruits at carotid, subclavian, axillary, brachial, renal, iliofemoral.
      1) Perform hyperabduction arm maneuver while auscultating subclavian, axillary, and brachial arteries.
      2) If dialysis fistula is present, assess for normal hyperdynamic bruit versus blunted flow signal (stenosis) or flow changes associated with aneurysm.

D. Considerations Across the Life Span

1. Children and young adults
   a. 15% of children aged 12 to 15 report symptoms of Raynaud disease; percentage is higher in females (18% vs. 12% males) and increases in later teens; no association with psychosocial factors such as economic level and school performance (Jones et al., 2003).
   b. Social factors: occupation, recreational activities, and tobacco and drug use are implicated in secondary phenomenon.
   c. Raynaud symptoms may be present for as long as 20 years prior to diagnosis of secondary causes, with conversion from primary disease to secondary phenomenon occurring in as many as 10% to 30% of cases (Hodges,1995).
   d. Systemic sclerosis (scleroderma) is rare in children; usually diagnosed between ages 35 and 65; frequently accompanied by family history of connective tissue disease (Klippel et al., 2001).
2. Women of childbearing age
   a. Increased prevalence in females (4:1 over males); usually diagnosed between ages 20 and 40 years (Coffman, 1996); affects as many as 20% of women of childbearing age (Barclay, 2004).
   b. For systemic sclerosis, female predominance most pronounced during mid to late childbearing years, with ratio of females to males 7 to 12:1 (Klippel et al., 2001).
   c. Raynaud's symptoms of skin blanching followed by cyanosis and/or erythema may affect nipples of breastfeeding mothers, causing painful breastfeeding.
      1) Associated with exposure to cold
      2) Treatment options: prevention or reduction of cold exposure, avoidance of vasoconstrictive medications, use of calcium channel blockers (nifedipine), aerobic exercise, biofeedback, calcium and magnesium supplements, evening primrose oil and fish oil (Barclay, 2004)
3. Elderly
   a. Primary disease is unusual in advanced years
   b. Assess for multiple secondary causes, especially atherosclerosis or prolonged use of walker
   c. Increased risk for injury results from cold exposure, falls

V. Pertinent Diagnostic Testing

A. Laboratory Tests

1. Once Raynaud phenomenon has been diagnosed based on presentation, laboratory evaluation is required to assess for possible secondary cause, especially in
   a. Men
   b. Women older than 40 years
   c. Patients who have associated signs of sclerodactyly, ulcers, gangrene
2. Basic laboratory tests
   a. Complete blood count
   b. Erythrocyte sedimentation rate (ESR)
   c. Antinuclear antibody (ANA)
   d. Urinalysis assesses for crystals, sediment, protein
   e. Chest radiographs assess for increased pulmonary markings, cardiac enlargement
   f. If any of these are abnormal, proceed with more extensive evaluation
3. ESR
   a. Measures speed with which red cells settle out of unclotted blood; during acute inflammation, asymmetric plasma proteins (e.g., fibrinogen, immunoglobulins) interact with red cells to cause stacking of cells; stacked cells fall to bottom of tube more quickly than normal cells.
   b. Normal value for most laboratory tests is greater than 20 mm/hr. Normally increases with age, pregnancy, anemia, and renal failure; normally decreases in heart failure.
   c. Elevation is seen in patients who have inflammatory process, infection, or neoplasia, but nonspecific.
   d. Important to obtain baseline at time of diagnosis because disease process may progress over time.
4. ANA
   a. Autoantibodies that react with a variety of nuclear antigens, including nucleic acids, histones, and parts of centromeres (Klippel et al., 2001)
   b. Normal value reported as titer of dilution of patient's serum that showed staining with fluorescein on a slide of human tumor cell, as well as pattern of staining.
      1) Normal titer greater than 1:40
      2) Patterns reported as homogeneous (SLE), speckled (scleroderma), nucleolar, peripheral, or centromere (CREST syndrome)
   c. Positive ANA titer usually indicates autoimmune disease but may be present in as many as 5% of healthy people, especially women (Klippel et al., 2001).
      1) 95% of patients who have SLE have positive titer.
      2) 25% of patients who have primary Raynaud's have positive ANA, but positive titer also associated with 63-fold increase in incidence of connective tissue disease (Hodges, 1995).
5. Other serum laboratory tests as indicated based on clinical suspicion: rheumatoid factor, lupus anticoagulant, complement levels, specific autoantibodies, hypercoagulopathy evaluation, lipid profile (when atherosclerosis is suspected), total protein (if elevated, obtain serum protein electrophoresis to assess for myeloma)

6. Electrocardiogram
   a. Assesses for arrhythmia
   b. If arrhythmia new, will need to be evaluated for possible myocardial infarction
7. Echocardiogram assesses for valve disease, cardiac enlargement and chamber function, and presence of thrombus as source of emboli.
8. Hand radiographs assess for subcutaneous calcium deposits (CREST syndrome) and/or prolonged narrowing of bone in distal fingertips.

B. Noninvasive Vascular Tests

1. Digital blood pressure with cold challenge
   a. May use blood pressure cuff or strain gauge.
   b. Double inlet cuff for local cooling is placed over the proximal phalanx of the test finger.
   c. Measure baseline digital artery pressure at rest in reference and test finger at normal ambient temperature and with digital cooling by circulation of water through cuff at 20°C, 15°C, 10°C, and 5°C for 5-minute intervals.
   d. Cuff is inflated above systolic level during cooling; pressure is measured after cuff is released following cooling.
   e. Results are expressed as the percentage of decrease in the cooled finger's systolic pressure on reperfusion as compared with pressure in the reference finger.
   f. Positive test: decrease in digital blood pressure of more than 20% considered positive for Raynaud's.
      1) Normal small digital pressure drop with decreasing temperature
      2) Vasospastic similar to normal until critical temperature is reached; then abrupt arterial closure occurs
      3) Obstructive similar to normal except much lower pressure seen at baseline and with cooling
   g. If baseline digital pressures are more than 30 mm Hg lower than brachial pressures at baseline, suspect atherosclerotic/stenotic process.
2. Pulse volume recording (PVR)
   a. Amplitude of PVR waveform normally decreases in cool environment; increases in warm environment.
   b. Primary Raynaud's: PVR flattens as patient is exposed to cold; restored to normal volume as patient rewarmed.
   c. PVRs will be flattened during cooling and rewarming in patients who have atherosclerotic occlusive disease.
3. Duplex ultrasound evaluation of extremity may be indicated for evaluation of secondary causes, especially atherosclerosis, aneurysm, arteriovenous fistula (refer to Chapter 10, Upper Extremity Arterial Occlusive Disease) (Schmidt, Drause, Schicke, & Wernicke, 2008).

C. Invasive Tests—Arteriography

1. Primary Raynaud disease: limited role, as diagnosis is usually established without invasive procedure (Gerhard-Herman & Creager, 2003).
2. Secondary phenomenon
   a. Gold standard for evaluation of upper extremity ischemia, trauma, arteritis, or occlusive disease
      1) Plaque, occlusions, emboli, aneurysms, traumatic injuries, arteriovenous malformations, and vasospasm are visualized.

2) Arteritis of aortic arch and major vessels shows individual or multiple areas of stenosis with no plaque or ulcerations.

b. Additional techniques used to improve visualization of small digital arteries.
   1) Hand warming
   2) Intra-arterial injection of vasodilators used to prevent vasospasm, which may occur at time of contrast injection
   3) Primary Raynaud disease may be distinguished from secondary Raynaud phenomenon with identification of cause

c. Collagen vascular disease: bilateral distal lesions with no findings of atherosclerotic changes; smooth, string-like arteries with or without segmental lesions; collateral circulation has "corkscrew" appearance (Bruni, 2004).

d. Provides surgeon/interventionist with a map with which to plan intervention, as well as identification of collaterals and distal vessel status.

e. Visualization of aortic arch and branches is important to identification of proximal lesions, aneurysms, and plaque.

f. One may perform maneuvers to evaluate thoracic outlet compression during examination.

g. Transfemoral route is preferred with use of the Seldinger technique.

D. Special Procedures

1. Nailfold capillary microscopy
   a. Microscopic visualization of cutaneous capillaries
   b. May assist in distinguishing primary Raynaud's from secondary Raynaud's associated with connective tissue disorders; primary disease will be normal.
   c. Place drop of grade B immersion oil on skin at base of fingernail; view area with stereoscopic microscope or hand-held ophthalmoscope set at 10 to 40 diopters, or with magnifying glass.
   d. Normal: capillaries are regularly spaced, hairpin loops.
   e. Abnormal: avascular areas with enlarged, deformed capillary loops are associated with scleroderma; disorganized capillaries with avascular areas and hemorrhage present in dermatomyositis and polymyositis.
2. Electromyogram (EMG) assesses for presence of nerve conduction delay in median and ulnar nerves caused by carpal tunnel syndrome or proximal cervical compression.
3. CT scan or MRI/MRA provides imaging of proximal upper extremity arterial circulation for diagnosis of secondary causes of Raynaud's symptoms.
   a. CT scanning: advances in technology (spiral CT, electron beam CT, spin echo) are expanding usage; increasing usefulness in imaging the thoracic outlet and aneurysms.
   b. MRA: gives full longitudinal and cross-sectional view of the vasculature; many advances are increasing its use; much less invasive than angiography (Bruni, 2004).

E. Diagnostic Criteria to Distinguish Primary from Secondary Raynaud Phenomenon.

Allen/Brown criteria proposed in 1932 for primary Raynaud disease:

1. Vasospastic attacks brought on by cold or emotional stimuli
2. Bilateral extremity involvement

TABLE 17-2 Clinical Features of Raynaud Disease

Primary Raynaud's	Secondary Raynaud's
1. Vasospastic attacks brought on by cold or stress; no underlying associated systemic disease	1. Clinical features of connective tissue disease, atherosclerosis, or other known related causes
2. Symptoms for >2 yrs, usually mild; spontaneous improvement in 15%; 38% progress to severe form	2. Symptoms intense and painful; progression or resolution depends on causative agent
3. Symmetric attacks involving both hands	3. Asymmetric attacks
4. Absence of tissue necrosis or gangrene; strong, symmetric peripheral pulses	4. Pitting scars or ulcers, ischemic skin lesions, digital gangrene
5. Normal nailfold capillaries	5. Evidence of microvascular disease on microscopy of nailfold capillaries
6. Normal erythrocyte sedimentation rate (ESR)	6. ESR may be elevated, depending on underlying disease state
7. Negative serologic examination, especially for antinuclear antibodies	7. Presence of autoantibodies (e.g., scleroderma associated with anticentromere, antitopoisomerase antibodies)
8. Age at onset: 14–40 yrs	8. Age at onset: >30 yrs
9. Affects females 4:1 over males	9. Variable depending on causative agent

Adapted from Wigley, F. M. (2002). Raynaud's phenomenon. *New England Journal of Medicine*, *347*(13), 1001–1008.

3. Gangrene absent or, if present, involves only skin of fingertips
4. No evidence of underlying disease that could cause vasospasm
5. History of symptoms for more than 2 years (see Table 17-2) (Coffman, 1996).

VI. Primary Prevention

A. Primary Disease

1. Awareness of familial tendency toward symptoms
2. Avoidance of triggers to prevent attacks
   a. Cold avoidance
   b. Stress reduction
3. Use of warm clothing, possibly more than appears appropriate for environment

B. Secondary Phenomenon

1. Awareness of predisposing risk factors
2. Avoidance of ergot-derivative medications
3. Avoidance of injury: should not use hand as a hammer; should make proper use of crutches, limit use of vibration equipment, exercise appropriate caution during participation in sports and high-risk occupations as listed
4. Prevention measures for atherosclerosis: maintain normal blood pressure and weight, exercise daily, stop smoking, eat heart-healthy diet

VII. Medical Management

A. Conservative Measures

1. No cure for primary disease; treatment is supportive.
2. Try to avoid medications for treatment of young fertile women, if possible.

3. Monitor frequency, severity, and duration of attacks through self-reporting.
4. Maintain total body warmth, as well as hand warmth.
   a. Loose-fitting, layered clothing should be worn.
   b. Head and feet should be covered—stockings/socks.
   c. Mittens are warmer than gloves.
   d. Air-conditioned environments should be avoided, if possible.
   e. Foot- or hand-warmers may be used: chemical packets that may be placed in shoes or mittens; battery-operated electric gloves/socks (avoid use near ulcers).
   f. Extra-depth, extra-width shoes may be worn to prevent constriction of feet; padded insoles.
5. Avoid pressure plus cold—holding cold steering wheel or beverages without gloves; use bottle openers.
6. Avoid smoking and use of tobacco products; nicotine causes vasoconstriction.
7. Reduce emotional stress.
8. Avoid use of drugs known to trigger attacks: ergot derivatives, beta blockers, sympathomimetic drugs, clonidine, serotonin-receptor agonists.

B. Pharmacotherapy for Vasospastic Disease

1. Indications
   a. Conservative therapy fails.
   b. Attacks interfere with daily activities or employment.
   c. Trophic digital lesions develop.
2. Calcium-channel blockers
   a. Most widely used agent for Raynaud's treatment
   b. Potent peripheral vasodilator; antiplatelet and anti–white cell activity (Belch & Ho, 1996; Thompson & Pope, 2005)
   c. Decreases frequency, duration, and severity of attacks in 66% of patients compared with placebo (Coffman, 1996; Wigley, 2002)
   d. Usual regimen: nifedipine 10 to 30 mg three times daily
   e. Slow-release products appear to be better tolerated with fewer side effects (Coffman, 1996)
   f. Diltiazem, 30 to 120 mg three times daily, is also beneficial
   g. Side effects: tachycardia, edema, flushing, headache, dizziness, constipation, orthostatic hypotension
3. Vasodilators: No significant effect compared to placebo or calcium channel blockers (Vinjar & Stewart, 2008).
4. Sympatholytic agents
   a. Increase digital capillary blood flow.
   b. Careful titration required to relieve symptoms but avoid side effects.
   c. Reserpine, 0.125 to 0.5 mg daily. Caution: do not give to patient with history of depression.
   d. Guanethidine, 10 to 50 mg daily
   e. Side effects: bradycardia, postural hypotension, dyspepsia, edema, lethargy, depression, impotence
   f. Alpha-adrenoceptor antagonist: prazosin, 2 to 8 mg daily; moderate effectiveness in two thirds of patients; improvement wanes over time (Coffman,1996).
   g. Other sympatholytic agents used: phenoxybenzamine, methyldopa

5. Nitroglycerine
   a. Direct-acting vasodilator
   b. Popular therapy, but studies show mixed results (Coffman, 1996)
   c. Quarter to half inch applied topically daily; may cause headache
   d. New nitroglycerine formulation, MQX-503, shows promise in improvement of the severity of Raynaud's symptoms (Chung et al., 2009)
6. Pentoxifylline
   a. Provides vasoactive activity plus increased flexibility of red blood cells to enter narrowed vessels; reduces blood viscosity.
   b. Popular therapy, but limited data to support use (Belch & Ho, 1996; Wigley, 2002).
   c. 400 mg three times daily; may cause dyspepsia.
7. Prostaglandins
   a. Prostacyclin and alprostadil (PGE1) have potent vasodilatory and platelet properties but are unstable and require intravenous administration; oral administration has not proved effective (Wigley, 2002).
   b. Iloprost, prostacyclin analogue, is more stable; may be given orally; intravenous administration more effective (Wigley, 2002).
      1) Infused daily for 6 hours for 3 to 5 days, not to exceed 2 ng/kg/min; dose gradually increased on day 1 until tolerated dose achieved; tolerated dose becomes maximum dose given daily.
      2) Benefit lasts for 6 weeks to 6 months.
      3) Shown to be more beneficial than nifedipine in healing digital ulcers (Belch & Ho, 1996).
      4) Side effects during infusion: hypotension, headaches, facial flushing, abdominal pain, nausea, vomiting, diarrhea
   c. Application of transdermal patch delivery system using PGE1 ethylester for 10 hours daily for 2 weeks showed improved skin perfusion and decreased attacks (Kahaleh, 2004).
8. Cilostazol (Pletal)
   a. Synthetic phosphodiesterase-III inhibitor; reversibly inhibits platelet aggregation
   b. Shown to effect vasodilatation of brachial arteries but has no effect on microvascular blood flow or frequency or severity of attacks in primary or secondary Raynaud's (Kahaleh, 2004)
   c. More effective for primary Raynaud disease than secondary Raynaud phenomenon (Rajagopalan et al., 2003)
   d. Multicenter study currently investigating effect of cilostazol in children with primary and secondary Raynaud's (http://www.clinicaltrials.gov)
9. Botox: Botulism toxin has been shown in clinical trials to be a safe and useful option for treatment of digital vasospastic ischemia (Fregene, Ditmars, & Siddiqui, 2009).
10. Other agents (Wigley, 2002)
    a. Fluoxetine: selective serotonin reuptake inhibitor (SSRI); single study indicated benefit at doses of 20 to 40 mg daily.
    b. Losartan: angiotensin II–receptor type I antagonist; one study showed benefit at doses of 25 to 100 mg daily.
    c. Investigational
       1) Cilostazol and sildenafil: phosphodiesterase inhibitors—small studies suggest some benefit for severe disease; more studied needed (De LaVega & Derk, 2009).
       2) Bosentan: endothelin-receptor inhibitor

3) Ketanserin: serotonin receptor antagonist
4) N-acetylcysteine: 2-year study supported positive benefit for patients with Raynaud phenomenon secondary to scleroderma (Salsano et al., 2005)

d. Nitric oxide, niacin derivatives, papaverine, cyclandelate, griseofulvin, arginine have not shown benefit compared with placebo (see Table 17-3).

C. Plasmapheresis

1. Defibrination process induces alterations in platelet function and reduces circulating immune complexes.
2. One study showed benefit in relieving symptoms of severe vasospasm compared with placebo or intravenous heparin (Coffman, 1996).

D. Temperature-Controlled Biofeedback

1. Patients immerse hands in 43°C water while body is maintained at 0°C.
2. Positive benefit lasting as long as 12 months reported by some authors (Hodges, 1995; Coffman, 1996); other studies unclear (Wigley, 2002).

E. Acute Ischemic Crisis (Wigley, 2002)

1. Initiate short-acting calcium-channel blocker (e.g., nifedipine 10 to 30 mg every 8 hours) and antiplatelet (aspirin) therapy.
2. Digital or wrist block with lidocaine or bupivacaine without epinephrine reduces pain, reverses vasospasm, and produces local chemical sympathectomy effect.
3. Intravenous iloprost (0.5 to 2 ng/kg/min for up to 5 days) reverses acute critical ischemia; not available in United States.
4. Intravenous heparin for 48 to 72 hours used for persistent critical ischemia and/or evidence of proximal arterial occlusive disease.
5. Digital sympathectomy may be used in refractory cases; see further discussion.

F. Medical Intervention for secondary Raynaud phenomenon, as appropriate for condition, may reduce frequency and severity of attacks. New lines of therapy are in development (Lambova & Muller-Ladner, 2009).

1. Phosphodiesterase type 5 inhibition (Caglayan et al., 2006).
2. Statin therapy has been shown to reduce incidence of digital ulcers (Abou-Raya, Abou-Raya, & Helmii, 2009).

VIII. Surgical Management

A. Sympathectomy: removes vasoconstrictor tone and relieves vasospasm in distal portion of limb.

1. Proximal resection of cervical dorsal sympathetic nerves may benefit 50% to 60% of patients with severe symptoms refractory to conservative and medical management (Coffman, 1996; Gerhard-Herman & Creager, 2003).
   a. Short-term pain relief, improved wound healing, and decreased tissue loss may be seen (Bruni, 2004).
   b. Relapses common within 6 to 24 months.

TABLE 17-3 Pharmacologic Treatment of Raynaud Phenomenon

Agent	Dose	Side Effects	Comments
Calcium-Channel Blockers			
Nifedipine	10–30 mg three times daily orally	Tachycardia, edema, flushing, headache, dizziness, constipation, orthostatic hypotension	Placebo-controlled trials indicate benefit
Sustained-release nifedipine	30–120 mg/d orally		
Amlodipine	5–20 mg/d orally		
Felodipine	2.5–10 mg twice daily orally		
Isradipine	2.5–5.0 mg twice daily orally		
Diltiazem[a]	30–120 mg three times daily orally		
Sustained-release diltiazem[a]	120–300 mg/d orally		
Sympatholytic Agent			
Prazosin	1–5 mg twice daily after first dose	Syncope, postural hypotension, dizziness, and palpitations possible	Efficacy often transient, may wane after several weeks
Angiotensin II-Receptor Type 1 Antagonist			
Losartan	25–200 mg/d orally	Dizziness, headache, fatigue, diarrhea	One placebo-controlled trial indicated benefit
Selective Serotonin-Reuptake Inhibitor			
Fluoxetine	20–40 mg/d orally	Insomnia, nausea, diarrhea, tremors	One placebo-controlled trial indicated benefit
Vasodilator			
Nitroglycerin	¼–½ in of 2% ointment applied topically per day	Headache, tachycardia, syncope, angina, rash, impotence, nausea, rebound hypertension	Popular therapy but little controlled data to support its use
Other Vasoactive Drug			
Pentoxifylline	400 mg three times daily orally	Dyspepsia, nausea, vomiting	Popular therapy but little controlled data to support its use
Prostaglandins			
Epoprostenol[b]	0.5–6 ng/kg of body weight/min	Flushing, diarrhea, headache, hypotension, rash Intravenously for 6–24 hr for 2–5 d	Used for critical ischemia; in-hospital infusion recommended
Alprostadil	0.1–0.4 μg/kg/min intravenously for 6–24 hr for 2–5 d		
Iloprost[c]	0.5–2 ng/kg/min intravenously for 6–24 hr for 2–5 d		

[a]Diltiazem is not as effective as the dihydropyridine class of calcium-channel blockers.
[b]The Food and Drug Administration has approved the use of epoprostenol for the treatment of pulmonary hypertension.
[c]Iloprost is not available in the United States.
Adapted from Table 2, Pharmacologic Treatment of Raynaud's Phenomenon, Wigley, F. M. (2002). Raynaud's phenomenon. *New England Journal of Medicine*, *347*(13), 1001–1008.

TABLE 17-4 Complications of Surgical Sympathectomy

Horner syndrome
Postsympathetic neuralgia
Atelectasis
Pleural effusion
Pneumonia
Pneumothorax
Winged scapula
Hemothorax
Subcutaneous emphysema
Sweating in the trunk or lower extremities
Intercostal neuralgia

c. A long-term study of 40 months showed excellent relief of symptoms initially with one third of patients studied achieving permanent improvement. Thoracoscopic approach recommended for severe cases (Thune, Ladegaard, & Licht, 2006).
d. Re-innervation occurs, perhaps because of presence of other sympathetic pathways to brachial plexus that are separate from cervicothoracic sympathetic trunk, or because of catecholamine hypersensitivity after denervation (Gerhard-Herman & Creager, 2003).
e. Patients without digital arterial occlusion do not benefit (Bruni, 2004).
f. Endoscopic and percutaneous techniques are being developed; these may prove beneficial with lower complication rates (see Table 17-4) (Bruni, 2004).

2. Digital sympathectomy
   a. Microsurgical technique used to strip adventitia from common and proximal digital arteries.
   b. Effective in relieving symptoms in both primary Raynaud's with severe disease and digital ischemia and secondary Raynaud's caused by trauma (Gerhard-Herman & Creager, 2003).
   c. Considered safe; can restore digital flow immediately, but limited to use in patients with severe disease, ulcers.
3. Lower extremity lumbar sympathectomy
   a. As high as 80% success for relief of toe symptoms, with longer-lasting results (Coffman, 1996).
   b. Limited usefulness: refractory vasospasm of lower extremity only accounts for 2% of all cases of lower limb vasospasm (Gerhard-Herman & Creager, 2003).
4. Radical microarteriolysis
   a. Extensive adventitiectomy and removal of periarterial scarring of the ulnar artery, palmar arch, and digital arteries
   b. Used successfully in small number of patients with severe Raynaud's secondary to scleroderma (Gerhard-Herman & Creager, 2003)

B. Operative Procedures and Wound Care as Indicated by Patient Condition

1. Trauma intervention
2. Surgical correction of fistulae, thoracic outlet compression, carpal tunnel syndrome, or atherosclerotic stenosis/occlusion (refer to Chapter 10, Upper Extremity Arterial Occlusive Disease)

3. Wound care and debridement: as many as 13% of patients with primary disease will have ulcerations, fissures, necrosis, and scarring (Coffman, 1996)
4. Digit amputation: 0.4% of patients with primary disease (Coffman, 1996)

IX. Nursing Management

A. Nursing Diagnoses

1. Knowledge deficit regarding disease process and vasospastic stimuli
2. Potential/actual impaired skin integrity related to altered circulation and vasospasm
3. Pain related to recurrent vasospastic attacks
4. Disturbed body image related to disease process
5. Impaired social function related to limiting effects of vasospastic attacks on work or recreational activities
6. Impaired health maintenance related to tobacco or drug/medication use

B. Expected Patient Outcomes

1. Verbalize understanding of triggers for vasospastic attacks.
2. Verbalize knowledge of primary or underlying secondary causes of vasospastic attacks.
3. Implement measures to prevent or limit attacks.
4. Maintain adequate tissue perfusion.
5. Determine comfort and function goals. Describe and implement measures to reduce pain.
6. Report changes in condition, especially skin breakdown and pain. Verbalize understanding of risk related to wounds (e.g., infection, digit loss).
7. Adhere to medication, wound care, or surgical treatment plan.
8. Function at acceptable level of activity; maintain economic stability.
9. Eliminate use of tobacco and/or drugs that may stimulate attacks.
10. State or demonstrate acceptance of condition and adjustment of lifestyle.

C. Interventions

1. Assessment: skin color and integrity, changes in skin color with provoking stimuli or during testing; all proximal and distal pulses; changes in skin that indicate systemic disease conditions (thickening, tightness, pallor, edema); thorough general physical assessment for underlying disease states.
2. Assess patient history for underlying causes: family history, past medical/surgical/trauma history, medication use, social history (including tobacco use, recreation, occupation).
3. Assess pain using pain rating scale; document frequency and severity of attacks and response to pain reduction measures, both pharmacologic and nonpharmacologic.
4. Patient education and counseling (see later discussion).
5. Provide warm, calm environment and warm hands and feet during attack; implement measures for relaxation.
6. Monitor patients (both those at risk and those with active disease or symptoms) for response to potential triggers (e.g., initiation of beta blocker therapy following myocardial infarction).

7. Provide appropriate limb/digit protection, which should prevent trauma, optimize skin hygiene, maintain warmth; use padding/mittens/sheepskin boots as needed; maintain arm at cardiac level (neither elevated nor dependent); avoid pressure on limb—minimize use of tourniquet, avoid constrictive dressings.
8. Implement appropriate wound care; monitor for response to treatment measures; include adjunctive measures to optimize healing: maintain nutrition, pain management, mobility.
9. Acknowledge patient's reactions to limitations as normal responses to adaptation; encourage patient to participate in plan of care and decision making for lifestyle changes (e.g., job transfer in case of vibration injury).
10. Encourage maintenance of independence, performance of activities of daily living, and daily exercise; discourage helplessness; collaborate with physical and occupational therapists as needed.
11. Perform postoperative care measures and monitoring as indicated by procedure and underlying disease process (refer to Chapter 10, Upper Extremity Arterial Occlusive Disease).

D. Evaluation

1. Frequency and severity of vasospastic attacks diminished
2. Skin integrity maintained
3. Triggers for vasospastic attacks avoided or removed
4. Pain rated less than 4 on scale of 1 to 10
5. Recommended lifestyle changes implemented
6. Social situation stabilized, including employment, independent function, relationships, stress reduction, and pursuit of enjoyable activities that do not induce attacks
7. Tobacco cessation maintained
8. Adherence to medical/surgical regimen documented, including all measures for treatment of underlying disease
9. Exercise regimen reported

X. Patient Education: primary prevention and health promotion

A. Primary Disease

1. Awareness of familial tendency toward symptoms
2. Avoidance of triggers to prevent attacks
   a. Cold (e.g., air conditioning, frozen food section of grocery store, winter sports, cold water)
   b. Stress
3. Use of warm clothing, possibly more than appears appropriate for environment, to maintain general body and extremity warmth

B. Secondary Phenomenon

1. Awareness of predisposing risk factors
2. Avoidance of cold/stress triggers, ergot derivatives, and beta blockers or other medications associated with symptoms
3. Avoidance of injury: should not use hand as a hammer; should make proper use of crutches, limit use of vibration equipment, exercise appropriate caution during participation in sports and high-risk occupations as listed

4. Prevention measures for atherosclerosis: maintain normal blood pressure and weight, exercise daily, stop smoking, eat heart-healthy diet

XI. Patient Education: secondary prevention and home care management

A. Acute Attack Measures

1. Take action immediately to decrease severity and length of attack
2. Warm body and extremities
   a. Go indoors or move away from cold air
   b. Run warm water over hands or feet or soak in bowl or tub of warm water. Avoid burns from water that is too hot
   c. Use chemical packets or electric socks or hand warmers
3. Take time to relax; de-escalate a stressful situation if possible

B. Prevention of Attacks

1. Keep body and extremities warm
   a. Wear layers of loose clothing; no constrictive clothing
   b. Cover head, hands, and feet
   c. Keep dry
   d. Use chemical or electric warmers; exercise caution with heating pads to avoid burns.
2. Avoid pressure plus cold (e.g., holding cold tools, steering wheels, iced drinks)
3. Quit smoking/tobacco use
4. Limit caffeine intake
5. Control stress
   a. Learn to recognize stressful situations
   b. Develop and practice relaxation techniques: deep breathing, yoga, stress management course
6. Exercise
   a. Daily exercise for 30 to 60 minutes
   b. Benefits: increases energy, promotes well-being, aids in maintenance of ideal weight, promotes restful sleep
7. Maintain general health
   a. Heart-healthy diet
   b. Regular medical examinations
   c. Adherence to medical plan of care
   d. General hygiene: mild soap, warm water; use of skin lubricants as needed; meticulous nail care
   e. Avoidance of trauma

C. Medication Education for Raynaud's and Treatment of Secondary Diseases

1. Expected effects: decreased severity and frequency of attacks
2. Recommended dose and regimen
3. Adverse side effects and potential drug interactions
4. Report problems and concerns to prescriber
5. Pain management: report adequacy of pain management plan and participate in pain control measures
6. Medications to avoid: ergot derivatives and beta blockers may precipitate attacks

D. Wound Care

1. Apply dressings and wound care agents as instructed
2. Inspect wounds daily
3. Avoid tape on skin
4. Notify health provider of new wounds or ulcers
5. Notify health provider of signs of infection or worsening of wound: unusual color, amount, or odor of drainage; increase in inflammation, redness, tenderness, or pain
6. Maintain adequate nutrition

E. Signs of Disease Progression

1. Increased frequency, severity, or length of attacks
2. Signs of other systemic disease: fever, rash, fatigue, weight loss, skin, hair, or nail changes; increased pain with use of limb; permanent color change of limb (cyanosis or pallor)
3. Development of ulcers, necrosis, or gangrene

F. Other Lifestyle Changes as Indicated

1. If symptoms are secondary to job-related trauma or vibration injury, patient may need job transfer, re-education services, and financial support during this process. Educate patient regarding services available.
2. If symptoms are due to participation in recreational activities (e.g., baseball, skiing, bowling), patient may need to substitute other activities. May benefit from sports medicine assessment and education.

G. Patient Resources

1. National Institute of Arthritis and Musculoskeletal and Skin Disease Information Clearinghouse (AMS Circle, Bethesda, MD 20892-3675 301-495-4484 or toll free @ 877-226-4267; www.nih.gov/niams)
2. Local chapters of scleroderma or lupus support groups (e.g., Lupus Foundation of America)

CASE STUDY

A 22-year-old White female presents to her primary care provider with chief complaint of painful digits when exposed to cold for the past 5 years. Symptoms of pallor and severe pain initially involved only index and middle fingers of both hands; fingers become blue and finally bright red when she is able to warm up her hands. All digits are now involved, with symptoms lasting as long as 30 minutes. Despite use of double gloves, she had to discontinue cross-country skiing, ice skating, and swimming and fishing; this is very distressing, as her fiance´ is an avid outdoorsman who enjoys these activities. Food preparation is becoming problematic because she cannot wash or prepare foods in cold water or cold conditions or shop in air-conditioned stores. She lives in Vermont and wears socks and mittens to bed year round except in July and August. For the past year, she has noted development of painful fissures on her fingertips during winter months, which are difficult to heal despite application of various emollients.

Past medical/surgical history: Migraine headaches; excision of large right ovarian cyst at age 20. Denies history of any other medical conditions or trauma.

Medications: OTC migraine medication or ibuprofen p.r.n

Allergies: Penicillin (rash)

Family history: Mother, 48, with history of hypothyroidism and intolerance to cold. Father, 50, with history of myocardial infarction at age 49, hypercholesterolemia and hypertension now controlled on medical regimen. Three sisters, aged 25, 20, 16; the 25-year-old has SLE, diagnosed at age 19.

Social history: Single, engaged. Recently graduated with degree in photography. Presently employed with local portrait studio but hopes to establish own business. Denies use of tobacco on regular basis but will occasionally smoke when dining out with friends. Denies use of illicit drugs. Three to five alcoholic beverages per week. Runs 3 miles four to five times per week for exercise; enjoys many other activities, such as cycling, kayaking, and hiking, but symptoms often limit ability to participate.

Review of systems: Denies changes in weight or appetite; no difficulty with sleep or excessive fatigue. Rare migraine headache with no associated visual disturbance, controlled with OTC medication taken with coffee. Denies exertional dyspnea or cough; no episodes of chest pain, pressure, or palpitations. Denies any food intolerance, history of anorexia/bulimia, constipation or diarrhea, bloating or gassiness. Menses regular on OCs. Sexually active, uses condoms. No prior history of STD. No history of seizure, tremor, weakness, or syncope. Mood generally stable; no prior history of anxiety or depression, although her present complaint and associated limitations provoke depressive thoughts.

Physical examination findings:

Height: 62 inches. Weight: 58 kg.
Vital signs: Temperature: 96.5°F; pulse: 64, regular; blood pressure: 104/66, right; 100/70, left.

Integument: Cool hands; small healed scars adjacent to lateral nail edge on left forefinger and right thumb. Skin otherwise intact without rashes or bruises. Normal texture and turgor. During examination, patient's fingers noted to become cooler and pale.

HEENT: Normocephalic. TMs pearly gray with normal light reflex; hearing intact.

PERRLA; EOMs full without nystagmus. Normal fundoscopic examination. Nares dry and patent. Oral mucosa moist without lesions; teeth in excellent condition. No thyromegaly or lymphadenopathy of cervical or supraclavicular chains.

Cardiovascular: Regular rate and rhythm; no murmurs, rubs, or gallops; S1, S2. All upper and lower extremity pulses 2+, equal and easily palpated. No dependent edema or varicosities. No bruits.

Respiratory: Chest clear; full excursion with normal contour and no areas of dullness to percussion.

Gastrointestinal: Soft, nontender with normally active bowel sounds in all quadrants; no organomegaly, bruits, palpable masses, or hernias.

Neurologic: Alert, oriented, appropriate but appears anxious. No tremors. DTRs brisk and equal in all extremities with equal strength. Normal cranial nerve examination.

Review Questions

1. Which findings on her physical examination suggest the possibility that this patient may not have primary Raynaud disease?
   a. Triphasic color change of fingers when exposed to cold followed by rewarming
   b. Normal skin texture
   c. Mother with thyroid disease and sister with lupus
   d. Healed scars on fingertips

2. Which laboratory tests are considered part of the basic evaluation for a young woman with symptoms of Raynaud's?
   a. Antinuclear antibody (ANA), erythrocyte sedimentation rate (ESR), complete blood count (CBC), and urinalysis
   b. Chest radiograph, echocardiogram, pulse volume recordings of upper extremities, and arteriogram
   c. Thyroid-stimulating hormone (TSH), chemistry panel including liver enzymes, cold agglutinins, partial thromboplastin time
   d. Lipid profile, creatinine, lupus antibody, electromyogram (EMG)
3. The patient is sent for noninvasive vascular studies to document the severity of her symptoms. Which test would be most helpful to diagnose primary Raynaud disease?
   a. Arterial duplex scan from subclavian to radial artery
   b. Allen test
   c. Digital blood pressures with cold challenge
   d. Pulse volume recording with hyperabduction of shoulder
4. The patient's basic laboratory tests all return normal and she has a positive noninvasive study. Her diagnosis is primary Raynaud disease. Because she already has significant limitation on activities with digital fissures, she is considered a candidate for medical intervention. Which class of drugs is most commonly used to treat Raynaud's symptoms?
   a. Beta blockers
   b. Calcium-channel blockers
   c. Ergot derivatives
   d. Narcotic analgesics
5. In providing education to this patient, which medications for migraine management should one tell her to avoid?
   a. Ergot derivatives
   b. Beta blockers
   c. Selective serotonin reuptake inhibitors (SSRI)
   d. Triptans
   e. (a) and (b)
   f. All of the above
6. This patient should be counseled to
   a. Avoid tobacco use
   b. Wear snug clothing to maintain general body warmth
   c. Relocate to a warmer climate to prevent all further attacks
   d. Give up all outdoor recreation

Answers/Rationales

1. d. Healed scars on fingertips. Ulcers are usually not present in patients with primary Raynaud disease, although, statistically, 38% of patients may progress to a severe form with painful digital fissures.
2. a. ANA, ESR, CBC, and urinalysis. Chest radiograph is also part of the initial evaluation to assess for abnormal pulmonary markings. If any of these test results are abnormal, further diagnostic evaluation is appropriate. However, if these results are normal, it is unlikely that the patient has a connective tissue disorder. Because 50% of patients with Raynaud's have primary disease, extensive diagnostic evaluation for secondary causes should be pursued based on history, clinical examination, and results of initial laboratory tests.
3. c. Digital blood pressures with cold challenge document diminished flow when hand is subjected to progressively colder water from 20°C to 5°C every 5 minutes. Systolic pressures are recorded in both a reference finger and the test finger. Results are expressed as the percentage

of decrease in the cooled finger's systolic pressure on reperfusion as compared with pressure in the reference finger. The test is considered positive for Raynaud's when there is a decrease in digital blood pressure of more than 20% in the cooled finger.

4. b. Calcium-channel blockers are the most widely used agent for Raynaud's treatment because they exhibit potent peripheral vasodilator effect, plus antiplatelet and anti–white cell activity. They have been shown to decrease frequency, duration, and severity of attacks in 66% of patients compared with placebo. The usual regimen is nifedipine, 10 to 30 mg three times daily.
5. e. Ergot derivatives and beta blockers are known to precipitate vasospastic attacks. SSRI, particularly fluoxetine, have been shown to have some benefit in symptom relief for Raynaud's attacks. Triptans are not contraindicated for patients with both migraine and Raynaud's.
6. a. Avoid tobacco use, because nicotine acts as a vasoconstrictor. Clothing should be loosely layered to maintain warmth, never constrictive. Although the incidence of Raynaud's is lower in warmer climates, relocation will not cure her disease and should be a personal choice. Exercise is encouraged to maintain general body health and sense of well-being; many outdoor activities may be continued with proper protection.

REFERENCES

Abou-Raya, A., Abou-Raya, S., & Helmii, M. (2009). Statins: Potentially useful in therapy of systemic sclerosis-related Raynaud's phenomenon and digital ulcers. *The Journal of Rheumatology, 35*(9), 1801–1808.

Anders, H. J., Sigi, T., & Schattenkirchner, M. (2001). Differentiation between primary and secondary Raynaud's phenomenon: A prospective study comparing nailfold capillaroscopy using an ophthalmoscope or stereomicroscope. *Annals of Rheumatoid Diseases, 60*(4), 407–409.

Bakst, R., Merola, J. F., Franks, A. G., Jr., & Sanchez, M. (2008). Raynaud's phenomenon: Pathogenesis and management. *Journal of the American Academy of Dermatology, 59*(4), 633–653.

Barclay, L. (2004). Raynaud's phenomenon of the nipple may cause painful breastfeeding. *Medscape Medical News.* Retrieved from http://www.medscape.com/viewarticle/473219

Belch, J. J. F., & Ho, M. (1996). Pharmacotherapy of Raynaud's phenomenon. *Drugs, 52*(5), 682–695.

Bruni, K. (2004). Upper extremity problems. In V. Fahey (Ed.): *Vascular nursing* (4th ed., pp. 311–334). St. Louis, MO: Saunders.

Caglayan, E., Huntgeburth, M., Karasch, T., Weihrauch, J., Hunzelmann, N., Krieg, T., ... & Rosendranz, S. (2006). Phosphodiesterase type 5 inhibition is a novel therapeutic option in Raynaud disease. *Archives of Internal Medicine, 166*(2), 231–233.

Chung, L, Shapiro, L, Florentino, D., Baron, M., Shanahan, J., Sule, S., ... Wigley, F. M. (2009). MQX-503, a novel formulation of nitroglycerin, improves the severity of Raynaud's phenomenon: A randomized, controlled trial. *Arthritis and Rheumatology, 60*(3), 870–877.

Coffman, J. D. (1996). Vasospastic diseases. In J. R. Young, J. W. Olin, & J. R. Bartholomew (Eds.), *Peripheral vascular diseases* (2nd ed., pp. 407–424). St. Louis, MO: Mosby.

Creager, M. A., & Dzau, V. J. (2005). Vascular disease of the extremities. In D. L. Kasper, A. S. Fauci, D. L. Longo, E. Braunwald, S. L. Hauser, & J. L. Jameson (Eds.), *Harrison's principles of internal medicine* (16th ed., pp. 1486–1490). New York: McGraw-Hill.

Czupryniak, A., Kaluzynska, A., Nowickim, M., Wiecke, B., Bald, E., & Owczarek, D. (2005). Raynaud's phenomenon and endothelial dysfunction in end-stage renal disease patients treated with hemodialysis. *Kidney and Blood Press Research, 28*(1), 27–31.

De Angelis, R., Salaffi, F., & Grassi, W. (2008). Health-related quality of life in primary Raynaud's phenomenon. *Journal of Clinical Rheumatology, 14*(4), 206–210.

De LaVega, A. J., & Derk, C. T. (2009). Phosphodiesterase – 5 Inhibitors for the treatment of Raynaud's: A novel indication. *Expert Opinion on Investigational Drugs, 18*(1), 23–29.

Fregene, A., Ditmars, D., & Siddiqui, A. (2009). Botulinum toxin type a: A treatment option for digital ischemia in patients with Raynaud's phenomenon. *Journal of Hand Surgery (American Volume), 34*(3), 446–452.

Gerhard-Herman, M., & Creager, M. A. (2003). Raynaud's phenomenon and other vasospastic disorders. In M. A. Creager, & E. Braunwald (Eds.). *Atlas of vascular disease* (2nd ed., pp. 173–188). Philadelphia, PA: Current Medicine, Inc.

Hodges, H. (1995). Raynaud's disease: Pathophysiology, diagnosis, and treatment. *Journal of the American Academy of Nurse Practitioners, 7*(4), 159–164.

Jones, G. T., Herrick, A. L., Woodham, S. E., Baildam, E. M., Macfarlane, G. J., & Silman, A. J. (2003). Occurrence of Raynaud's phenomenon in children ages 12–15 years. *Arthritis and Rheumatism, 48*(12), 3518–3521.

Kahaleh, M. B. (2004). Raynaud phenomenon and the vascular disease in scleroderma. *Current Opinions in Rheumatology, 16*(6), 718–722.

Klippel, J. H., Crofford, L. J., Stone, J. H., & Weyand, C. M. (2001). *Primer on the rheumatic diseases* (12th ed.). Atlanta, GA: The Arthritis Foundation.

Kropman, R. F. (2004). Raynaud's phenomenon of the penis. *The Journal of Urology, 171*, 1630.

Lambova, S. N., & Muller-Ladner, U. (2009). New lines of therapy of Raynaud's phenomenon. *Rheumatology International, 29*(4), 355–363.

Rajagopalan, S., Pfenninger, D., Somers, E., Kehrer, C., Chakrabarti, A., Mukherjee, D., ... Kaplan, M. J. (2003). Effects of cilostazol in patients with Raynaud's syndrome. *American Journal of Cardiology, 92*(11), 1310–1315.

Salsano, R., Letizia, C., Proletti, M., Rossi, C, Proietti, A. R., Rosato, E., & Pisarri, S. (2005). Significant changes of peripheral perfusion and plasma adrenomedullin levels in N-acetylcysteine long term treatment of patients with sclerodermic Raynaud's phenomenon. *International Journal of Immunopathology and Pharmacology, 18*(4), 761–770.

Schmidt, W. A., Drause, A., Schicke, B., & Wernicke, D. (2008). Color Doppler ultrasonography of hand and finger arteries to differentiate primary from secondary forms of Raynaud's phenomenon. *The Journal of Rheumatology, 35*(8), 1591–1598.

Syed, R. H. & Moore, T. L. (2008). Methylphenidate and dextroamphetamine-induced peripheral vasculopathy. *Journal of Clinical Rheumatology, 14*(1), 30–33.

Thompson, A. E. & Pope, J. E. (2005). Calcium channel blockers for primary Raynaud's phenomenon: A meta-analysis. *Rheumatology, 44*(2), 145–150.

Thune, T. H., Ladegaard. L., & Licht, P. B. (2006). Thoracoscopic sympathectomy for Raynaud's phenomenon – a long term follow-up study. *European Journal of Vascular and Endovascular Surgery, 32*(2), 198–202.

Vinjar, B. & Stewart, M. (2008). Oral vasodilators for primary Raynaud's phenomenon. *Cochrane Database of Systematic Reviews, 16*(2), Art. No.: CD006687.

Wigley, F. M. (2002). Raynaud's phenomenon. *New England Journal of Medicine, 347*(13), 1001–1008.

RELEVANT WEB SITES

www.arthritis.org

www.nih.clinicaltrials.gov

Questions and answers about Raynaud's phenomenon, National Institute of Arthritis and Musculoskeletal and Skin

Diseases, National Institute of Health. Available at: http://www.niams.nih.gov/hi/topics/raynaud/ar125fs.htm

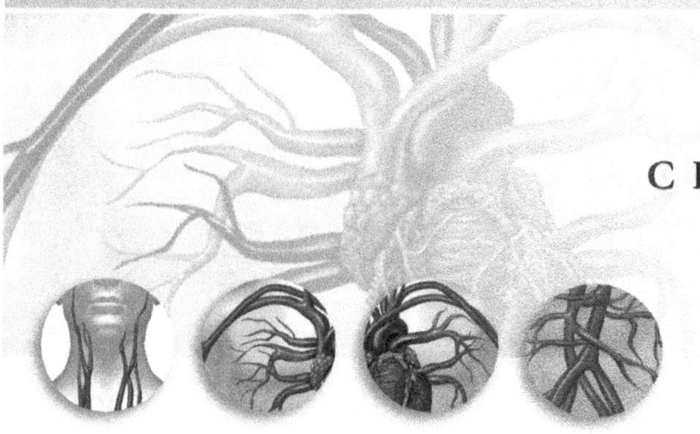

CHAPTER 18

Thoracic Outlet Syndrome

Tiffany Street

First Edition Author: *Catherine Wiegand*

OBJECTIVES

1. Define thoracic outlet syndrome.
2. Differentiate between neurogenic, arterial, and venous symptoms.
3. Discuss conservative medical management and surgical intervention for treatment of thoracic outlet syndrome.
4. Identify nursing implications relevant to patients with thoracic outlet syndrome.

Introduction

Thoracic outlet syndrome (TOS) is a complex set of symptoms caused by abnormal compression of the neurovascular bundle in the thoracic outlet area. Entrapment of the neurovascular structures in the past has been described by a series of names, such as costoclavicular compression, hyperabduction syndrome, cervical rib syndrome, and first rib syndromes. Peet coined the term "thoracic outlet syndrome" in 1956 to indicate all compressions of the neurovascular bundle (Urschel & Razzuk, 1998). The name itself may be confusing because the area of compression between the scalene muscles and the first rib is correctly called the thoracic inlet. Currently, however, the term "thoracic outlet syndrome" is used to describe patients with compression of the subclavian vein, subclavian artery, and brachial plexus which are the three components of the thoracic outlet area. Compression usually occurs as a result of congenital or acquired changes in the surrounding bony or soft tissue. There are three major classifications of TOS: neurogenic, arterial, and venous.

The most common form of TOS is neurogenic and accounts for 95% of all TOS patients. These patients are usually young adults, and women predominate at approximately a ratio of 4:1 to men. Arterial TOS is rare and occurs in less than 5% of patients. Venous TOS is also uncommon and occurs in 2% to 3% of patients. These patients frequently present with a thrombotic event. Venous presentation is often a result of congenital anomalies of the costoclavicular space and a result of repetitive activities such as overhead shoulder movements, throwing, or swimming (Sanders, 2010).

The wide variability of patient symptoms, including vascular and neural signs, diffuse symptoms, and the lack of diagnosis-specific tests to confirm the diagnosis of TOS make it difficult to diagnose correctly. Patients may present with a variety of signs and symptoms rather than one specific symptom. Symptoms may be neurogenic, arterial, venous, or mixed (Stoney & Cheng, 1995).

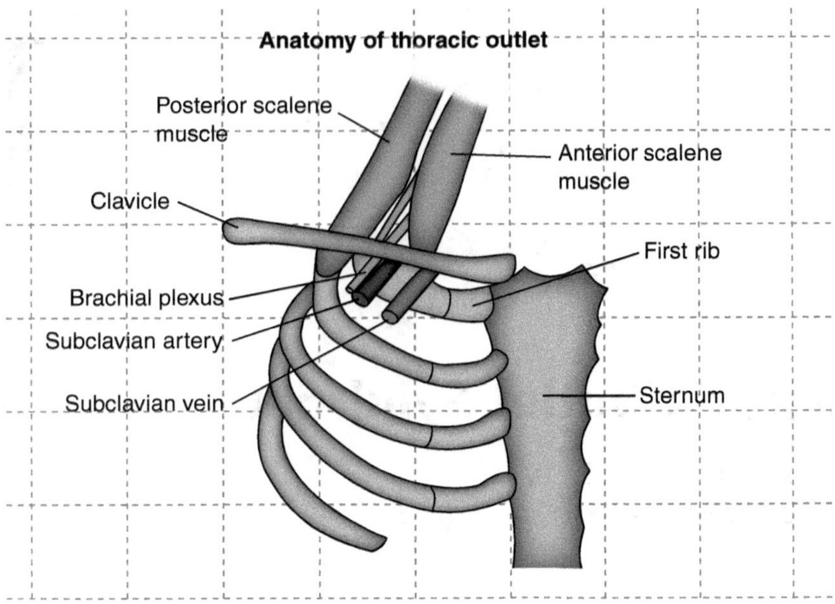

FIGURE 18-1. Anatomy of the thoracic outlet.

I. Anatomy (Fig. 18-1) (Atasoy, 1996; MacKinnon & Novak, 2002; Stoney & Cheng, 1995)

A. First Rib forms the floor of the outlet. This rib is relatively flat, approximately 3 in long, with two transverse processes on the anterior surface. Located between the two groves is a tubercle for the attachment of the scalenus anticus muscle. The first rib forms the framework to which muscles and ligaments attach.

B. Clavicle with the Subclavius muscle forms superior portion.

C. Scalene Muscles are secondary respiratory muscles and raise the first rib and slightly rotate and bend the neck.

1. Scalenus anticus (anterior scalene muscle) muscle originates from the anterior tubercles of the transverse processes of C3 to C6 and inserts in the scalene tubercle on the first rib.
2. Scalenus medius (middle scalene muscle) muscle is the largest and longest and originates from the posterior tubercles of the transverse processes of the last six cervical vertebrae. It inserts inferiorly between the subclavian artery groove and the tubercle on the first rib. It is in close proximity to the posterior brachial plexus.
3. Scalenus minimus, if present (30% to 50%), arises from the transverse process of C6 to C7 and inserts in the fascial support of the pleura and first rib.

D. Neurovascular Bundle

1. Subclavian artery exits the chest by arching over the first thoracic rib posterior to the scalene anticus and anterior to the scalenus medius muscle. It lies just anterior to the brachial plexus.

2. Subclavian vein normally passes anterior to the scalene anticus and through the costoclavicular space between the first rib and the head of the clavicle.
3. Brachial plexus forms from the nerve roots C5 to T1. It gains access to the axilla by passing posterior to the anterior scalene muscle in close association with and superior to the subclavian artery. C8 and T1 nerve roots, which contribute to the medial cord and ulnar nerve, are commonly affected by pressure of the underlying first rib.

E. Cervical Bands (congenital myofascial bands/ligaments)

1. Can extend from the transverse process of C7 or from the tip of a cervical rib and attach to the scalene tubercle of the first rib.
2. Composed of posterior fibers of the anterior scalene and medial fibers of the middle scalene muscle, which lie either with the body of the scalenus medius or on the anterior surface of the muscles.
3. David B. Ross, MD has classified extensively up to nine separate types of bands, the most common of which are as follows:
   a. Type 3 (the most common), which is critical in compression of C8 and T1 branches of the brachial plexus.
   b. Type 5 (the second most common), which may have its lower insertion in the first rib.
   c. Type 4 (less commonly seen), which is a powerful band capable of compressing both nerve and artery.

F. Cervical Ribs

1. If a cervical rib is present, the brachial plexus may be displaced and impinge on the apex of the interscalene triangle.
2. Can be a natural anomaly that may be a complete bony structure or a fibrous band that stretches to the first rib from the cervical transverse process.
3. Cervical ribs occur in approximately 0.45% to 1.5% of the general population and up to 5% of patients with TOS (Sanders, 2010).
4. Female to male ratio is approximately 2:1 (Kieffer & Ruotolo, 1995).

G. Sites of Compression

1. Interscalene triangle bordered by the anterior scalene muscle, the middle scalene muscle, and first rib inferiorly. The subclavian artery and the three trunks of the brachial plexus traverse this space. The middle scalene muscle is a key factor in neurogenic compression.
2. Costoclavicular space bordered by the clavicle, first rib with the costoclavicular ligament anteriorly, and the edge of the middle scalene muscle posteriorly. The subclavian artery, vein, and brachial plexus are located in this space. Neurovascular compression in this space may occur as a result of a congenital or acquired changes in the clavicle first rib, structural changes in muscles, or changes in shoulder position or trauma.
3. Subcoracoid space beneath the pectoralis muscles, the coracoid process, and ribs posteriorly. The brachial plexus travels through this area and can be affected by hyperabduction of the arm.

II. Pathophysiology (MacKinnon & Novak, 2002)

A. Neurogenic Compression

1. Pathophysiology is complex and may vary depending on the specific predisposing and causative factors. Severity of the condition depends on the duration and magnitude of compressive forces.
2. Mechanical and ischemic factors lead to acute and chronic inflammation
3. Intraneural edema and pressure lead to breakdown of blood–nerve barrier.
4. Pressure cannot escape the peripheral diffusion barrier.
5. Connective tissue thickening occurs.
6. Demyelination of nerve (focal and then more diffuse) occurs.
7. Nerve fibrosis occurs with axonal degeneration, which leads to symptoms and clinical findings.

B. Arterial Compression

1. Secondary to significant and longstanding compression
2. Frequently associated with presence of cervical rib
3. Congenital or acquired abnormalities of first rib, congenital bands, and hypertrophic muscles play a part but are less common than neurogenic factors (Kieffer & Ruotolo, 1995)
4. Arterial wall becomes thick and fibrotic
5. Inflammatory changes fix artery to surrounding structures
6. Poststenotic dilatation and associated chronic compression can progress to aneurysmal changes
7. Localized intimal damage of vessels can lead to thrombosis, subclavian artery occlusion, and ischemia
8. Platelet aggregation can lead to microembolization, distal ischemia, and Raynaud syndrome (Kieffer & Ruotolo, 1995)

C. Venous Compression

1. External pressure on vein results in compression.
2. Thick subclavian muscle, costocoracoid ligament, anterior scalene muscle, and bands create compression.
3. Inflammatory reaction from continuous compression can lead to endothelial injury and venous stasis (MacKinnon & Novak, 2002).
4. Thrombosis of subclavian vein is often referred to as Paget–Schroetter syndrome.

III. Etiology/Predisposing Factors (Atasoy, 1996; MacKinnon & Novak, 2002; Martinez, 1999; Stoney & Cheng, 1995)

A. Mechanical Factors are primary causes of impaired nerve function

1. Postural abnormalities of the shoulder girdle
   a. Prolonged positioning leads to chronic nerve irritation
   b. Decreased muscle length
      1) Pectoralis minor
      2) Scalene muscles
      3) Sternocleidomastoid
      4) Serratus anterior

c. Increased muscle length
   1) Middle trapezius
   2) Lower trapezius
2. Muscle imbalance/strain
   a. Increased pressure of certain compression sites
      1) Overuse of muscles
         a) Upper trapezius
         b) Levator scapulae
      2) Underuse of muscles
         a) Middle trapezius
         b) Lower trapezius
         c) Serratus anterior

B. Trauma

1. 60% to 70% of patients have had injury to neck and shoulder girdle area (Atasoy, 1996; Martinez, 1999).
2. Whiplash-type injuries may precipitate compression (Kieffer & Ruotolo, 1995).

C. Occupational Demand

1. Repetitive movements
2. Heavy lifting, particularly if associated with repeated vigorous abduction movement

IV. Assessment

In the absence of a specific gold standard test for TOS, an accurate clinical history and evaluation are paramount in assessing patients.

A. History (Atasoy, 1996; Machleder, 1994; MacKinnon & Novak, 2002)

1. Subjective findings. Symptoms are usually insidious in nature.
   a. Neural symptoms
      1) In all types the most common symptoms are pain and paresthesia weakness with an easily fatigued arm.
      2) Patients reported feelings of clumsiness and dropping things (Urschel & Razzuk, 1998).
      3) Symptoms can be aggravated by hyperabduction, elevation of the arm.
      4) Pain is usually dull and aching and may progress to such a severity that strong analgesic agents are required for relief.
      5) Upper plexus involvement may include pain in side of neck radiating to mandible and face, earache, and occipital headaches. Left upper chest pain can mimic angina pectoris.
      6) Dizziness, vertigo, and blurred vision have been reported in some patients with upper plexus compression (woods).
      7) Lower plexus symptoms include pain in supraclavicular area, back of neck, and scapular and rhomboid region. Pain can radiate along posterior axilla and inner aspect of arm down to ulnar nerve distribution.
      8) Combined, usually is a mixture of symptoms.
      9) Neural compression can cause vasomotor changes in the extremity. Changes include coldness and blanching of the hand.

b. Vascular symptoms
  1) Arterial
    a) Rare but most common manifestation is hand ischemia as a result of microembolization (pain, pallor, coldness, paresthesia)
    b) Can be associated with less dramatic symptoms
    c) Many times goes unrecognized because it occurs in younger populations without atherosclerotic risk factors
    d) Mild symptoms are of exertional arm pain
    e) Moderate to severe symptoms of exertional arm pain and even ulceration of the digits
  2) Venous symptoms
    a) Most common presenting symptom is arm edema
    b) Also can have shoulder pain, extremity heaviness and dilated subcutaneous veins in the chest or arm

2. Objective findings
  a. Detailed history of trauma
  b. Attention to activity or injuries that involve stretching of plexus or hyperabduction, such as typing, painting, lifting, whiplash-type injuries
  c. Sleeping postures with arms above the head and elbows flexed may cause complaints of numbness and tingling
  d. Pain history, including aggravating activities, alleviating factors

B. Physical Examination

1. Inspection
  a. Patient posture
  b. Neck and shoulders for bony prominence, apparent muscle spasms
  c. Hands for color temperature, muscle strength, and atrophy of small muscles
  d. Range of motion of neck and shoulder
2. Palpation
  a. Palpate for supraclavicular tenderness elicited by palpating over the anterior scalene muscle, which may reproduce the patient's pain and numbness.
  b. Palpate for a pulsatile mass. It may not indicate an aneurysm, but the artery may be pushed forward by an abnormal bony structure.
  c. Palpate peripheral pulses, including brachial and radial. If nonpalpable pulses, obtain Doppler examination for signals.
3. Auscultation
  a. Take blood pressure in both arms.
  b. Listen for bruits over the supraclavicular fossa.
4. Postural maneuvers/provocative tests (Machleder, 1994; MacKinnon & Novak, 2002; Stoney & Cheng, 1995)

  False-positive and false-negative results make monitoring of pulse unreliable in firm diagnosis. Tests that reproduce the patient's symptoms may provide more accurate information.

  a. EAST (elevated arm stress test; Dr. Roos). Arm elevation for 3 minutes with 90-degree shoulder abduction and external rotation and elbow flexed at 90 degrees. Patient opens and closes the hand rapidly. This test has positive results with reproduction of symptoms including pain, paresthesia, and weakness within 60 seconds.
  b. Adson test. Patient's arm is down at the side, head is turned toward the affected side, patient takes deep breath, and radial pulse is monitored. Test is modified with head turned toward unaffected side. Test result is

positive if radial pulse is obliterated. This test is considered nonspecific in diagnosis of neurogenic TOS.

c. Roos maneuver. Supraclavicular compression of the brachial plexus at the scalenus anticus level. With compression, symptoms may be reproduced.
d. Halsted test (costoclavicular test). Patient assumes a military pose with shoulder backward and downward to narrow the costoclavicular space. The radial pulse is monitored and test result is positive with obliteration of pulse.
e. Wright test. Hyperabduction external rotation of shoulder to 180 degrees. The radial pulse is monitored and a positive test result is indicated with obliteration of radial pulse.

C. Differential Diagnosis (Stoney & Cheng, 1995)

1. Several disorders can have similar presenting symptoms and must be considered in the differential diagnosis of TOS. This list includes the following:
   a. Cervical disc disease
   b. Carpal tunnel syndrome
   c. Ulnar nerve entrapment
   d. Causalgia
   e. Paraspinal muscle myofibrositis
   f. Soft tissue disorders/tumors
   g. Rotator cuff syndrome
   h. Angina pectoris
   i. Raynaud disease
   j. Mitral valve prolapse

V. Considerations Across the Life Span (Machleder, 1994; Stoney & Cheng, 1995)

A. TOS is usually a condition that affects young adults in the third to fifth decade (Stoney & Cheng, 1995).

B. TOS can affect people in their 60s but is usually associated with trauma.

C. Ratio of Female to Male is usually 4:1 (Stoney & Cheng, 1995).

D. Arterial TOS Patients are usually young and report a history of vigorous arm activity.

E. Venous Thrombosis tends to occur more in young men and is associated with strenuous work (MacKinnon & Novak, 2002).

VI. Pertinent Diagnostic Testing

A. General Testing

1. Plain chest x-rays (posteroanterior and lateral) help determine apical lung pathology.

2. C-spine films provide information related to the presence of cervical ribs, elongated C7 transverse process, clavicular fractures, other bony abnormalities, or signs of degenerative disc disease.
3. Magnetic resonance imaging (MRI) or computed tomography (CT) scan may be indicated in the presence of upper plexus disease to rule out cervical disc compression.

B. Testing for Neurogenic TOS

1. Electromyelogram (EMG)/nerve conduction studies (NCS) determine impairment of nerve conduction function of the brachial nerve at the thoracic levels. It may assist with differential diagnosis of cervical disc disease or carpal tunnel syndrome.
   a. Measurement taken when motor conduction velocity is slow across the supraclavicular transaxillary segment of ulnar nerve component of the medial core of the brachial plexus.
   b. Normal is considered 60 to 72 m/sec. Less than 60 m/sec is suspicious for TOS (Urschel & Razzuk, 1998).
2. Somatosensory-evoked potential F-wave studies evaluate the brachial plexus.
   a. Stimulation of distal part of the upper limb and recordings are in the supraclavicular fossa.
   b. Results vary and may produce normal results even in the presence of TOS.
3. These tests have a low level of sensitivity for TOS

C. Testing for Arterial TOS

1. Arterial duplex of the subclavian and axillary arteries demonstrate aneurysmal changes or elevated velocities correlating with a compressive stenosis. TOS maneuvers include the arm at rest and in a horizontal and hyperextended position.
   a. May quantify the postural changes in arterial circulation and localize the arterial occlusion
2. Assess collateral circulation. CT with intravenous contrast-enhanced angiography is helpful to obtain the diagnosis and can assist with surgical planning.
   a. Can identify the exact point of compression and extent of arterial pathology
   b. Has replaced conventional angiography as the main radiographic study in most institutions
3. Arteriogram is performed when patient has evidence of arterial involvement, such as supraclavicular bruit or evidence of microemboli.
   a. "Gold standard"
   b. Should include from the aortic arch to the digital vessels
   c. Can demonstrate distal arterial occlusion and presence of collateral flow

D. Testing for Venous TOS

1. Venous duplex can be used to detect venous thrombosis.
2. Venogram, which is diagnostic for subclavian vein thrombosis. Films should be done in resting and hyperextended arm positions to confirm subclavian axillary vein stenosis or occlusion.

E. Other

1. Electrocardiogram and cardiac echocardiograms, which are conducted to eliminate conditions such as mitral valve prolapse and coronary artery disease

VII. Medical/Conservative Management

A. Neurogenic: Success with conservative treatment of TOS ranges from 50% to 90%. Goal is to decrease compression on the brachial plexus and improve muscle imbalance.

1. Patient education
   a. Pathology of nerve compression
   b. Impact of activities of daily living on symptoms
   c. Aggravating symptoms
   d. Relieving strategies individualized to patients
   e. Encouragement and support to follow recommended medical regimen and exercise program
2. Activity
   a. Activity may need to be modified, especially in highly irritable conditions.
   b. Evaluate sleep patterns.
      1) Support cervical spine with neck pillows
      2) May use neck rolls
   c. Encourage patients to maintain work if possible. Occupational modifications, work reassignment, or leave may be needed.
   d. Weight reduction, if applicable, may help relieve muscle strain.
3. Physical therapy (MacKinnon & Novak, 2002)

   Goal is to restore movement of shoulder girdle and provide more space for neurovascular structures.
   a. Posture correction with muscle-specific exercises
      1) Neck exercise to increase range of motion
      2) Stretching exercises should be low force and longer duration. Target muscles are upper trapezius, levator scapulae, scalene, and sternocleidomastoid
      3) Strengthening started after adequate pain-free range of motion is achieved. Target is middle/lower trapezius, serratus anterior, and lower rhomboids
      4) Swimming has been found to be a useful modality in some individuals but may aggravate symptoms in others
      5) Supervised program is recommended for 2 to 3 weeks to ensure that proper techniques are used
      6) Home exercise program may take up to 6 months for impact to be noted
      7) Exercises that are too aggressive may lead to noncompliance and be labeled as failure
   b. Massage
      1) Used to produce muscle relaxation
      2) Provides symptom relief and comfort
   c. Thermal treatment
      1) Moist ice packs in acute case
      2) Moist heat in chronic pain

4. Medications
   a. Anti-inflammatory agents provide relief from inflammatory reaction/swelling that occurs with nerve compression.
   b. Muscle relaxants
      1) Affect central nervous system and include carisoprodol (Soma), methocarbamol (Robaxin), and cyclobenzaprine HCl (Flexeril)
      2) Affect spinal cord and include baclofen (Lioresal), chlorzoxazone (Parafon), and metaxalone (Skelaxin)
   c. Analgesics
      1) Pain control can be long term and significant problems occur with patients with chronic nerve entrapment.
      2) Over-the-counter medications are recommended (acetaminophen) but may not be helpful after time.
      3) Analgesics should be used in combination with other pain relief modalities, such as heat, massage, and diversional interventions.
      4) Narcotic medications should be used as last resort and should be monitored carefully to prevent dependence.
      5) Medications may need to be alternated to minimize tolerance to one specific agent.
   d. Antidepressants may be helpful in select cases, especially with sleep pattern disturbances
5. Other modalities
   a. Transcutaneous electrical nerve stimulator (TENS)
   b. Braces, which maintain posture in presence of weak muscles, have been used for short-term relief of assistance
   c. Nerve blocks, such as brachial plexus and anterior scalene muscle blocks, may grant temporary relief
6. Psychological support
   a. Living with chronic pain is stressful to patient and family.
   b. Can lead to emotional strain and financial strain if unable to work.
   c. Affects body image/role performance in family.
   d. Counseling/education should be offered to patient and family members.
   e. Specific social services may be needed.
   f. Referral to psychologist or psychiatrist may be indicted if patients have severe depression or express suicidal ideation.
7. Rehabilitation
   a. Work evaluation may be required for a patient to continue in the same job or determine if work reassignment is required.
   b. Evaluation of the activities of the job should include overall ergonomics.
   c. Evaluation of need for lifting, working with arms above the head, repetitive motions is noted.
   d. Close communication with occupational nurse case managers is necessary.
   e. Work reassignment may be required to prevent continued injury.
   f. Vocational rehabilitation nurses are a prime resource to assist an individual in continuing to work.

B. Arterial

1. An exercise program is contraindicated in arterial TOS.
2. Overall treatment is surgical intervention.

C. Venous

1. In acute phase, the immediate treatment is that of an acute deep venous thrombosis
   a. Anticoagulation with unfractionated heparin followed by conversion to oral warfarin for 2 to 4 months
   b. Thrombolysis is frequently used to restore patency.
2. An exercise program is contraindicated.
3. May be followed by surgical decompression

VIII. Surgical Management

Goal is complete decompression of the thoracic outlet with excision of the first rib, cervical bands, and cervical ribs, if present, to relieve constriction on the neurovascular bundle.

A. **Indications for Surgery** (Martinez, 1999; Urcshel & Razzuk, 1998)

1. Decision for surgery is multifactorial
2. Failure of carefully supervised exercise program
3. Increasing decree of disability
4. Clinical deterioration
5. Evidence of arterial insufficiency or aneurysm
6. Venous thrombosis

B. **Surgical Approaches**—Various combinations of surgical approaches are available, including first rib resection, scalenectomy

1. Supraclavicular approach: The incision is parallel and 2 cm above the clavicle in the supraclavicular fossa.
   a. Advantages
      1) Access to interscalene triangle is easier via this approach
      2) Exposure to the posterior two thirds of first rib
      3) Direct visualization of all four nerve roots
      4) Identification of anatomic relationship between bony and fascial structures brachial plexus
      5) Removal of cervical rib, if present
   b. Disadvantages
      1) Access to costoclavicular space and subcoracoid space is poor
      2) Incomplete decompression of cervical bands
2. Transaxillary approach is used for rib resection in presence of neurologic symptoms. A transverse incision is made across the axilla to provide safe access to the first rib.
   a. Advantages
      1) Good access to costoclavicular space
      2) Possibility of complete resection of first rib
   b. Disadvantages
      1) Deep limited exposure. Limitations of exposure can lead to injury of long thoracic nerve and vascular structures
      2) Inability to perform cervical rib resection, if needed
   c. Endoscopic-assisted transaxillary approach (Martinez, 1999) was developed to address issues of inadequate visualization.
      1) Provides direct visualization of structures, including anatomic variations (i.e., cervical bands)

2) Magnifies basic anatomic structures
3) Allows minimally invasive approach

3. Scalenectomy is the division of scalenus anticus and resection of lower portion of muscle at the attachment of the first rib.
    a. Advantages
        1) Used frequently in arterial TOS and with history of trauma.
        2) Complications of this procedure are rare.
        3) May be used in combination with first rib resection to provide complete decompression.
    b. Disadvantages
        1) Phrenic nerve injury possible
        2) Procedure alone usually is not sufficient for decompression of thoracic outlet
4. Other approaches, such as the posterior and infraclavicular, have been reported for first rib resections. They are not widely used, and outcome data are not readily available.
5. Arterial reconstruction
    a. May be required with arterial TOS.
    b. Alternatives may include placement of prosthetic graft, patch, angioplasty, and stent.
    c. Postoperative considerations would be same for any patient undergoing arterial reconstruction.

C. Potential Complications of Surgical Intervention (Stoney & Cheng, 1995)

1. Nerve injury
    a. Brachial nerve injury is serious. Permanent damage is rare, but arm paralysis has been reported.
    b. Long thoracic nerve damage can result in winging of the scapula.
    c. Phrenic nerve injury can be identified on chest film with elevation of hemi-diaphragm. Treatment is conservative.
2. Vascular injury
    a. Subclavian artery or subclavian vein can be entered inadvertently and repaired intraoperatively.
3. Thoracic duct injury
    a. Lymphatics can be damaged during the procedure.
    b. When identified, lymphatics are ligated. Small collection may need to be managed in the postoperative period.
4. Pleural complications
    a. Most common complication is small tear in the pleura, which can lead to pneumothorax.
    b. Small drain can be used or chest tube may be needed for larger injury.
5. Wound infection
    a. Uncommon after this type of procedure
    b. Treated with local wound care and antibiotic therapy

D. Results—Successful treatment is often reported based on pain relief and return to work/activities. Excellent result is one in which there is complete pain relief and return to work at same job (Urschel & Razzuk, 1997).

1. Mortality is extremely low. No reports of deaths were identified in the literature reviewed.

2. Success outcomes vary. Between 70% and 95% of patients have good or positive outcomes (Machleder, 1993).
3. Approximately 5% of patients have poor results.
4. Symptoms can persist or recur (Mingoli et al., 1995).
   a. Scar tissue formation
   b. Remnants of first rib
   c. Chronic myofibrositis and paraspinal muscle spasms (Martinez, 1999)

IX. Nursing Diagnosis

A. Conservative Care

1. Alteration in comfort related to chronic pain of TOS
   a. Expected outcome: appropriate management of pain levels
   b. Nursing intervention
      1) Assess pain level on specific scale (e.g., scale of 0 to 10).
      2) Identify aggravating and alleviating factors.
      3) Set pain level target with patient.
      4) Avoid blood pressure, IV, venipuncture in affected arm.
      5) Discuss effect of chronic pain on ADL and family role.
      6) Use nonmedication strategies as appropriate.
         a) Modify activity to avoid repetitive motion, heavy lifting
         b) Provide alternative measures, including breathing techniques, relaxation, positioning, diversion therapy, heat, and massage
      7) Reinforce physical therapy exercise program
      8) Administer medication as appropriate, including muscle relaxants and nonsteroidal anti-inflammatory agents
   c. Evaluation of nursing care
      1) Pain level on scale at or less than identified target
2. Anxiety related to threat of self-image, chronic pain, uncertainness of treatment options
   a. Expected outcome: management of anxiety-related physical and behavioral symptoms
   b. Nursing interventions
      1) Assess anxiety level and causative factors
      2) Identify manifestations of anxiety
      3) Educate on identified knowledge deficit that may aggravate anxiety
      4) Reinforce effective coping strategies
      5) Assist in setting realistic goals for symptom relief
   c. Evaluation of nursing care
      1) Recognize anxiety and coping patterns
      2) Identify potential anxiety relief techniques
3. Potential alteration in family processes related to illness of patient and potential change in roles
   a. Expected outcome: support in management of family environment
   b. Nursing interventions
      1) Encourage participation by family members/significant others in process

2) Assess current family dynamics
3) Identify potential needed resources
4) Educate to alleviate knowledge deficit
5) Refer to appropriate social service agencies as appropriate
6) Encourage and support questions and open dialogue of family members

c. Evaluation of nursing care
1) Verbalize potential coping strategies to relieve situational stressors
2) Refer to appropriate agencies, if needed

4. Potential sleep pattern disturbance
a. Expected outcome, experience an optimal balance of rest and activity
b. Nursing intervention
1) Provide measures to induce sleep, such as soft music, back rub, warm showers
2) Use support mechanism such as neck rolls, pillows for proper positioning at night
3) Limit number of daytime naps
4) Reduce or eliminate environmental distractions

c. Evaluation of nursing care
1) Verbalize effective measures for personal environment
2) Verbalize improvement in night-time sleep pattern

5. Knowledge deficit related to disease processes, treatment options, and pain control
a. Expected outcome
1) Express understanding of causes of TOS, aggravating factors, and alleviating factors
2) Describe needed alterations in lifestyle
3) Discuss medications, including dose indications and potential adverse reactions

b. Nursing intervention
1) Assess current knowledge level.
2) Assess readiness to learn, including learning barriers, cultural influences, current pain level, and anxiety.
3) Review anatomy, probable etiology.
4) Discuss management of aggravating activities.
5) Identify with patient mechanism to alleviate pain.
6) Review and reinforce information about medications.

c. Evaluation of nursing care
1) Verbalize understanding of TOS.
2) Identify strategies to minimize symptoms.
3) Take medication as ordered and report any adverse events.

B. Postoperative Care

1. Alteration in comfort related to postoperative pain from surgical incision
a. Expected outcome: adequate control of acute postoperative pain
b. Nursing intervention
1) Assess pain level on specific scale (e.g., 0 to 10 scale); reassess after implementation of pain management techniques.
2) Identify aggravating and alleviating factors.
3) Set pain level target with patient.

4) Use nonmedication strategies as appropriate, including breathing techniques, relaxation, positioning, and diversion therapy.
5) Administer medication as appropriate.

c. Evaluation of nursing care
   1) Pain level on scale of 10 is 4 or less or at identified target

2. Ineffective airway clearance related to pain and potential ineffective cough
   a. Expected outcome: exhibits adequate respiratory function
   b. Nursing intervention
      1) Assess lung sounds and respiratory rate, temperature at regular intervals (potential for atelectasis and pneumonia)
      2) Encourage lung expansion
         a) Cough and deep breathing frequently
         b) Use incentive spirometer, if indicated.
         c) Ambulate at regular intervals.
      3) Maintain adequate hydration
      4) Review postoperative chest film and report abnormal findings to physician
   c. Evaluation of nursing care
      1) Demonstrate effective coughing and deep breathing.
      2) Maintain patent airway and clear lung sounds.
3. Potential neurodeficit related to neurocompromise
   a. Expected outcome: absence of neurocompromise
   b. Nursing interventions
      1) Monitor ulnar, radial, and palmar arch pulses.
      2) Assess color warmth and movement of fingers/hand.
      3) Assess sensory motor function of affected arm.
      4) Elevate arm on pillow in presence of edema.
   c. Evaluation
      1) Motor sensory function intact
4. Potential alteration in peripheral tissue perfusion
   a. Expected outcome: maintenance of adequate circulation and perfusion to affected extremity
   b. Nursing intervention
      1) Assess arterial and venous circulation.
         a) Monitor radial pulse, color, warmth, movement, numbness, and tingling.
         b) Examine for edema, venous distention.
      2) Position for comfort in neutral position, may elevate on pillow
   c. Evaluation of nursing care
      1) Circulation intact
5. Potential for infection
   a. Expected outcome: free from infection
   b. Nursing intervention
      1) Monitor vital signs at regular intervals
      2) Monitor laboratory work, especially WBC as indicated
      3) Maintain aseptic technique in dressing changes and management of drains
      4) Assess IV sites and drain sites
   c. Evaluation of nursing care
      1) Temperature within normal limits
      2) Wound healing without evidence of infection

X. Patient Teaching

A. Conservative Management

1. Encourage participation by family/significant others.
2. Define TOS.
3. Discuss effect of chronic pain on ADL and family role.
4. Discuss alterations and methods to adjust lifestyle; identify strategies to deal with symptom management.
5. Reinforce and encourage physical therapy exercises to be continued at home after initial instruction in physical therapy department.
6. Discuss diet: high protein, low animal fat.
7. Discuss activity, balance of activity, and rest.
8. Discuss medication, including pain cycle use, dose, and adverse effects.

B. Preoperative

1. Complete required preoperative testing (laboratory work, ECG, and others as indicated)
2. Discuss hospital admission process (registration, surgery, postoperative unit)
3. Anticipate postoperative course, including nursing assessments, medication administration, and length of stay
4. Encourage questions for clarification and understanding
5. Provide support to patient and family/significant others

C. Postoperative

1. Wound care
   a. Observe for changes and note swelling, redness, drainage, or bleeding
   b. May shower, wash with soap and water, pat dry
   c. Wear deodorant only above incision line until wound healed
2. Medications, including pain cycle use, dose, adverse effects
3. Activity
   a. Activity as tolerated
   b. No driving until first postoperative visit
   c. May use arm for simple activities (e.g., brushing teeth, eating), but maintain below shoulder level until given instructions on postoperative exercise
   d. Do not carry purse or backpack with affected arm until postoperative visit.
4. Diet
   a. High-protein diet is needed for wound healing
   b. Low animal fat
5. Signs and symptoms of infection
   a. Observe for signs of redness or drainage from surgical incision
   b. Report elevated temperature
   c. Maintain good handwashing
   d. Take acetaminophen or ibuprofen for fever, unless specifically contraindicated. Discuss with physician or nurse
6. Follow-up appointments
   a. Usually 1 to 2 weeks after discharge
   b. Notify sooner for any questions or unusual findings
   c. Postoperative exercise instructions usually given at first postoperative visit

CASE STUDY

EJ is a 29-year-old woman who was referred to the vascular surgeon for evaluation of possible TOS. With the exceptions of her current problems, her past medical history is negative. Current medications include birth control pills and over-the-counter treatment for arm pain and headaches. She states that the acetaminophen is no longer effective.

She started teaching 6 months previously, which required increased computer work and arm elevation to write on the board. She is a harp player and plays or practices five nights a week for minimum of 1 hour duration.

Current symptoms include pain in the upper right arm for 2 years, but the pain has worsened since starting teaching. She has paresthesia when playing harp. She also states that she is having increasing numbers of headaches and neck pain.

Objective evaluation exhibited the following findings: A young female, 5′7″ tall and 127 lbs, with a slight frame. She is right handed. Blood pressures are equal bilaterally. There is no bruit noted over the supraclavicular fossa. Brachial, radial, and ulnar pulses are 2+ at rest and elevation. Hands are pink and warm and have strong hand grasp. No evidence of micro-embolization or venous distention. There is tenderness over the supraclavicular area, and her symptoms are reproducible with pressure.

Review Questions

1. What provocative maneuvers during physical examination can assist in the diagnosis of TOS?
2. List three disorders that must be considered in the differential diagnosis of TOS.
3. Diagnostic testing, including chest x-ray, C-spine films, EMG/NCV, and MRI were completed, and the diagnosis of neurogenic TOS on the right side was made. At this time, patient had not exhausted medical treatment.

   Patient education should include what conservative measures to improve symptoms and control pain?
4. Patient did well with exercise for 2 years. Now returns with complaint of increased pain in lower arm, numbness in the fourth and fifth digits of right hand. She states that she has clumsiness and seems to have difficulty with fine motor movement necessary to play the harp.

   On physical examination, her right hand is cool at rest and pale when elevated. Pulses are 1+ at rest and absent with elevation. Medications now include Tylenol #3, which she states she is taking at night to help her sleep and once or twice a day as needed. An arterial duplex scan is positive for diminished flow during TOS maneuvers.

   What were the indications for surgery?
5. Patient underwent a right transaxillary rib resection and was discharged on the second postoperative day. What should her discharge teaching include?

Answers/Rationales

1. (a) EAST (elevated arm stress test; Dr. Roos). Arm elevation for 3 minutes with 90-degree shoulder abduction and external rotation and elbow flexed at 90 degrees. Patient opens and closes the hand rapidly. The test result is positive with reproduction of symptoms; (b) Adson test. With the patient's arm at the side and his or her head turned toward the affected side, the patient takes a deep breath and the radial pulse is monitored. Test is modified with head turned toward unaffected side. Test result is positive if radial pulse is obliterated. This test is considered nonspecific in diagnosis of neurogenic TOS; (c) Roos maneuver. Supraclavicular

compression of the brachial plexus at the scalenus anticus level. With compression, symptoms may be reproduced; (d) Halsted test (costoclavicular test). Patient assumes a military pose with shoulder backward and downward to narrow the costoclavicular space. The radial pulse is monitored and test result is positive with obliteration of pulse; (e) Wright test. Hyperabduction external rotation of shoulder to 180 degrees. The radial pulse is monitored and a positive test result is indicated with obliteration of radial pulse.

2. Any of the following:

Cervical disc disease	Carpal tunnel syndrome
Ulnar nerve entrapment	Causalgia
Rotator cuff syndrome	Paraspinal muscle myofibrositis
Mitral valve prolapse	Angina pectoris
Raynaud disease	Soft tissue disorders/tumors

3. (a) Physical therapy to restore movement of shoulder girdle and provide more space for neurovascular structures. Should include postural correction and strengthening exercises. This starts with a supervised program and continues in a home exercise program; (b) Massage to produce muscle relaxation and comfort; (c) Heat in chronic TOS is recommended as pain relief and to help reduce spasms; (d) Medications, which may include anti-inflammatory agents, muscle relaxants, and analgesics. Antidepressant drugs may be helpful in some patients; (e) Analgesics, if necessary, should start with over-the-counter medication before narcotics are initiated. They should be used in combination with other pain control modalities; (f) Pain control measures should include alternatives to medications, such as biofeedback, diversion, and relaxation therapy; (g) Psychological support should be offered to patient and family because TOS can affect body image, role in family, and financial and social status of the entire family.
4. (a) Increase in neurogenic symptoms: pain in lower arm extending down to digits, "clumsiness," and decreased fine motor movement of fingers; (b) Evidence of an arterial component: cool hand, pale on elevation, diminished pulses at rest and absent with elevation; (c) Increasing requirements for medication for pain control. Decreasing quality of life.
5. (a) Wound care: Observe for changes and note swelling, redness, drainage, or bleeding. May shower, wash with soap and water, and pat dry. Wear deodorant only above incision line until wound healed; (b) Activity: Activity as tolerated; no driving until first postoperative visit. May use arm for simple activities (i.e., brush teeth, eat, but maintain arm below shoulder level until given instructions on postoperative exercise). Do not carry purse or backpack with affected arm until postoperative visit; (c) Diet: Low animal fat, high-protein diet is needed for wound healing; (d) Signs and symptoms of infection: Observe for signs of redness or drainage from surgical incision. Report elevated temperature. Maintain good handwashing. May take acetaminophen or ibuprofen for fever, unless specific contraindications. Discuss with physician or nurse; (e) Rehabilitation: May be slow and should not be rushed. Work evaluation may be required for patient to continue in the same job or determine if work reassignment is required.

REFERENCES

Atasoy, E. (1996). Thoracic outlet compression syndrome. *Orthopedic Clinics of North America, 27*(2), 265–303.

Kieffer, E., & Ruotolo, C. (1995). Arterial complications of thoracic outlet syndrome. In R. Rutherford (Ed.), *Vascular surgery* (4th ed., pp. 992–999). Philadelphia, PA: W.B. Saunders.

Machleder, H. (1993). Vascular disease of the upper extremity and the thoracic outlet syndromes. In W. Moore (Ed.), *Vascular surgery: A comprehensive review* (pp. 597–605). Philadelphia, PA: W.B. Saunders.

Machleder, H. (1994). Thoracic outlet disorders: Thoracic outlet compression syndrome and axillary vein thrombosis. In F. Veith, R. Hobson, R. Williams, & S. Wilson (Eds.), *Vascular surgery principles and practice* (2nd ed.). New York, NY: McGraw Hill.

MacKinnon, S., & Novak, C. (2002). Thoracic outlet syndrome. *Current Problems in Surgery, 39*, 1070–1145.

Martinez, B. (1999). Thoracic outlet syndrome: Endoscopic transaxillary first rib resection and thoracodorsal sympathectomy for causalgia. In R. White & T. Fogarty (Eds.), *Peripheral endovascular interventions* (2nd ed., pp. 531–538). New York, NY: Springer.

Mingoli, A., Feldhaus, R. J., Farina, C., Cavallari, N., Sapienza, P., di Marzo, L., & Cavallaro, A. (1995). Long-term outcome after transaxillary approach for thoracic outlet syndrome. *Surgery, 118*(5), 840–844.

Sanders, R. J. (2010). Thoracic outlet syndrome, general considerations. In J. L. Cronenwett & K. W. Johnston (Eds.), *Rutherford's vascular surgery* (7th ed., pp. 1865–1877). Philadelphia, PA: Saunders.

Stoney, R., & Cheng, S. (1995). Neurogenic thoracic outlet syndrome. In R. Rutherford (Ed.), *Vascular surgery* (4th ed., pp. 976–992). Philadelphia, PA: W.B. Saunders.

Urschel, H., & Razzuk, M. (1997). Upper plexus thoracic outlet syndrome: Optimal therapy. *Annals of Thoracic Surgery, 63*, 935–939.

Urschel, H., & Razzuk, M. (1998). Neurovascular compression in thoracic outlet: Changing management over 50 years. *Annals of Surgery, 228*(4), 609–617.

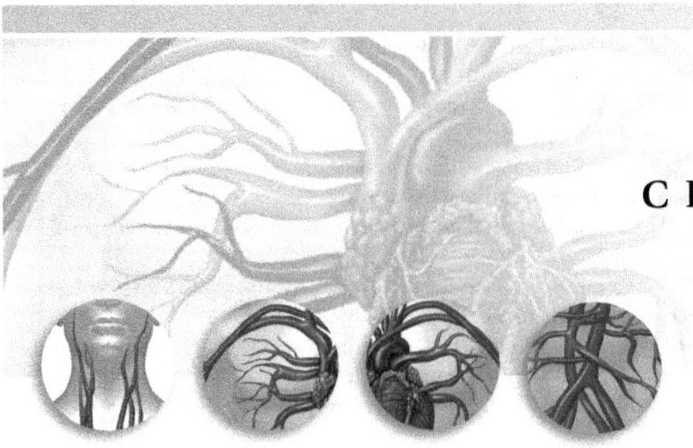

CHAPTER 19

Superficial Thrombophlebitis and Deep Vein Thrombosis

Melody Heffline
M. Kate Schmidt
First Edition Authors: *Kim Zurat and Karla Mees*

OBJECTIVES

1. Describe the clinical significance of superficial and deep venous thrombosis.
2. Identify the risk factors for both superficial thrombophlebitis (STP) and deep vein thrombosis (DVT).
3. Identify diagnostic tests and procedures frequently used in the evaluation and treatment of venous thromboembolism.
4. Discuss the medial and surgical treatments for both STP and DVT.
5. Describe treatment modalities and essential elements of nursing care in management of thromboembolism.

Introduction

Venous thromboembolism is a major health problem. The Center for Disease Control (CDC) estimates the prevalence of venous disease to affect between 300,000 and 600,000 annually in the United States; of those 200,000 to 400,000 are diagnosed with DVT and 100,000 to 200,000 of those individuals will embolize to the pulmonary system. Around 30,000 to 60,000 of patients, who sustain pulmonary emboli (PE), will die (Office of the Surgeon General [US], 2008).

Venous thrombosis (clot formation) can occur in the superficial or deep venous systems. Superficial thrombus is clot formed in the superficial system producing pain, swelling, and erythematous streaking. Superficial venous thrombosis (SVT) are common affecting at least 125,000 people annually, with the incidence higher in women during pregnancy and in the postpartum period. The overall incidence has risen with the increased use of intravenous catheters and occurs more frequently when plastic catheters are inserted in the lower extremities (Ferri, 2011). STPs are generally treated symptomatically and rarely extend into the perforating veins and into the deep venous system.

DVT carries a higher risk of morbidity and mortality than STPs. One of the most serious complications is PE which occurs in more than one third of patients with DVT (Hirsh, Guyatt, Albers, Harrington, & Schunemann, 2008).

Venous disease also has a tremendous impact on the quality of life for thousands of Americans and presents a significant economic burden to the health care system. Increased awareness and early detection is important to reduce long-term sequelae and potential extension of the disease with the accompanied increased risk of death.

I. Anatomy (see also Chapter 3, Anatomy and Physiology of the Vascular System)

A. Deep Venous System

1. Names correspond to the named arteries
2. Includes larger, deep veins
3. Lie below fascia and bound by muscle fascia
   a. Abdomen
      1) Inferior vena cava, mesenteric, renal, hepatic (in order of flow)
   b. Lower extremity
      1) Tibial, peroneal, popliteal, femoral, iliac
   c. Upper extremity
      1) Radial, ulnar, brachial, axillary, subclavian, jugular, innominate, superior vena cava

B. Superficial Venous System

1. Smaller veins, closer to the skin
2. Lie within subcutaneous tissue
   a. Lower extremity
      1) Greater saphenous
      2) Lesser saphenous
   b. Upper extremity
      1) Cephalic
      2) Basilic

C. Perforating Veins

1. Connect the deep and superficial venous systems by penetrating through the fascia (see Fig. 19-1)

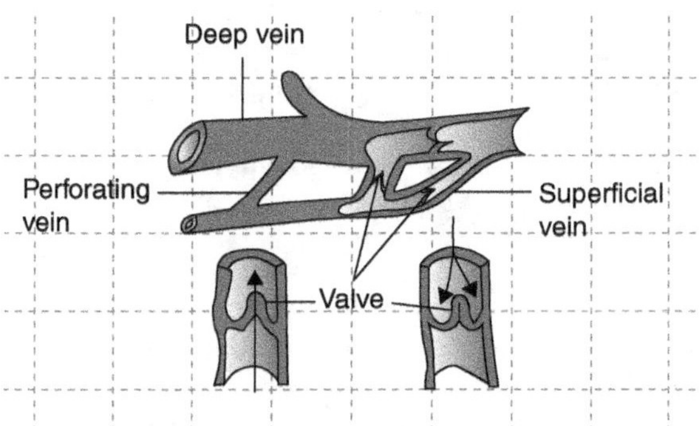

FIGURE 19-1. Anatomy of the venous system.

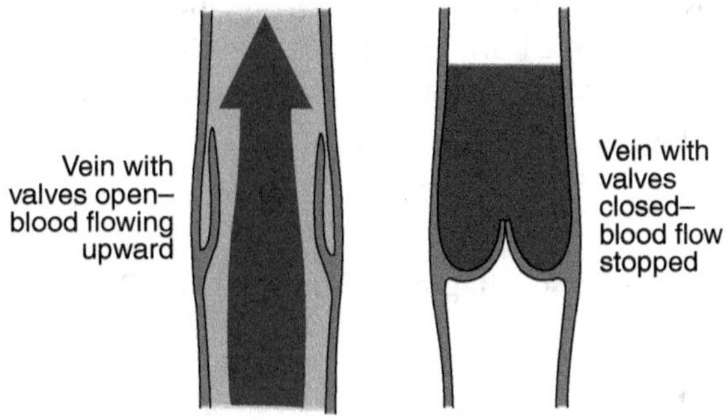

FIGURE 19-2. Venous valvular function.

D. Vein Structure

1. Tunica intima
   a. Innermost layer
   b. Endothelium, connective tissue, basement membrane
2. Tunica media
   a. Smooth muscle and classic fibers
3. Tunica externa
   a. Thin layer of connective tissue containing graduated and collagenous fibers

E. Valves (see Fig. 19-2)

1. One-way valves located within the veins
2. Open in diastole and closed in systole
3. Larger number of valves in distal veins (peroneal, tibial, popliteal); few in femoral and iliac; vena cava has no valves
4. Provide unidirectional blood flow back to heart (McCance & Huether, 2010)

II. Pathophysiology

A. Inflammatory response triggered by the clotting cascade (tissue factor pathway)

B. Coagulation Cascade (tissue factor pathway)

1. Initiated by vascular injury
   a. Exposes the connective tissue matrix leading to platelet adhesion and formation of hemostatic plug
   b. Tissue factor collaborates with secreted platelet factor and activated platelets to activate the clotting system to form fibrin clots
   c. The fibrin/platelet clot contracts to form a more permanent plug
   d. Regulatory pathways are activated (fibrinolysis) to limit the size of the plug and begin the healing process

C. Virchow Triad

1. Three factors that result in DVT known also as Virchow triad
   a. Local venous trauma
   b. Stasis of venous blood flow
   c. Systemic coagulation abnormalities (McCance & Huether, 2010)

2. Risk factors for STP and DVT
   a. Trauma is common cause of STP—either a direct blow or iatrogenic injury (e.g., intravenous line or cannula with infusion of substances caustic to the vein wall)
      1) Hypertonic solution: potassium chloride
      2) Injurious compounds: antibiotics, barbiturates, benzodiazepines, chemotherapeutic agents
      3) Needle insertion, which causes local inflammatory response
      4) Incidence of catheter related is 0.1%, 100 out of 100,000 (Ferri, 2011)
      5) Sclerotherapy of varicose vein is an example of beneficial effects of traumatic thrombophlebitis: a hypertonic agent is injected into the telangiectasia or varix to cause local inflammation and subsequent permanent scarring with closure of the vessel
   b. Infection

D. Potential Outcomes of a VTE

1. Superficial VTE
   a. Extension into deep vein system
      1) Lower extremity: at the saphenofemoral junction thrombus moves from greater saphenous vein into common femoral vein; at lesser saphenous vein thrombus moves into popliteal vein
      2) Upper extremity: thrombus moves from cephalic into axillary and subclavian vein
      3) 20% of STP cases are associated with occult DVT (Ferri, 2011)
   b. Signs and symptoms of superficial VTE
      1) Subcutaneous vein is palpable, tender; cord present with erythema and edema of the overlying skin and subcutaneous tissue
      2) Induration, redness, and tenderness are localized along the course of the vein. This linear appearance rather than circular appearance is useful to distinguish thrombophlebitis from other conditions (cellulitis, erythema nodosum)
      3) No significant swelling of the limb
      4) Low-grade fever may be present; high-grade fevers are suggestive of septic phlebitis
   c. Suppurative thrombophlebitis: infectious process, usually at intravenous puncture site
      1) Serious, potentially lethal; requires rapid treatment
      2) Usual pathogens: *Staphylococcus aureus* was the most common pathogen, found in 65% to 78% of the cases of superficial suppurative thrombophlebitis before 1970; now the most cases are caused by *Enterobacteriaceae,* especially Klebsiella–Enterobacter spp. Usually acquired nosocomially and often resistant to multiple antibiotics (Ferri, 2011)
      3) Signs and symptoms
         a) Pus at intravenous line site (fever), elevated white blood cell count, intense pain at site (Hingorani & Ascher, 2009)
         b) Superficial suppurative thrombophlebitis may be difficult to identify because local findings of inflammation may be absent. Fever is present in >70% of cases but rigors are rare
         c) Local finding (warmth, erythema, tenderness, swelling, lymphangitis) are present in only one third of patients (Ferri, 2011)

d. Migratory thrombophlebitis
   1) Multiple STPs at various sites most common in lower extremities
   2) May be associated with carcinoma and may precede diagnosis of the carcinoma by several years
   3) Workup for occult malignancy may be warranted (Hingorani & Ascher, 2009)
   4) Other causes of migratory STP
      a) Hypercoagulable states: protein C resistance, deficiencies of anti-thrombin III, protein C, and protein S
      b) Estrogen therapy and birth control pills
      c) Vasculitis: patients who have Buerger disease may develop "phlebitis migrans"; also seen in patients who have polyarteritis nodosa
      d) Mondor disease: STP of the thoracoepigastric vein of the breast and chest wall. Thought to be associated with breast carcinoma or hypercoagulable state but some reported with no identifiable cause. Term also applied to SVT of dorsal vein of the penis. Treatment consists of conservative measures with warm compresses and NSAIDs (Hingorani & Ascher, 2009)
      e) If multiple STPs occur in younger patient, suspect inflammatory vasculitis process; in an older patient, suspect malignancy

2. DVT
   a. Pulmonary embolism, possibly fatal (refer to Chapter 20, Pulmonary Embolism)
   b. Increased risk of long-term morbidity from post-thrombotic syndromes and chronic venous insufficiency (refer to Chapter 21, Chronic Venous Disease and Venous Ulcers)
      1) Chronic changes in size, shape, and skin texture of the lower extremity caused by increased ambulatory venous pressure
      2) Limb initially develops chronic swelling; over time, shape changes to that of an inverted champagne bottle because of distal leg skin sclerosis of subcutaneous fat layer (lipodermatosclerosis)
      3) Nonhealing venous ulcers may form on medial and lateral malleolar surface because of effects of high venous pressure and absence of skin elasticity
      4) 20% to 50% of patients with DVT develop post-thrombotic syndrome characterized by leg edema, pain, venous ectasia, skin induration, and ulcerations. Patients with extensive DVT and those with more severe post-thrombotic manifestations 1 month after DVT have poor long-term outcomes (Ferri, 2011)
   c. High costs related to diagnosis, hospital readmissions, treatment of VTE, and long-term complications
   d. Phlegmasia alba dolens
      1) Advanced iliofemoral venous thrombosis commonly seen in pregnant women
      2) Limb is swollen, pale, cool; nonpalpable pulses
      3) Appearance of leg is caused by "severe perivenous inflammatory reaction extending to the peri-arterial sympathetic nerve fibers, producing arterial spasm or compression" (Walsh & Rice, 2004)
   e. Phlegmasia cerulean dolens (also known as venous gangrene)
      1) Near-total occlusion of venous outflow with increased venous pressure inhibiting arterial inflow

2) Seen in advanced carcinomas, especially of the pelvis or abdomen
3) Gangrene may result from combined arterial insufficiency with severe venous congestion
4) Patient complains of sudden deep pain, massive edema, and cyanosis of the limb (Walsh & Rice, 2004)

III. Etiology/Precipitating Risk Factors

A. Age

1. Most consistently associated with increased risk of DVT
2. Increases by factor of 200 between ages 20 and 80 with relative risk of 1.9 for each 10 year increase in age
3. Appears related to several age-associated factors
   a. Decreased mobility
   b. Increased number of major thrombotic risk factors
   c. Age-related hypercoagulability
   d. Changes in the venous system

B. Surgery

1. Multifactorial
   a. Perioperative immobilization with resulting venous stasis
   b. Activated coagulation
   c. Transient depression of fibrinolysis
   d. Increases in thrombin activation
   e. Elevated levels of plasminogen and activator inhibitor
2. Degree of risk varies by
   a. Age of the patient
   b. Length and type of procedure
   c. Presence of other thrombotic risk factors
3. Incidence of DVT based on type of surgery
   a. 25% general surgery
   b. 32% retropubic prostatectomy
   c. 22% and 14% for gynecological procedures with and without malignancy
   d. 22% for elective neurosurgical procedures
   e. 45%, 51%, and 47% among those having surgery for hip fracture, hip arthroplasty, and knee arthroplasty, respectively (Meissner, 2009)
4. Postoperative patients at risk during entire period of immobility, especially after discharge when support for ambulation and activity may be lessened

C. Hormones

1. Oral contraceptives
   a. Those that contain both estrogen and progestin increase the risk of a blood clot by 2 to 8 fold
   b. The risk may be even greater with patches that contain transdermal contraceptives, since the amount of estrogen absorbed can be 60% higher
   c. The absolute risk of women of fertile age using oral contraceptives is fairly low at 2 to 8 per 10,000 person-years, substantially lower that the risk faced by older men and women (US Dept of HR, 2008)

   d. The highest risk of VTE occurs during the first year of use (Walsh & Rice, 2004)
   e. Risk remains until the third month following discontinuation (McBane & Heit, 2009)
2. Hormone replacement therapy (HRT)
   a. The relative risk of HRT is reported to be comparable to that of oral contraceptives despite a significantly lower amount of estrogen (Walsh & Rice, 2004)
3. Pregnancy
   a. Risk of VTE increases 3 to 6 fold during pregnancy and is evenly distributed across all three trimesters
   b. Rate of VTE after pregnancy is 172 to 199 per 100,000 deliveries
   c. Risk is higher after cesarean section than vaginal delivery
   d. Risks may be related to
      1) High estrogen levels
      2) Venous stasis
      3) Pelvic trauma with delivery
      4) Acquired hypercoagulability related to elevated procoagulants variables such as fibrinogen, von Willebrand factor, and factor VIII as well as decreased natural anticoagulants such as protein S
   e. Risk factors associated with thrombosis during pregnancy include
      1) Increasing age (>35 years)
      2) Immobility
      3) Obesity
      4) Previous DVT
      5) African Americans appear to have a greater risk than Caucasians (McBane & Heit, 2009)

D. Cancer

1. Incidence of VTE in patients with an active malignancy may be as high as 11% (McBane & Heit, 2009)
2. Tumors secrete clotting factor—tissue thromboplastin—like substance
3. High risk for development of thrombophlebitis
   a. Risk of venous thrombosis after surgery for malignancy is 2 to 5 fold increased risk for postoperative VTE than surgery for nonmalignant conditions (Caprini & Arcelus, 2007)
   b. Decreased fibrinolytic activity
   c. Compression or infiltration of vein by tumor
   d. Increased age
   e. Greater likelihood of needing surgical procedure
   f. Exposure to chemotherapeutic agents
   g. Multiple invasive procedures and indwelling catheters
4. Patients with cancer have a >2 fold increased risk for VTE recurrence than those without cancer (Caprini & Arcelus, 2007)
5. Active cancers account for 20% of incidental VTE occurring in the community
6. Highest rates of venous thrombosis occur in carcinomas involving the kidney, stomach, pancreas, brain, and lymphoma
7. Lowest rates occurred in cancers of the head/neck, bladder, breast, esophagus, uterus, and cervix (Walsh & Rice, 2004)

8. Idiopathic venous thrombosis associated with 7.6% of malignancy; recurrent venous thrombosis associated with 17.1% incidence of malignancy (Mcbane & Heit, 2009)

E. Immobilization: bed rest of 72 hours or longer

1. Venous return is compromised due to lack of calf muscle pump activity
2. Blood pools in the extremities, increasing the risk of clot formation
3. Can be secondary to surgery, trauma, illness, or stroke resulting in paralysis

F. Heart Disease

1. Promotes stasis and emboli formation
2. Congestive heart failure; elevated central venous pressure and patients are often less mobile
3. Atrial fibrillation, cardiomyopathy, myocardial infarction, prosthetic heart valve, and valvular heart disease

G. Dehydration/Sepsis (relative hypercoagulable state)

H. Venipuncture/Numerous Central Catheters

I. Pulmonary Disease: severe chronic obstructive pulmonary disease with increased right heart pressure/failure reducing venous return

J. Previous History of DVT, PE, or Venous Disease

1. 30% develop recurrence within 10 years
2. 20% with optimal therapy will have extension or recurrence (Caprini & Arcelus, 2007)

K. Morbid Obesity

1. Increased incidence of DVT noted in patients weighing 20% above ideal weight for age, sex, and frame size, but obesity is not yet identified as an independent risk factor
2. Impaired fibrinolytic system
3. Increased immobility

L. Medications: chemotherapy and hormone therapy

M. Varicose Veins: the most frequent predisposing risk factor for SVT is presence of varicose veins, which occurs in 62% of patients (Hingorani & Ascher, 2009).

1. Varicosities adjacent to venous ulcers are more likely to become phlebitic.
2. Greater and lesser saphenous vein varicosities more often involved.
3. Spontaneous bleeding from grapelike clusters of telangiectasias near ankle can occur because of high venous pressure in these small superficial vessels. Small ulcers may then occur at the site of bleeding.

N. Inherited Factors

1. Antithrombin III deficiency
2. Protein C & S deficiency
3. Factor V Leiden mutation
4. Prothrombin 20210 mutation
5. Dysfibrinogenemia

O. Travel

1. Association between travel and VTE controversial
2. Association appears related to duration of travel
3. Most individuals with VTE associated with prolonged travel have additional risk factors (Mcbane & Heit, 2009)

P. Others

1. Myeloproliferative disorders
2. Polycythemia vera

IV. Primary Prevention

A. Ambulatory/Outpatient Setting

1. Assess for presence of risk factors
2. Promote education regarding risk factors
3. Promote healthy lifestyle
4. Special coagulations studies
   a. May be obtained if there is a family history of thrombophlebitis, especially in family members under the age of 40 with no other risk factors for DVT
   b. May be used to assess if patient is a high risk for development of thrombophlebitis
5. Nonpharmacologic methods for VTE prophylaxis
   a. Exercise
      1) Walking as much as possible
      2) Dorsi/plantar flexion of feet with prolonged sitting or bed rest to promote venous return
6. Nonpharmacologic methods for VTE prophylaxis
   a. Early mobilization
      1) Routine part of postoperative care
      2) Sole prophylaxis in lower-risk patients (<40 years of age without additional risk factors having minor surgery; less than 45 minutes) (Caprini & Arcelus, 2007)
   b. Graduated compression stockings, 15 to 20 mm Hg pressure
      1) Less effective than other methods
      2) Recommended as an adjunct for most moderate or higher-risk patients
      3) In the absence of palpable dorsalis pedis or posterior tibial pulses, an ABI is required
      4) Contraindicated in patients with ABI <0.5
   c. Intermittent pneumatic compression (IPC)
      1) Recommended in combination with compression stocking after neurosurgery (Ferri, 2011)

2) Has been recommended in multiple trauma patients when anticoagulation is not feasible, especially in the setting of active bleeding (Mcbane & Heit, 2009)
3) Research suggests IPC can reduce risk in general surgical patients; strong evidence for use of IPC as sole therapy in moderate risk patients and as adjunctive therapy in high risk patients but more research is needed (Caprini & Arcelus, 2007)

d. Consider inferior vena cava filter placement, if other forms of prophylaxis are contraindicated

B. Pharmacologic Methods for VTE Prophylaxis

1. Low-dose unfractionated heparin (UFH)
   a. Facilitates the binding of antithrombin III with the activated clotting factors thrombin, factor IXa and Xa
   b. Subcutaneous administration, usually with twice-daily injections; typical dose is 2,500 to 5,000 units
   c. Half-life is 0.5 to 2.5 hours
   d. Use is decreasing because of the availability of low-molecular-weight heparin (LMWH)
2. LMWH
   a. Lovenox (enoxaparin), Fragmin, (dalteparin), Innohep (tinzaparin)
   b. Facilitates the binding of antithrombin III with activated clotting proteins, catalyzing inactivation of thrombin and other clotting factors
   c. Can be administered subcutaneously as an outpatient or inpatient
3. Direct thrombin inhibitor
4. Factor Xa inhibitor
5. Oral vitamin K antagonist: warfarin may be recommended prophylactically for high-risk patients with a history of previous VTE
6. Oral direct thrombin inhibitor

C. Surgical Hospitalized Patients: example of an institution-specific protocol for DVT prevention (see Table 19-1)

V. Assessment

A. Risk Factors

1. Family history of venous thrombosis and or familial thrombophilia
2. Acquired thrombophilia
3. Assess for predisposing factors contributing to venous thrombosis as listed above

B. Patient History

1. Subjective
   a. Focused history of patient, previous episodes of thrombophlebitis
   b. Family history of venous thrombophlebitis or familial thrombophilia
   c. Symptoms and duration of symptoms
   d. Pain assessment, severity and location
2. Objective
   a. Thrombophlebitis documented by diagnostic testing

TABLE 19-1 Prevention of Deep Vein Thrombosis (DVT) in Hospitalized Patients

Type of Patient	Prevention Measures
1. Low risk (no history of DVT, minor surgery, under 40)	Early Ambulation
2. Moderate risk (past history of DVT, orthopedic surgery, hip fracture)	1. Low dose UFH* 2. Preoperative LMWH started 12–24 hrs preoperatively 3. Graduated compression stockings and pneumatic compression device 4. Warfarin started pre- or postoperative with International Normalized Ratio (INR) goal 2.5, range 2–3
3. Higher risk (history of DVT, abdominal surgery, bed rest, immobilization)	1. UFH or LMWH, weight based 2. Pneumatic compression device and graduated compression stockings 3. Warfarin with INR goal 2.5, range 2–3
4. High risk (general surgery patient with wound complications)	1. Pneumatic compression device 2. Graduated compression stockings 3. Evaluate risks and benefits of anticoagulation 4. Consider inferior vena caval filter if other forms of prophylaxis contraindicated
5. Very high risk (recent DVT, major abdominal surgery, neuro surgery, multiple trauma, prolonged immobility/bed rest)	1. Low dose UFH 2. LWMH, weight based 3. Pneumatic compression device and graduated compression stockings 4. Warfarin with INR goal 2.5, range 2–3 5. Inferior vena caval filter

*Anticoagulation monitoring not required for low-dose subcutaneous heparin, but platelet count should be checked every 2 to 3 days to assess for heparin-induced thrombocytopenia (HIT).

b. STP: unilateral limb swelling along an erythematous, tender, palpable cord. If limb is generally swollen or STP is in high, suspect coexistent DVT

C. Clinical Diagnosis of DVT is Unreliable

1. Many DVTs are clinically silent or asymptomatic, especially if obstruction is only partial, thrombus is small or collateral vessels have developed around complete obstruction (Walsh & Rice, 2004)
2. Up to 70% of patients presenting with complaints consistent with DVT will not have the disease and many patients with DVT will be asymptomatic (Lohr, Kin, & Krallman, 2009)
3. Homan sign (pain in the upper calf during forced dorsiflexion of the foot) is insensitive and nonspecific
4. Other nonspecific signs and symptoms: leg cramps, redness, cyanosis, varicose vein distention

D. Physical Examination

1. Inspection
   a. Swelling, erythema, streaking, cord
      1) Compare contralateral limb
      2) Distended neck or chest veins in upper extremity and/or central thrombosis

3) Presence of dilated superficial veins
4) Presence of cyanosis or inflammation

b. Varicosities or signs of chronic venous disease (skin changes, ulceration)
c. Oral mucosa for evidence of petechiae or bleeding

2. Palpation
   a. Assess pulses
   b. Amount of edema: measure circumference of both limbs at similar levels and document
   c. Skin: check for warmth, erythema
   d. Palpable cord
   e. Liver or spleen enlargement
3. Auscultation
   a. Lung and cardiac examination for tachypnea, tachycardia, or murmurs
4. Vital signs
   a. Temperature: presence of a fever
   b. Blood pressure: hypo- or hypertension
   c. Respiratory rate: tachypnea, congestion
   d. Heart rate, rhythm and sounds for presence of arrhythmia, tachycardia, or murmurs
5. Height and weight
6. Homan sign: limited usefulness because of lack of sensitivity and specificity

E. Differential Diagnosis (Ferri, 2011)

1. SVT
   a. Lymphangitis
   b. Cellulitis
   c. Erythema nodosum
   d. Panniculitis
   e. Kaposi sarcoma
2. DVT
   a. Postphlebitic syndrome
   b. STP
   c. Ruptured Baker's cyst
   d. Cellulitis or lymphangitis, Achilles tendonitis
   e. Hematoma
   f. Muscle or soft tissue injury, stress fracture
   g. Varicose veins, lymphedema
   h. Arterial insufficiency
   i. Abscess
   j. Claudication
   k. Venous stasis

F. Considerations Across the Life Span

1. Young adulthood
   a. Participation in contact sports
   b. Oral contraceptive
   c. Alcohol, tobacco, or illicit drug use
   d. Compliance
   e. Presence of other disease

f. Diabetes
g. Cancer
h. Recent surgery or trauma, high-risk occupations such as long distance drivers or travelers, and sedentary office workers
i. Consider familial hypercoagulability if no other known risk factors present
j. Nutritional status and dietary habits, especially vegetarianism
k. Other medications and potential interactions with anticoagulants

2. Women of childbearing age
   a. Oral contraceptive use
   b. Conception planned
      1) Warfarin crosses placenta and causes neural tube birth defects
      2) Consider low-dose UFH or LMWH, which does not cross the placenta; if on warfarin (Coumadin) prior to conception for previous thromboembolic event, may need therapeutic dosing of LMWH throughout pregnancy rather than low dose
   c. Alcohol, tobacco, or illicit drug use
   d. Compliance
   e. Nutritional status and dietary habits
   f. Other medications and potential interactions with warfarin
3. Elderly
   a. HRT
   b. Safety issues
      1) History of falls
      2) Home environment
      3) Presence of support system
      4) Memory issues
      5) Increased risk of bleeding
      6) Compliance
   c. General health and nutrition status: may require a lower dose of warfarin
   d. Use of alcohol, tobacco, or illicit drugs
   e. Other medications
      1) Interaction with warfarin
      2) Clues to treatment for medical comorbidities

VI. Pertinent Diagnostic Testing

A. Noninvasive

1. Duplex ultrasound (also refer to Chapter 5, Vascular Diagnostic Studies)
   a. First-line test; ≥95% sensitive and specific for proximal DVT
   b. Real-time sonography allows visualization of veins and thrombi in transverse and longitudinal views, including "floating" thrombi that could embolize (Walsh & Rice, 2004)
   c. Detects venous flow in both gray scale and color; can assess for antegrade and retrograde (reflux) flow direction
2. Computed tomography
   a. Not usually ordered to diagnose thrombophlebitis, but thrombophlebitis may be visualized
   b. Useful in pelvic or abdominal DVT diagnosis

B. Invasive

1. Ascending venography
   a. Seldom performed because of high sensitivity of duplex scan, cost, and potential complications of invasive procedure
   b. Involves placement of catheter in the dorsum of the foot, radiopaque contrast medium injection and use of x-ray
   c. Provides accurate visualization of the veins and thrombi
   d. Criteria for DVT diagnosis: intraluminal filling defect seen in multiple views
   e. Useful for equivocal duplex scans
   f. Complications: pain at injection site; hyperosmolar contrast may cause damage to endothelium of vessel and lead to STP or DVT; hypersensitivity reaction, renal failure, and potential for skin necrosis due to extravasation of contrast at the injection site

C. Other Less Commonly Used Diagnostic Tests

1. Air or impedance plethysmography (refer to Chapter 5, Vascular Diagnostic Studies); used when other testing modalities are not available
2. Nuclear scan with radioactive isotope, fibrinogen I-125 (Walsh & Rice, 2004)
   a. Identifies fibrinogen attached to thrombi
   b. Injection of radioactive fibrinogen is followed in 12 to 24 hours by nuclear scan
   c. Highly accurate for DVT, including tibial and peroneal vessel thrombi
   d. Disadvantages: costly, unable to detect thrombi that do not contain fibrinogen, time delay for diagnosis

D. Laboratory Tests

1. Baseline tests before initiation of treatment
   a. Complete blood cell count with platelet count
   b. Activated partial thromboplastin time (APTT)
   c. Prothrombin time (PT)
   d. INR
   e. Fecal occult blood to detect gastrointestinal bleeding
   f. Creatinine
   g. Fibrinogen levels if plan tPa
2. Special coagulation testing when indicated
   a. Familial thrombophilia
      1) Factor V R 5060Q (Leiden) gene mutation
      2) Prothrombin 20210
      3) Homocysteine level
      4) Protein S level (must draw before initiating warfarin)
      5) Protein C level (must draw before initiating warfarin)
      6) Antithrombin III level (must draw before initiating UFH/LMWH)
      7) Activated protein C resistance
   b. Acquired thrombophilia
      1) Antiphospholipid antibodies
      2) Antinuclear antibodies
3. D-dimer (refer to Chapter 20, Pulmonary Embolism)
4. Fibrin degradation: indicative of the presence of active clotting

VII. Medical Management

A. SVT

1. Prevention of SVT (Geerts et al., 2008)
   a. Rotate intravenous sites every 3 days.
   b. Dilute irritating intravenous infusions (e.g., potassium chloride).
   c. Change intravenous tubing routinely under sterile conditions.
   d. Avoid insertion of three-way stopcocks directly into hub of catheter.
2. Treatment of SVT (Hofmann, 2009)
   a. Remove in-dwelling cannulae immediately.
   b. Early use of extremity may speed recovery.
   c. Treat pain with moist heat, elevation of limb, and oral or topical nonsteroidal anti-inflammatory medication for symptom relief unless contraindicated.
   d. Consider appropriate prophylaxis for DVT as indicated by risk factors.
   e. Frequent evaluation of site.
   f. Symptoms usually subside in 2 to 3 weeks.
   g. For spontaneous SVT may use LMWH, UFH, or vitamin K antagonist for 4 weeks. Not recommended to use oral anticoagulants and anti-inflammatory agents together.
3. Suppurative STP: inflammation and thrombosis in the setting of bacteremia (Mermel et al., 2009)
   a. Monitor for signs of systemic illness
   b. Culture catheter
   c. Start empiric antibiotic therapy while awaiting culture results: vancomycin is drug of choice where MRSA is prevalent
   d. Antibiotics per culture sensitivity until cellulitis resolved, or up to 6 weeks for bacteremia
   e. Uncomplicated exit sites should be treated with topical antimicrobial agents on the basis of culture; mupirocin for *S. aureus* and ketoconazole or lotrimin for *Candida*
   f. For trauma patients, prevention of suppurative STP is critical because of high rate of contamination of lines in first rescue efforts; all intravenous lines removed in first 24 hours
4. STP associated with varicose veins
   a. Treatment directed at symptomatic relief: moist heat, rest, limb elevation, anti-inflammatory agents if not contraindicated
   b. Activity encouraged
   c. Compression support stocking if tolerated: may need to wait until initial pain and inflammation subside
   d. Special coagulation studies if known recurrence

B. Deep Vein Thrombosis (Ageno et al., 2012; Hirsh et al., 2008)

1. Preliminary considerations
   a. Baseline laboratory tests before initiation of treatment
      1) APTT, PT (INR), complete blood cell count, creatinine, glomerular filtration rate (GFR)
      2) Other coagulation studies may be ordered. Results of some studies may be affected by degree of clot burden and results may not be accurate in the acute phase of thrombosis. Should be drawn prior to starting any anticoagulation therapy if used

b. Assess for contraindication to anticoagulation therapy
   1) History of HIT: will change choice of anticoagulants used
   2) Recent gastrointestinal bleed or hemorrhagic cerebrovascular accident within past 3 months
   3) Allergy
   4) Recent major surgery

2. Intravenous UFH (Guyatt, Akl, Crowther, Gutterman & Shuünemann, 2012; Holbrook et al., 2012)
   a. Mechanism of action
      1) Heparin and antithrombin inactivate thrombin (factor IIa) and factors IXa, Xa, XIa, XIIa to stop clot propagation and decrease risk of embolization
      2) Thrombolytic system begins to lyse thrombus naturally. UFH has no effect on existing thrombus
      3) Half-life: 60 to 90 minutes
      4) Does not cross placental barrier: safe in pregnancy
   b. Dosing guidelines
      1) Initial bolus 80 units/kg and infusion of 18 units/kg
      2) Discontinue heparin infusion when INR at therapeutic range for 2 days with overlapping warfarin. Warfarin initiated on day 1 of treatment
      3) Rate of recurrent thrombus found to be significantly lower with weight-based dosing
   c. Monitoring UFH
      1) APTT used to measure activity of thrombus activators and inhibitors. Endpoint is amount of time in seconds for the generation of a fibrin clot.
      2) Usual target range 1.5 to 2.5 time control. Due to institutional monitoring variations, APTT range should be based on responsiveness of the reagent and coagulometer used (Ansell et al., 2008).
      3) Obtain baseline APTT and platelet count prior to initiation and follow daily platelet count to assess for HIT.
   d. Rapid achievement of therapeutic APTT critical for prevention of recurrent DVT
      1) In patients without significant comorbid risk factors for bleeding (e.g., renal or liver failure), supratherapeutic APTT is not associated with increase in clinically significant bleeding
      2) Goal is to achieve therapeutic APTT within first 24 hours using weight-based dosing
   e. Contraindications: allergies to heparin, LMWH, previous history of HIT, recent history of bleeding/active bleeding, hemophilia, shock
   f. Complications associated with UFH
      1) Hemorrhagic: bleeding risk varies between 0% and 2% depending on underlying disease, other medications, and intensity/duration of therapy. Most common sites include GI tract, urinary tract, soft tissue, and oropharynx. Co-morbid conditions, particularly cancer, heart, renal or liver disease, and recent surgery or trauma increase risk of bleeding. Risk of bleeding increases with concomitant use of thrombolytic agents or GP IIb/IIIa inhibitors. Reversal of UFH is accomplished with protamine sulfate. Dose is 1 mg for every 100 units of heparin administered over the previous 4 hours. Administered IV slowly to prevent hypotension.

2) Nonhemorrhagic: heparin-induced thrombocytopenia (HIT) is a rare but serious complication occurring due to the development of heparin-specific antibodies binding to the platelet membrane. Results in drop in platelet count due to platelet aggregation. Mild thrombocytopenia may occur between days 2 and 6 of treatment. This usually resolves with discontinuation of UFH. More severe reductions in platelet count seen between days 4 and 15 may lead to significant decreases in platelet count of 30% to 40% from baseline with levels below 100,000. Skin necrosis from thrombosis may occur (Warkentin, Grienacher, Koster, & Lincoff, 2008).
3) Other: anaphylaxis, bronchoconstriction, urticaria, alopecia, osteoporosis (with long-term use such as during pregnancy)

3. LMWH (Holbrook et al., 2012)
   a. Mechanism of action: produces major anticoagulant effect by activating antithrombin. Produce a more predictable anticoagulant response than heparin. Half-life of 3 to 6 hours after injection with peak levels in 3 to 5 hours. Half-life is dose dependent; cleared by kidneys.
   b. Dosing and monitoring
      1) No monitoring is recommended in routine patients. Patients treated during pregnancy should be monitored with anti-Xa levels and dose adjusted for weight gain. Levels must be drawn 3 to 5 hours after injection during the peak of action. Target anti-Xa levels are dependent on the agent used and the dosing regimen, for example, q12h dosing versus q24h dosing.
      2) Dosing: weight based. Weight-based dosing recommended in obese rather than fixed dose. For severe renal disease (CrCl <30 mL/min) recommendation is for UFH or reduction in LMWH dose by 50%.
      3) Reversal: protamine sulfate 1 mg per 100 anti-Xa units of LMWH for LMWH given within 8 hours. Administer second dose of 0.5 mg per 100 anti-Xa units if bleeding continues.
   c. Contraindications: same as for heparin
   d. Complications: bleeding, HIT less frequency than with UFH, osteoporosis less likely than with UFH
4. Fondaparinux (Garcia, Baglin, Weitz, & Samama, 2012; Holbrook et al., 2012)
   a. Synthetic pentasaccharide, anti-Xa activity higher than LMWH, half-life about 17 hours; safe for patients with HIT
   b. Administered SQ once daily in fixed doses, no laboratory monitoring
   c. Prophylactic dose is 2.5 mg daily. Treatment of DVT or PE 7.5 mg for weight 50 to 100 kg. Decrease to 5 mg for <50 kg, increase to 10 mg for >100 kg.
   d. Contraindicated in severe renal disease (CrCl <30 mL/min), dose reduction of 50% with CrCl <50 mL/min.
   e. No reversal. May administer recombinant factor VIIa for uncontrolled bleeding.
   f. Complications: no reports of HIT; may cause urticarial reactions, local skin necrosis.
5. Intravenous direct thrombin inhibitor (Garcia et al., 2012)
   a. Agents: lepirudin, desirudin, bivalirudin, argatroban. Used in patients who have suspected or confirmed HIT

b. Dosing and monitoring
   1) Reduced dose in renal disease with CrCl <60 mL/min but >30 mL/min for lepirudin or desirudin and monitor with APTT. Do not use lepirudin or desirudin with CrCl <30 mL/min.
   2) Argatroban not used with hepatic dysfunction. Monitor with factor X levels due to variable effect on INR. Cannot stop infusion until INR reaches therapeutic level with oral vitamin K antagonist to decrease risk of thrombosis. Factor X levels <45% associated with INR value >2. Factor X levels safer than aiming for INR of 4 or greater before stopping infusion.

6. Oral direct thrombin inhibitors: dabigatran (Pradaxa) (Ageno et al., 2012; Prescriber's Letter, 2013; Schulman et al., 2009)
   a. Predictable anticoagulant effect with fixed dosing
   b. No monitoring required, no reversal agent
   c. Half-life 17 to 21 hours
   d. Approved for stroke prevention in atrial fibrillation and prophylaxis for DVT in elective hip or knee arthroplasty
   e. Avoid in patients with severe renal failure. Check renal function at baseline and yearly
   f. US approval for prevention of stroke in nonvalvular afib and available only in 150 mg doses dosed twice daily. Off-label use for prevention of VTE posthip and knee replacement
   g. Canada approved for stroke prevention and VTE prevention posthip or knee replacement. For stroke prevention dosed 150 mg twice daily under age 80. Over age 80, 110 mg twice daily. For VTE prevention posthip/knee 220 mg daily for 10 days postknee and 28 to 35 days posthip. Initial dose 110 mg if started 1 to 4 hours postoperatively. Consider 150 mg daily for patients over age 75 with initial dose 75 mg.
   h. Dosing based on balance between efficacy and bleeding risk. Major risk is bleeding.
   i. Must be used within 4 months of opening bottle. Store in original package only. Take at least 2 hours before antacids.
   j. P-glycoprotein inhibitors may increase dabigatran levels, for example, dronedarone, ketoconazole, verapamil, quinidine, amiodarone, clarithromycin. P-glycoprotein inducers may decrease dabigatran efficacy. Avoid P-glycoprotein inducers, for example, rifampin, carbamazepine, St. John's wort.

7. Vitamin K antagonists (Ageno et al., 2012)
   a. Warfarin (Coumadin): inhibits synthesis of vitamin K-dependent proteins (factors II, VII, IX, X and proteins C and S) involved in the coagulation process; highly water soluble and rapidly absorbed from GI tract; circulates bound to plasma proteins; accumulates in the liver.
   b. Produces anticoagulant and antithrombotic effects; anticoagulant effect occurs 12 to 24 hours after first dose; antithrombotic effect occurs 2 to 7 days after steady state has been achieved. Time to steady state related to long half-life of warfarin (36 to 42 hours) and long half-life of some factors (up to 90 hours).
   c. Dosing
      1) Initiate UFH/LMWH and start warfarin on same day
      2) Adjust doses based on INR with testing beginning at baseline and after two or three doses or oral anticoagulation therapy

3) Overlap UFH/LMWH therapy for 5 days or until INR therapeutic for 2 days to allow for further reduction in factor II and X
4) Initial dosing may range from 5 to 10 mg; not recommended to use high initial dosing in elderly, debilitated, malnourished, CHF, liver disease, recent major surgery, or taking medications known to increase sensitivity to warfarin

d. Monitoring
1) INR used to monitor stability; consistent measure from one laboratory to another
2) Monitoring may be done through office point-of-care testing by advanced practice nurse, pharmacist, or nurse via protocol; self-testing may be done by qualified patients with scheduled reporting
3) Contraindications
a) Same as for other anticoagulants; use with caution in patients with drainage tubes, malabsorption disorders, dietary deficiencies, gastrointestinal ulcers, renal or liver dysfunction
b) Absolute: pregnancy—warfarin may cause teratogenic effect in the first trimester; crosses placental barrier and may cause fetal bleeding; for high-risk women with mechanical valves vitamin K antagonist may be used after 13th week with LMWH or UFH resumed close to delivery

e. Complications
1) Bleeding: proportional to elevation of INR and other risk factors; may be corrected with use of vitamin K, preferably administered orally; dose dependent on levels of INR and presence/absence of significant bleeding. Oral administration achieves reversal in approximately 24 hours. Low doses <5 mg are usually sufficient. Parenteral administration achieves quicker reversal but may lead to difficulty in achieving therapeutic levels after bleeding under control due to long half-life. For INR >5 but <9 and no significant bleeding, omit one or two doses and lower dose, monitor more frequently until stabilized. For serious bleeding, omit dose and supplement vitamin K reversal with FFP.
2) Food and drug interactions: associated with alteration in vitamin K availability/intake, reduced warfarin absorption, changes in warfarin protein binding, effects on drug metabolism. Vigilance and stability in dietary intake and concomitant medications is required. Any changes in medication warrant testing to monitor for interactions.
3) Skin necrosis: usually observed on third to eighth day; caused by extensive thrombosis of venules and capillaries in subcutaneous fat; may also cause limb gangrene due to outflow obstruction of venous circulation. Treated with discontinuation of warfarin, resumption of heparin, comfort measures, surgical debridement. May require skin grafting or amputation of limb if severe.

8. Direct Factor Xa inhibitor rivaroxaban (Xarelto) (Ageno et al., 2012; Guyatt et al., 2012; Prescriber's Letter, 2013)

a. Dosing
1) Prevention of DVT 10 mg daily beginning 6 to 10 hours postoperatively for 2 weeks after total knee arthroplasty and 5 to 6 weeks after total hip replacement. Take with food.
2) Treatment of DVT/PE 15 mg twice daily for 3 weeks and then 20 mg daily. Take with food.

b. No monitoring necessary, no reversal agent
c. Not for use in patients with CrCl <15 mL/min, hepatic disease with coagulopathy. Monitor renal function periodically.
d. Do not use with strong CYP3A4 inducers or inhibitors, for example, ketoconazole, itraconazole, voriconazole, posaconazole, fluconazole protease inhibitor, clarithromycin, erythromycin.

9. Length of therapy
   a. First episode: 3 to 6 months depending on location of thrombus, presence of reversible risk factor; long-term treatment recommended for unprovoked proximal DVT when no risk of bleeding and good anticoagulant monitoring is available
   b. For recurrent DVT or thrombophilia, therapy may be lifelong

C. Supportive Measures

1. Graduated compression stockings to reduce swelling and promote venous return
2. Elevation of the affected extremity 10 to 20 degrees above heart level
3. Progressive ambulation as allowed; avoid or delay for significant limb edema

D. Thrombolysis of DVT (Gogainiceanu et al., 2009)

1. Dissolution of intraluminal thrombus via chemical lysis to restore vessel patency; recommended use in selected patients with extensive proximal DVT, such as ilio-femoral, with low risk of bleeding; directly infused into the venous thrombus via multi-side-hole catheter
2. Balloon angioplasty and stents recommended for correction of underlying venous lesions
3. Indications
   a. Phlegmasia cerulea dolens resulting in compromised arterial circulation
   b. Extensive ilio-femoral DVT
4. Benefits
   a. Lysis of thrombus may prevent late destruction of venous valves thereby reducing the risk of chronic postphlebitic syndrome (chronic swelling, ulceration)
   b. Performed percutaneously with direct catheter placement into thrombosed area under local anesthesia
   c. Rapid acting and rapidly cleared from the body: half-life 5 to 8 minutes, administered by IV infusion
5. Disadvantages
   a. High risk of systemic bleeding complications; risk of bleeding differs with respect to underlying disorders and co-morbid conditions; appears to be associated with 1.5 to 2-fold increase in risk of major bleeding
   b. Definitions of major bleeding differ among studies: most ominous bleed is intracerebral
   c. Frequent angiograms needed to check extent of thrombolysis requiring increased contrast load and risk of subsequent contrast-induced nephropathy
   d. Intensive care monitoring required
6. FDA-approved thrombolytic agents
   a. Streptokinase

1) First agent approved
2) Disadvantages: not as rapid in clot lysis as other agents, frequent hypersensitivity reactions; seldom used

b. Urokinase
1) More effective than streptokinase in clot lysis but less effective in restoring venous flow than recombinant tissue plasminogen activator (tPa)

c. Recombinant tissue plasminogen activator (tPa)
1) More rapid and complete thrombus dissolution than urokinase
2) Shortest treatment time

7. Contraindications to thrombolytic therapy
a. Absolute: active bleeding, cerebrovascular disease/event or procedure within past 2 months
b. Relative: recent major surgery or trauma (within 10 days), postpartum, cardiopulmonary resuscitation with rib fractures, thoracentesis, paracentesis, lumbar puncture, any condition requiring maintenance of normal clotting or healing
c. Potentially serious bleeding: uncontrolled coagulation defects, severe hypertension, pregnancy, any condition with potential bleeding risk (refer Chapter 20, Pulmonary Embolism, for patient-care guidelines)

VIII. Interventional Management (Vedantham, 2009; Walsh & Rice, 2004)

A. DVT Thrombectomy

1. General/spinal anesthesia
2. May be done percutaneously or through incision; thrombus removed by fragmentation and aspiration of clot
3. Requires anticoagulation with heparin and warfarin once hemostasis is achieved
4. Usually performed in conjunction with thrombolytic therapy
5. Indications: same as for thrombolysis, DVT not responsive to medical intervention
6. Best outcome if performed within 2 to 3 days of thrombus formation

B. Vena Cava Filter Placement

1. Indications
a. Unable to use anticoagulant therapy due to contraindications
b. Prevention of pulmonary embolization of thrombus (originating in the lower extremity or pelvic veins) in high-risk patient
c. Recurrent thromboembolism despite adequate anticoagulation
d. Patient undergoing pulmonary embolectomy
e. Chronic recurring pulmonary embolism
f. Elderly patients at risk of falling with severe consequences if receiving anticoagulation therapy
g. Free-floating proximal thrombus
h. Mentally unstable patient
i. Low cardiac reserve or pulmonary hypertension
j. Massive pulmonary embolism
2. See Chapter 20, Pulmonary Embolism for devices, insertion technique, and complications

C. Saphenofemoral Junction Ligation for SVT

1. Indication: prevention of DVT when superficial venous thrombophlebitis extends into the saphenofemoral junction
2. Surgical procedure with a small groin incision under local or general anesthesia, ligation or disassociation of the superficial saphenous vein from the deep femoral vein
3. Outpatient procedure or 1-day hospital stay depending on patient circumstances

D. Suppurative STP (Mermel et al., 2009)

1. Surgical resection limited to patients with purulent superficial veins or when infection extends beyond vessel wall or failure of conservative therapy
2. Wound left open for secondary healing
3. Skin graft may be needed once infection resolved and patient stable

E. Varicose Vein STP: phlebectomy for recurrent episodes; refer to Chapter 21, Chronic Venous Disease and Venous Ulcers for various techniques

IX. Upper Extremity DVT (Munoz et al., 2008; Persson, Arnhjort, Larfars, & Rosfors, 2006)

A. DVT of Axillary, Subclavian, Brachiocephalic

1. Precipitating factors similar to lower extremity, but may also include
   a. Increased use of subclavian vein for central line
   b. Use of irritating intravenous solutions or drug abuse
   c. Muscular effort of arms, especially in athletes such as swimmers, weightlifters, rowers, painters, wrestlers (Paget–Schroetter syndrome)
   d. Thoracic outlet syndrome
   e. Pacemaker wires
   f. Tumor
   g. Congenital venous malformations
2. Signs and symptoms
   a. May be asymptomatic
   b. Pain and local tenderness
   c. Warmth
   d. Edema
   e. Supraclavicular fullness
   f. Palpable cord
   g. Increased venous pattern on chest wall
   h. Upper limb cyanosis
3. Complications
   a. Chronic venous insufficiency
   b. Upper limb ulceration
   c. Phlebitis
   d. Thoracic duct obstruction
   e. Superior vena cava syndrome
   f. Brachial plexopathy
   g. Pulmonary embolism

4. Diagnosis established by
   a. Clinical history and physical examination
   b. Venous duplex ultrasound
   c. Venography
   d. Magnetic resonance venography: valuable for central veins
   e. CT venography: useful in detecting external compression of the venous system
5. Medical management: elevation, moist heat, anticoagulation, and/or thrombolytic agent
6. Interventional/surgical management
   a. Superior vena cava filter
   b. Venous thrombectomy (early re-thrombosis common)
   c. Transaxillary first rib resection: most useful for thoracic outlet syndrome or effort thrombosis after initial thrombolytic or anticoagulation therapy

B. Superior Vena Cava Syndrome (Sajid, Ahmed, Desai, Baker, & Hamilton, 2007)

1. Most common causes
   a. Bronchogenic cancer
   b. Lymphoma
   c. Metastatic tumor from breast or testicles
   d. Radiation therapy
   e. Central line placement, especially Swan–Ganz, Hickman, or transthoracic pacemakers
   f. Other causes: aortic aneurysm, polyarteritis nodosa, pericardial hematoma, congenital anomaly
2. Pathophysiology
   a. Extrinsic compression from slowly progressive tumor that eventually obstructs superior vena cava
   b. Direct invasion of vessel or acute thrombosis causes sudden, dramatic symptoms
3. Signs and symptoms
   a. Upper extremity and facial edema, including conjunctival edema
   b. Dilation of superficial veins on chest, neck, or arms
   c. Cough, hoarseness, shortness of breath with stridor due to laryngeal edema
   d. Dysphagia due to esophageal edema
   e. Dizziness, headache, visual complaints, somnolence, change in mental status (including coma)
   f. Symptoms worse with lying, stooping, bending
4. Diagnosis
   a. Venous duplex may be done initially but venography confirms diagnosis
   b. Chest radiography and CT scan identify underlying problem
   c. Biopsy through a percutaneous approach for tumor/mass
5. Treatment
   a. Bed rest, diuretics, head elevation
   b. Steroids for laryngeal and esophageal edema
   c. Anticoagulation and/or thrombolysis if thrombosis of superior vena cava has occurred
   d. Surgical reconstruction may be attempted in some cases

X. Nursing Management/Diagnoses

A. Alteration in tissue perfusion related to venous thrombosis as evidenced by swelling

1. Expected patient outcomes
   a. Patient will have decreased swelling
   b. Patient will have continued arterial flow
2. Interventions
   a. Leg/arm elevation above the level of the heart
   b. Graduated compression stockings
   c. Anticoagulation as indicated
   d. Avoid prolonged sitting or standing when allowed out of bed
3. Evaluation
   a. Measure circumference of affected limb
   b. CMS checks (circulation, motion, and sensation)

B. Alteration in tissue perfusion related to venous thrombosis as evidenced by pain

1. Expected patient outcomes
   a. Patient will be pain free
   b. Patient will be able to perform activities of daily living
2. Interventions
   a. Analgesia as needed
   b. Graduated compression stockings
   c. Bed rest/elevation of affected limb
   d. Position for comfort (do not gatch bed at knees and avoid extreme flexion of hips)
3. Evaluation
   a. Assess pain using a scale of 1 to 10 every 4 to 8 hours
   b. Note usage of analgesia and response
   c. Observe activity level the patient is able to tolerate
   d. Obtain physical and occupational therapy consults as needed to help patient return to normal activities of daily living

C. Potential for injury/bleeding related to anticoagulation

1. Expected patient outcomes
   a. Patient will show no signs of bleeding
2. Interventions
   a. Avoid intramuscular injections
   b. Recommend use of electric razors and soft toothbrushes
   c. Apply pressure to all venipuncture sites for 3 to 5 minutes
   d. Check IV site with each physical assessment
   e. Monitor PTT/PT/INR/platelet count
3. Evaluation
   a. Assess for signs of epistaxis, bleeding gums, melena, hematuria, bruising, and petechiae with each physical assessment
   b. Monitor for internal bleeding as noted by a change in vital signs
      1) Increased heart rate
      2) Decreased blood pressure
      3) Pallor

XI. Patient/Family Education

A. Disease Prevention/Health Promotion and Secondary Prevention

1. Discuss etiology/pathophysiology of venous thrombosis
2. Identify/discuss and evaluate patient/family understanding of risk factors
3. Explain treatment goals

B. Prevention of Subsequent Thrombosis/Embolism/ Post-Thrombotic Syndrome

1. Wearing compression garment
2. Maintenance of baseline activities of daily living
3. Elevate as necessary

C. Medication Education

1. Tablet strength, color, how many, and how often to take
2. INR goal: define, give expected range (2 to 3), and explain that adjustments may be necessary periodically
3. Side effects
   a. Bleeding/easily bruised
   b. New rash
   c. Seek medical attention if any side effects occur
4. Interactions with other medications
   a. No aspirin/anti-inflammatory drug unless prescribed by health care provider
   b. Multiple drug interactions with warfarin
5. Subcutaneous injection technique teaching if self-administering LMWH
6. Discuss estrogen therapy risks with medical provider

D. Symptom Management

1. Infection: call health care provider
2. Increased pain, swelling, warmth, erythema: go to emergency department
3. Pulmonary embolism
   a. Chest pain, rapid pulse, diaphoresis, anxiety, fainting, hemoptysis
   b. Call 911
4. Bleeding
   a. Major: call 911 or go to emergency department
   b. Minor: alert health care provider
5. Unilateral paralysis, numbness, facial droop, vision/speech change, loss of coordination, or change in mental status: seek emergency care, call 911

E. Home Care Considerations

1. Diet: issues involving vitamin K
   a. Diet should be consistent and moderate
   b. Provide list of foods moderate to high in vitamin K
      1) Green leafy vegetables are high in vitamin K
      2) Green tea and tobacco are very high in vitamin K and should be avoided
   c. Avoid alcohol use
   d. Encourage patient to check with health care provider before using any herbal remedies

2. Activity
   a. Walk regularly, may also jog, swim, cycle, or engage in low-impact sports after acute phase of thrombosis
   b. Avoid prolonged sitting/standing
   c. Elevate legs whenever nonambulatory
   d. Avoid crossing legs and constrictive clothing
3. Compression garment should be measured and fitted by an experienced professional
4. Safety precautions
   a. Protect the feet
   b. Exercise caution when using sharp items (e.g., scissors, broken glass)
   c. Wear a helmet when riding a bicycle
   d. Wear or carry identification that indicates anticoagulation therapy
   e. Seek immediate care for serious injury or head injury
   f. Avoid contact sports
5. Home environment
   a. Ability to come in for routine INR checks
   b. Ability to administer own medications accurately
   c. Assess for risk of falls
   d. Self-testing for select patients based on diagnosis, dexterity, and compliance
6. Notify health care provider
   a. Changes in medication, diet, missed dose
   b. Questions or symptoms

CASE STUDY

A 22-year-old female, Ms. K., with no significant past medical history, sustains severe trauma to her right knee in a skiing accident. She undergoes knee reconstruction. A tourniquet is placed above the affected knee during the surgical procedure to minimize operative bleeding. Twenty-four hours after the procedure, the patient reports increased pain and swelling of her right leg.

Physical examination includes the following:

- Integument: warm, red right leg above the level of her dressing with increased swelling compared with previous postoperative examination. Incision is intact and without erythema or evidence of wound infection. All other skin intact and normal
- Cardiovascular: apical pulse 84, regular rate and rhythm, no murmurs, rubs, or gallops, blood pressure 138/74, palpable pulses throughout with moderate edema from right foot to mid-thigh level
- Respiratory: clear bilaterally, even respirations, rate 20
- Gastrointestinal: hypoactive bowel sounds, no masses or tenderness
- Neurologic: alert and oriented × 3, appears in mild distress, tearful; sensation and motion of extremities normal, negative Homan sign
- Additional vital signs: temperature: 37.8°C
- Pain scale rating: 9 on scale of 1 to 10

Social history: independent with activities of daily living; single, lives with two roommates in a one-story apartment and attends local college; nonsmoker, drinks socially on the weekends; has taken birth control pills for the last 4 years.

Family history: mother, father, one brother alive and well; mother had two miscarriages, reasons unknown.

Laboratory values reveal the following:

Hematocrit 36 (normal)
Hemoglobin 14 (normal)
Creatinine 0.7 (normal)
Oxygen level 99% pulse oximetry (normal)
Platelets 176,000 (normal)

Initial diagnosis: suspicious for right leg postoperative DVT

Review Questions

1. What signs and symptoms are suspicious for venous thrombosis?
   a. Pain
   b. Swelling
   c. Homan sign
   d. a and b
2. What diagnostic test would the provider order next?
   a. Antithrombin III
   b. Venous duplex ultrasound
   c. CT scan
   d. Venography
3. What was the most important precipitating factor that resulted in her DVT?
   a. Immobilization
   b. Systemic coagulation abnormalities
   c. Birth control pills
   d. Venous stasis
   e. Venous trauma
   f. d and e.
4. What immediate care measures need to be instituted to aid in preventing a pulmonary embolism?
   a. Elevation of the affected extremity
   b. Anticoagulation with warfarin
   c. Anticoagulation with heparin or low-molecular-weight heparin
   d. Compression therapy
5. What teaching and instructions need to be included in her discharge plan?
   a. Continued avoidance of all tobacco products
   b. Discontinuation of birth control pills
   c. Compression therapy
   d. Medication teaching
   e. All of the above

Answers/Rationales

1. d. a and b. Pain, swelling, and tenderness are typically seen with venous thrombosis; however, the signs and symptoms can vary depending on the extent and location of the clot. Physical findings may be completely absent (silent DVT) when there is minimal obstruction or adequate collateral flow. Homan sign is an unreliable indicator for presence of DVT.
2. b. Venous duplex ultrasound. Acute leg pain and swelling may have many causes, especially in this postoperative patient with total knee reconstruction. Diagnosing DVT is difficult on

clinical grounds alone. Noninvasive studies have become the most useful tools in diagnosing a DVT; duplex ultrasound is ordered most frequently because of its high sensitivity and specificity of >95% for proximal vessels. A CT scan can show a DVT, but it is not the first-line choice. Venography is invasive and therefore is used less than other diagnostic tests, although it is still the most reliable. Venography may be indicated in patients suspected of having DVT if there is an inconclusive test in a patient who has a strong clinical suspicion for DVT. Because of its risk, discomfort, and expense, venography should only be used when it is imperative to establish a definitive diagnosis. Checking the antithrombin III level will not help diagnose the DVT. It will only tell if the patient has a clotting abnormality. Ms. K. was sent for a duplex ultrasound, which confirmed a right popliteal to femoral DVT.

3. f. Venous stasis and venous trauma. The tight tourniquet placed around the patient's leg during surgery, combined with severe trauma, probably injured the leg veins and also caused blood stasis. Although the patient is young and probably has a low propensity for thrombosis, the vessel injury/stasis in this setting was of sufficient magnitude to precipitate a DVT. Oral contraceptives and immobilization are predisposing risk factors to the development of DVT. However, Virchow triad (stasis of venous blood, local venous trauma, and coagulation abnormalities) is still believed to be of primary importance in the formation of thrombus in the systemic veins.

4. c. Anticoagulation with heparin or low-molecular-weight heparin. This patient needs immediate anticoagulation to prevent propagation of the thrombus or embolism. Treatment consists of therapeutic-dose UFH or LMWH for at least 5 days, overlapped with and followed by treatment with Coumadin for 3 to 6 months. Lethal pulmonary embolism most often originates in the femoral or iliac veins, and thrombosis in this area absolutely requires anticoagulation. Isolated calf vein or tibial vein thromboses rarely lead to clinically detectable pulmonary embolus; thus this type of thrombus may not require full anticoagulation therapy. Elevation is recommended to help prevent swelling and will help with comfort measures; the more the leg swells, the more it hurts but it will not prevent pulmonary embolism. Compression therapy is used after the acute phase of thrombosis to help with the swelling and to prevent long-term postphlebitic complications. Ms. K's INR is 2.6 on postoperative day 4, and she is being discharged.

5. e. All of the above. Patient and family education and understanding of the treatment, prevention, and risk factors associated with DVT is of primary importance. Anticoagulation therapy instruction should focus on its purpose, side effects, drug interactions, dietary and physical activity restrictions, and the need for continued follow-up and frequent blood tests. Inform the patient of the risks of smoking and taking oral contraceptives in someone who has had a DVT, as well as the risk of recurrence in certain situations (e.g., air travel). The risks associated with alcohol consumption and warfarin therapy should be reviewed, especially because this patient admits to social drinking. Inform the patient that the graduated compression stocking needs to be worn to promote venous blood return, decrease leg swelling, and help prevent the long-term complications of postphlebitic syndrome. Education is critical to the success of a patient's overall treatment plan. Taking the time to instill an understanding of why interventions and life-style modifications are necessary will help the patient comply for better short-term and long-term health.

REFERENCES

Ageno, W., Gallus, A., Wittkowshy, A., Crowther, M., Hylek, E., & Palareti, G. (2012). Oral anticoagulant therapy; Antithrombotic therapy and prevention of thrombosis 9th ed: American college of chest physicians evidence-based clinical practice guidelines. *Chest, 141*(2 Suppl.), 44S–88S.

Ansell, J., Hirsh, J., Hylek, E., Jacobson, A., Crowther, M., & Palareti, G. (2008). Pharmacology and management of the vitamin K antagonists: American college of chest physicians evidence-based clinical practice guidelines. *Chest, 133,* 160S–198S.

Caprini, J., & Arcelus, J. (2007). Venous thromboembolism prophylaxis in the general surgical patient. In J. Bergan (Ed.), *The vein book* (pp. 369–380). Burlington, MA: Elsevier.

Ferri, F. J. (2011). *Ferri's clinical advisor 2011: Instant diagnosis and treatment* (pp. 310–312; 1084). St. Louis, MO: Elsevier, Mosby.

Garcia, D., Baglin, T., Weitz, J., & Samama, M. (2012). Parenteral anticoagulants antithrombotic therapy and prevention of thrombosis, 9th ed: American college of chest physicians evidence-based clinical practice guidelines. *Chest, 141*(2 Suppl.), 24S–43S.

Geerts, W., Bergqvist, D., Pineo, G., Heit, J., Samama, C., Lasses, M., & Colwell, C. (2008). Prevention of venous thromboembolism: American college of chest physicians evidence-based clinical practice guidelines (8th ed.). *Chest, 133,* 381S–453S

Gogainiceanu, P., Johnston, C. J., Kahlid, U., Holt, P., Hincliffe, R., Loftus, I., & Thompson, M., (2009). Indications for thrombolysis in deep venous thrombosis. *European Journal of Vascular and Endovascular Surgery, 38,* 192–198.

Guyatt, G., Akl, E., Crowther, M., Gutterman, D., & Shuünemann, H. (2012). Executive summary: Antithrombotic therapy and prevention of thrombosis, 9th ed: American College of Chest Physician evidence-based clinical practice guidelines. *Chest, 141*(2 Suppl.), 7S–46S.

Hingorani, A., & Ascher, R. (2009). Superficial venous thrombophlebitis. In *Handbook of venous disorders: Guideline of the American venous forum* (pp. 314–319). London, UK: Hodder Arnold.

Hirsh, J., Bauer, K., Donati, M., Gould, M., Samama, M., & Weitz, J. (2008). Parenteral anticoagulants: American college of chest physician evidence-based guidelines (8th ed.). *Chest, 133,* 141S–159S.

Hirsh, J., Guyatt, G., Albers, G., Harrington, R., & Schunemann, H. (2008). Antithrombotic and thrombolytic therapy: American college of chest physicians, evidence-based clinical practice guidelines (8th ed.). *Chest, 133,* 110S–112S.

Hofmann, L. (2009). Therapies for acute and chronic deep venous thrombosis. *Clinical Advances in Hematology & Oncology, 7,* 301–303.

Holbrook, A., Schulman, S., Witt, D. M., Vandvik, P. O., Fish, J., Kovacs, M., . . . Guyatt, G. H. (2012). Evidence-based management of anticoagulant therapy: Antithrombotic therapy and prevention of thrombosis, 9th ed: American college of chest physician evidence-based clinical practice guidelines. *Chest, 141*(2 Suppl.), 152S–177S.

Lohr, J., Kin, D., & Krallman, K. (2009). Diagnostic algorithms for acute deep vein thrombosis and pulmonary embolism. *Handbook of venous disorders: Guideline of the American venous forum* (pp. 208–220). London, UK: Hodder Arnold.

Mcbane, R., & Heit, J. (2009). Current recommendations for prevention of deep vein thrombosis. In *Handbook of venous disorders: Guideline of the American venous forum,* (pp.277–291). London, UK: Hodder Arnold.

McCance, K., & Huether, S. (2010). *Pathophysiology: The biologic basis for disease in adults and children* (6th ed., pp. 952–988 & 1091–1141). Maryland Heights, MO: Mosby.

Meissner, M. (2009). The epidemiology of and risk factors for acute deep venous thrombosis. In *Handbook of venous disorders: Guideline of the American venous forum,* (pp.94–104). London, UK: Hodder Arnold.

Mermel, L., Allon, M., Bouza, E., Craven, D., Flynn, P., O'Grady, N., . . . Warren, D. (2009). Clinical practice guidelines for the diagnosis and management of intravascular catheter-related infection: 2009 update by the infectious disease society of America. *Clinical Infectious Diseases, 49,* 1–45.

Munoz, F., Mismetti, P., Poggio, R., Valle, R., Barron, M., Guil, M., & Monreal, M. (2008). Clinical outcome of patients with upper-extremity deep vein thrombosis. *Chest, 133,* 143–148.

Office of the Surgeon General (US); National Heart, Lung, and Blood Institute (US). The Surgeon General's Call to Action to Prevent Deep Vein Thrombosis and Pulmonary Embolism. Rockville, MD: Office of the Surgeon General (US); 2008. Available from http://www.ncbi.nlm.nih.gov/book/NBK44189

Persson, L., Arnhjort, T., Larfars, G., & Rosfors, S. (2006). Hemodynamic and morphologic evaluation of sequelae of primary upper extremity deep venous thrombosis treated with anticoagulation. *Journal of Vascular Surgery, 43,* 1230–1235.

Prescriber's Letter. (2013). Comparison of oral antithrombotics, *Prescriber's Letter,* Detail document #290201, Retrieved from www.PrescribersLetter.com, accessed June 28, 2013.

Sajid, M., Ahmed, N., Desai, M., Baker, D., & Hamilton, G. (2007). Upper limb deep vein thrombosis: A literature review to streamline the protocol for management. *Acta Haematologica, 118,* 10–18.

Schulman, S., Kearon, C., Kakkar, A. A., Mismetti, P., Schellong, S., Eriksson, H., . . . Goldhaber, S. (2009). Dabigatran versus warfarin in the treatment of acute venous thromboembolism. *New England Journal of Medicine, 361,* 2342–2352.

Vedantham, S. (2009). Deep venous thrombosis: The opportunity at hand. *American Journal of Radiology, 193,* 922–927.

Walsh, M. E., & Rice, K. L. (2004). Venous thromboembolic disease. In V. Fahey (Ed.), *Vascular nursing* (4th ed., pp. 365–398) St. Louis, MO: Saunders.

Warkentin, R., Greinacher, A., Koster, A., & Lincoff, A. (2008). Treatment of heparin-induced thrombocytopenia: American college of chest physicians evidence-based clinical practice guidelines (8th ed.). *Chest, 133,* 340S–380S.

SUGGESTED READINGS

Bregenzer, T., Conen, D., Sakmann, P., & Widmer, A. F. (1998). Is routine replacement of peripheral intravenous catheters necessary? *Archives of Internal Medicine, 158*(2), 151–156.

Geerts, W., Pineo, G., Heit, J., Berquist, D., Lassen, M., Colwell, C., & Ray, J. (2004). Prevention of venous thromboembolism: The seventh ACCP conference on antithrombotic therapy. *Chest, 126,* 338–400.

Heit, J. (2009). The epidemiology of venous thromboembolism in the community: Implications for prevention and management. In J. Bergan (Ed.), *The vein book* (pp. 323–330) Burlington, MA: Elsevier.

Ligush, J., & Johnson, G. (1996). Superficial thrombophlebitis. In P. Gloloviczki & J. S. T. Yao (Eds.), *Handbook of venous disorders: Guidelines of the American venous forum* (pp. 235–243). London, UK: Chapman & Hall Medical.

Schulman, S., Beyth, R., Kearon, C., & Levine, M. (2008). Hemorrhagic complications of anticoagulant and thrombolytic treatment: American college of chest physicians evidence-based clinical practice guideline (8th ed.). *Chest, 133,* 257S–298S.

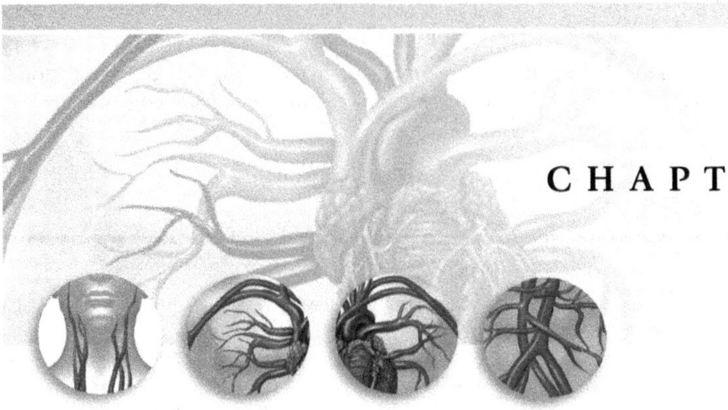

CHAPTER 20

Pulmonary Embolism

Michelle Tinkham
Patrica A. Lewis
First Edition Authors: *Patricia A. Lewis and Karla Mees*

OBJECTIVES

1. List three risk factors for pulmonary embolism.
2. Discuss methods of prevention of venous thromboembolism.
3. Describe pertinent diagnostic testing modalities for pulmonary embolism.
4. Identify key elements in educating the patient who is treated for pulmonary embolism.

Introduction

A venous embolus is a detached blood clot or thrombus that travels through the venous circulation, generally lodging in a more proximal vessel or site distant from the original source. A pulmonary embolus (PE) is a thrombus that lodges in a segment of the pulmonary arterial system, thereby causing either complete or partial obstruction of pulmonary blood flow that may result in a significant decrease of oxygenation. Most pulmonary emboli originate in the veins of the lower extremities in the form of deep venous thrombosis (DVT), but other sources include the pelvic veins and the right side of the heart. Pulmonary infarction is the term used to describe a local area of necrosis in lung tissue resulting from vascular obstruction. This is an uncommon complication of PE, although some studies have shown that pulmonary infarction is more likely when the lung is already infected or congested prior to the development of pulmonary embolism (Roach & Laufman, 1955).

Pulmonary embolism is the third leading cause of death from cardiovascular disease, exceeded only by ischemic heart disease and stroke, and may be the most common preventable cause of death in the world (Wheeler & Anderson, 1996). Twenty per cent of DVT cases lead to fatal pulmonary embolism (Rosendaal, 1999). The 7-day survival rate for those diagnosed with pulmonary embolism is 59% (Heit et al., 2001). Although true incidence of the disease is unknown because of low autopsy rate and lack of diagnoses, 94,000 cases of pulmonary embolism are identified annually (Heit et al., 2001). "Most patients with DVT will develop pulmonary embolism and the majority of cases will be clinically unrecognized. Untreated, approximately one third of patients who survive an initial pulmonary embolism will die from a future embolic episode. This is true whether the initial (clot) is small or large. Most patients who die from pulmonary embolism have not had any diagnostic workup, nor have they received any prophylaxis for the disease" (Feied &

Handler, 2000). It is estimated that the overall financial burden of pulmonary embolism is over \$1.5 billion/year in associated health care costs or \$30,000 per incident whereas the preventative costs are only \$3,000 per patient (American Thoracic Society, 2010).

However, even though the reported number of cases of pulmonary embolism is significantly less than the true incidence, there has been a documented 37% decline in nonfatal PE while at the same time diagnosis of DVT has increased by 108% (Wheeler & Anderson, 1996). This is thought to be due to improved diagnosis and treatment of DVT, with wider acceptance of prophylaxis and public education regarding prevention.

I. Anatomy

A. Pulmonary Artery

1. Composed of elastic connective tissue, smooth muscle, and fibrous connective tissue
2. Large elastic vessel with thinner muscle layer (media) than systemic circulation
3. Originates at right ventricle
4. Lower pressure and resistance than systemic circulation; average pulmonary artery pressure +25/10 mm Hg, and mean of 15 mm Hg
5. Carries unoxygenated blood to the lungs
6. Divides and enters the lung at the hilus with each main bronchus and branches with the bronchus at every division (see Fig. 20-1)
7. Facilitates gas exchange, delivers nutrients to lungs, filters out clots, air, and other debris (McCance & Heuther, 1998)

B. Large Size of inferior vena cava and right heart chambers prevents emboli from adhering to vessel wall prior to pulmonary circulation

II. Pathophysiology

A. Direct Consequence of DVT (refer to description in Chapter 19, Superficial Thrombophlebitis and Deep Vein Thrombosis)

1. 90% from deep veins of legs as demonstrated by Virchow through dissection studies (Wheeler & Anderson, 1996)
2. 10% from inferior vena cava, upper extremity, and right side of heart
3. Most common site of origin is iliofemoral system (Abrams, 1997)

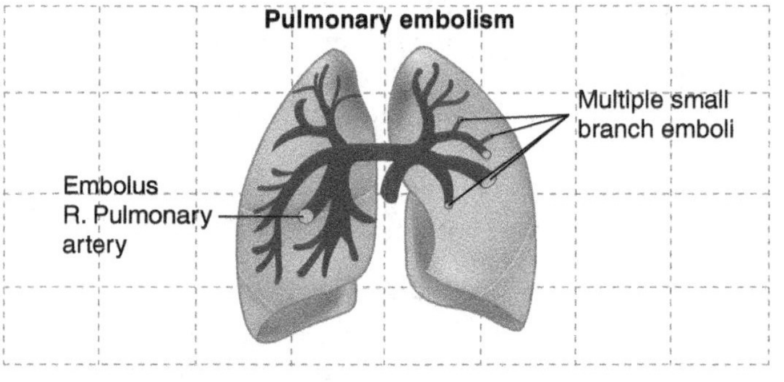

FIGURE 20-1. Pulmonary embolism and infarction.

4. Superficial thrombophlebitis (STP) generally does not lead to PE unless thrombus extends from greater saphenous vein (GSV) beyond saphenofemoral junction (SFJ) into common femoral vein

B. Nonthrombotic Emboli: <10% of PEs

1. Air embolism
   a. Displaces blood in the arterioles and capillaries
   b. Leads to ischemia and necrosis
2. Amniotic fluid
   a. Displaces blood and reduces oxygen, nutrient, and waste exchange
   b. Introduces antigens, cells, and proteins
   c. Causes inflammation and coagulation
3. Bacterial/septic embolism
   a. Subacute bacterial endocarditis the most common cause
      1) Vegetation is dislodged from infected valve and injected into circulation
4. Fat embolism
   a. Trauma induced, often fracture of large long bone (femur)
      1) Globules of fat/bone marrow are released
      2) Platelets adhere to fat
   b. Can cause adult respiratory distress syndrome
5. Foreign matter
   a. Enters bloodstream through trauma, intravenous or intra-arterial lines, or drug particulate, including illicit drug use
   b. Coagulation cascade is initiated
   c. Thromboemboli form around the particle; ischemia can occur (McCance & Huether, 1998)

C. Effects of PE

1. Produces area of lung that is ventilated but underperfused (ischemia and organic dysfunction)
   a. Increased physiologic dead-space ventilation
   b. Reflex bronchospasm in affected area as a result of histamine or serotonin release from the clot
      1) Thought to be compensatory in the occluded area since it reduces the unevenness of ventilation and perfusion
      2) In adjacent lung tissue, bronchospasm may result in considerable hypoxemia
2. Pulmonary hypertension results from large area of reduced flow through pulmonary vascular bed
   a. Two thirds of vascular bed must be obliterated prior to development of pulmonary hypertension (Abrams, 1997)
   b. One large embolus or multiple recurrent emboli (showers)
3. Infarction
   a. Localized area of ischemic necrosis of lung tissue
   b. Uncommon because of lung's dual blood supply (pulmonary and bronchial)
   c. Associated with occlusion of medium-size lobar or lobular artery and insufficient collateral flow from the bronchial circulation
   d. Pleural friction rub and small pleural effusion are signs (Abrams, 1997)
4. Pain: secondary to ischemia

D. Size of Embolus Determines Outcome/Symptoms

1. Small embolus in patient with healthy lung may be asymptomatic or very subtle/nonspecific
2. Small embolus in patient with lung disease (chronic obstructive pulmonary disease, cancer) may cause severe hypoxia
3. Multiple small emboli (emboli shower) may have similar effect on lung function, oxygenation as one large embolus
4. Massive PE: "Saddle" embolus
   a. Complete occlusion of bifurcation of main pulmonary artery
   b. Complete obstruction of outflow from right ventricle
   c. Sudden shock with severe chest pain, tachycardia, hypotension, cyanosis, stupor, syncope
   d. Death within 30 minutes before medical intervention can be initiated

III. Etiology/Precipitating Factors

A. All Risk Factors for development of DVT (Virchow triad) as listed in Chapter 19, Superficial Thrombophlebitis and Deep Vein Thrombosis

1. Venous Stasis
   a. Age: risk progressively increases over 40; threefold increase in risk after age 70 (Caprini, Arcelus, Hasty, Tamhane, & Fabrega, 1991)
   b. Immobilization: bed rest, travel, sedentary work
   c. All surgery, especially orthopedic
   d. Obesity: increased intra-abdominal pressure plus relative sedentary lifestyle
   e. Pregnancy and postpartum state, estrogen therapy: hormonal changes affect vessel wall
   f. Acute CVA
   g. Spinal cord injury
2. Vessel wall injury
   a. Postsurgical or trauma patient: especially chest, abdomen, pelvic, or leg injury
   b. Pelvic or hip fractures
   c. Intravenous therapy, central venous catheters
3. Hypercoagulability
   a. Malignancy
   b. Pregnancy (hormone fluctuation)
   c. Polycythemia: associated with other pulmonary conditions or congenital heart defects
   d. Genetic disorders of coagulability (refer to Chapter 19, Superficial Thrombophlebitis and Deep Vein Thrombosis)
   e. Tobacco use
   f. Myocardial infarction
   g. Nephrotic syndrome
   h. Dehydration
   i. Inflammatory bowel disease
   j. Buerger disease
   k. Lupus anticoagulant/anticardiolipin antibody
   l. Disseminated intravascular coagulation (DIC)
   m. Medications: chemotherapy, estrogen/oral contraception

B. High-Risk Disorders

1. Congestive heart failure is single most important condition predisposing to DVT/PE (Abrams, 1997)
2. Postoperative state
   a. Hip surgery
   b. Extensive abdominal or pelvic surgery for malignancy
3. Postpartum
4. History of DVT or PE
5. Varicose veins
6. Long bone fractures
7. Abdominal infection
8. Diabetes mellitus
9. Sickle cell anemia
10. Chronic lung disease
11. Malignancy: tumors secrete clotting factor

C. Prevention of PE in surgical and trauma patients (refer to Table 19-1 in Chapter 19, Superficial Thrombophlebitis and Deep Vein Thrombosis)

IV. Assessment

A. Risk Factors

1. Family history of thromboembolism
2. Assess for conditions predisposing to venous thrombosis as listed above

B. Primary Prevention

1. Smoking cessation
2. Public education
   a. Awareness of risk factors
   b. Promotion of a healthy lifestyle: maintain appropriate weight, exercise/mobility
   c. Smoking cessation
   d. Control hypertension
3. Assess for presence of risk factors
4. Familial coagulation studies if positive family history
   a. Factor V Leiden
   b. Protein C
   c. Protein S
   d. Prothrombin 20210 gene mutation
   e. Activated protein C resistance
   f. Homocysteine
   g. Nonpharmacologic modalities
      1) Exercise: "ambulate or elevate!", ankle rotation, plantar flexion/extension increases venous return
      2) Graduated compression stockings for patients with history of DVT, venous insufficiency or ulcer, or varicose veins
         a) 20 to 30 mm Hg compression if no prior history of DVT and normal vascular studies

b) 30 to 40 mm Hg compression with positive history of DVT, ulcer, abnormal vascular examination/studies

5. Prevent VTE during air travel: Drink lots of water, move around, avoid alcohol, wear compression hose (Goldhaber & Morrison, 2002)

C. Prevention for hospitalized general medical patients with one or more risk factors

1. Ambulate/exercise as able or appropriate
2. Graduated compression support stocking (18 to 20 mm Hg) if patient has normal arterial examination
3. Weight-based unfractionated heparin or low-molecular-weight heparin (LMWH)
4. PE prevention for surgical and trauma patients (refer to Table 19-1 in Chapter 19, Superficial Thrombophlebitis and Deep Vein Thrombosis)

D. Patient History

1. Signs and symptoms variable, subtle, and nonspecific
   a. General health state of patient: small PE may cause significant distress if patient has underlying cardiovascular or pulmonary disease; other patients may be asymptomatic if relatively healthy
   b. Size of embolus/occlusion: massive PE may lead to acute right heart failure and cardiopulmonary arrest and death
   c. Sudden unexplained hypotension, chest pain, or respiratory distress suggests possibility of pulmonary embolism (Wheeler & Anderson, 1996)
   d. Diagnosis of PE often unsuspected: two thirds of deaths from PE occur within 1 hour of embolism and are undiagnosed (Cardin & Marinelli, 2004)
2. Classic subjective symptoms in order of frequency (Thompson & Hales, 2004)
   a. Dyspnea: 73%
   b. Pleuritic chest pain, especially exacerbated by movement or breathing: 66%
   c. Cough: 37%
   d. Hemoptysis: 13%
   e. Restlessness/anxiety
   f. Lightheadedness/fainting
   g. Increased respiratory and heart rate
   h. Sweating (Goldhaber & Morrison, 2002)
3. Objective patient history
   a. Documented history of a pulmonary embolism
   b. Recent history of a DVT
   c. Family history of thrombophilia

E. Physical Examination/Objective Findings

1. Most common signs, in order of frequency (Thompson & Hales, 2004)
   a. Tachypnea/hypoxemia: 70%; caused by mismatch of alveolar ventilation without pulmonary flow in that area
   b. Rales: 51%

c. Tachycardia: 30%
d. Fourth heart sound: 24%
e. Accentuated pulmonic component of the second heart sound: 23%
f. Frequency of these findings was the same for patients without PE: no particular clinical finding is sensitive or specific enough to establish diagnosis

2. Inspection
    a. Neuro: anxiety, level of consciousness/faint or syncope
    b. Skin: diaphoretic, flushed or pale evidence of shock; cyanosis
    c. Respiratory: labored breathing, orthopnea, cough/hemoptysis, acute cor pulmonale
    d. Cardiovascular: distended neck veins
    e. Extremities: peripheral edema (especially unilateral), bulging varicosities, erythema
3. Palpation
    a. Pulses usually normal unless edema diminishes ability to palpate or patient in shock
    b. Presence and amount of edema
    c. Skin temperature/low-grade fever, diaphoresis
4. Percussion
    a. Chest: areas of dullness indicate consolidation/fluid collection
    b. Abdomen: assess for masses
5. Auscultation
    a. Vital signs
    b. Tachycardia
    c. Tachyon
    d. Hypotension/shock
    e. Cardiac: murmur, rub, arrhythmia, bruits
    f. Lung sounds: rales, pleural friction rub, diminished lung sounds
    g. Abdomen: bowel sounds will be diminished if in shock
6. Shock
    a. Indicates massive PE in healthy patient or submassive PE in patient with pre-existing cardiopulmonary disease
    b. Associated with fivefold increase in mortality (Cardin & Marinelli, 2004)
    c. Mechanism: blockage of pulmonary outflow tract by emboli, resulting in severe right ventricular hypertension and failure

F. Considerations Across the Life Span for Increased Risk

1. Young adulthood: contact sports; oral contraception; alcohol, tobacco, and illicit drug use; compliance; presence of other diseases (e.g., diabetes, cancer); nutritional status; other medications (interactions with anticoagulants)
2. Women of childbearing age: oral contraception; planned conception (warfarin crosses placenta and causes birth defects); alcohol, tobacco, and illicit drug use; compliance; other medications such as steroid therapy; varicose veins
3. Elderly: hormone replacement therapy; safety issues: increased risk of falls, home environment, support systems, memory loss, increased bleeding risk; general health/nutritional status (may require a lower dose); use of alcohol, tobacco, and illicit drugs; polypharmacy/medications; prior episodes of DVT/PE; stroke/paralysis; surgery/trauma

V. Pertinent Diagnostic Testing

A. Critical Bedside Laboratory Tests Used for Rapid Diagnosis

1. Chest x-ray after injection of contrast (American Thoracic Society, 2010): 80% are abnormal but nonspecific in majority of patients
   a. Important in identifying other cardiac or pulmonary problems which may resemble PE
   b. Pulmonary infarct shows triangular, wedge-shaped defect
   c. Lung markings (primarily blood vessels) are diminished in area supplied by clotted artery
   d. Right heart enlargement
   e. Atelectasis, pleural effusion, pulmonary infiltrates, elevated hemidiaphragm may be seen
2. Electrocardiogram (ECG)
   a. May show nonspecific changes in T-wave, S-T segment, or axis deviation: if present, may indicate right heart strain secondary to pulmonary arterial obstruction
   b. Useful to evaluate for myocardial infarction, arrhythmia, or other cardiac causes of symptoms
3. Arterial blood gases (ABG)
   a. Low arterial oxygen (PO_2) highly suspicious for PE, especially if chest x-ray normal
   b. Usually show hypoxemia, hypocapnia, respiratory alkalosis, but not always seen, so ABGs do not play major role in diagnosis
   c. Normal does not exclude PE but makes diagnosis less likely
   d. Pulse oximetry is of little diagnostic value, but if <95% at time of diagnosis, patient is at increased risk of complications (e.g., respiratory failure, cardiogenic shock, and death)
4. Noninvasive venous studies (venous duplex ultrasound or impedance plethysmography)
   a. Positive study for DVT very helpful in establishing diagnosis and origin or PE
   b. Eliminates need for transport for invasive testing if positive
5. D-dimer assay (Thompson & Hales, 2004)
   a. A degradation product of fibrin, which is broken down by natural fibrinolysis
   b. Quantitative indicator for active clotting process; elevated eightfold after DVT/PE, but also may be increased in presence of infection, cancer, surgery, heart failure, kidney failure
   c. Negative (<500 ng/mL) essentially excludes PE in healthy patients with low clinical suspicion and nondiagnostic ventilation/perfusion (V/Q) scan
   d. Positive (>500 ng/mL) does not provide specific diagnostic information, especially if there is history of malignancy, recent trauma, or surgery within past 3 months: lacks specificity, especially in advanced age (Thompson & Hales, 2004)
   e. Sensitivity and negative predictive value is high: 85% using SimpliRED test (rapid RBC agglutination testing used at bedside). This increased to 99% if patients had low probability of PE from clinical assessment (Thompson & Hales, 2004)

f. Reliance on D-dimer for PE diagnosis is limited
   1) Test methodology and assays vary
   2) D-dimer analyses using enzyme-linked immunosorbent assays (ELISA) yield best sensitivities (95%) for excluding PE/DVT
   3) A negative rapid ELISA is as useful as normal lung scan and negative venous duplex scan to exclude PE

6. Nuclear medicine lung scan (American Thoracic Society, 2010)
   a. Shows where blood does not flow
   b. Good for seeing smaller lung arteries

B. Noninvasive Testing

1. V/Q scan
   a. Assesses airflow and pulmonary circulation to identify areas that may have normal air exchange but abnormal blood flow indicative of obstruction
   b. Ventilation scan requires inhalation of radioactive gases or aerosols followed by imaging to detect nonventilated area
   c. Perfusion scan requires injection of radioactive material (albumin with technetium or iodine) followed by imaging to detect area of nonperfusion suggestive of blocked artery
   d. Pre-existing lung disease (atelectasis, pneumothorax, emphysema, chronic pulmonary lung disease) may cause false-positive results: need to compare chest x-ray and patient history
   e. A normal ventilation scan with abnormal perfusion scan is associated with high probability of PE
   f. When clinical suspicion for PE is high, and V/Q scan read as high probability for PE, accuracy is 96% (Wheeler & Anderson, 1996)
   g. When clinical suspicion low and V/Q is normal, likelihood of PE very low (2% to 9%)
   h. Many patients have indeterminate results: further evaluation with invasive studies needed
2. Spiral computed tomography (CT): test of choice in many institutions
   a. Employs continuous movement of patient through scanner with concurrent rotating rapid scanning
   b. More accurate when intravenous contrast material used
   c. Detection of proximal vessel emboli easier than in segmental arteries; limited ability to detect emboli beyond segmental arteries
3. MRI: has been used to make diagnosis but not cost effective or safe in critically ill patients; respiratory and cardiac artifact limit imaging
4. Echocardiography (ECHO)
   a. Evaluates for acute cor pulmonale
   b. When PE causes >50% pulmonary artery obstruction, severe pulmonary artery hypertension leads to distention of right ventricle and severe right heart failure
   c. 80% of patients with known PE have abnormal ECHO
   d. ECHO has been used to monitor improvement of obstruction, especially during treatment with fibrinolytic agents

C. Invasive Testing: pulmonary angiography

1. Gold standard for diagnosis of PE, but not often performed (see Limitations)

2. Allows visualization of pulmonary arteries via catheterization of groin, injection of contrast material, and x-ray
3. Internal filling defect in pulmonary artery confirms diagnosis
4. Limitations
   a. Invasive procedure using contrast material: need to note allergies
   b. Critically ill patient needs to be monitored: may be difficult and dangerous
   c. Especially risky for patients with right heart failure, severe pulmonary hypertension, and respiratory failure; mortality from procedure <2%
   d. High level of technical expertise; expensive
   e. Not suitable for routine use or screening

D. Other Testing: Consider screening for familial/genetic hypercoagulabilities as discussed in Chapter 19 (Superficial Thrombophlebitis and Deep Vein Thrombosis)

VI. Medical Management of Pulmonary Embolism

A. Treatment Goals

1. Maintain adequate cardiac and respiratory function until blockage resolves, usually within 10 to 14 days
2. Prevent recurrence of thrombosis or other embolic events

B. Prompt, Accurate Diagnosis with immediate stabilization using supportive care and anticoagulation therapy required for maximal outcome

1. Elevate head of bed >30 degrees
2. Oxygen via nasal cannula, mask, or both
3. Intubation and mechanical ventilation if needed for severe respiratory distress
4. Intravenous access: large bore needle if possible
5. Small doses of opiates (intravenous morphine, 1 to 2 mg) for discomfort and anxiety; avoid larger doses which may lead to respiratory depression
6. Cautious administration of intravenous fluids to avoid exacerbation of right heart failure
7. Graduated compression stockings
8. Medications to control/stabilize blood pressure, manage dysrhythmias, maintain normal volume status

C. Baseline Laboratory Values Prior to Initiation of Treatment

1. Activated partial thromboplastin time (aPTT), prothrombin time (PT) with international normalization ratio (INR), complete blood count (CBC), creatinine
2. Special coagulation studies, if necessary
3. ABG
4. Stool for occult blood

D. Heparin

1. Cornerstone of treatment for PE (Wheeler & Anderson, 1996)
   a. Stops progression of thrombosis
   b. Associated with less than 5% recurrence rate of PE

c. Emboli dissolve over course of several days because of natural fibrinolytic mechanisms
d. In cases of incomplete lysis, chronic pulmonary hypertension may result
2. Intravenous unfractionated heparin standard treatment
a. Important to reach therapeutic level as quickly as possible to prevent reoccurrence of PE: 1.5 to 2.5 times baseline aPTT
1) Initial bolus of 120 to 140 units/kg: 5,000 to 10,000 units
2) Infusion of 20 units/kg/hr: usually 1,000 to 2,000 units/hr
3) Check aPTT every 6 hours until stable, adjust heparin as necessary (Feied & Handler, 2000)
4) Close monitoring for first 24 to 72 hours required to prevent under- or over-anticoagulation. "The most common mistake that occurs is to give too little heparin initially when the heparin requirement is high, and too much heparin later, when the heparin requirement is generally low" (Walsh & Rice, 2004).
3. LMWH
a. "With proper dosing, several LMWH products have been found safer and more effective than unfractionated heparin both for prophylaxis and for treatment of DVT and PE" (Feied & Handler, 2000)
b. If creatinine is >2.0 or the platelet count is <100,000, alert the medical provider to discuss use of unfractionated heparin
c. No need to check aPTT, as there is no correlation with LMWH

E. Fondaparinux (Arixtra): factor Xa inhibitor, FDA approved 2001

1. Action
a. Selectively catalyzes factor Xa by antithrombin III without inhibiting thrombin
b. Does not bind to platelet factor 4; does not affect platelet aggregation
2. Current use
a. Prophylaxis of DVT that could lead to PE in patients undergoing hip fracture repair or hip or knee replacement surgery or abdominal surgery (PEGASUS Trial Study, 2005)
b. Dosage for DVT prevention hip and knee replacement: 2.5 mg subcutaneous injection daily for 5 to 9 days, up to 11 days
c. Dosage for prevention of DVT hip fracture surgery: 2.5 mg subcutaneous injection daily for 29 to 33 days
d. Dosage for prevention of DVT in abdominal surgery: 2.5 mg subcutaneous injection 6 hours after surgery for 5 to 9 days
3. Use in PE (The Matisse Investigators, 2003)
a. Fondaparinux and enoxaparin have similar safety and efficacy profile in treatment of PE
b. Dosage for DVT/PE treatment: 5 mg (patient weight <50 kg); 7.5 mg (50 to 100 kg); 10 mg (>100 kg) for 5 to 9 days
c. Continue treatment until therapeutic oral anticoagulation is complete
4. Potential advantages
a. Fewer bleeding complications
b. Minimization/elimination of biological variability, immunogenic reactivity, and pathogenic contamination (less potential for hypersensitivity reactions)
c. Shown to be as safe and effective as LMWH (Buller et al., 2004)
d. Cost: $18.09 for 2.5 mg dose
e. Once-daily dosing; dose does not need to be calculated

5. Disadvantages/adverse reaction
   a. Not recommended for patients with severe renal insufficiency, low body weight, active major bleeding, bacterial endocarditis, or thrombocytopenia
   b. Common injection site bleeding, rash, pruritus, fever
   c. Serious major bleeding, thrombocytopenia, aminotransferase elevation, anemia
   d. Drug interactions: many; avoid other anticoagulants, vitamin A, herbal products such as ginkgo, green tea, devil's claw, St. John's wort

F. Warfarin Oral Anticoagulation

1. Initiated on day 1 of heparin therapy if possible, usually 5 to 15 mg
2. Adjust subsequent daily dose according to the INR, with goal of 2 to 3
3. Overlap heparin and warfarin for 5 to 7 days or until INR stable at therapeutic goal for 48 hours to allow for depletion of vitamin K-dependent clotting factors
4. Anticoagulate with warfarin for 3 to 6 months (Feied & Handler, 2000)
5. If the individual has a familial or acquired thrombophilia, recurrent thromboembolism or ongoing risk factors, anticoagulation may be lifelong (refer to Chapter 19, Superficial Thrombophlebitis and Deep Vein Thrombosis for chronic anticoagulation management)

G. Fibrinolytic Therapy

1. Dissolution of clot via chemical lysis of fibrin component, resulting in rapid removal of intraluminal thrombus and restoration of vessel patency
2. Potential benefits
   a. Prompt dissolution of physiologically compromising occlusion of pulmonary circulation: may be life-saving; clot lysis usually occurs in 80% to 90% of cases
   b. Faster recovery
   c. Prevention of recurrent thrombus formation
   d. Rapid restoration of hemodynamic function
   e. Compared to use of conventional heparin alone, improved long-term right ventricular function and less pulmonary hypertension (Wheeler & Anderson, 1996)
3. Disadvantages
   a. High risk of systemic bleeding complications: double or triple compared to heparin (Erdman, Rodvold, & Friedenberg, 1997)
   b. Most serious is intracranial bleeding: 1% incidence (Wheeler & Anderson, 1996)
   c. Intraperitoneal bleeding may be life threatening
   d. Close monitoring: intensive care if patient unstable
   e. Cost of medication
   f. Studies have not shown improved overall mortality compared to heparin (Erdman et al., 1997)
4. Proposed indications
   a. Massive/submassive PE with hemodynamic compromise
   b. Massive PE without hemodynamic compromise
   c. Submassive PE in patients who cannot tolerate further cardiopulmonary compromise
   d. Heparin treatment failures
   e. Extensive proximal DVT

5. Contraindications to thrombolytic therapy (Erdman et al., 1997)
   a. Absolute: active bleeding, cerebrovascular disease/event or procedure within past 2 months
   b. Relative: recent major surgery or trauma (within 10 days), postpartum, cardiopulmonary resuscitation with rib fractures, thoracentesis, paracentesis, lumbar puncture, any condition requiring maintenance of normal clotting or healing
   c. Potentially serious bleeding: uncontrolled coagulation defects, severe hypertension, pregnancy, any condition with potential bleeding risk
6. FDA approved fibrinolytic agents
   a. Streptokinase: first agent approved but is no longer manufactured
   b. Urokinase: urokinase is not currently available since Abbokinase is no longer manufactured and Kinlytic is not yet FDA approved
   c. Recombinant tissue plasminogen activator (rt-PA)
      1) 100 mg as continuous infusion over 2 hours
      2) More rapid and complete thrombus dissolution compared to urokinase
      3) Shortest treatment time
      4) Alteplase is only FDA approved for pulmonary embolism (Jaff et al., 2011)
7. Precautions and guidelines for patient care
   a. Minimizing bleeding
      1) Careful patient selection/evaluation with attention to neurologic history
      2) Laboratory monitoring prior to infusion: CBC, platelet count, aPTT, and PT, and tests for coagulation defects (e.g., fibrin degradation products); repeat as indicated during and after therapy
      3) Fecal occult blood sample prior to therapy
      4) Minimal venipuncture and arterial puncture
      5) Short infusions via pulmonary artery catheter (usually inserted in groin) directed into thrombus; adequate pressure on site once catheter removed
      6) If possible, avoidance of lytic agents as emergency treatment: can be used successfully as an elective procedure via peripheral vein with less bleeding risk (Wheeler & Anderson, 1996)
      7) Avoid administration of heparin: if heparin recently given, wait until aPPT is less than 1.5 control. Once lytic therapy complete, do not resume heparin until aPPT <80 seconds (Walsh & Rice, 2004)
   b. Monitor for adverse effects
      1) Hemorrhage: major bleeding occurs in approximately 20% (Erdman et al., 1997). Lytic agents have short half-life: discontinuation results in rapid cessation of lytic activity. If blood replacement required, whole blood, packed red cells, fresh-frozen plasma, or cryoprecipitate may be given. If bleeding continues, 5 g doses of E-aminocaproic acid (EACA) may be given
      2) Allergic reaction: mostly associated with streptokinase, although mild allergic reactions to other agents have been reported; urticaria, itching, flushing, nausea, headache, alteration of blood pressure. Treat with antihistamines
      3) Fever: seldom greater than 104°F; 30% with streptokinase; 15% with other agents. Treat with acetaminophen
      4) Hypotension: associated with rapid or high-dose infusions of any lytic agents; treat by slowing infusion

5) Thrombocytopenia: reported in 10% of rt-PA infusions; discontinue if platelet count falls below 75,000/mm^3

c. Guidelines for patient care (Erdman et al., 1997)
   1) Minimal repositioning of patient
   2) Discontinue parenteral medications
   3) Substitute oral medications when possible
   4) Avoid invasive procedures
   5) Apply compression at venipuncture sites
   6) Avoid any other anticoagulants
   7) Avoid use of platelet-active drugs, aspirin-containing drugs, antiplatelet agents, and dextran

VII. Surgical Management

A. Inferior Vena Cava Filter Placement

1. Indications (see Table 20-1)
2. Percutaneous insertion technique in radiology (Feied & Handler, 2000)
   a. Local anesthetic and small incision in groin
   b. Catheter is introduced into the femoral vein
   c. Radiopaque contrast is administered and filter is placed in the inferior vena cava, with apex near the level of the lowest renal vein at approximately L2 and L3
   d. Requires anticoagulation with heparin and followed by lifelong warfarin
3. Devices
   a. Permanent
      1) Greenfield filter: either stainless steel or titanium; only device shown to maintain patency of inferior vena cava and avoid renal vein occlusion (Greenfield & Proctor, 1996)
      2) Nitinol filter
      3) Bird's nest filter
      4) Vena Tech
      5) TrapEase
      6) SiteFlo (Siskin & Cho, 2011).
   b. Retrievable filter: may be removed between 14 and 41 days of placement or remain in place as permanent filter; reported technical success rate of 93% (Morris, Rogers, Najarian, Bhave, & Shackford, 2004)
      1) ALN
      2) G2

TABLE 20-1 Indications for Insertion of a Vena Cava Filter

Deep Vein Thrombosis (DVT) or Pulmonary Embolism (PE) in patients with contraindication or complication to anticoagulants
Prevention of PE in patients undergoing surgery, cancer, or trauma
Failure of anticoagulants
IVC or iliofemoral thrombus

Siskin, G., & Cho, K. (2011). Inferior vena cava filters. Retrieved from http://emedicine.Medscape.com/article/419796-overview, accessed November 30, 2012.

3) Eclipse
4) Gunther-Tulip
5) Celect
6) OptEase
7) Option (Siskin & Cho, 2011)

4. Potential complications (Walsh & Rice, 2004)
   a. Recurrent PE
   b. Venous insufficiency
   c. Air embolism
   d. Occlusion of device with bilateral venous outflow obstruction
   e. Improper placement or migration
   f. Hematoma at the insertion site

B. Pulmonary Embolectomy

1. Indications: usually only for life-threatening situations, although some centers suggest improved surgical technique and careful patient selection may expand use of this procedure (Aklog, Williams, Byrne, & Goldhaber, 2002)
   a. Massive PE; patient pre-terminal
   b. Thrombolytic therapy unavailable or contraindicated
   c. Most patients die before they can be transported to operating room or stabilize and no longer require procedure
   d. Rarely used electively for patients with chronic PE where clot did not naturally lyse
2. Procedure
   a. Balloon-tipped catheter is inserted into the pulmonary artery via incision in groin
   b. The clot is removed by withdrawal of the inflated catheter
   c. Immediately followed by vena caval filter placement and anticoagulation
   d. Rheolytic thrombectomy: high-velocity saline solution to create a strong Venturi effect, followed by aspiration of the clot with catheter or syringe
   e. Open surgical embolectomy: used for patients with adequate systolic arterial pressure but profound right ventricular failure; beating heart bypass technique (Aklog et al., 2002; Cardin & Marinelli, 2004)

VIII. Nursing Diagnosis

A. Alteration in tissue perfusion related to pulmonary arterial obstruction as evidenced by dyspnea, tachypnea, and tachycardia

1. Expected patient outcomes: patient will maintain end-organ perfusion
2. Interventions
   a. Supplemental oxygen and/or mechanical ventilation as indicated
   b. Elevate head of bed; unaffected lung positioned down to allow for increased blood flow to area of continuous perfusion/ventilation (e.g., if PE in left lung, patient lies on right side)
   c. Assist patient with activities of daily living
   d. Turn, cough, and deep breathe
   e. Hydrate patient cautiously, avoiding overhydration and exacerbation of right heart failure

3. Evaluation
    a. Monitor oxygen saturation either continuously or with each assessment and p.r.n.
    b. Auscultate lung and heart sounds with each assessment and p.r.n.
    c. Check vital signs as frequently as level of acuity indicates is appropriate
    d. Observe for dyspnea, tachycardia, diaphoresis, anxiety, or other symptoms of distress with any activity

B. **Alteration** in comfort related to obstruction of pulmonary circulation

1. Expected patient outcomes
    a. Patient will be pain free
    b. Patient will be able to perform activities of daily living
2. Interventions
    a. Position of comfort and optimal oxygenation (good lung down)
    b. Analgesia p.r.n.
    c. Support chest with a pillow when coughing
    d. Activity as tolerated
3. Evaluation
    a. Assess pain on a scale of 1 to 10 minimally every 8 hours and p.r.n.
    b. Observe/record frequency of requests for pain medication
    c. Observe tolerance of activity: increased pain, tachycardia, hypertension
    d. Observe/record response to analgesia

C. **Anxiety** related to dyspnea, pain, and unknown treatments/diagnostics

1. Expected outcomes
    a. Patient will appear physically calm/comfortable and express feeling less anxious
    b. Patient will verbalize understanding of related tests and medical/nursing treatments
2. Interventions
    a. Administer medication as indicated for control of anxiety in acute stage of illness
    b. Provide patient/family education regarding disease process, treatment, diagnostics, and expected outcomes
    c. Provide calm atmosphere
    d. Use open-ended questions with patient
    e. Allow patient and family to verbalize feelings
3. Evaluation
    a. Assess for physical signs of anxiety hourly and p.r.n. during acute illness; then every 8 hours once stable
    b. Assess feelings as patient verbalizes emotions
    c. Note patient's interactions with others

IX. Patient Teaching

A. Disease Prevention/Health Promotion and Secondary Prevention

1. Define PE to patient/family and explain why this occurred, with discussion of specific situation if known (e.g., thrombus formation associated with recent air travel)

2. Identify patient's risk factors
3. Explain treatment goals
   a. Prevention of subsequent thrombosis/embolism
   b. Maintenance of activities of daily living or pre-illness level of function
   c. Avoidance of complications of therapy
   d. INR goal: define and give expected range (usual 2 to 3)
4. Anticoagulant medication education
   a. Tablet strength, color, how many, and how often to take
   b. Side effects
      1) Easy bruisability
      2) Medical attention for new rash or significant bleeding
   c. Interactions with other medications
      1) No ASA unless prescribed by care provider
      2) Multiple drug and food interactions with warfarin
      3) Discuss any new OTC or prescription products prior to starting
   d. Subcutaneous injection technique if self-administering heparin or LMWH
   e. Discuss estrogen therapy risks with medical provider
5. Symptoms to watch for and what to do
   a. Infection: call medical provider
   b. Increased pain, swelling, warmth, erythema of leg: seek emergency care, call 911
   c. Chest pain, rapid pulse, sweating, anxiety, fainting, hemoptysis: seek emergency care, call 911
   d. Unilateral paralysis, numbness, facial droop, vision or speech change, loss of coordination, change in mental status: seek emergency care, call 911
   e. Bleeding
      1) Major: call 911 or go to emergency room
      2) Minor: alert health care provider

B. Home Care Considerations

1. Diet
   a. Vitamin K: can have a negative effect on warfarin
      1) Diet should be consistent and moderate
      2) Give list of foods that are moderate to high in vitamin K
         a) Green leafy vegetables are high in vitamin K
         b) Green tea and tobacco are very high in vitamin K and should be avoided
   b. Avoid alcohol use
   c. Maintain desired weight (BMI between 19 and 25)
   d. Check with health care provider before using any herbal remedies
2. Activity
   a. Walk regularly/daily: may also jog, swim, cycle
   b. Avoid prolonged sitting or standing
   c. Elevate legs when nonambulatory
   d. Avoid crossing legs
3. Avoid constrictive clothing and footwear: compression support hose should not be overly binding and is best obtained from experienced compression garment fitter
4. Safety precautions
   a. Protect the feet
   b. Exercise caution when using sharp items such as scissors, broken glass, and so forth

c. Wear a helmet when riding a bicycle
d. Wear or carry identification that indicates anticoagulation therapy
e. Seek immediate care for serious injury or head injury
5. Home environment and support system concerns
a. Ability to come in for routine laboratory/INR
b. Ability to administer own medications accurately
c. Review fall risks and recommend necessary changes or precautions
6. Call nurse or medical provider for
a. Changes in medication, diet, missed dose
b. Questions or symptoms they have

X. Research and Further Study (American Thrombosis Society, 2010)

A. Genetic Factors: link being discovered between genetics and blood clotting problems

B. Information on Blood Clotting Process: improving

C. Improved Diagnostic Tools

D. New Anticoagulant Agents: options that can be used when main frontline agents are contraindicated

CASE STUDY

J.D. is a 54-year-old tree service owner who suffered a back injury after falling out of a tree. He did not seek immediate medical attention but placed himself on bed rest for 5 days and took acetaminophen 1,000 mg three times daily for pain. Mr. D. subsequently presented to the emergency room with chest pain and dyspnea. He is on no other medications and denied any other health issues. He specifically denied any bleeding problems. Immediate examination upon presentation includes the following:

Integument: diaphoretic; otherwise, skin intact without bruises or rash
Cardiovascular: apical pulse 120, regular without murmurs, S1, S2. B/P 130/70; uniform mild edema of right lower extremity from proximal thigh to ankle, radial and pedal pulses +4
Respiratory: rate 24, even and labored; chest clear bilaterally with no areas of dullness to percussion
Gastrointestinal: bowel sounds present in all four quadrants; no organomegaly, bruits, or masses
Neurologic: no deficits; alert, oriented, and appropriate but appears anxious with rapid speech and restlessness
Social history: independent ADLs; lives with his wife in a one-story home; two daughters who live close; smokes 1 pack per day for past 40 years; drinks 1 to 3 beers after work daily
Family history: mother, age 81, and two maternal uncles, both deceased, have history of DVT

Laboratory values reveal the following:

Hgb: 14 (normal)
Platelets: 180,000 (normal)
Creatinine: 1.0 (normal)
ABGs SaO_2: 88 (abnormal)
ECG tachycardia with nonspecific T-wave and ST segment changes

Initial diagnosis: pulmonary embolism and right lower extremity DVT suspected

Review Questions

1. What signs and symptoms are suspicious for thromboembolism?
   a. Dyspnea with tachypnea and labored respirations
   b. Chest pain
   c. Tachycardia
   d. Anxiety
   e. All of the above
2. What diagnostic test is most helpful in establishing the diagnosis of PE?
   a. Electrocardiogram
   b. Arterial blood gas
   c. Chest x-ray
   d. Venous duplex ultrasound
   e. D-dimer assay
3. Mr. D. is sent for a spiral CT scan to confirm the diagnosis of PE, rather than a ventilation/perfusion (V/Q) scan. What conditions might lead to an erroneous V/Q scan result?
   a. Chronic obstructive pulmonary disease (COPD)
   b. Myocardial infarction
   c. Atherosclerosis
   d. Spinal stenosis
4. What immediate care measures are essential in ensuring Mr. D's safety and maintenance of normal gas exchange?
   a. Trendelenburg position
   b. Administration of oxygen and 1 mg of morphine sulfate
   c. 1 L of normal saline rapidly infused over 30 minutes
   d. Graduated compression stockings
5. In treating Mr. D's pulmonary embolism, the most common mistake is to give too little anticoagulation initially when the heparin requirement is high, and too much heparin later, when the heparin requirement is lower. True or False?
6. What laboratory tests are recommended prior to initiation of heparin therapy?
   a. CBC with platelet count
   b. Creatinine
   c. Stool for occult blood
   d. Familial coagulopathy tests
   e. All of the above
7. Patient and family teaching at the time of Mr. D's discharge should emphasize:
   a. Avoidance of all green leafy vegetables
   b. Smoking cessation and use of a medication bracelet
   c. Limited walking for 3 months
   d. Discussion of anticoagulation side effects and his work responsibilities
   e. a and b
   f. b and d

Answers/Rationales

1. e. All of the above. While all of the presenting symptoms are nonspecific and could indicate other disorders (such as myocardial infarction), the most classic subjective symptom is dyspnea, followed by pleuritic chest, cough, hemoptysis, restlessness. Objective findings include tachypnea with hypoxia, tachycardia, rales, and the presence of a fourth heart sound.
2. d. Venous duplex ultrasound. A positive venous ultrasound which demonstrates presence of deep vein thrombosis is very helpful in establishing diagnosis of PE and eliminates need for further invasive testing. The information obtained on other tests may be supportive but is not confirmatory, although a negative D-dimer assay essentially rules out the possibility of a PE in a patient who is otherwise at low risk and has low index of suspicion (which is NOT Mr. D). While pulmonary angiogram remains the gold standard for absolute diagnosis of PE, it is invasive and may be very risky in a critically unstable patient.
3. a. COPD. Mr. D. has a history of smoking for 40 years and likely has either emphysematous changes of his lungs or COPD. Both of these conditions, as well as pneumothorax or atelectasis which could have occurred when he fell out of the tree, can lead to false-positive V/Q results.
4. b. Administration of oxygen and 1 mg of morphine sulfate. He has hypoxemia and is anxious; treating both will stabilize his respiratory and cardiac function, allowing his tachypnea and tachycardia to resolve. Close monitoring for further deterioration is essential: continuous pulse oximetry, cardiac monitoring, cautious administration of fluids to prevent worsening right heart failure but access via a large bore IV in case of rapid decline. Head of bed should be elevated with positioning so that the good (unaffected) lung is down to maximize blood flow to perfused lung tissue. Graduated compression stockings are recommended but are not immediately essential to stabilize the patient.
5. True. Heparin remains the cornerstone of treatment for PE. Early (within first 24 hours) achievement of a therapeutic aPPT (1.5 to 2.5 baseline) has been shown to stop progression of thrombosis and lower recurrence rate. However, continuing high infusion rates beyond 72 hours results in higher risk for bleeding complications.
6. e. All of the above. Mr. D. needs to be assessed for presence of anemia and platelet abnormality prior to anticoagulation to establish a baseline in case he should develop bleeding complications or platelet abnormality as a reaction to heparinization. His anticoagulation therapy would require dose adjustment in the presence of renal insufficiency, and he may not be a candidate for anticoagulation if he has an occult GI bleed. Since his mother and two uncles have a history of venous thrombosis, he (and other family members) should also be assessed for genetic hypercoagulability, although this is not immediately essential since he has several other obvious risk factors for venous thrombosis.
7. b and d. Helping Mr. D understand the risk factors for recurrence of PE can be life saving. They are specifically smoking and his family history, as well as possibility of future work-related trauma. He cannot change his family history, but he needs information regarding important lifestyle changes, including smoking and alcohol cessation, ambulation, leg elevation when not walking, avoidance of trauma, maintenance of desired weight, and a consistent diet. His high-risk occupation should be frankly discussed to investigate possible changes to provide a safer environment. In addition, he needs to be given information on how to contact his health care providers, seek emergency care if needed, and have as complete an understanding of anticoagulation effects and need for follow-up care as possible, with social support systems in place as his circumstances require.

REFERENCES

Abrams, G. D. (1997). Disturbances in circulation. In S. A. Price, & L. M. Anderson (Eds.), *Pathophysiology: Clinical concepts of disease process* (5th ed., pp. 92–107). St. Louis, MO: Mosby-Year Book.

Aklog, L., Williams, C. S., Byrne, J. G., & Goldhaber, S. Z. (2002). Acute pulmonary embolism: A contemporary approach. *Circulation, 105,* 1416–1419.

American Thoracic Society. (2010). Chapter 16: Pulmonary embolism in breathing better in America. Retrieved from http://www.thoracic.org/education/breathing-in-america/index.php, accessed November 30, 2012.

Buller, H. R., Davidson, B. L., Decousus, H., Gallus, A., Gent, M., Piovella, F., . . . Matisse Investigators. (2004). Fondaparinux or enoxaparin for the initial treatment of symptomatic deep venous thrombosis: A randomized trial. *Annals of Internal Medicine, 140*(11), 867–873.

Caprini, J. A., Arcelus, J. I., Hasty, J. H., Tamhane, A. C., & Fabrega, F. (1991). Clinical assessment of venous thromboembolic risk in surgical patients. *Seminars in Thrombosis and Hemostasis, 17*(Suppl. 3), 304–312.

Cardin, T., & Marinelli, A. (2004). Pulmonary embolism. *Critical Care Nurse Quarterly, 27*(4), 310–322.

Erdman, S. M., Rodvold, K. A., & Friedenberg, W. R. (1997). Thromboembolic disorders. In J. T. Dipiro, R. L. Talbert, G. C. Yee, G. R. Matzke, B. G. Wells, & L. M. Posey (Eds.), *Pharmacotherapy: A pathophysiologic approach* (3rd ed., pp. 399–434). Stamford, CT: Appleton & Lange.

Feied, C., & Handler, J. (2000). Pulmonary embolism. Emedicine-Instant Address to the Minds of Medicine. Retrieved from http://www.emedicine.com/EMERG/topic490.html

Goldhaber, S., & Morrison, R. (2002). Pulmonary embolism and deep vein thrombosis. *Circulation, 106,* 1436–1438.

Greenfield, L. J., & Proctor, M. C. (1996). Diagnosis and management of pulmonary embolism. *The Annals of Thoracic Surgery, 61*(3), 1037–1038.

Heit, J. A., Silverstien, M. D., Mohr, D. N., Petterson, T. M., Lohse, C. M., O'Fallon, W. M., & Melton, L. J., III. (2001). The epidemiology of venous thromboembolism in the community. *Thrombosis and Haemostasis, 86,* 452–463.

Jaff, M., McMurtry, M. S., Archer, S. L., Cushman, M., Goldenberg, N., Goldhaber, S. Z., . . . Zierler, B. K. (2011). Management of massive and submassive pulmonary embolism, iliofemoral deep vein thrombosis, and chronic thromboembolic pulmonary hypertension. *Circulation, 123,* 1788–1830.

McCance, S. L., & Huether, S. E. (1998). *Pathophysiology: The biological basis for disease in adults and children* (3rd ed., pp. 968–1023). St. Louis, MO: Mosby.

Morris, C. S., Rogers, F. B., Najarian, K. E., Bhave, A. D., & Shackford, S. R. (2004). Current trends in vena caval filtration with the introduction of a retrievable filter at a level I trauma center. *Journal of Trauma, 57*(1), 32–36.

PEGASUS Trial Study. (2005). Clinical trial results. Retrieved from http://www.trialresultscenter.org/study7632-PEGASUS.htm, accessed August 17, 2013.

Roach, H. D., & Laufman, H. (1955). Relationship between pulmonary embolism and pulmonary infarction: An experimental study. *Annals of Surgery, 142*(1), 82–91.

Rosendaal, F. R. (1999). Venous thrombosis: A multicausal disease. *The Lancet, 353*(9159), 1167–1173.

Siskin, G., & Cho, K. (2011). Inferior vena cava filters. Retrieved from http://emedicine.Medscape.com/article/419796-overview, accessed November 30, 2012.

The Matisse Investigators. (2003). Subcutaneous fondaparinux versus intravenous unfractionated heparin in the initial treatment of pulmonary embolism. *New England Journal of Medicine, 349,* 1695–1702.

Thompson, B. T., & Hales, C. A. (2004). Clinical manifestations and diagnostic strategies for acute pulmonary embolism. Retrieved from http://www.uptodate.com

Walsh, M. E., & Rice, K. L. (2004). Venous thrombosis and pulmonary embolism. In V. Fahey (Ed.), *Vascular nursing* (4th ed., pp. 365–397). Philadelphia, PA: W.B. Saunders.

Wheeler, H. B., & Anderson, F. A. (1996). Pulmonary embolism. In P. Gloviczki, & J. S. T. Yao (Eds.), *Handbook of venous disorders* (pp. 274–291). London, UK: Chapman & Hall.

SUGGESTED READINGS

American Thoracic Society. (1999). The diagnostic approach to acute venous thromboembolism. *American Journal of Respiratory and Critical Care Medicine, 160,* 1043–1066.

Autar, R. (1996). Nursing assessment of clients at risk of deep vein thrombosis (DVT): The autar DVT scale. *Journal of Advanced Nursing, 23*(4), 763–770.

Berg, D. E. (1992). Components and defects of the coagulation system. *Nurse Practitioner Forum, 3*(2), 62–71.

Breen, P. (2000). DVT: What every nurse should know. *RN, 63*(4), 59–62.

Dolovich, L. R., Ginsberg, J. S., Douketis, J. D., Holbrook, A. M., & Cheah, G. (2000). A meta-analysis comparing low-molecular-weight heparins with unfractionated heparin in the treatment of venous thromboembolism. *Archives of Internal Medicine, 160,* 181–187.

Geerts, W. H., Heit, J. A., Clagett, G. P., Pineo, G. F., Colwell, C. W., Anderson, F. A., Jr., & Wheeler, H. B. (2001). Prevention of venous thromboembolism. Sixth ACCP Consensus Conference on Antithrombotic Therapy. *Chest, 119*(1), 132S–175S.

Goldhaber, S., Fanikos. (2004). Prevention of deep vein thrombosis and pulmonary embolism. *Circulation, 110*, e445–e447.

Grady, D., Wenger, N. K., Herrington, D., Khan, S., Furberg, C., Hunninghake, D., . . . Hulley, S. (2000). Postmenopausal hormone therapy increases risk for venous thromboembolic disease. *Annals of Internal Medicine, 132*(9), 689–696.

WEB SITES

Anonymous. (1996). Low-molecular-weight heparin may reduce hospital stays. Mayo clinic health oasis. Retrieved from http://www.mayohealth.org/mayo/9701/htm/heparin.htm

Anonymous. (1998). Pulmonary embolism-what you know may save your life. Mayo clinic health oasis. Retrieved from http://www.mayohealth.org/mayo/9807/htm/pulmonary.htm

Anonymous. (2000). Ask the Mayo physician. Mayo clinic health oasis. Retrieved from http://www.mayohealth.org/mayo/askphys/qa970604.htm

Beer, A. E. Thrombophilia: Inherited and acquired. Reproductive Medicine Program, Finch University of Health Science, Chicago Medical School. Retrieved from http://www.repro-med.net/papers/thromb.html

Beer, A. E., Kwak-Kim, J., Ntrivalas, E., & Chung, H. S. Acquired thrombophilia antiphospholipid antibody syndrome category 2 immune problems. Reproductive Medicine Program, Finch University of Health Science, Chicago Medical School. Retrieved from http://www.repro-med.net/papers/apa.html

Gallus, A. S. (1998). Treatment of deep leg vein thrombosis. Australian Prescriber, *21*, 64–66. Retrieved from http://australianprescriber.com/magazines/vol21no3/vein_thrombosis

Kujovich, J., & Goodnight, S. (1999). Factor V Leiden thrombophilia. Gene Clinics, University of Washington, Seattle. Retrieved from wysiwyg://78/http://www.geneclinics.org/profiles/factor-v-leiden/details.html

Peripheral Venous Disorders. Columbia University college of p & s complete home medical guide. Retrieved from http://cpmcnet.columbia.edu/texts/guide/hmg16_0007.html

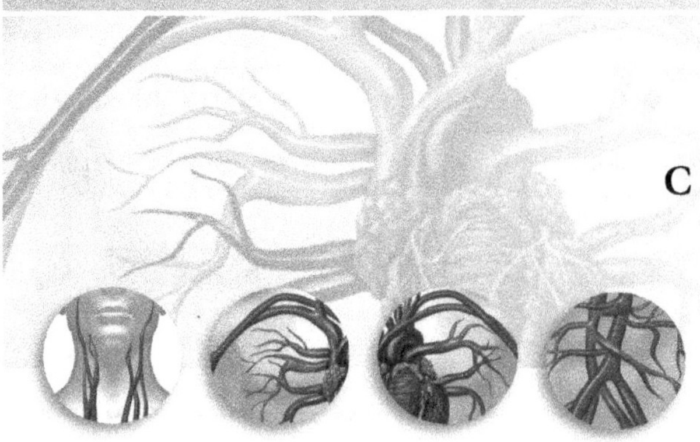

CHAPTER 21

Chronic Venous Disease and Venous Ulcers

Section 1: *Carolyn Robinson*
Section 2: *Monica Melo*

OBJECTIVES

1. Define the pathophysiology of chronic venous disease.
2. Describe methods for classification of venous disease.
3. Describe diagnostic testing for venous disease.
4. Describe the most common invasive interventions for venous disease.
5. Identify the nursing implications relevant to chronic venous disease.
6. Describe the common findings associated with venous ulceration.
7. Identify common diagnostic testing associated with venous disease/ulceration.
8. Identify appropriate interventions for venous ulcers.
9. Describe methods of long-term self-care for venous disease/ulceration and prevention of recurrence.

Introduction

Chronic venous disease (CVD) includes a spectrum of clinical presentations ranging from uncomplicated telangiectasias and varicose veins to venous ulceration (Meisner, 2004). Venous disorders can be congenital or acquired. Chronic venous insufficiency (CVI) results from chronic venous hypertension related to dysfunction of the vein walls or valves (Hurie & Wakefield, 2012). Venous hypertension usually is the result of obstruction to venous flow, dysfunction of venous valves, and or failure of the venous pump (Alguire & Mathes, 2013).

Section 1: Chronic Venous Disease

A. Incidence

1. CVD affects approximately 2.5 million people in the United States. Approximately 20% develop leg ulcers.

2. Varicose veins affect up to 40% of adults and are more common in obese people, and in women who have had more than two pregnancies.
3. The prevalence of varicose veins vary widely from 2% to 56% in men and from 1% to 60% in women

B. Epidemiology

1. Older age
2. Family history
3. Female gender: pregnancy, especially multiparity
4. Standing occupation
5. Constipation/low-fiber diet
6. Obesity: BMI >30 kg/m^2
7. Smoking
8. Oral contraceptives/HRT
9. Physical activity
10. Injury
11. History of phlebitis/clot (Dean & Spruiell, 2011)

C. Classification

1. Primary: degenerative process in normally formed vessel walls and valves without an identifiable mechanism of venous dysfunction
2. Secondary: result of a precursing event such as deep venous thrombosis (DVT). As the occluded venous segments recanalize after a DVT, chronic luminal changes occur along with partial obstruction and reflux leading to venous hypertension (Davies & Lumsden, 2011)

D. Venous Anatomy

1. The muscular fascia which surrounds the calf and leg muscles is separated into the superficial and deep compartments. The superficial compartment includes all tissues between the skin and muscular fascia. The deep compartment includes the muscles and deep veins which lie beneath the muscular fascia. The veins are divided into three systems: the superficial veins, the deep veins, and the perforating veins (Oğuzkurt, 2012).
2. Superficial venous system
   a. Drains the skin and subcutaneous tissue
   b. The superficial veins lie in the subcutaneous tissue
   c. Great saphenous vein
      1) Originates along the medial edge of the foot
      2) Ascends along the medial leg joining the common femoral vein below the inguinal ligament
      3) Communicates with the deep system through perforating veins
   d. Small saphenous vein
      1) Originates at the lateral edge of the foot
      2) Ascends along the posterior calf joining the popliteal vein at or just below the knee (Kaufman, 2004)
3. Deep venous system
   a. Contained in the deep muscle compartments
   b. Intramuscular (within the muscle)
   c. Intermuscular (between the muscle groups)

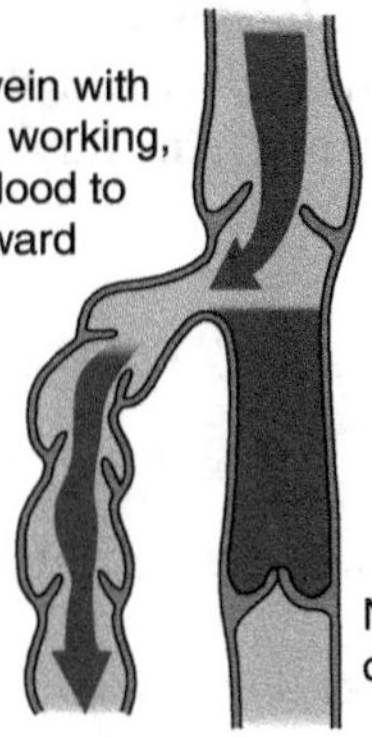

FIGURE 21-1. Normal vein valve closure and varicose vein.

   d. Responsible for 90% of venous return through the action of the foot, calf, and thigh muscle pumps (Meisner, 2004)
   e. Drain the lower extremity muscles (Meisner, 2005)
4. Perforating veins: connect the superficial with the deep veins and are found in the anterior, lateral, medial, and posterior thigh and calf (Moneta, 2013)

E. Vein Functions

1. Competent vein: blood flow returns normally to the heart
2. Incompetent vein: blood flows in the wrong direction
3. Reflux: blood flows backward in the vein

F. Chronic Vein Abnormalities (Moneta, 2013)

1. Telangiectasias (spider veins) are dilated intradermal venules less than 1 mm in diameter (Dean & Spruiell, 2011).
2. Reticular veins are dilated bluish subdermal veins 1 to 3 mm in diameter.
3. Varicose veins are dilated, elongated, tortuous, subcutaneous veins 3 mm or greater in size (see Fig. 21-1).

I. Pathophysiology/Etiology

A. Normal Venous Function

1. Calf muscle pump
   a. Approximately 90% of the venous return in the legs occurs in the deep veins by the action of the foot, calf, and thigh muscle pumps (Meisner, 2005).
   b. Propels blood toward the heart when the legs are moved or the calf muscle is tensed. Does not work when the person stands perfectly still (Hall, 2011).
   c. The ejection fraction of the calf pump is approximately 65% as compared to the thigh pump which is 15% (Meisner, 2004) (see Fig. 21-2).
2. Gastrocnemius and soleal muscles
   a. Systolic phase: calf muscle contraction closes valves of the perforator veins, propelling blood out of the deep veins toward the heart
   b. Diastolic phase: calf muscle relaxes. Pressure in the deep veins and the sinuses decreases and the blood flows via perforators from the superficial system into the deep system (Dean & Spruiell, 2011)

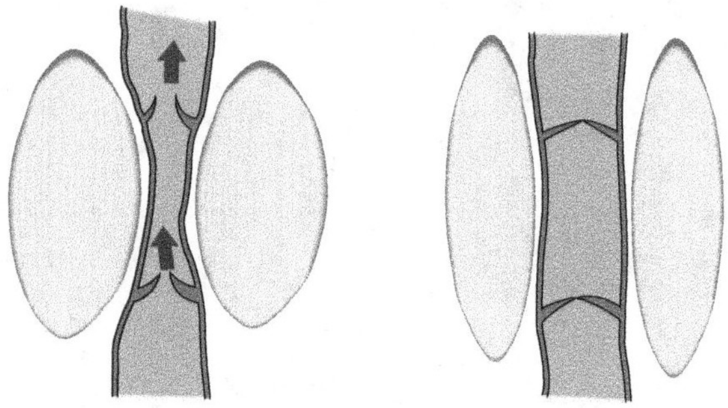

FIGURE 21-2. Calf pump muscle effect on venous valves.

3. Venous valves
   a. Usually bicuspid. Direct blood flow from distal to proximal and from the superficial to the deep system
   b. Arranged to only allow blood to flow toward the heart (Hall, 2011)

B. Abnormal Venous Function

1. Calf muscle pump (venous pump)
   a. Systolic phase: Incompetent perforators allow direct flow of blood from the deep into the superficial veins. Ambulatory venous pressure is increased.
   b. Diastolic phase: functions similar to a normal limb.
2. Reflux
   a. Pathologic retrograde flow of blood
   b. Occurs when the valves are absent or incompetent either by degenerative processes or an episode of DVT
   c. Retrograde flow during calf muscle relaxation prevents the usual reduction in pressure (Meisner, 2004)

II. Assessment

A. Risk Factors (Hurie & Wakefield, 2012)

1. Congenital: factor VII excess, protein C deficiency, protein S deficiency, factor V Leiden, antithrombin deficiency, prothrombin
2. Acquired: HICV infection, age, immobilization, malignancy, heparin-induced thrombocytopenia, Behcet disease, nephrotic syndrome, antiphospholipid antibodies, myeloproliferative disorders, polycythemia vera, paroxysmal nocturnal hemoglobinuria, inflammatory bowel disease
3. Situational: surgery, trauma, pregnancy, oral contraceptives, hormone replacement therapy
4. Mixed: hyperhomocysteinemia, increased factor VIII levels, increased factor XI levels

B. Patient History

1. Subjective findings: leg aching, heaviness, burning, itching, fatigue, stinging, throbbing, venous claudication, edema, and in serious cases,

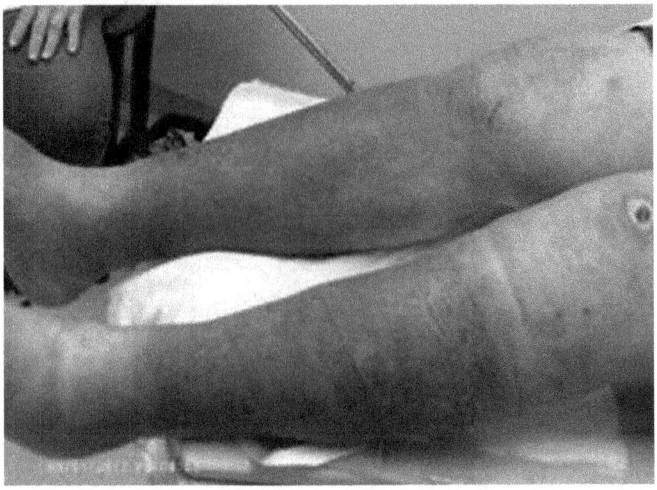

FIGURE 21-3. Hyperpigmentation changes associated with chronic venous disease.

ulcerations. Symptoms are aggravated by dependency and worse at the end of the day (Dean & Spruiell, 2011; Kachroo et al., 2012).

2. Social: ETOH use, nicotine, and illicit drug use. Employment, daily activities, living situation, support systems.
3. Medications: prescribed and OTC

C. Physical Examination (Dean & Spruiell, 2011)

1. Inspection: Compare legs
   a. Edema: initially seen at the ankle progressing to the calf as the disease progresses. May be pitting initially; however, as the disease progresses, the area becomes fibrotic with woody induration.
   b. Hyperpigmentation: brownish coloration in the gaiter area (ankle to mid-calf) denoting extravasated intact or fragmented erythrocytes and hemosiderin (see Fig. 21-3).
   c. Dermatitis: seen in the posteromedial gaiter area. Generally well demarcated, erythematous, dry and scaly.
   d. Lipodermatosclerosis: localized chronic inflammation and fibrosis of the skin and subcutaneous tissue in the lower leg (Moneta, 2012).
   e. Atrophie blanche or "white atrophy": White, macular areas overlying the distal lower extremity as the CVI becomes more advanced.
2. Examination
   a. Vital signs including height and weight
   b. Pulse examination
   c. Measure circumference of both legs just above the ankle, at the widest part of the calf, and the widest part of the thigh

D. Scoring Tools for Classification of Venous Disease

CEAP classification (Eklöf et al., 2004): developed to communicate the results of a comprehensive venous evaluation classifying venous disease by severity, cause, site, and specific abnormality. As the diagnosis and treatment modalities for venous disease changed, the original classification has been modified. Venous disease can be reclassified at any time and should be followed by date. Venous disease is often classified using only the C classification.

Basic CEAP classification

1. Clinical classification
   - C_0: no visible or palpable signs of venous disease
   - C_1: telangiectasias or reticular veins
   - C_2: varicose veins
   - C_3: edema
   - C_{4a}: skin pigmentation or eczema
   - C_{4b}: lipodermatosclerosis or atrophie blanche
   - C_5: healed venous ulcer
   - C_6: active venous ulcer
   - S: symptomatic, including ache, pain, tightness, skin irritation, heaviness and muscle cramps and other complaints attributable to venous dysfunction
   - A: asymptomatic
2. Etiologic classification
   - Ec: congenital
   - Ep: primary
   - Es: secondary (post-thrombotic)
   - En: no venous cause identified
3. Anatomic classification
   - As: superficial veins
   - Ap: perforator veins
   - Ad: deep veins
   - An: no venous location identified
4. Pathophysiological classification

   Basic CEAP
   - Pr: reflux
   - Po: obstruction
   - Pr,o: reflux and obstruction
   - Pn: no venous pathophysiology identified

   Advanced CEAP is the same as basic CEAP with the addition of locators for venous pathology

E. Venous Severity Scoring System (VCCS) (see Table 21-1)
(Vasquez & Munschauer, 2011; Vasquez et al., 2010)

1. Developed to be more sensitive to changes in patient disease status over time.
2. Scores the venous disease based on categories: pain, varicose veins, venous enema, skin pigmentation, inflammation, induration, active ulcer, ulcer size, ulcer duration, and use of compression.

III. Diagnostic Testing

A. Noninvasive Testing

1. Duplex ultrasonography
   - a. Test of choice for diagnosing venous insufficiency (Dean & Spruiell, 2011).
   - b. Obstruction: seen with loss-of-flow signal; chronic reveals smaller diameter of vein and is partially compressible; acute shows distension of vein and is not compressible. Characteristics of the intraluminal obstruction are different.

TABLE 21-1 Venous Severity Scoring System (VCCS)

None (0)	Mild (1)	Moderate (2)	Severe (3)
Pain	Occasional pain or discomfort not interfering with daily activities	Daily pain or discomfort interfering with but not preventing daily activities	Daily pain limiting most regular daily activities
Varicose veins	Few scattered (isolated branch varicosities or clusters) includes corona phlebectatica	Confined to calf or thigh	Involves calf and thigh
Venous edema	Limited to foot and ankle	Extends above ankle but below knee	Extends to knee and above
Skin pigmentation	Limited to perimalleolar area	Diffuse over lower one third of calf	Wider distribution above lower one third of calf
Inflammation	Limited to perimalleolar area	Diffuse over lower one third of calf	Wider distribution above one third of lower calf
Induration	Limited to perimalleolar area	Diffuse over lower one third of calf	Wider distribution above one third of lower calf
Active ulcer duration	<3 mos	>3 mos <1 yr	>1 yr
Active ulcer	<2 cm diameter	2–6 cm diameter	>6 cm diameter
Use of compression	Intermittent	Most days	Full compliance

Vasquez, M. A., Rabe, E., McLafferty, R. B., Shortell, C. K., Marston, W. A., . . . Rutherford, R. B. (2010). Revision of the venous clinical severity score: Venous outcomes consensus statement: Special comminication of the American Venous Forum Ad Hoc Outcomes Working Group. *Journal of Vascular Surgery*, *52*(5):1387–1396. doi:10.1016/jvs.2010.06.161 (2010).

c. Valvular insufficiency: seen when patient performs a Valsalva maneuver or compression of a vein above the probe, as reflux in a vein. Normal reflux is less than 1 second.

2. Magnetic resonance venography (MRV) and Computed Tomographic Venography (CTV)
   a. Valuable technique for assessing veins in regions inaccessible or poorly accessible to sonography (Glockner & Lee, 2010).
   b. Both allow for large fields of view with cross-sectional images that provide superb soft tissue detail and levels of contrast that permit clear delineation between veins and adjacent structures (Bismuth, Shah, & Karmonik, 2011).
3. Air plethysmography (APG) (Hurie & Wakefield, 2012)
   a. Physiologic study used to assure venous reflux, calf muscle pump function, and venous obstruction
   b. Measures calf volume change in response to gravity and exercise as a reflection of reflux (Meisner, 2004)
   c. Can be useful in determining who will benefit most from surgical therapy
4. Photoplethysmography (PPG) (Meisner, 2004)
   a. Simplest noninvasive test. Provides little quantitative information.
   b. Based on transmission of infrared light into the skin and measurement of backscattered light by an adjacent photoreceptor.

IV. Nonsurgical Management (the most common are discussed)

A. Supportive (Dean & Spruiell, 2011)

1. Leg elevation: when sitting, the legs should be higher than the hips and when lying, the legs should be higher than the heart.

TABLE 21-2 Compression Stocking Classification

Class	Pressure	Support	Indication
OTC	<15 mm Hg	Minimal	Asymptomatic, used for comfort
I	15–20 mm Hg	Mild	Minor varicosities, tired aching legs, minor ankle, leg, or foot swelling
II	20–30 mm Hg	Moderate	Moderate to severe varicosities. Following vein ablation
III	30–40 mm Hg	Firm	Severe varicosities, severe swelling Management of active ulceration Following DVT, postsurgery
IV	>40 mm Hg	Extra firm	Lymphedema

Eidt, J. F. (2012). *Open surgical techniques for lower extremity vein ablation*. Retrieved from www.uptodate.com, accessed June 28, 2013.

2. Calf exercises with flexion and extension movements at the level of the ankle.
3. Meticulous skin care. Regular use of moisturizing lotions, creams. Exfoliating with a urea or alpha-hydroxy acid containing lotion for hyperkeratotic or ichthyotic skin.
4. Periodic use of topical glucocorticoid for eczematous stasis dermatitis.

B. Compression

1. To be effective, stockings must fit firmly with diminishing compression as the garment ascends the leg, avoiding a proximal constricting band.
2. Graduated external compression should provide a counterbalance to the graduated hydrostatic pressure change within the superficial veins.
3. Prescription stockings measured to fit properly are recommended.
4. Prescription garment can be designed to provide compression at the ankle ranging from 20 to 60 mm Hg. 20 to 30 mm Hg is usually sufficient for people with primary varicose veins.
5. Knee length is generally enough.
6. Stockings lose their elasticity with wear and washing. It is important to educate the patient in proper caring of the garment, to replace it every 6 months (see Table 21-2).

C. Pharmacology: The use of medications in the treatment of venous insufficiency has been studied in Europe but not in the United States.

1. Agents that may be useful (Dean & Spruiell, 2011)
   a. Phlebotropic agents
      1) Horse chestnut seed extract, hydroxyrutosides, micronized flavonoid fraction, maritime oxandrolone and danazol pine bark extract, calcium dobesilate, centella asiatica, aminaftone, and grape seed extract
   b. Fibrinolytic agents
      1) Stanozolol, oxandrolone, danazol, defibrotide, sulodexide, mesoglycan
   c. Hemorheologic agents
      1) Pentoxifylline
   d. Antiplatelet agents
      1) Aspirin

V. Invasive Management: A complete ultrasound evaluation of the venous system is done prior to intervention to identify reflux.

A. Sclerotherapy (Dean & Spruiell, 2011)

1. Indications
   a. Telangiectasias: cosmetic
   b. Small superficial varices that do not drain into an incompetent vein
   c. Superficial venous malformations
2. Technique
   a. Sclerosing agent (e.g., hypertonic saline, sodium tetradecyl [diluted or concentrated]) injected using a fine needle into the vessel
   b. Results in inflammatory injury to the endothelium, thrombosis, and obliteration of the vein
   c. Compression applied for 3 to 21 days, depending on provider preference
3. Risks
   a. Inadvertent intra-arterial injection
   b. Unexpected anaphylaxis
4. Complications
   a. Hyperpigmentation most common
   b. Additional complications have been listed but are rare

B. Radiofrequency Ablation (RFA)

1. Removes refluxing saphenous vein from circulation
2. Indicated for symptomatic GSV or SSV reflux with or without reflux at their corresponding deep system junctions
   a. Nontortuous major saphenous tributaries such as the accessory saphenous, anterior thigh circumflex branch, and the vein of Giacomini (Acquista & Diietzek, 2011)
   b. Can be performed in a physician's office
   c. Delivers temperature-controlled energy directly to the vein wall immediately contracting the luminal diameter and effects a fibrotic seal of the treated vein
   d. Contraindications include nonpalpable pedal pulses, ABI <0.7, active local or systemic infection, aneurysmal segments, and AV malformation of the vein planned for treatment
   e. Adverse effects: paresthesia (most common), skin burns, phlebitis, DVT, pulmonary embolism, hematoma, ecchymosis, and hyperpigmentation (Dean & Spruiell, 2011)
   f. Post procedure: compression, ace wraps or graduated high thigh compression is recommended to reduce bruising and swelling in the postoperative period. The patient is encouraged to walk immediately after the procedure and 5 to 10 minutes every hour when awake. Prolonged sitting and standing should be avoided and the legs should be elevated above the heart when lying. Bruising is common and may take 6 weeks to resolve. Normal activities can be resumed in 3 to 4 days. A DVT study is recommended in 48 to 72 hours post procedure to assess for DVT (Eidt, 2012)

C. Laser Ablation

1. Minimally invasive procedure performed in a physician's office or clinic

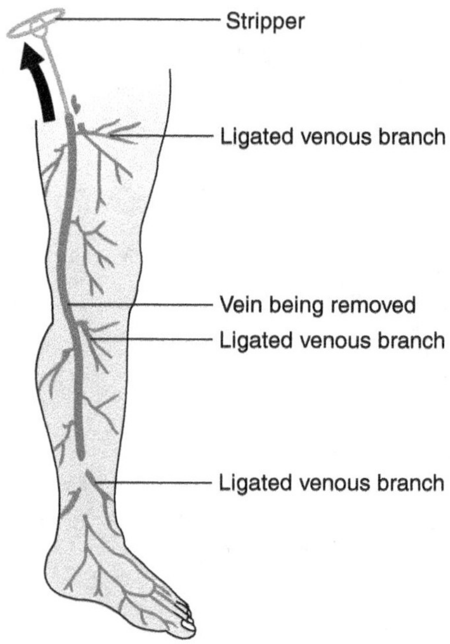

FIGURE 21-4. Vein ligation and stripping.

2. A laser fiber is inserted through the skin and directly into the affected vein. The laser heats the lining within the vein, damaging it and causing it to collapse, shrink, and eventually disappear
3. Typically is used to treat large varicose veins in the legs
4. Takes less than 30 minutes to perform
5. Creates a nonthrombotic vein occlusion by delivering laser energy directly to the vein walls
6. Contraindications: same as RFA
7. Adverse effects: bruising, pain, hyperpigmentation, paresthesia, burns, phlebitis, and induration along the treated vein (Dean & Spruiell, 2011)

D. High Ligation Greater Saphenous Vein (GSV) (see Fig. 21-4)

1. Performed in the operating room under local or general anesthesia as an outpatient
2. Through a groin incision (possibly on both sides), the tissue is dissected down to the GSV/femoral vein junction
3. The GSV is then clamped and tied off
4. The connection between the superficial system (the GSV) and the deep system (the femoral vein) is severed
5. Adverse effects include bruising and hematoma, possible nerve injury, wound infection, and rarely DVT and pulmonary embolism (Dean & Spruiell, 2011)
6. Post procedure care
   a. Generally does not require an overnight stay
   b. Dressings and compression generally not removed for 48 hours
   c. Compression is required for 2 to 6 months. If there is deep venous insufficiency, lifetime compression is recommended
   d. The patient is advised to watch for redness, swelling, pus, fever, and other signs of infection

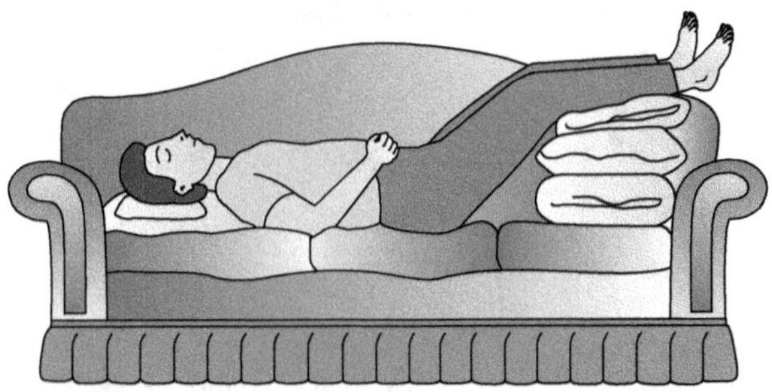

FIGURE 21-5. Proper technique for elevating legs/feet.

VI. Nursing Diagnosis

A. Alteration in Tissue Perfusion Related to Increased Venous Pressure and Obstruction

1. Expected patient outcomes
   a. Decreased edema
   b. Improved perfusion evidenced by decreased skin changes
2. Interventions
   a. Avoid heavy lifting
   b. Elevate legs higher that heart (see Fig. 21-5)
   c. Effective compression supportwear replaced every 6 months
   d. Proper application and care of compression
   e. Fragrance free moisturizers
   f. Regular exercise, especially walking
   g. Weight management
   h. Smoking cessation
3. Evaluation
   a. Patient edema controlled
   b. No progression in skin changes

B. Potential for Skin Breakdown and Tissue Loss Related to Venous Hypertension

1. Expected patient outcome
   a. Patient will remain free of leg ulcers
2. Interventions
   a. Excellent skin care
   b. Avoid hot showers, tub baths
   c. Daily cleansing nonsoap mild cleansers to remove crusting
   d. Early recognition and treatment of dermatitis
   e. Fragrance free, lanolin free moisturizers
   f. Education on ulcer recognition
   g. Regular use of compression
   h. Regular leg elevation every 1 to 2 hours for 10 minutes
   i. Avoid scratching or bumping legs
   j. Early ulcer care
3. Evaluation
   a. Patient will recognize the signs of impending tissue loss
   b. Patient will be adherent to the use of compression

C. Alteration in Comfort Related to Edema and Venous Hypertension

1. Expected outcome
   a. Decrease in leg discomfort
2. Interventions
   a. Leg elevation
   b. Compression
   c. Avoid prolonged period of standing
   d. Avoid habit-forming drugs for analgesia
   e. Referral for surgical intervention if symptoms are not controlled
3. Evaluation
   a. Adherence to plan of care
   b. Discomfort is controlled

VII. Patient/Family Education

A. Disease Prevention/Health Promotion

1. Educate the patient at each visit on the importance of edema control and skin care
   a. Leg elevation 10 to 15 minutes every 2 to 4 hours
   b. Adherence to compression
   c. Avoidance of constrictive clothing
   d. Regular exercise program
   e. Weight management
   f. Avoidance of nicotine products
   g. Avoidance of prolonged standing
   h. Use nonsoap cleansers
   i. Use of fragrance free, lanolin free moisturizers

B. Home Care Considerations

1. Educate at each visit
   a. Maintain a healthy lifestyle
   b. Lower extremity protection
      1) Avoid constrictive clothing
      2) Use and care for compression garments as advised
      3) Use nonsoap cleansers
      4) Use fragrance free, lanolin free moisturizers
      5) Avoid scratching
      6) Arrange furniture to reduce the risk of injury to skin
      7) Avoid use of tapes on skin
      8) Review all medications, indication and dosage
      9) Avoid heavy lifting
   c. Wound management
      1) Early recognition of skin breakdown
      2) Apply wound care products as instructed
      3) Monitor wound for color changes, increased odor, pain, swelling, or drainage
      4) Avoid over-the-counter products without health provider recommendations
      5) Notify health care provider of changes in condition

CASE STUDY

JD is a 42-year-old Caucasian male with complaints of burning, aching, throbbing varicosities, right leg greater than the left. He works 40 to 60 hours weekly in construction and has never worn compression. He notices that his legs swell during the day returning to normal size at night.

Past medical history is significant for sinus allergies. Past surgical history: none. Social habits: current cigarette smoker. 50 pack/year history ETOH: beer on the weekends. Illicit drug use: occasional marijuana. Medications: loratadine

Physical Examination: HT: 62" Wt. 275 lb. BP right arm 142/80, Left arm 138/78, Pulse 80, Respirations 16.

Lower extremities: Left calf circumference 52 cm ankle: 43 cm. Right calf circumference: 49 cm ankle 40 cm. There are bulging varicosities on the left medial thigh and calf. There is brawny pigmentation in the medial malleolar area. The skin is very dry. There are varicosities on the right medial calf and thigh not as prominent as the left. His feet and arm warm. Dorsalis pedis and posterior pulses are 2+ bilaterally.

Review Questions

1. What is the first step in treating this gentleman?
   a. Knee high compression garments 20 to 30 or 30 to 40 mm Hg at all times when out of bed
   b. RFA of bilateral varicosities
   c. Healthy life style changes: smoking cessation, weight loss, skin care.
   d. High ligation of varicosities
   e. a and c
2. What patient teaching is needed?
   a. Application and care of the compression garments
   b. Smoking cessation and dietary changes
   c. Proper leg elevation for optimizing venous drainage
   d. Excellent skin care
   e. All of the above
3. What follow-up is recommended?
   a. Schedule a bilateral venous insufficiency study with clinic follow-up in 3 months
   b. Primary medicine for risk factor modification
   c. a and b

Answers/Rationales

1. e. The first step in treating a patient with varicosities is conservative management with compression. It is important to assess for both deep and superficial venous insufficiency before planning a procedure.
2. e. The proper application and care of compression garments is very important to control edema and reduce the risk of complications for the compression.
3. a. Venous insufficiency study is indicated to evaluate the deep and superficial venous system. If there is deep venous insufficiency, ongoing long-term compression will be required. Ongoing risk factor modification includes regular exercise, smoking cessation, weight reduction, low fat diet, and limb elevation.

Section 2: Venous Ulcers

VIII. Venous Ulcer Assessment Findings (Doughty & Holbrook, 2007; Kelchi & Johnson, 2012)

A. Ulcer Characteristics (see Figs. 21-6 and 21-7)

1. Tend to be in the medial malleolar area/inner ankle/"gaitor" area
2. Tend to have large amounts of drainage
3. May have significant amounts of yellow fibrin/slough tissue
4. Red granulation tissue
5. Irregular edges
6. Usually painful, especially with leg dependency

B. Periwound/Lower Extremity Examination

1. Hemosiderosis
   a. Caused by the breakdown of hemosiderin from extravasated red blood cells
   b. Brownish discoloration of the skin, often starts medially and progresses proximally and laterally
   c. Causes weakness and dryness of the skin
2. Edema
   a. Often related to deep venous insufficiency or alterations in mobility
   b. Located between ankle and calf

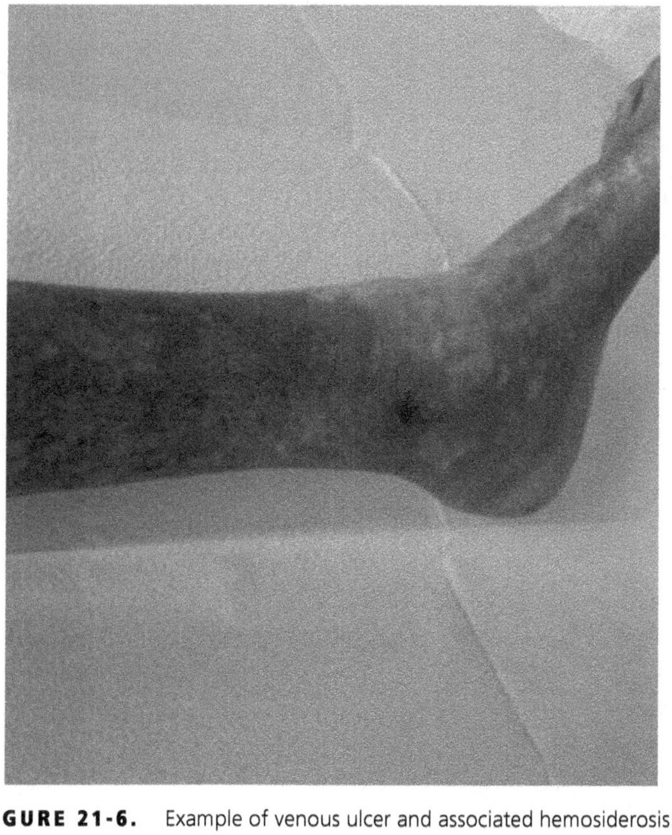

FIGURE 21-6. Example of venous ulcer and associated hemosiderosis.

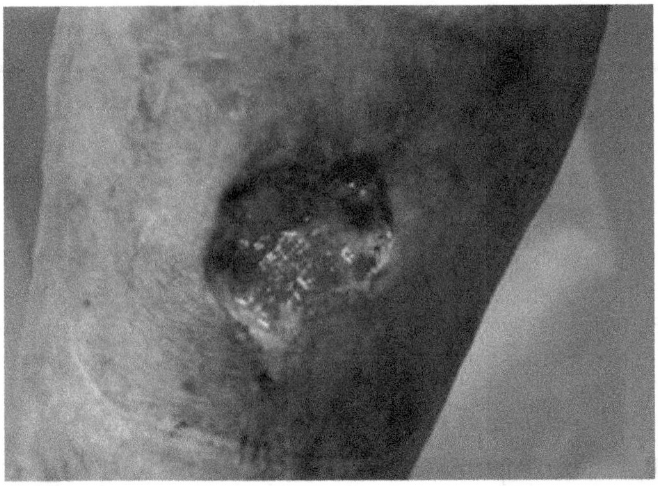

FIGURE 21-7. Example of venous ulcer with fibrin and granulation tissue.

   c. Tends to worsen throughout day from leg dependency, improves with elevation
   d. "Brawny edema": firm edema, nonpitting, accompanied by hemosiderin staining
3. Lipodermatosclerosis
   a. Hardening of the tissues in the ankle area (see Fig. 21-8)
   b. Causes an inverted champagne bottle appearance to the lower limb
4. Atrophie blanche
   a. White plaques noted within hemosiderin stained areas not caused by prior ulceration
   b. High risk areas for ulceration
5. Dermatitis
   a. Itching, scaling, crusting: can be severe
   b. Caused by hemosiderin deposits and possibly reactions to topical agents
6. Varicosities
   a. May be branches of greater or lesser saphenous vein
   b. Telangiectasias/spider veins often present in foot and ankle areas

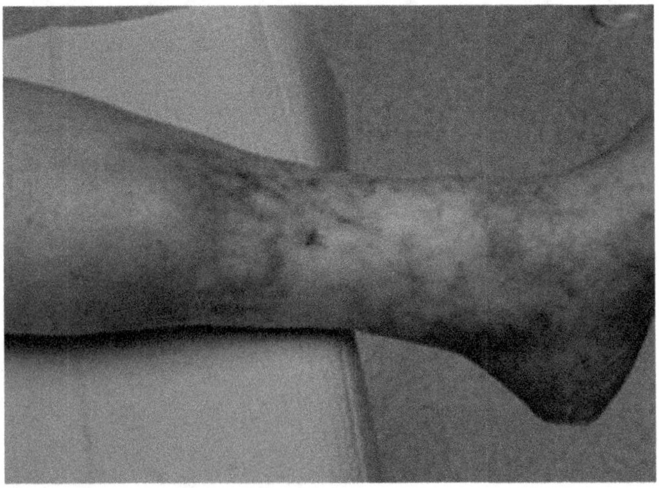

FIGURE 21-8. Lipodermatosclerosis secondary to chronic venous disease.

7. Pulses
   a. Generally palpable unless concomitant arterial disease also present
   b. May be difficult to palpate in the presence of edema or lipodermatosclerosis

IX. Diagnostics

A. Ankle–Brachial Index (ABI) (Doughty & Holbrook, 2007; Kelchi & Johnson, 2012)

1. Should be performed prior to compression therapy
2. ABI >0.8: should be able to tolerate therapeutic compression
3. ABI 0.5 to 0.8: compression needs to be used cautiously, at a lower level of compression, and the patient monitored frequently
4. ABI <0.5: static compression should be avoided

B. Venous Ultrasound (Kelchi & Johnson, 2012)

1. Standard venous ultrasound to rule out acute DVT
2. Standing venous ultrasound to identify areas of reflux from incompetent venous valves: potential areas for surgical intervention

C. Venogram (Marston, Fish, Unger, & Keagy, 2011; Raju, Darcey, & Neglen, 2010)

1. Can identify iliac vein stenosis, which is implicated in delay of venous ulcer healing
2. Iliac stent placement can be performed at the time of the study
3. Decreases venous hypertension symptoms in patients with deep system reflux

X. Treatment: reduce or eliminate causative factors

A. Compression (Doughty & Holbrook, 2007; Kelchi & Johnson, 2012; O'Meara, Cullum, Nelson, & Dumville, 2012)

1. Increases venous return
2. Decreases edema
3. Static
   a. Elastic: applies consistent compression whether walking or at rest
      1) Multilayer wraps: Need to check ABI and rule out arterial insufficiency prior to use. Change once or twice a week. Use in combination with other topical therapies for maximal effectiveness.
      2) Single-layer elastic wraps: Can be used for treatment or long-term therapy. Generally applied with 50% overlap in a spiral or figure-eight pattern.
      3) Compression stockings: Need to be measured by a certified fitter when edema is at minimum. Need to be replaced every 4 to 6 months. Various donning aids available to assist in application. Therapeutic strength ranges for CVI are 15 to 20, 20 to 30, and 30 to 40 mm Hg.

b. Inelastic
   1) Works best with ambulatory patients
   2) Supports calf muscle pump to promote venous return
   3) Need to be reapplied within a short time period during initial wraps: as edema reduces, the wraps can fall down and will lose compression
      a) Unna boot: consists of an inelastic layer of gauze impregnated with zinc and glycerine, can also contain calamine. This is wrapped beginning at the toes to the knee, with the foot dorsiflexed at a 90-degree angle to leg. Generally two layers of this material are applied without tension, starting at the toes with each layer. An elastic bandage or a self-adherent wrap are usually used to provide an elastic layer and prevent soilage of clothing from the zinc.
      b) Orthotic wraps/strapping devices: several options available consisting of inelastic materials or short-stretch type bandages. Straps of device wrap around calf and are secured to themselves with hook and loop closure. May be easier to apply than stockings and can be adjusted throughout day as needed.
      c) Short-stretch bandages: Often used in lymphedema treatment. Bandages are reusable but can slip out of place due to lack of elasticity. Can be used with patients with ABIs 0.5 or higher.

4. Dynamic (Comerota, 2011; Kelchi & Johnson, 2012)
   a. Intermittent pneumatic compression pumps
      1) Can treat lymphedema and edema related to CVI
      2) Generally each leg has several pockets which inflate and deflate sequentially, moving fluid from the feet and legs toward the torso
      3) Should be used for 1 to 2 hours at a time, once or twice daily
      4) Can generally be used in patients with lower ABIs that cannot tolerate sustained compression
5. Contraindications to compression therapy (Doughty & Holbrook, 2007)
   a. ABI less than 0.5
   b. Acute congestive heart failure

B. Elevation (Doughty & Holbrook, 2007)

1. Above level of the heart
2. At least 1 to 2 hours per day (can divide into 3 to 4 half-hour sessions)
3. Can elevate foot of bed with pillow between mattress and box spring or use a wedge pillow while sleeping
4. Avoid prolonged sitting or standing in one position

C. Provide Systemic Support for Healing

1. Ensure adequate nutrition and oxygenation
   a. Mesoglycan and rutosides may improve ulcer healing rates (Belcaro et al., 2008; Gohel & Davies, 2009; Tufano et al., 2010)
2. Encourage tight glycemic control in diabetic patients
3. Control pain
   a. Oral analgesics
   b. Topical anesthetics during dressing changes as needed

4. Medications
   a. Doxycycline (Sadler, Wallace, & Stacey, 2012; Serra et al., 2013)
      1) May decrease matrix metalloproteases (MMPs) in wound fluid
      2) Anti-inflammatory effects
   b. Pentoxifylline (Jull, Arroll, Parag, & Waters, 2012)
      1) May enhance microcirculation by decreasing blood viscosity and improving erythrocyte flexibility
   c. Horse chestnut seed extract (Kelchi & Johnson, 2012)
      1) Reduces pain and edema

D. Apply Appropriate Topical Therapy (i.e., Dressings) (Hess, 2013a, 2013b; Rolstad & Ovington, 2007)

1. Remove necrotic tissue
2. Autolytic debridement
   a. Hydrogels
   b. Hydrocolloids
   c. Honey dressings
   d. Polymer gel pads
3. Enzymatic debridement
   a. Collagenase
   b. Sharp debridement

E. Identify and Eliminate Infection (Kelchi & Johnson, 2012; Leaper, 2011; McVeigh, 2011; O'Meara, Al-Kurdi, Ologon, & Ovington, 2010; Stotts, 2007)

1. Wound culture
   a. All wounds are contaminated
   b. Signs of clinically significant infection include increased pain, erythema, induration, edema, purulent or malodorous drainage, and friability of granulation tissue. Lack of wound progress may also indicate critical colonization or infection.
2. Topical antiseptics and antibiotics
   a. Normal, routine cleansing should consist of washing the wound and periwound with noncytotoxic cleansers
   b. Antiseptics can be used when bioburden needs to be reduced
   c. Antiseptics include chlorhexidine, gentian violet, and hypochlorous acid solutions
   d. Antibacterial preparations can be used short term for infection; should not be used routinely
   e. Mupirocin is generally effective on gram positive bacteria, including MRSA
   f. Gentamicin is generally effective on gram negative bacteria
   g. Bacitracin and polymyxin B sulfate–bacitracin zinc–neomycin are effective on both gram positive and gram negative bacteria, but are common allergenic substances
   h. Metronidazole effective against aerobic bacteria
3. Silver dressings
   a. Effective against bacteria, fungi, and some viruses
   b. Manages malodor
   c. Low bacterial resistance at present
   d. Available in many forms, including creams, gels, hydrocolloids, alginates, and foams

e. Different forms have varying lengths of effectiveness (refer to manufacturer guidelines)

4. Systemic antibiotics

F. Fill Dead Space and Absorb Excess Exudate

1. Foam dressings
2. Calcium alginates
3. Hydrofibers/hydroconductive dressings
4. Polymer absorption dressings
5. Negative pressure wound therapy

G. Maintain a Moist Wound Surface

1. Hydrocolloids
2. Hydrogels
3. Nonadherent porous dressings

H. Provide Thermal Insulation

I. Protect the Healing Wound and Periwound

1. Treat periwound dermatitis with steroid cream or ointment (Kelchi & Johnson, 2012)
2. Protect periwound from maceration (Hunter et al., 2013; Letizia, Uebelhor, & Paddack, 2010)
   a. Skin barrier ointments
   b. Zinc-based ointments
   c. Polymer acrylate (skin prep wipe or spray)
   d. Control exudate with appropriate dressing selection
3. Compression therapy should be uninterrupted when wound is healed, that is, should transition from wraps to stockings without a delay

J. The "Stalled Wound"

1. Lack of progress after 4 weeks
2. Wound culture to identify occult infection
3. Biopsy of wound to rule out malignancy, vasculitic ulcer, and so forth
4. Consider advanced wound therapies (Frantz, Broussard, Mendez-Eastman, & Cordrey, 2007)
   a. Collagen dressing
   b. Negative pressure wound therapy
   c. Skin substitutes
   d. Ultrasound mist therapy
   e. Electrical stimulation
   f. Amniotic membrane allograft
   g. Referral to plastic surgeon for skin grafting (Labropoulos, Wang, Lanie, & Khan, 2012)

XI. Documentation (Kelchi & Johnson, 2012)

A. Testing Performed and Results

B. Wound Characteristics: location, size, wound margins, wound bed tissue, periwound skin appearance, signs/symptoms of infection

C. Periwound Assessment

D. Treatment Performed

E. Patient Response

F. Patient Education Performed

XII. Long-Term Maintenance and Prevention of Recurrence

(Doughty & Holbrook, 2007; Kelchi & Johnson, 2012) (also see discussion above within discussion of CVD)

A. Compression Stockings should be replaced every 4 to 6 months, according to manufacturer's guidelines

B. Skin Care Measures

1. Use of mild, fragrance-free soaps
2. Daily moisturizing to keep skin supple
3. Promptly seek attention from health care provider for recurrent ulcers

C. Exercise/Walking/Aquatic Exercise

D. Weight Management

E. Venous Surgery

CASE STUDY

Mrs. B is a 67-year-old female with a long history of varicose veins, which started becoming prominent during pregnancy. She developed progressive skin changes over the years, starting with edema and a brown discoloration spreading from her medial ankle to mid-calf area. Over time she noted that the skin feels hard to the touch, and is often flaky and itchy. She has compression stockings that she was measured for approximately 10 years ago, and her newest pair is 2 years old. Approximately 3 weeks ago, she bumped her leg on the car door when going to work as a cashier in a local department store, causing an open wound. She has tried to heal this with triple antibiotic ointment, but has noted increasing redness and irritation. The wound is becoming larger and more painful, with increasing amounts of drainage.

An ABI was ordered and the result was 0.9 bilaterally. A venous ultrasound was performed and was negative for DVT, but did demonstrate reflux in the GSV.

Review Questions

1. Which of the following interventions would be appropriate to institute at the initial visit for Mrs. B?
   a. Wound culture
   b. Dakin solution wet to dry daily
   c. Silvadene and dry gauze twice daily
   d. Multi-layer compression wrap with foam dressing to wound
   e. a and d

2. Mrs. B's wound culture was positive for MSSA and she was started on appropriate systemic antibiotics. Which other interventions would be appropriate to combine with compression therapy at this time?
   a. Silver alginate dressing
   b. Cadexomer iodine dressing
   c. Hydrocolloid dressing
   d. Hydrogel sheet
   e. a or b
   f. c or d

3. Which of the following would be appropriate for treatment of the irritated periwound area?
   a. Triple antibiotic ointment
   b. Steroid cream or ointment
   c. Tincture of benzoin
   d. Betadine solution

4. Mrs. B responded well to all your interventions and has completely healed. What should your next step(s) be?
   a. Instruct her in appropriate skin care measures
   b. Discuss opportunities for leg elevation during the day
   c. Recommend a water exercise program in your area
   d. Measure for new compression stockings and instruct her that they must be replaced every 4 to 6 months
   e. All of the above

Answers/Rationales

1. e. Both a and d are indicated given the presenting findings. Given the increasing redness, pain, and drainage, a wound culture is indicated to guide systemic therapy for infection. Mrs. B's ABI is within range to tolerate multi-layer compression. Dakin solution would not be a recommendation. Silvadene would address infection, but would not be appropriate with a multi-layer compression wrap. The use of compression therapy is the key to treating venous ulceration.

2. e. A silver alginate would reduce bacterial burden as well as absorb the significant amount of drainage that would be expected. Cadexomer iodine has also been shown to effectively control bacteria in venous ulcers. Both hydrocolloids and hydrogels are contraindicated due to the amount of drainage the patient is experiencing, even if they were silver-impregnated.

3. b. Steroid cream or ointment would be effective in reducing the periwound dermatitis that may have been exacerbated by the patient's use of topical antibiotics. Patients with venous sufficiency are particularly prone to contact/allergic dermatitis, and are likely to experience a reaction to triple antibiotic ointment. Neither tincture of benzoin nor betadine is indicated to treat periwound inflammation.

4. e. All of these interventions are appropriate to recommend to Mrs. B. Because she was measured for compression stockings approximately 10 years ago, a new measurement of her legs to assure proper fit is required. Her compression stockings were also well past the recommended timeframe for replacement. Leg elevation, exercise, and good skin care measures are also important components of care for venous ulcer patients.

REFERENCES

Acquista, E., & Diietzek, A. M. (2011). Endovenous radiofrequency ablation of the saphenous vein. Mechanism of action, procedural technique, and review of clinic outcomes. In M. G. Davies & A. B. Lumsden (Eds.), *Chronic venous insufficiency, contemporary endovascular management* (Vol. 1, pp. 47–62). Minneapolis, MN: Cardiotext Publishing, LLC.

Alguire, P. C., & Mathes, B. M. (2013). *Pathophysiology of chronic venous disease.* From UpToDate. Retrieved from www.uptodate.com, accessed June 29, 2013.

Belcaro, G., Cesarone, M. R., Ledda, A., Cacchio, M., Ruffini, I., Ricci, A., ... Grossi, M. G. (2008). 5-year control and treatment of edema and increased capillary filtration in venous hypertension and diabetic microangiopathy using O-(β-hydroxyethyl)-rutosides: A prospective comparative clinical registry. *Angiology, 59*(Suppl. 1), 14S–20S. doi:10.1177/0003319707312683

Bismuth, J., Shah, D. J., & Karmonik, C. (2011). The role of computed tomography and magnetic resonance in venous imaging. In M. G. Davies & A. B. Lumsden (Eds.), *Chronic venous insufficiency, contemporary endovascular management* (Vol. 1, pp. 35–46). Minneapolis, MN: Cardiotext Publishing, LLC.

Comerota, A. J. (2011). Intermittent pneumatic compression: Physiologic and clinical basis to improve management of venous leg ulcers. *Journal of Vascular Surgery, 53*, 1121–1129.

Davies, M. G., & Lumsden, A. B. (2011). *Chronic venous insufficiency.* Minneapolois, MN: Cardiotext Publishing, LLC.

Dean, S. M., & Spruiell, S. S. (2011). Chronic venous insufficiency and varicose veins. In M. R. Jaff & C. J. White (Eds.), *Vascular disease diagnostic and therapeutic approaches* (pp. 459–517). Minneapolis, MN: Cardiotext Publishing, LLC.

Doughty, D., & Holbrook, R. (2007). Lower-extremity ulcers of vascular etiology. In R. A. Bryant & D. P. Nix (Eds.), *Acute & chronic wounds: Current management concepts* (3rd ed., pp. 258–306). St. Louis, MO: Mosby.

Eidt, J. F. (2012). *Open surgical techniques for lower extremity vein ablation.* Retrieved from www.uptodate.com, accessed June 28, 2013.

Eklöf, B., Rutherford, R. B., Bergan, J. J., Carpentier, P. H., Gloviczki, P., Kistner, R. L., . . . Wakefield, T. W. (2004). Revision of the CEAP classification for chronic venous disorders: Consensus statement. *Journal of Vascular Surgery, 40*(6), 1248–1252.

Frantz, R. A., Broussard, C. L., Mendez-Eastman, S., & Cordrey, R. (2007). Devices and technology in wound care. In R. A. Bryant & D. P. Nix (Eds.), *Acute & chronic wounds: Current management concepts* (3rd ed., pp. 427–460). St. Louis, MO: Mosby.

Glockner, J. F., & Lee, C. U. (2010). Magnetic resonance venography. *Applied Radiology, 39*(6). Retrieved from http://www.appliedradiology.com/Issues/2010/06/Articles/AR_06-10_Glockner/Magnetic-resonance-venography.aspx, accessed June 28, 2013.

Gohel, M. S., & Davies, A. H. (2009). Pharmacological agents in the treatment of venous disease: An update of the available evidence. *Current Vascular Pharmacology, 7*, 303–308.

Hall, J. E. (2011). *Guyton and hall textbook of medical physiology* (12th ed.). Philadelphia, PA: Saunders.

Hess, C. T. (2013a). Venous etiology clinical pathways integrated with evidence-based decisions: Part 1. *Advances in Skin & Wound Care, 26*(4), 192.

Hess, C. T. (2013b). Venous etiology clinical pathways integrated with evidence-based decisions: Part 2. *Advances in Skin & Wound Care, 26*(5), 240.

Hunter, S. M., Langemo, D., Thompson, P., Hanson, D., Anderson, J., Oh, I. E., ... Roth, D. L. (2013). Observations of periwound skin protection in venous ulcers: A comparison of treatments. *Advances in Skin & Wound Care, 26*(2), 62–66. doi:10.1097/01.ASW.0000426714.57540.c4

Hurie, J. B., & Wakefield, T. W. (2012). Approach to and management of chronic venous insufficiency. In S. Rjagopalan, S. M. Dean, E. R. Mohler, & D. Mukherjee (Eds.), *Manual of vascular diseases* (2nd ed., pp. 439–464). Philadelphia, PA: Wolters Kluwer/Lippincott Williams & Wilkins.

Jull, A. B., Arroll, B., Parag, V., & Waters, J. (2012). Pentoxifylline for treating venous leg ulcers. *Cochrane Database of Systematic Reviews, 11*, CD000265. doi:10.1002/14651858.CD000265.pub3

Kachroo, S., Boyd, D., Bookhart, B. K., LaMori, J., Schein, J. R., Rosenberg, D. J., & Reynolds, M. W. (2012). Quality of life and economic costs associated with postthrombotic syndrome. *American Journal of Health-System Pharmacy, 69*(7), 567–571.

Kaufman, J. (2004). Lower-extremity veins. In J. Kaufman & M. Lee (Eds.), *Vascular and interventional radiology* (pp. 445–468). Philadelphia, PA: Mosby.

Kelchi, T. J., & Johnson, J. J. (2012). Guideline for the management of wounds in patients with lower-extremity venous disease: An executive summary. *Journal of Wound, Ostomy and Continence Nursing, 39*(6), 598–606. doi:10.1097/WON.0b013e31827179e9

Labropoulos, N., Wang, E. D., Lanier, S. T., & Khan, S. U. (2012). Factors associated with poor healing and recurrence of venous ulceration. *Plastic & Reconstructive Surgery, 129*, 179–186.

Leaper, D. (2011). Topical antiseptics in wound care: Time for reflection. *International Wound Journal, 8*(6), 547–549.

Letizia, M., Uebelhor, J., & Paddack, E. (2010). Providing palliative care to seriously ill patients with nonhealing wounds. *Journal of Wound Ostomy Continence Nursing, 37*(3), 277–282.

Marston, W., Fish, D., Unger, J., & Keagy, B. (2011). Incidence of and risk factors for ileocaval venous obstruction in patients with active or healed venous leg ulcers. *Journal of Vascular Surgery, 53*, 1303–1308.

McVeigh, H. (2011). Topical silver for preventing wound infection. *International Journal of Evidence-Based Healthcare, 9*, 454–455.

Meisner, M. (2004). Pathophysiology of varicose veins and chronic venous insufficiency. In M. Meissner, & J. W. Hallett Jr. (Ed.), *Comprehensive vascular and endovascular surgery* (p. 571). Philadelphia, PA: Mosby.

Meisner, M. H. (2005). Lower extremity venous anatomy. *Seminars in Interventional Radiology.* Retrieved from http://www.ncbi.nlm.nih.gov/pmc/articles/PMC3036282/, accessed June 29, 2013.

Moneta, G. (2012). *Classification of lower extremity chronic venous disorders.* From UpToDate. Retrieved from www.uptodate.com, accessed June 28, 2013.

Moneta, G. (2013). *Classification of lower extremity venous disorders.* From UpToDate. Retrieved from www.uptodate.com, accessed June 28, 2013.

Oğuzkurt, L. (2012). Ultrasonographic anatomy of the lower extremity superficial veins. *Diagnostic and Interventional Radiology, 18*(4), 423–430. doi:10.4261/1305-3825.DIR.5321-11.1

O'Meara, S. O., Al-Kurdi, D., Ologon, Y., & Ovington, L. G. (2010). Antibiotics and antiseptics for venous ulcers. *Cochrane Database of Systematic Reviews*, (1), Art. No.: CD003557. doi:10.1002/14651858.CD003557.pub3

O'Meara, S. O., Cullum, N., Nelson, E. A., & Dumville, J. C. (2012). Compression for venous leg ulcers. *Cochrane Database of Systematic Reviews*, (11), Art. No.: CD000265. doi:10.1002/14651858.CD000265.pub3

Raju, S., Darcey, R., & Neglen, P. (2010). Unexpected major role for venous stenting in deep reflux disease. *Journal of Vascular Surgery, 51*, 401–409.

Rolstad, B. S., & Ovington, L. G. (2007). Principles of wound management. In R. A. Bryant & D. P. Nix (Eds.), *Acute & chronic wounds: Current management concepts* (3rd ed., pp. 391–426). St. Louis, MO: Mosby.

Sadler, G., Wallace, H., & Stacey, M. (2012). Oral doxycycline for the treatment of chronic leg ulceration. *Archives of Dermatological Research, 304*(6), 487.

Serra, R., Gallelli, L., Buffone, G., Molinari, V., Stillitano, D. M., Palmieri, C., & de Franciscis, S. (2013). Doxycycline speeds up healing of chronic venous ulcers. *International Wound Journal*, doi:10.1111/iwj.12077

Stotts, N. A. (2007). Wound infection: Diagnosis and management. In R. A. Bryant & D. P. Nix (Eds.), *Acute & chronic wounds: Current management concepts* (3rd ed., pp.161–175). St. Louis, MO: Mosby.

Tufano, A., Arturo, C., Cimino, E., DiMinno, M. N., DiCapua, M., Cerbone, A. M., & Di Minno, G. (2010). Mesoglycan: Clinical evidences for use in vascular diseases. *International Journal of Vascular Medicine, 2010*, 390643. doi:10.1155/2010/390643

Vasquez, M. A., & Munschauer, C. E. (2011). Chronic venous insufficiency: Comprehensive treatment guided by investigation and classification. In M. G. Davies & A. B. Lumsden (Eds.), *Chronic venous insufficiency, contemporary endovascular management* (Vol. 1., pp. 9–24). Minneapolis, MN: Cardiotext Publishing, LLC.

Vasquez, M. A., Rabe, E., McLafferty, R. B., Shortell, C. K., Marston, W. A., ... Rutherford, R. B. (2010). Revision of the venous clinical severity score: Venous outcomes consensus statement: Special communication of the American Venous Forum Ad Hoc Outcomes Working Group. *Journal of Vascular Surgery, 52*(5):1387–1396. doi:10.1016/jvs.2010.06.161

SUGGESTED READINGS

Eberhardt, R. T., & Raffetto, J. D. (2005). Contemporary reviews in cardiovascular medicine: Chronic venous insufficiency. *Circulation, 111*, 2398–2409. doi:10/1161/01.CIR.0000164199.72440.08

Harlander-Locke, M., Lawrence, P., Jimenez, J. C., Rigberg, D., DeRubertis, B., & Gelabert, H. (2012). Combined treatment with compression therapy and ablation of incompetent superficial and perforating veins reduces ulcer recurrence in patients with CEAP 5 venous disease. *Journal of Vascular Surgery, 55*, 446–450.

Ramundo, J. M. (2007). Wound debridement. In R. A. Bryant & D. P. Nix (Eds.), *Acute & chronic wounds: Current management concepts* (3rd ed., pp. 176–192). St. Louis, MO: Mosby.

Word, R. (2010). Medical and surgical therapy for advanced chronic venous insufficiency. *The Surgical Clinics of North America, 90*(6), 1195–1214. doi:10.1016/j.suc.2010.08.008

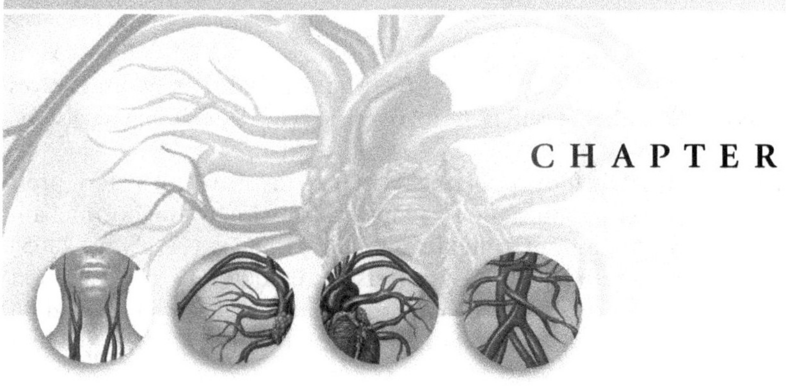

CHAPTER 22

Diabetic Foot Management

Robyn Strauss
Cynthia Christensen

OBJECTIVES

1. Describe the pathophysiology of diabetes mellitus that leads to the formation of foot problems in this patient population.
2. Identify the essential elements of a complete assessment of the diabetic foot, with and without ulceration.
3. List appropriate nursing recommendations for primary and secondary prevention of diabetic foot ulcerations.

Introduction/Overview

Diabetes mellitus is a genetic disorder of carbohydrate metabolism characterized by hyperglycemia and glucose intolerance, resulting from defects in insulin production, insulin action at the tissue level, or both. This disease, which affects both the microvascular and macrovascular circulation, is common in the United States. Diabetes affects 25.8 million people (8.3% of the US population) (Centers for Disease Control and Prevention (CDC), 2011). The incidence of new cases for people over age 20 is 1.9 million per year, with the greatest increase in prevalence expected in the elderly (252% for women; 537% for men) over the next five decades.

- In contrast to the 2007 National Diabetes Fact Sheet, which used fasting glucose data to estimate undiagnosed diabetes and prediabetes, the 2011 National Diabetes Fact Sheet uses both *fasting glucose and A1C levels* to *derive estimates for undiagnosed diabetes and prediabetes.* These tests were chosen because they are most frequently used in clinical practice.
- Minority groups are more likely to have diabetes than Caucasians. After adjusting for population age differences, 2007 to 2009 national survey data for people aged 20 years or older indicate that 7.1% of non-Hispanic Whites, 8.4% of Asian Americans, 11.8% of Hispanics, and 12.6% of non-Hispanic Blacks had diagnosed diabetes. Among Hispanics, rates were 7.6% for both Cubans and for Central and South Americans, 13.3% for Mexican Americans, and 13.8% for Puerto Ricans.
- Compared to non-Hispanic White adults, the risk of diagnosed diabetes was 18% higher among Asian Americans, 66% higher among Hispanics, and 77% higher among non-Hispanic Blacks. Among Hispanics compared to non-Hispanic White adults, the risk of diagnosed diabetes was

about the same for Cubans and for Central and South Americans, 87% higher for Mexican Americans, and 94% higher for Puerto Ricans. Native Americans, including Alaskan Natives, are also 2.2 times more likely to have diabetes than non-Hispanic Whites of similar age (CDC, 2011).
- Many people with diabetes will develop foot problems related to their disease. A foot problem is the most common reason that diabetic patients require admission to the hospital and is the number one cause of lower leg amputations in the United States (Frykberg, 2005). The annual incidence of lower extremity leg and foot ulcers is 200,000. There are approximately 65,000 lower extremity amputations in diabetic patients annually and in 2006, more than 60% of nontraumatic lower-limb amputations occurred in people with diabetes (CDC, 2011).
- 50% to 70% of all nontraumatic lower leg amputations occur in diabetic. Of these amputations, 85% are performed for complications of foot ulcers, 5% to 15% of all people with diabetes will require an amputation at some time in their lives. Fifty percent of diabetics who undergo amputation of one leg will go on to loose the other leg within 5 years (Yao & Pierce, 2001).

Patient education and proper foot care can reduce the amputation rate by 80% and hospitalizations by 65%. The three leading components that define the pathophysiologic triad of diabetic foot ulcers are ischemia, neuropathy, and altered response to infection (Frykberg, 2003).

I. Anatomy/Pathology

A. Predisposition to the Development of Foot Disorders Due to Vascular and Neuropathic Complications Common to the Disease

1. Enhanced vulnerability of the foot to damage by environmental trauma.
2. Arterial insufficiency resulting in ischemia may produce pathology in the lower extremity by tissue necrosis, or may adversely affect the ability to heal or fight infection.
3. Loss of pain and temperature sensation.
4. Decreased resistance to infection.

B. Anatomic Change in Shape of Foot: Charcot foot.

1. Two theories explain change in structure (Sommer & Lee, 2001)
    a. Neurotraumatic theory: bony destruction due to loss of pain sensation and proprioception combined with repetitive and mechanical trauma to foot.
    b. Neurovascular theory: joint destruction due to autonomically stimulated vascular reflex that leads to hyperemia (arteriolar–venular shunting) and periarticular calcium loss (osteopenia); trauma also contributes to change.
2. Muscle imbalance leads to increased pressure on heel and plantar surfaces.
3. Microfractures and ligament laxity result, causing progressive bony destruction.
4. Tarsometatarsal (Lisfranc) joint most common site for arthropathy (Sommer & Lee, 2001).
    a. 70% midfoot
    b. 15% forefoot or rearfoot.
5. 50% of patients can recall a precipitating trauma, for example, ankle sprain.

II. Pathophysiology

A. Hyperglycemia

1. Chronic hyperglycemia and insulin resistance in insulin-sensitive target tissues causes major complications related to cardiovascular, peripheral vascular, retinal or renal comorbid conditions.
2. Diabetes accelerates development of all atherosclerotic complications causing vascular complications in microvessels (eye, kidney, and nervous system) and macrovessels (heart and peripheral circulation).
3. Changes in myo-inositol, polyol pathway, (producing excess sorbitol) NA/K/ATPase and phosphoinositol metabolism leads to accumulation of products toxic to nerve tissue. Water accompanies the sorbitol into these tissues, causing the nerve cell to expand. The result is decreased nerve conduction speed and eventual irreversible nerve damage. Decreased myo-inositol alters myelin synthesis, also decreasing NA/K/ATPase activity.
4. When blood glucose levels are elevated, a glucose molecule attaches itself to hemoglobin in a red blood cell. The longer the glucose remains above normal, the more glycosylated hemoglobins form. Raised levels of glycosylated hemoglobin, which binds oxygen to itself causes tissue hypoxia. Protein glycosylation results in decreased joint mobility, leading to high foot pressures (Frykberg, 2005).
5. Impedes outflow of leukocytes thus lowering resistance to infection and probably impairs host defense against infection. Functional abnormalities of neutrophils occur.

B. Neuropathy: 60% of patients with diabetes present for longer than 5 to 10 years have neuropathy (Frykberg, 2005).

1. Peripheral neuropathy
   a. Distal symmetrical polyneuropathy most common form involving sensory, motor, and autonomic nerve fibers
      1) Paresthesia: symptoms of tingling or buzzing
      2) Dysesthesia: more severe manifestation of sensory nerve fiber destruction, causing sensations ranging from mildly painful "pins and needles" to intense burning pain like "hot poker"
      3) Hyperesthesia: an exaggerated sensitivity in the skin
   b. Changes in nerve cell axon causes a "dying back" of the nerve with distal neurons being affected producing a "stocking-glove" distribution. Loss of myelinated and unmyelinated nerve fibers.
   c. Involvement of large sensory and motor fibers diminishes light touch and proprioception, the latter resulting in ataxic gait and unsteadiness, weakness of intrinsic muscles of hand and feet.
   d. Involvement of small fibers diminishes pain and temperature perception.
   e. Motor nerve impairment may cause muscle atrophy leading to foot deformation and maldistribution of pressure over surface of foot.
2. Autonomic neuropathy
   a. Pseudomotor neuropathy: produces asymptomatic anhydrosis in "stocking glove" distribution causing absence of sweating leading to dry, cracked, fissured skin.
   b. Vasomotor instability may produce arteriovenous shunt in foot possibly due to abnormal sympathetic innervation resulting in lower tissue oxygen tension.

C. Peripheral Vascular Disease

1. Changes in vessel walls, both in media and intima consist of deposits of platelets, smooth muscle cells, lipids, cholesterol, and calcium.
2. Small vessel or microangiopathy with involvement of the tibial and peroneal arteries and their smaller branches below the knee (infrageniculate) most common. However, the dorsalis pedis has been found to be spared, rendering revascularization to the foot a most viable option for this population.
   a. Thickening of capillary basement membrane makes it highly permeable to fluid and protein.
   b. Plasma becomes more viscous, erythrocyte and platelet aggregation increase, and fibrinogen levels rise while fibrinolytic activity fall causing formation of microthrombi and/or total occlusion of the capillary.
3. Large vessel or macroangiopathy: Thrombus formation and occlusions can cause gangrene in large segment of lower extremity depending on level and degree of vascular occlusion.
4. Hypoxia resulting from macrovascular and microvascular disease causes
   a. Increased flow
   b. Peripheral edema
   c. Neuropathic edema
   d. Endothelial dysfunction
   e. Impaired nitric oxide production (Frykberg, 2005)

D. Diabetic Foot Ulcers

1. Progressive loss of peripheral nerve function leading to loss of protective sensation
2. Progressive loss of blood supply
3. Infection
   a. Mild infection: monomicrobial organism; usually gram-positive cocci (*Staphylococcus aureus* and Group B beta hemolytic streptococci) found most frequently
   b. Severe infection: polymicrobial; gram-negative rods and anaerobes from deeper wounds
   c. Anaerobes frequent due to anoxia in poorly vascularized tissues
   d. Up to 30% incidence of methicillin-resistant S. *aureus* (MRSA) (Frykberg, 2003)
   e. Destroys tissue and leads to microthrombi resulting in gangrene and amputation
   f. Ulceration is rarely caused by infection, but open ulcers serve as a portal of entry for pathogenic bacteria
   g. Culturing wounds that are not clinically infected not recommended; cultures of deep or limb-threatening infections is reliable for isolation of causative organism (Frykberg, 2003)

III. Etiology or Precipitating Factors

A. Chronic Hyperglycemia

1. Tight control of diabetes reduces risks for development of foot ulcers, infection, and hospitalization of foot problems. The DCCT and EDIC Diabetes Control and Complications Trial (NIH Publication No. 08-3874,

2008) landmark 9-year multicenter randomized clinical trial was designed to compare intensive with conventional diabetes therapy with regard to their effects on the development and progression of early vascular and neurologic complications of IDDM. The results show that tight control could reduce retinopathy by 70%, peripheral neuropathy by up to 60%, and nephropathy by up to 50% in patients with Type I diabetes. This was achieved by maintaining HgbA1C at or below 7.2% (NIH Publication No. 08-3874, 2008).

2. In March 2009, the long awaited results of the Normoglycemia in Intensive Care Evaluation–Survival Using Glucose Algorithm Regulation (NICE–SUGAR) were released. This created intense controversy in the area of glycemic control in the critically ill. NICE–SUGAR was powered to finally address the question of "does tight glycemic control in the intensive care unit (ICU) decrease mortality?"
3. NICE–SUGAR was a much larger study conducted in multiple countries at 41 different centers and was specifically powered to detect an absolute risk reduction similar to that of the original Leuven study. It included a heterogeneous population of medical and surgical patients, treating physicians, nurses, and other caregivers. It is unlikely that an intuitive culture for intensive insulin target (IIT) and nutrition was nurtured in this setting. In addition, insulin infusions were started through central lines and other venous access types as well. Furthermore, a variety of glucose determination methods were used to target glycemic control. Patients in this study were not started on a dextrose infusion on day 1, nor were they placed on combined enteral and parenteral nutrition to achieve a caloric goal. This study reported a significant 3% increase in mortality in the IIT group. Even though there was no increased morbidity with tighter glycemic ranges, there was no protective effect, which the original Leuven study had initially found (Scurlock, Raikhelkar, & Mechanick, 2010).
4. Multiple variables were not reproduced in the study aims of the NICE–SUGAR trial and several factors were not able to be controlled for. The various instruments to measure serum blood glucose, variation of control targets, serum blood glucose measurement access (arterial or venous line), variation of caregiver knowledge related to treatment algorithm, all lead to varied results in the ICU-managed diabetic patient (Scurlock et al., 2010).
5. However, tight glycemic control was associated with a lower rate of septicemia and significantly increased risk of hypoglycemia (Scurlock et al., 2010).
6. Obesity was linked to poor control of diabetes and risk factor for heel problems and Charcot joint.

B. Neuropathy (see Fig. 22-1)

1. Sensory: loss of sensation in feet primarily responsible for initial foot wound and failure to heal.
    a. Painless trauma
        1) Mechanical
            a) Blisters and calluses from ill-fitting shoes
            b) Home surgery on corns and calluses or cutting toenails too close
        2) Chemical
            a) Use of irritating topical and keratolytic agents
            b) Corrosive chemicals

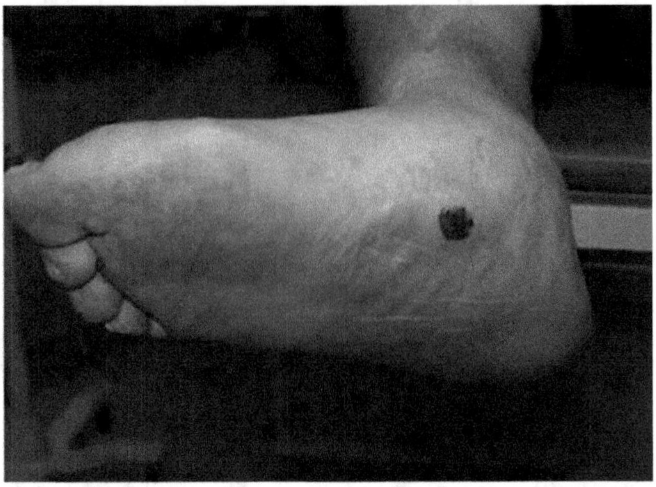

FIGURE 22-1. Neuropathic foot medial callus.

3) Thermal
   a) Bathing in hot water
   b) Use of heating pads, hot water bottles, heaters, and so forth.
   c) Frostbite
2. Motor: foot deformities from motor fiber destruction
   a. Muscle atrophy secondary to motor nerve impairment causes change in configuration of foot and leads to new pressure points.
      1) Depression of metatarsal heads that shift plantar fat pad
      2) Hammer toes: buckling of toe into swan neck deformity caused by weakness of small muscles of foot; toes no longer stabilized on ground; leads to increased pressure over metatarsal head, elevated interphalangeal joint (middle knuckle) and tips of toes
      3) Claw toes: more buckling and greater deformity than hammer toes; fixed flexion of interphalangeal joint with callus or ulcers on toe tips and dorsum of interphalangeal joints
      4) Pes cavus: abnormally high arch or dome that extends between first metatarsal head and calcaneus; leads to decreased area of contact of forefoot with ground while walking and results in abnormal increased pressure with callus formation under metatarsal heads
      5) Fibrofatty padding depletion: reduction of thickness of fat pad over metatarsal heads; cushion no longer able to pad normal walking pressures
      6) Hallux valgus: deformity of first metatarsophalangeal joint with lateral deviation of hallux; medial aspect of foot more prominent and prone to ulcerate from tight shoes
   b. Charcot foot
      1) Bone and joint damage to midfoot leads to collapse
      2) Rocker-bottom deformity: displacement of tarsus downward
      3) Convexity of medial midfoot: talonavicular joint displaced
      4) Bony prominence leads to difficult-to-heal ulceration on plantar foot
      5) If the ankle is involved, the hindfoot becomes unstable
      6) If the collapse is acute with marked swelling, erythema, and pain, it is difficult to distinguish from osteomyelitis or cellulitis
   c. Foot drop/peroneal paralysis: lesion in lateral peroneal nerves

3. Autonomic
   a. Denervation of sweat glands leads to cracking of dry skin and serves as portal for bacterial invasion, especially if hygiene poor
   b. Fissures are common on heels or in calloused skin
   c. Loss of sympathetic tone results in arteriovenous shunting and insufficient nutrient flow

C. Skin and Nail Problems

1. Skin
   a. Dry, cracked
   b. Stasis dermatitis: pruritus leads to self-inflicted wounds from scratching
   c. Dependent edema: multiple etiologies; leads to blisters from tight shoes
   d. Tinea pedis: chronic skin breakdown and source of infection; often interdigital
2. Nails
   a. Onychomycosis: chronic fungal nail; may lead to complete destruction with detachment, odor, and purulent drainage
   b. Neglected nail care: promotes fungal changes and ulceration of surrounding soft tissue
   c. Improper nail trimming: cutting skin, creation of residual spikes, or attempting to trim nails on insensate foot may lead to infection
   d. Involved nail: exaggerated C-shape with curvature of lateral edges into skin may require permanent removal to prevent recurrent infection or pain

D. Peripheral Vascular Disease: inadequate blood flow to meet demands of infection/wound healing

IV. Assessment

A. Risk Factors/Primary Prevention

1. Smoking
2. Hyperglycemia
3. Hyperlipidemia
4. Age
5. Duration of diabetes
6. Hyperinsulinemia (insulin acts as a growth hormone-like substance and high insulin levels may stimulate growth of smooth muscle cells on these plaques)
7. Medications
   a. Vasopressors, for example, dopamine: vasoconstriction effects
   b. Inotropic drugs
   c. Beta blockers: can impair peripheral circulation from unopposed alpha; vasoconstriction effects.

B. Ulcer History/Foot Injuries

1. Direct mechanical injury: skin is broken or penetrated
2. Ischemia injury: can result from very low pressures over 1 to 12 hours. Usually occurs over side of foot and is the result of shoes that are too tight

3. Repetitive stress
   a. Most frequent cause of injury to insensitive foot due to constant, repeated, moderate repetitive pressure to plantar surface while walking long distances
   b. High pressure point area will become blister and eventually forms ulcer

C. Spreading Infection

1. Infection is present in majority of foot ulcers and is a frequent precursor to amputation (Frykberg, 2003)
2. The patient does not change gait in the early stages of trauma as it is not perceived as painful and continues to walk on foot, thus spreading infection throughout the soft tissues
   a. Chronic osteomyelitis
   b. Necrotizing fasciitis
   c. Gangrene
   d. Synergistic necrotizing cellulitis

D. Patient History

1. Subjective findings
   a. Patient's chief complaint
      1) Main reason for hospitalization is infection and impending loss of limb
      2) Outpatient treatment/management possibly consists of debridement, wound care, antibiotics, and close follow up
      3) History of events causing wound and development of ulcer
      4) Painful or nonpainful wound
      5) Previous treatment or therapy for problem; antibiotics
      6) History of vascular disease
         a) Intermittent claudication: walk for several minutes, legs cramp, need to stop until the discomfort stops, then walk again for several more minutes and pain comes back causing individual to stop again.
         b) Rest pain: persistent pain caused by nerve and vessel ischemia; decreases with dependency of lower extremities; aggravated by heat, elevation, and exercise. Patients get relief by sitting up and dangling legs.
         c) Nocturnal ischemic pain: form of ischemic neuritis usually precedes rest pain. Occurs at night during sleep with little perfusion of lower extremities; relieved by standing up or dangling feet over edge of bed or taking a few steps.
      7) History of neuropathy
         a) Signs and symptoms of numbness, pain, or tingling in legs and feet.
         b) Walking tends to relieve neuropathic pain.
      8) History of diabetes duration and control: method of self-monitoring at home, frequency of diabetic complications (DKA and hypoglycemia), current treatment of diabetes including medications, meal plan, and diabetes self-management training.
   b. Foot care behaviors at home
   c. Previous ulcer: 70% risk of new ulcer if previous ulcer within past 5 years (Frykberg, 2005)

d. Other: history of other diabetic complications (e.g., retinopathy, nephropathy, heart disease)

2. Objective findings
   a. Types of injury
      1) Direct mechanical injury
      2) Ischemic injury
      3) Repetitive stress
      4) High pressure point area will become blister and eventually form an ulcer
   b. Metabolic control: HgbA1c
   c. Metabolic disorders/autoimmune disorders
   d. Medications which impede wound healing
      1) Steroids
      2) Nonsteroidal anti-inflammatory drugs
      3) Antineoplastics
   e. Vital signs and laboratory values indicating hypertension or infection (delineation of wet or dry gangrene): elevated blood sugars, white blood cell count, and presence of fever or chills
   f. Nutritional assessment: vitamin/mineral deficiencies
   g. Tumors
   h. Family history
      1) Hypertension
      2) Hyperlipidemia
      3) Noninsulin-dependent diabetes mellitus
      4) Insulin-dependent diabetes mellitus
      5) Atherosclerotic cardiovascular disease and age of onset
   i. Social history
      1) Occupation if working
      2) Tobacco use in any form
      3) Alcohol use or abuse
      4) Compliance-related issues/barriers to care: family support, money to buy food, blood sugar testing supplies, or appropriate shoes
      5) Medication history
      6) Length of time on oral hypoglycemics
      7) Length of time on insulin
      8) Antibiotics for current problem
         a) All current drugs including OTC and herbal supplements, past use of beta-blockers or vasopressors

E. Physical Examination

1. Inspection
   a. Presence of wound or ulcer (neuropathic diabetic ulcers are usually found on the plantar surface of the foot, punched out margins with hyperkeratotic rim, round dry lesions, may be covered with green-brown eschar. Ischemic ulcers result usually from trauma to the foot, wound appearance is usually smooth with punched out margin, and pale and unhealthy granulation tissue)
      1) Size and depth of ulcer, staging of ulcer if applicable (Stages 1 to 4)
      2) Diameter
      3) Drainage

4) Color of drainage
5) Gas bubbles present
6) Edema of surrounding tissues
7) Cellulitis
8) Abscess
9) Fluctuation
10) Inspect between toes

b. Color
   1) Pale, bluish, mottled, or dusky tone of feet indicate poor circulation
      a) Note color changes of extremity in relation to position change
      b) Pallor on elevation, prolonged filling time, and dependent rubor are hallmarks of significant lower extremity vascular insufficiency. Feet will pale on elevation after 30 seconds especially in soles, heel, and toes. Then dangle legs; normally color will return to toes in 10 seconds
      c) Dependent rubor after 2 minutes indicates severe ischemia
   2) Redness or early inflammation or irritation. the normal responses to infection, vessel dilation, heat, and redness are not always seen in the diabetic patient
   3) Dark brown patches may be vascular abnormalities
   4) Dark brown scars, indicate past lesions

c. Hair loss on lower extremities

d. Shape of foot or change in shape—foot drop or abnormal gait.

e. Hygiene
   1) Cleanliness
   2) Condition of stockings and shoes. Look at signs of wear inside the shoe

f. Condition of toenails and presence of fungal infections

2. Palpation
   a. Pulses bilaterally, amplitude as well as deficits
      1) Popliteal, posterior tibial, dorsalis pedis
      2) Noncompressible arteries are common in diabetes due to arterial calcification
   b. Skin temperature: compare one side to the other; note any line of coolness. "Hot spots" are among first signs of inflammation but may not always be present
   c. Assess for pedal edema or edema of surrounding area of ulcer
   d. Note any crepitus indicating gas gangrene and nonclostridial gangrene

3. Percussion
   a. Decreased vibratory sensation indicate peripheral neuropathy; normally perceived for 20 to 25 seconds
   b. Achilles deep tendon reflex: decreased or absent in presence of peripheral neuropathy

4. Auscultation: may have fixed tachycardia or orthostatic hypotension with autonomic neuropathy

F. Wound Classification

1. Even though several scales are currently utilized, American Diabetes Association (ADA) does not recommend a specific classification scheme (Frykberg, 2005)

2. Meggitt–Wagner: most commonly used scale worldwide (Frykberg, 2005)
   a. Grade 0: preulcer lesions, healed ulcers, presence of bony deformities
   b. Progresses to grade 5: gangrene of entire foot
   c. Does not address ischemia or infection
3. University of Texas classification system
   a. Used to document depth, presence of infection, and vascular impairment
   b. Validated to predict amputation as depth of wound progresses from grade 0 to 3 and through four stages
      1) Stage A: no infection
      2) Stage B: infection
      3) Stage C: peripheral vascular disease
      4) Stage D: infection plus peripheral vascular disease
4. ADA consensus recommendations for diabetic wound evaluation (Frykberg, 2005)
   a. History of trauma: penetrating, blunt, or burn
   b. Duration of wound: acute versus chronic
   c. Progression of local or systemic symptoms: improving, stable, or deteriorating
   d. Prior treatment of wounds and effectiveness of interventions

G. Considerations Across the Life Span

1. Young adulthood: neuropathic changes can develop in young adults with type I DM if disease poorly controlled for extended period of time
2. Women of childbearing age: diabetic foot ulcers unlikely in gestational diabetes due to short duration of illness
3. Elderly: highest risk for ulceration due to longevity of disease process and other co-morbidities, especially atherosclerosis

V. Diagnostic Study Findings

A. Laboratory

1. Glucose, electrolytes, HbA1c to determine diabetic control
2. Acetone if indicated or insulin-dependent diabetes mellitus
3. Creatinine and microalbumin to detect nephropathy from longstanding or uncontrolled diabetes
4. Albumin and total lymphocyte count to determine nutritional status
5. Lipid profile: hyperlipidemia connected with poor glycemic control and development of atherosclerosis in the coronary vessel as well as carotids and renal arteries
6. Complete blood count and sedimentation rate: detect infection

B. Radiologic

1. X-ray to rule out subcutaneous gas, foreign body, fracture, osteomyelitis, Charcot foot; chronic osteomyelitis: x-ray shows mottled lytic lesions
2. Observe x-ray for arterial and medial calcification which is not related to atherosclerotic occlusive disease but may prevent accurate ankle blood pressure measurement
3. Bone scan or MRI to differentiate osteomyelitis from Charcot foot

C. Special

1. Test for loss of protective sensation. Assess peripheral neuropathy with Semmes-Weinstein 5.07 (10 g) monofilament wire system test.
   a. Used to evaluate neural sensory threshold and quantify the severity of peripheral neuropathy.
   b. Twelve test sites: most common sites of diabetic ulcer.
   c. Filament lightly pressed against skin just to point of flexing the filament: failure to detect the filament's pressure indicates increased/high risk for ulcer formation.
2. For all patients with diabetes, perform an annual comprehensive foot examination to identify risk factors predictive of ulcers and amputations.
3. Additional testing for protective sensation includes any one of the following
   a. Vibration using 128-Hz tuning fork
   b. Pinprick sensation
   c. Ankle reflexes
   d. Vibration perception threshold (American Diabetes Association (ADA), 2011)
4. Transcutaneous Oxygen Tension Determination ($TcPO_2$). Electrodes placed directly on the skin, the measured $TcPO_2$ levels reflect the perfusion of the skin. In general, the $TcPO_2$ is approximately 80% of the arterial oxygen tension (PO_2). The normal $TcPO_2$ value in a patient breathing room air is greater than 55 mm Hg. A value greater than 30 mm Hg suggests the presence of adequate tissue perfusion for wound healing to occur. Most patients with ischemic foot ulcers have a $TcPO_2$ on the dorsum of the foot of less than 10 mm Hg.
5. If a diabetic ulcer probes to bone there is direct correlation with osteomyelitis (Grayson, Gibbons, Balogh, Levin, & Krachmer, 1995).
6. Vascular studies
   a. Ankle–arm indices; ankle–brachial indices: Ankle–arm index of the affected limb of less than 0.5 has high risk of ischemia and is in need of revascularization in order to heal wound
   b. Vascular laboratory criteria for prediction of foot lesion healing: ABI normal is 1.0. Probability for wound healing and degree of ischemia is directly proportional to declining values. Must also assess wave forms to observe a correlation relationship
   c. Arterial Doppler waveform analysis
      1) Diagnostic pressures in Doppler testing are higher in diabetics because of greater degree of atherosclerosis and calcification in vessels and need for higher pressure to compress these arteries
      2) Toe pressure should always be measured in the diabetic secondary to noncompressible larger vessels. Normal brachia/toe pressure indices is 0.7
   d. Arteriography and/or digital subtraction angiography: for locating blockage and determining feasibility of vascular surgery
      1) Carries risk and should be used only as preoperative diagnostic technique. May also be helpful to have stenting prior to surgery (usually of larger iliac and femoral arteries) as well to enhance or eliminate need for surgery
      2) Check creatinine and hydrate well if procedure is required

e. Magnetic Resonance Angiography (MRA): one of the most advanced developments in magnetic resonance imaging is the MRA which can evaluate blood flow and identify blockages in arteries and veins (refer to Chapter 5, Vascular Diagnostic Studies)
   1) Minimally invasive, no radiation exposure
   2) Selected patients per practitioner

VI. Medical Management

A. Offloading: use of an orthotic device allows the patient to ambulate on a limited basis as well as provide pressure relief to the heel in bedbound patients.

1. Devices redistribute plantar pressures evenly, protect vulnerable margins, protect the sheering effect when patients push with their heels to sit up as well as shift pressure to area of the foot that can bear more stress.
2. Examples include commercial boot for heel offloading and the wedge shoe to prevent pressure on the forefoot.
3. May also require crutches, wheelchair, or bedrest (total non–weight bearing rarely practical)

B. Infection Control

1. Up to one fourth of diabetic foot wounds contain anaerobes as well as aerobes. Assure that gram-positive and negative coverage is extended.
2. Deep tissue cultures are the best way to assess bacterial growth. Surface swabbing is inconclusive.
3. An infected diabetic foot ulcer can lead to limb loss in a matter of days, but not all ulcers are infected.
   a. Many wounds have bacterial colonization, with the distinction between this and infection being difficult
   b. Clinical signs are the most reliable indicators. The presence of swelling, pus, and loss of control of blood glucose levels usually dictates the need for antibiotics
4. Pain in a numb foot is a worrisome finding.
5. With severe infection, there may be crepitus owing to gas formation and fluctuance indicating abscess.
6. The most common organisms include staphylococci, streptococci, gram-negative organisms, and anaerobes. MRSA has become an increasing problem.
7. Osteomyelitis should be suspected in a deep ulcer if a sinus tract is present or the ulcer fails to heal (Deery & Sangeorzan, 2001; Shaw & Boulton, 2001)

C. Edema Reduction: leg elevation above the level of the heart if tolerated by patient level of pain related to ischemia in the lower extremity.

D. Enzymatic Debriding Agents: enzymes or solutions applied to devitalized tissue in the wound for the purpose of selective debridement. Able to lyse fibrin, denatured collagen, elastin but not normal tissue.

E. **Total Contact Cast:** complete offloading of wound with medication placed at wound site. Covered with plaster casting. Disadvantage: unable to visualize wound and reassess ability to heal.

F. **Autolysis:** involves the use of moisture-retentive dressings

1. Occlusive, semi-occlusive and nonocclusive that cover the wound and allow enzymes normally present in wound fluids to self-digest devitalized tissue.
2. Conservative approach and may require 3 to 7 days to accomplish.
3. Effective, inexpensive, and painless.
4. Autolysis with occlusion is contraindicated when infection is present

VII. Surgical Management

A. Goals of Diabetic Foot Surgery

1. Establish drainage
2. Remove infected necrotic soft tissue or bone
3. Correct deformity
4. Reduce risk of ulceration or amputation
5. Restore stability and alignment
6. Preserve function
7. Achieve cosmetically acceptable result
8. Prevent major limb amputation (Edmonds, Foster, & Sanders, 2004)

B. Types of Procedures (Edmonds et al., 2004)

1. Elective
   a. Correction of defect in a patient with intact sensation, adequate perfusion, and well-controlled diabetes
   b. Risks and benefits similar as for nondiabetic patient
   c. Example: bunion correction
2. Prophylactic
   a. Procedures necessary to prevent further problems or ulcerations/wounds
   b. "At risk" foot: neuropathic, insensate, deformity
   c. Examples: stable Charcot foot with residual deformity that cannot be accommodated by shoe or brace; correction of hammer toe deformity; lengthening of Achilles tendon
3. Emergent
   a. Usually present with serious foot infection; signs of systemic infection present or not present
   b. Rapid assessment to distinguish between limb-threatening versus life-threatening wound
   c. Requires immediate hospitalization for treatment of infection and surgery; antibiotics alone usually inadequate to control infection
      1) Incision and drainage
      2) Wound exploration
      3) Debridement of necrosis

4) Revascularization
5) Amputation

C. Indications for Revascularization via dorsalis pedis artery bypass or popliteal to dorsalis pedis artery bypass graft with and without superficial femoral artery balloon angioplasty (refer to Chapter 9, Lower Extremity Arterial Disease).

1. Tissue necrosis in the presence of moderate-to-severe ischemia (limb salvage) (Pomposelli & Campbell, 2002)
   a. Ischemic heel ulcers
   b. Ischemia complicated by foot infection
2. Presence of an outflow artery in direct continuity with the foot (Yao & Pierce, 2001)
3. Multilevel occlusive disease with poor distal runoff
4. Disabling rest pain (Dale, 1985)
5. Active infection must first be controlled before dorsalis pedis bypass. Adequate control implies resolution of cellulitis, lymphangitis, and edema; especially in areas of proposed incisions required to expose the distal artery of saphenous vein

D. Contraindications for Revascularization

1. Bedridden patient with no hope of ever ambulating/bearing weight (Dale, 1985); may vary depending on surgeon's discretion and patient's risk assessment.
2. Advanced disease states: for example, malignancy in a patient for whom predicted death is within 6 months may be more amendable to primary amputation (Dale, 1985).
3. Relative contraindications
   a. Careful consideration should be used in patients with unstable or irreversible pulmonary, cardiac, hepatic, or cerebral disease states
   b. If comorbid disease states are stable or reversible, a vascular repair under spinal anesthesia is indicated
   c. Preoperative evaluation with specific comorbid risk factor analysis is warranted
   d. Absence of autologous venous conduit: prosthetic graft material is not ideal for distal bypasses (below the knee), although composite or prosthetic grafts have been used if other options are limited (Hughes et al., 2004; Yao & Pierce, 2001)

E. Preoperative Evaluation

1. Thorough physical examination with aggressive management of diabetes and medical comorbidities
   a. Cardiovascular, renal, peripheral vascular, and infectious disease consults may be indicated
   b. Nutritional status
2. Noninvasive arterial examination
3. Perform contrast angiography with digital subtraction to include complete infrapopliteal circulation including foot vessels. Anteroposterior and lateral foot views should be included to differentiate branch vessels and to visualize all stenosis (Yao & Pierce, 2001). MRA may be used as an alternative

F. Technical Considerations, Results, and Risks of Distal Bypass Procedures

1. Proximal bypass to the popliteal or proximal tibioperoneal arteries may restore foot pulses, but these are often not robust enough to normalize arterial pressure in the target area and subsequently heal a diabetic heel ulcer.
   a. Peroneal bypass: not in continuity with the foot vessels; reserved for rare instances where there is no dorsalis pedis or posterior tibial artery or insufficient venous conduit; more distal reconstruction often needed to heal wounds of the forefoot (Yao & Pierce, 2001).
   b. Autogenous vein grafting to the dorsalis pedis artery with subsequent anastomosis to tarsal, plantar, and malleolar or paramalleolar arteries: skin bridging with preliminary subcutaneous graft tunneling will avoid ischemia owing to tension (Pomposelli & Campbell, 2002; Yao & Pierce, 2001).
2. Results
   a. Five-year patency rates to the pedal arteries are reported to be 68% to 80% with limb salvage of 87% to 90% (Pomposelli & Campbell, 2002; Roddy et al., 2001).
   b. Review experience of lower extremity revascularization in a largely diabetic population of nearly 1,000 patients observed 5 years or longer: a total of 962 vein grafts were performed on 843 patients, of which 83% (795 grafts) were in patients with diabetes. Minimum follow-up was 5 years and extended up to 9 years. The dorsalis pedis or plantar/tarsal arteries served as the outflow artery in 271 (35%) of the diabetic patients. Cumulative primary graft patency was 74.7% overall, with no difference among patients with and without diabetes (diabetic, 75.6% vs. nondiabetic, 71.9%; $P = $ NS). Most importantly, 5-year limb salvage and survival rates were virtually identical in diabetic and nondiabetic patients. The overall limb salvage rate was 87.1% (diabetic, 87.3% vs. nondiabetic, 85.4%; $P = $ NS). Survival at 5 years was 58.1% in the entire cohort (diabetic, 58.2% vs. nondiabetic, 58.0%; $P = $ NS) (Akbari et al., 2000).
   c. These data strongly emphasize that concern for long-term mortality, limb loss, and graft patency in diabetic patients is unwarranted and should not prevent aggressive attempts at distal bypass required for limb salvage.
3. Risks: graft infection, repeat operations, postoperative lymphedema, limb loss, and death often related to high cardiovascular risks (Nehler, Hiatt, & Taylor, 2003).
4. Distal bypass graft failure and outcomes (Domenig et al., 2005).
   a. Early failure: occurs within 30 days of surgery and usually results in amputation; further intervention to maintain graft patency is futile.
   b. Late failure: occurs after 30 days postoperatively; rate of amputation is lower owing to higher rate of successful graft revision and lower occurrence of critical limb ischemia.

G. Management of Gangrene/Necrosis

1. Wet gangrene: odorous wet wound with swelling, necrosis, and erythema.
   a. Acute immediate need to remove gangrenous area surgically to salvage limb

   b. Gas (crepitus or crackling of soft tissues) is a serious finding requiring immediate surgical drainage of all affected areas and intravenous antibiotics
   c. Initiate intravenous antibiotics with hospitalization and workup for limb salvage, revascularization, or amputation
2. Dry gangrene: chronic dry black eschar
   a. Protect and keep dry until workup of limb salvage completed.
   b. Revascularization may be needed, after which the gangrenous area can be surgically debrided or amputated.
   c. Auto-amputation (digit falls off without surgical intervention) of dry gangrenous toe is painless and safe as long as digit remains dry.

H. Amputation of Diabetic Foot (refer to Chapter 25, Amputation)

1. Nonemergent
   a. Neuropathic feet with structural impairment leading to recurrent nonhealing wounds
   b. Intact circulation and controlled infection
2. Emergent
   a. Gangrene, severe soft tissue infection, osteomyelitis, peripheral vascular disease, trauma
   b. Level of amputation determined by extent of healthy tissue and blood supply
3. Ideal wound healing criteria (Edmonds et al., 2004)
   a. Tissue oxygen perfusion ($TcPO_2$) >30 mm Hg
   b. Toe pressured >60 mm Hg or toe–brachial index >0.60
   c. Ankle–brachial index >0.50
   d. Serum albumin >3.0 g/dL
   e. Serum protein >6.0 g/dL
   f. Total lymphocyte count >1,500
   g. Medically stable with diabetes and infection under control
4. Types of foot amputations
   a. Digital: used for fixed deformity, osteomyelitis, recurrent tip ulcers
   b. Ray: excision of toe and metatarsal; may lead to new pressure point ulceration
   c. Transmetatarsal and midfoot, including Lisfranc and Chopart
   d. Procedures for Charcot foot: ostectomy of prominent plantar, medial, or lateral bones; arthrodesis to stabilize neuropathic joints via open reduction and internal fixation

VIII. Wound Care

A. Assessment

1. Presence of infection: if infection is suspected, avoid occlusive dressings
2. Amount of wound drainage
3. Size of wound, including depth and tunneling
4. Wound base: granulation tissue, fibrinous slough, necrosis, eschar, bone
5. Periwound skin: erythematous, warm, pale or cool, cyanotic, tender, thin or dry, calloused
6. Limb: insensate, edematous, pale, cool, cyanotic, warm, or erythematous

B. Phases of Wound Healing: wound healing is a physiologic process that involves a series of sequential yet overlapping stages.

1. Homeostasis occurs immediately at the time of injury. During hemostasis a provisional matrix seals the injury site and initiates the process of wound healing.
2. Inflammation is triggered by a variety of mediators released from injured tissue cells and capillaries, activated platelets and their cytokines, and the by-products of hemostasis.
3. The wound surface is covered with new skin, and vascular and structural integrity is restored as granulation tissue fills the defect.
4. Remodeling is responsible for maturation of the granulation tissue into mature connective tissue, scar, or both.
5. A thorough understanding of wound healing physiology is an important prerequisite to providing care that optimizes wound healing and prevents unnecessary complications.
6. Wound dressings are now considered interactive products able to affect the microenvironment of the wound to promote rapid wound healing.

C. Wound Goals and Treatments: management goals to consider

1. The etiology of the wound
2. Contributing factors and local wound care
3. Practical, consistent, and takes into consideration the overall health and lifestyle of the patient
4. Management goals or patient outcomes may vary depending on the general health of the host and the severity of the injury
5. Odor control: odor management is achieved through control of bacteria levels. It includes removal of devitalized tissue and modulating the amount of exudate in the wound

D. Select Primary Dressing Based on Exudates and Wound Bed Appearance

1. Dry: apply moist dressing, such as wound gel
2. Mild-to-moderate drainage: light absorbent, such as hydrocolloid
3. Heavily draining: absorbent, such as alginate
4. Fibrinous slough: autolytic debridement or chemical debridement agent
5. Hard, dry eschar: may require sharp surgical debridement before dressing application

E. Wound and Limb Protection

1. Pain management: a significant decrease in pain perception has been reported with moisture-retentive dressings. Moisture also limits mechanical damage to tissues during dressing removal. Always premedicate before dressing removal, with the exception being the insensate foot.
2. Periwound protection: use of skin sealant and barriers before dressing application.
3. Off-load pressure from wound and limb as listed in Medical Management.
4. Keep extremity warm; use protective socks and closed-toe shoes if possible.

5. If the patient can wear shoes, select extradepth, extrawidth shoes with orthotic linings to off-load pressure points.
6. Perform close monitoring for signs/symptoms of infection or change in appearance.

IX. Nursing Diagnoses

A. Impairment of Skin Integrity Related to Diabetic Foot Disease (Datta, 2001; Fahey & Schindler, 2004; Gibson, 2001; MacVittie, 1998)

1. Assessment for defining characteristics
   a. Change in appearance of wound and surrounding tissues
   b. Change in vital signs
   c. Increased weakness
2. Expected outcome: infection will not spread and wound will heal preventing amputation of area and lower leg
3. Nursing interventions
   a. Assess wound and provide wound care as directed
   b. Do not use tape on skin but apply tape to gauze wrap
   c. Protect affected extremity with bed cradle, use of heel guards, offloading
   d. Monitor vital signs for increased signs of infection
   e. Administer IV antibiotics as directed
   f. Absolute need to refrain from walking on infected area; will need wheelchair, crutches, or bed rest
   g. Nutrition: consults dietitian for proper diet; weight loss diet not appropriate at this time.
4. Evaluation of nursing care
   a. All changes in status are recorded and reported immediately.
   b. Medicines and dressing changes are performed in timely manner.

B. Alteration in Tissue Perfusion Relating to Impaired Peripheral Vascular Function (Bryant, 2001; Fahey & Schindler, 2004; MacVittie, 1998)

1. Assessment for defining characteristics
   a. Change in pulse quality, capillary refill time
   b. Change in skin color, temperature
2. Expected outcome: patient will maintain tissue perfusion
3. Nursing interventions
   a. Avoid smoking: refer to smoking cessation program
   b. Avoid vasoconstrictive drugs
   c. Avoid constricting clothing, crossing of legs, tight bandages
   d. Avoid long periods of standing or sitting that may cause tourniquet effect on circulation resulting in pooling of blood and edema of dependent tissues; muscle action facilitates venous return
   e. Monitor for cool skin, tingling, pallor, poor capillary refill time, the presence of petechiae, and mottling of limbs
4. Evaluation of nursing care: skin remains intact, warm, and with appropriate color, with brisk capillary refill and pulses intact

C. Disturbance in Self-Concept Related to Wounds and Treatments (Fahey & Schindler, 2004; Gibson, 2001; MacVittie, 1998)

1. Assessment for defining characteristics
   a. Disease state requires changes of lifestyle, long-term prognosis is uncertain
   b. Mood change or depression
   c. Self-destructive or unhealthy health behaviors
2. Expected outcome: patient will have a positive body image
3. Nursing interventions
   a. Assess level of acceptance and adaptation of patient and significant others
   b. Encourage verbalization of fears and life changes
   c. Explain procedures and tests involved; allow patient to verbalize fears
   d. Refer for counseling as needed
   e. Establish a trusting relationship
   f. Promote social interaction
4. Evaluation of nursing care
   a. Patient is able to take responsibility for life style changes needed
   b. Patient and significant other acknowledge ongoing care and treatment needed

D. Potential Knowledge Deficit of Management of Diabetes; Impairment in Metabolic State

1. Assessment for defining characteristics
   a. Chronic hyperglycemia
   b. Obesity
   c. Hypertension
   d. Self-management of diabetes
2. Expected outcomes
   a. Diabetes will be under acceptable control
   b. Patient will take responsibility for self-management at home
3. Nursing interventions
   a. Monitor blood glucose and electrolytes; I & O, daily weights
   b. Correct factors that precipitate development of diabetic ketoacidosis
   c. Avoid fluctuations in blood sugar to prevent hyperglycemia and hypoglycemia
   d. Assess need for referral for psychosocial counseling
   e. Assess and review medication administration, importance of dietary regulation, and weight control
   f. Teach and reinforce importance of home glucose monitoring
   g. Consult with dietitian if needed
4. Evaluation of nursing care
   a. Blood sugar remains in normal range (70 to 110 mg/dL)
   b. Patient expresses understanding of medication and administration
   c. Patient expresses understanding of diabetes and its complications, glucose monitoring, diet, and weight control (American Diabetes Association(ADA), 2004b; Gibson, 2001; MacVittie, 1998)

E. Potential for Infection Related to Diabetes

1. Assessment for defining characteristics
   a. Change in vital signs
   b. Change in skin integrity or wound appearance

2. Expected outcome: infection will resolve; patient will remain free of infection
3. Nursing interventions
   a. Assess for fever, cellulitis, wound drainage, and elevated white blood cell count
   b. Use aseptic technique for dressing changes
   c. Administer antibiotics as directed
4. Evaluation of nursing care
   a. Patient remains afebrile
   b. Wound size decreases and is without drainage, redness, increased warmth, or odor (Fahey & Schindler, 2004; Gibson, 2001; MacVittie, 1998)

X. Patient Teaching

A. Disease Prevention/Health Promotion

Since diabetes often causes the feet to become less sensitive and not feel pain, you have to look at your feet to find a problem.

1. Using a good light, inspect your feet and between the toes every day for blisters, corns, cuts, and sores. Use a mirror to see the bottoms of your feet or have a family member help you (see Fig. 22-2).
2. Do not soak your feet as soaking dries out the skin, but do wash your feet every day with mild soap and warm water. Test the water with your elbow before putting your feet in.
3. Dry the feet well but carefully, especially between the toes, by blotting with the towel; be gentle.
4. Use a nonperfumed, moisturizing lotion on your feet immediately after washing and drying them to seal in the moisture. Do not put lotion between the toes, as this area must be kept dry. Report any sign of fungal infection immediately.
5. Clippers should be used to cut your toenails, but it is recommended that someone trained in diabetic foot care cut your toenails. You may use a cardboard emery board and file straight across the nail, but do not use scissors or a metal file.

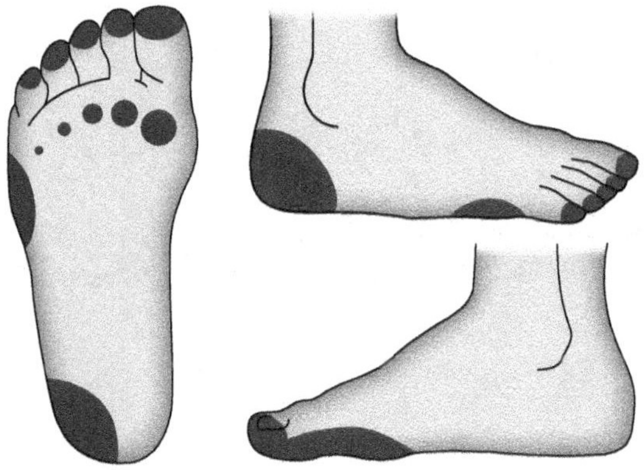

FIGURE 22-2. Pressure areas on the foot.

6. Do not use any type of corn remover products or over–the-counter medicines on your feet. Never perform any kind of "bathroom surgery" on your feet such as cutting or trimming corns and calluses.
7. If your feet feel cold at night, wear loose-fitting socks; do not using a heating pad or hot water bottle on your feet.
8. Wear high-grade cotton socks that fit well; do not wear mended stockings and those with thick seams. Socks should not fit too tightly on your legs so avoid knee-high hose and circular garters. Change your socks every day and always wear socks with your shoes.
9. Shoes should fit properly and protect your feet. Buy new shoes in the afternoon; do not depend on new shoes to stretch out. Avoid pointed toed shoes that squeeze the toes. Check your feet carefully and frequently if wearing new shoes. Avoid cut out or opened toed shoes, especially sandals with a strap between the toes.
   a. Protect your feet in the summer from sunburn and in the winter from frostbite.
   b. Feel inside your shoes with your hand before putting them on. Check for rough or torn linings, protruding nails, or foreign objects.
10. Never go barefoot! Always wear some type of footwear to protect your feet.
11. Always wash your hands before and after changing a dressing. Wrap the gauze lightly around the dressing and tape the gauze. Never put tape directly on your skin.
12. Do not smoke or use tobacco products as they decrease the blood supply to your feet.
13. No matter how minor you think it is always report any sign of foot problems or injury to your doctor or nurse immediately (American Diabetes Association (ADA), 2004a).

CASE STUDY

C.C. is an 84-year-old Hispanic male, living alone, presenting with a 1-month history of right foot pain and an open area on the bottom of his foot. He has been cleansing the area daily with alcohol, applying antibiotic ointment, and covering it with a band aid. He has come to the wound clinic because the sore has begun to develop an odor and the patient is worried that something is wrong. He had fractured his ankle approximately 2 years ago and it healed in an abnormal shape. He denied any PMH except for "circulation problems." PSH includes a left fifth toe amputation secondary to an accidental cut. He has smoked ½ pack of cigarettes per day for 40 years, takes no medications.

Assessment: VS: Temperature 98.6°F, Heart Rate 96, Respirations16, and Blood Pressure 136/70. Pedal pulses not palpable on the right, trace dorsalis pedis on the left, minimal edema in the right foot. The right foot is deformed medially with a pressure area at the proximal arch. There is an open area 1 cm round × 5 mm deep with a pale base and white fibrinous center. A thick callous surrounds the perimeter.

Laboratory values: white blood cell count and basic metabolic panel within normal limits except for a glucose of 278. ABIs were R = 0.80, L = 1.02, biphasic flow noted in the right DP, left DP and PT; triphasic flow in the right PT; waveforms symmetrically reduced.

X-ray was negative for infection.

Review Questions

1. What further testing should be done initially?
   a. Foot culture
   b. HgbA1c
   c. Bone scan
   d. Arteriogram
2. What type of wound care should be done for this ulcer?
   a. Continue current treatment
   b. Wet to dry saline gauze four times a day
   c. Cleanse with saline, continue antibiotic ointment daily
   d. Cleanse with saline, apply enzymatic debriding agent daily
3. What are the predisposing factors for this ulcer?
   a. Smoking history
   b. Abnormal gait
   c. Diabetes
   d. All the above
4. What is the most likely cause of C.C.'s foot ulcer?
   a. Mechanical injury
   b. Ischemic injury
   c. Repetitive stress injury
   d. Infective process
5. What is the best way to decrease the effects of neuropathy associated with diabetes?
   a. Perform daily foot examinations
   b. Tight control of hypertension
   c. Tight control of hyperglycemia
   d. Wear proper footwear
6. Along with proper wound care, what other medical management technique should be used for C.C.?
   a. Addition of a multivitamin
   b. Soaking the foot for 30 minutes a day
   c. Orthotic device for offloading the foot
   d. Foot massage
7. What is one important factor to C.C.'s ability to heal his wound?
   a. He lives alone
   b. His BP is 136/70
   c. History of tobacco abuse
   d. History of left fifth toe amputation

Answers/Rationales

1. b. Because of the elevated glucose, an HgbA1cshould be done to assess for diabetes.
2. d. Neither a nor c will accomplish the debridement needed for this wound. Wet to dry saline gauze will debride the ulcer but is labor intensive and compliance is low. An enzymatic agent will debride the fibrin allowing granulation tissue to grow. Home nursing care should be arranged to provide this skilled service.
3. d. All of these are risk factors for ulceration.
4. c. The abnormal foot pattern and gait, along with the callous around the perimeter of the ulcer describes a repetitive stress injury.

5. c. Tight control of hyperglycemia with an HgbA1c at or below 7% reduces retinopathy, nephropathy, and peripheral neuropathy (ADA, 2011).
6. c. An offloading device is needed to reduce pressure at the ulcer site and promote blood flow to the area for healing.
7. c. Tobacco abuse decreases the blood supply to the extremities by increasing platelet aggregation and plaque propagation.

REFERENCES

Akbari, C. M., Pomposelli, F. B., Jr., Gibbons, G. W., Campbell, D. R., Pulling, M. C., Mydlarz, D., & LoGerfo, F. W. (2000). Lower extremity revascularization in diabetes: Late observations. *Archives of Surgery, 135*, 452–456.

American Diabetes Association (ADA). (2004a). Preventive foot care in people with diabetes. *Diabetes Care, 27*, s63–s64; doi:10.2337/diacare.27.2007.S63

American Diabetes Association(ADA). (2004b). Standards of medical care for patients with diabetes mellitus. *Diabetes Care, 27*, s15–s35; doi:10.2337/diacare.27.2007.S15

American Diabetes Association (ADA). (2011) Standards of medical care in diabetes-2011. *Diabetes Care, 34*(Suppl. 1), S11–S61.

Bryant, G. (2001). Stump care. *American Journal of Nursing, 101*(2), 67–71.

Centers for Disease Control and Prevention (CDC). (2011). National diabetes fact sheet: National estimates and general information on diabetes and prediabetes in the United States, 2011. Retrieved from http://www.cdc.gov/diabetes/pubs/pdf/ndfs_2011.pdf, accessed February 29, 2012.

Dale, W. A. (1985). *Management of vascular surgical problems.* New York, NY: McGraw-Hill.

Datta, D. (2001). Amputation, rehabilitation and prosthetic developments. In J. Beard & P. A. Gaines (Eds.), *Vascular and endovascular surgery* (pp. 89–102). London, UK: W.B. Saunders Company.

Deery, H. G., & Sangeorzan, J. A. (2001). Saving the diabetic foot with special reference to the patient with chronic renal failure. *Infectious Disease Clinics of North America, 15*(3), 953–981.

Domenig, C. M., Hamdan, A. D., Holzenbein, T. J., Kansal, N., Aulivola, B., Skillman, J. J., . . . Pomposelli, F. B., Jr. (2005). Timing of pedal bypass failure and its impact on the need for amputation. *Annals of Vascular Surgery, 19*(1), 56–62.

Edmonds, M. E., Foster, A. V. M., & Sanders, L. J. (2004). *A practical manual of diabetic foot care.* Malden, MA: Blackwell Publishing.

Fahey, V. A., & Schindler, N. (2004). Arterial reconstruction of the lower extremity. In V. A. Fahey (Ed.), *Vascular nursing* (4th ed., pp. 251–285). St. Louis, MO: W.B. Saunders.

Frykberg, R. G. (2003). An evidence-based approach to diabetic foot infections. *The American Journal of Surgery, 186*(5A), 44S–54S.

Frykberg, R. G. (2005). A summary of guidelines for managing the diabetic foot. *Advances in Skin & Wound Care, 18*(4), 209–214.

Gibson, J. (2001). Lower limb amputation. *Nursing Standard, 15*(28), 47–52.

Grayson, M. L., Gibbons, G. W., Balogh, K., Levin, E., & Krachmer, A. W. (1995). Probing to bone in infected pedal ulcers. A clinical sign of osteomyelitis in diabetic patients. *Journal of the American Medical Association, 273*, 721–723.

Hughes, K., Domenig, C. M., Hamdan, A. D., Schermerhorn, M., Aulivola, B., Blattman, S., . . . Pomposelli, F. B., Jr. (2004). Bypass to plantar and tarsal arteries: An acceptable approach to limb salvage. *Journal of Vascular Surgery, 40*(6), 1149–1157.

MacVittie, B. A. (1998). *Vascular surgery.* St.Louis, MO: Mosby.

Nehler, M. R., Hiatt, W. R., & Taylor, L. M. (2003). Is revascularization and limb salvage always the best treatment for critical limb ischemia? *Journal of Vascular Surgery, 37*(3), 704–708.

NIH Publication No. 08-3874. (2008). DCCT and EDIC: The diabetes control and complication trial and follow-up study. National Diabetes Information Clearing House. Retrieved from http://diabetes.niddk.nih.gov/dm/pubs/control/DCCT-EDIC_508.pdf, accessed July 20, 2013.

Pomposelli, F. B., & Campbell, D. R. (2002). Vascular surgery for the diabetic foot. In A. Veves, J. M. Giurini, & F. W. LoGerfo (Eds.), *The diabetic foot* (pp. 411–428). Totowa, NJ: Humana Press.

Roddy, S. P., Darling, R. C., Chang, B. B., Kreienberg, P. B., Paty, P. S., Lloyd, W. E., & Shah, D. M. (2001). Outcomes with plantar bypass for limb-threatening ischemia. *Annals of Vascular Surgery, 15*(1), 79–83.

Scurlock, C., Raikhelkar, J., & Mechanick, J. I. (2010). Critique of normoglycemia in intensive care evaluation: Survival using glucose algorithm regulation (NICE-SUGAR)- a review of recent literature. *Current Opinion in Clinical Nutrition & Metabolic Care, 13*(2), 211–214.

Shaw, J. E., & Boulton, A. J. (2001). The diabetic foot. In J. D. Beard & P. A. Gaines (Eds.), *Vascular and endovascular surgery* (pp. 105–125). London, UK: W.B. Saunders Company.
Sommer, T. C., & Lee, T. H. (2001). Charcot foot: The diagnostic dilemma. *American Family Physician, 64*(9), 1591–1598.
Yao, J. S., & Pierce, W. H. (2001). *Current techniques in vascular surgery.* New York, NY: McGraw-Hill.

RELEVANT WEBSITES

Diabetes.org
Diabetesaction.org

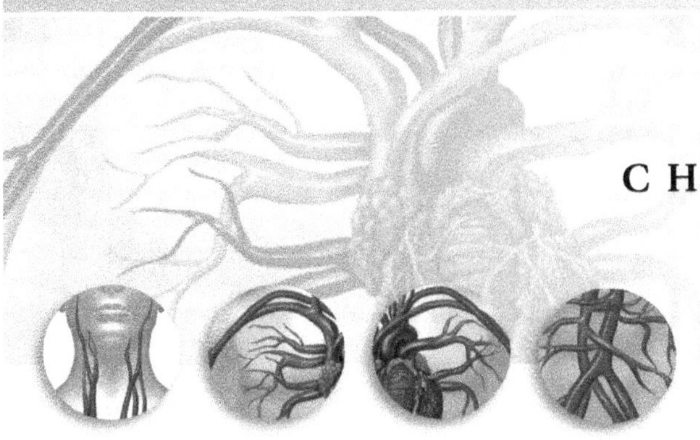

CHAPTER 23

Lymphedema

Patricia A. Lewis
M. Eileen Walsh

OBJECTIVES

1. Describe normal lymphatic flow.
2. Identify criteria used to diagnose primary and secondary lymphedema.
3. Describe medical and surgical management of lymphedema.
4. Discuss nursing interventions related to patient teaching, disease prevention, home care and self-care.

Introduction

Lymphedema is swelling of a body part due to the accumulation of protein-rich interstitial fluid or lymph in the skin and subcutaneous tissues (Mohler & Mondry, 2013). Lymphedema most often affects an extremity, but it may develop in the face or head, chest wall, abdomen, pelvis, or genitalia. Lymphedema is caused by imbalances in the microcirculation or disruptions that result in an inability of the lymphatic vessels to adequately transport lymph fluid back to the central circulation. The process is characterized by nonpitting edema and predisposes an individual to recurrent infections, such as lymphangitis and cellulitis. It is important to distinguish lymphedema from other forms of edema, such as venous stasis or dependent edema secondary to heart failure.

The world-wide incidence of lymphedema is estimated at over 150 million, with more than 1% Americans affected (Felty & Rooke, 2004), although the true incidence may be higher due to under-reporting and nonrecognition by both patients and health care providers. "Accurate estimates of the incidence of lymphedema are difficult to find because of

- The lack of a standard clinical definition of the condition
- Very few consistent surveys have appeared in the literature
- The occurrence of lymphedema is so dependent on the patient's genetic predisposition to develop the condition
- The patient's general health and lymphatic system health, including the nature and extent of lymphatic trauma" (Weiss, 2007).

Lymphedema can result from a congenital anomaly, dysfunction, or from an acquired disease. Primary lymphedema refers to cases of unknown etiology or congenital abnormality; secondary lymphedema refers to cases with a known cause such as infection, trauma, malignancy, or surgery. Filariasis caused by a parasite is the most common cause of lymphedema world-wide, and affects more than 100 million people. In nonindustrialized countries, the most common cause of lymphedema is cancer and cancer therapy (Gloviczki & Wahner, 2000).

The natural course of the disease is a progressive increase in the size of the affected body area over the lifetime of the individual. Chronic lymphedema can be a cosmetic deformity as well as a disabling condition. Although lymph vessels and nodes were first mentioned in medical literature dating back to Hippocrates and Aristotle, it has long been a neglected topic in medicine until recent advances in physiologic investigation have led to improvements in diagnosis and management (Gloviczki, 2000). There is no cure for lymphedema; however, therapeutic interventions can lessen the degree of swelling and aide in preventing progression and complications.

I. Anatomy and Normal Lymphatic Function

A. Lymph Fluid

1. Clear, colorless fluid
2. Formed by transudation of fluid into tissue spaces
3. Composition
   a. Protein: approximately half of all proteins are transported from interstitium into systemic circulation via lymph flow every 24 hours
   b. Water: serves as transport medium for cellular products
   c. Cellular components: varies depending on location; includes white blood cells/lymphocytes, cancer cells, bacteria, viral cells, cellular debris from phagocytosis, and protein breakdown
   d. Fatty acids: lipids are absorbed by intestinal tract travel via lymphatics to enter blood circulation; fats and other digestive byproducts cause a milky appearance of lymph fluid or chyle in mesenteric system. Approximately 4 to 5 lbs are produced every 24 hours
4. Lymphocytes circulate to fight infection
5. Lymph fluid is filtered through lymph nodes, which remove bacteria, debris, and chemicals

B. Lymphatic System: recognized in 18th century as an integrated system responsible for absorption by Drs. William and John Hunter (Gloviczki, 2000)

1. Lymphatic vasculature: main function is to transport interstitial fluid and protein lost from the capillary system; transport infectious material and debris, back into venous circulation
   a. Initial lymphatics (also called terminal, superficial, or capillaries) (Foeldi, 2012)
      1) Found in skin and mucus membranes, blind-ended sinuses lined by single layer of lymphatic endothelial cells
      2) Located in all tissues and organs except CNS and cornea
      3) Structure similar to venous capillary except for
         a) Presence of large openings between cell junctions in capillary
         b) Openings allow fluids and large solutes (proteins) to enter capillary
         c) Overlapping design creates one-way valve: allows entry of fluids and proteins, but substances cannot flow back out

d) Opening of flaps stimulated by variations in tissue pressure and contraction of fibrils attached to exterior cell walls and surrounding connective tissue (Kelly, 2002)

b. Lymphatic pre-collectors
   1) Thicker: less permeable but still capable of absorption
   2) Valves expedite movement of fluid from superficial capillaries toward deeper transport vessels

c. Lymphatic ducts: also known as collectors, lymphatics, or valved vessels
   1) Carry lymph toward trunk, run parallel to deep arteries and veins
   2) Walls contain contractile smooth muscle similar to veins but have thinner walls and valves at shorter intervals
   3) Two major collecting channels
      a) Superficial (epifascial) system: collects 80% of fluid from skin and subcutaneous tissue. In lower extremity, this system has 10 to 15 large lymphatic channels located mainly along greater saphenous vein
      b) Deep lymphatic system: drains subfascial structures (bone, muscles, deep blood vessels); follows tibial, popliteal, and femoral vessels in leg
      c) In the extremities, two systems merge at the inguinal nodes (legs) or axillary nodes (arms)
      d) Lymph transported through iliac and para-aortic channels (legs) or axillary channels (arms) and nodes into lymphatic trunks of deep lymphatic circulation system

d. Thoracic duct: major lymph trunks connect into thoracic duct
   1) Also collects chyle from mesenteric lymph vessels via cisterna chili, saclike chamber originating around L2 vertebra that collects lymph from lumbar and intestinal trunks
   2) Average output of 1.5 L/day (Schirger & Gloviczki, 1996)
   3) Lymph from left jugular, subclavian, and bronchomediastinal trunks and all trunks below diaphragm empties into venous system at the left jugulo-subclavian junction (angle between the left subclavian vein and left jugular vein)
   4) Lymph from right side of head, neck, chest, and right arm empties into right lymphatic duct in the right chest 25% of the total lymph load

2. Distribution of lymph tissue and organs
   a. Areas at greater risk of injury or infection have increased distribution of lymphatics and nodes
   b. Issues: include tonsils and connective tissue nodules located beneath epithelial linings in the body
   c. Organs: include lymph nodes, thymus, and spleen; facilitate lymphocyte production and distribution
   d. Lymph nodes
      1) 600 to 700 small, ovoid organs encapsulated by dense connective tissue with connection to blood vessels, lymphatics, and nerves
      2) Major groups of lymph nodes at base of each lymphatic duct, arranged in groups or chains
      3) Facilitate lymph drainage from local limb or regional structure
         a) Sentinel lymph node: initial draining node in a region
      4) Filter waste and aid in regulation of protein concentration in lymph fluid

C. Lymph Circulation: concept of lymph formation and movement began with Starling's description of hydrostatic and oncotic pressure (Foeldi, 2012; Gloviczki, 2000; Mohler & Mondry, 2013)

1. Microcirculation lymph flow allows for continuous movement from bloodstream to tissues and back into bloodstream through lymphatics and depends on:
   a. Diffusion: passive movement of molecules from area of high concentration to lower concentration
      1) Two factors affecting diffusion are molecular size (small molecules diffuse more rapidly) and temperature (higher temperature increases rate of diffusion)
      2) Osmosis: net diffusion of water across cell membrane; fluid follows proteins into or out of lymph vessel
      3) Hydrostatic pressure: resistant force preventing too much fluid from entering a solution; elastic properties of skin play an important role in maintaining tissue hydrostatic pressure
   b. Filtration: hydrostatic pressure forces water across membrane from area of high pressure to lower pressure; occurs at arterial capillary end where blood pressure is higher than tissue pressure
   c. Reabsorption: occurs as result of osmosis; osmotic pressure forces water toward the solution containing higher solute concentration. Osmotic pressure is lowest at venous end of capillary, allowing water and solutes to be pulled into venous system
   d. Approximately 24 L of fluid moves out of plasma and into interstitial space daily
      1) 85% to 90% reabsorbed directly into venous capillaries
      2) 10% to 15% (2 to 4 L) enters lymphatic vessels for return to central venous circulation
2. Precollectors move fluid via capillary absorption plus contraction of valves
3. Deep vessels are divided into segments called lymphangions; each segment moves fluid via intrinsic contractions
   a. Vessels contract 6 to 10 times/min at rest; 60 to 100 times/min during exercise
   b. Stimulated to contract segmentally and empty via several mechanisms
      1) Sympathetic, parasympathetic, and sensory nervous stimulation: located in lymph vessels and nodes; regulate contractile function
      2) Contraction of adjacent muscles (see Fig. 23-1)
      3) Pulsation of adjacent arteries

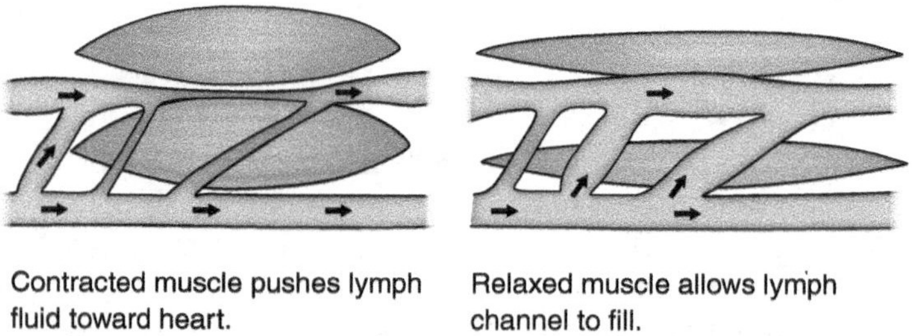

FIGURE 23-1. Effect of muscle contraction on lymph circulation.

4) Alteration in abdominal and thoracic pressure during respiration
5) Lower blood capillary pressure in deep veins
6) Lymph vessel volume: as one segment (lymphangion) fills to maximum volume, receptors signal start of a contraction due to tension on inner wall, pushing fluid into next lymphangion
7) Mechanical stimulation or traction: external pressure such as compression/support garment or massage

4. Lymph nodes
   a. Lymph flows into node via deeper afferent vessels; flows out toward venous system after filtration via efferent vessels
   b. Nodes also help regulate protein concentration in lymph fluid, thus aiding control of hydrostatic pressure to maintain equilibrium in surrounding tissues
   c. It is very difficult for lymph fluid to pass through a region following lymph node dissection and formation of scar tissue
5. Thoracic duct flow is facilitated by same mechanisms as deep lymphatics, with increased flow stimulated by drop in intrathoracic pressure during abdominal breathing creating a suction effect that pulls lymph fluid into chest

II. Pathophysiology

A. Malformation or Obstruction of Lymphatic Vessels and Nodes

1. Increases osmotic pressure within lymphatics; fluid will not be drawn into vessels, allowing accumulation in subcutaneous and interstitial spaces.
2. Inability of lymphatics to collect and drain interstitial fluid and protein results in dilation of lymphatics and edema.
3. Unlike general edema conditions (such as congestive heart failure), rate of capillary filtration is normal in patients with lymphedema (Mohler & Mondry, 2013).

B. Stages of Lymphedema Progression: International Society of Lymphology, 1985 (Kerchner, Fleischer, & Yosipovitch, 2008; Mohler & Mondry, 2013; Newton, 2011)

1. Based on two criteria
   a. Softness or firmness of tissue (fibrosis)
   b. Effect of elevation
2. Stage 0: swelling not evident, subclinical or latent condition; may feel heaviness in limb; may be present for months to years before overt symptoms occur
3. Stage I: reversible
   a. Extracellular fluid collects within interstitium and can easily be squeezed out
   b. Pitting edema; resolves with extremity elevation
   c. Skin is normal in appearance, soft, and elastic
4. Stage II: irreversible
   a. Concentrated proteins in the interstitial fluid act as foreign material, stimulating chronic inflammatory response and proliferation of connective tissue (Kelly, 2002)

b. Fibrosclerotic tissue forms as collagen deposits increase (Witte & Witte, 2000)
   1) Fibrous tissue impairs endothelial cell function
   2) Diffusion and osmosis are hindered, leading to abnormal control of hydrostatic pressure
   3) Initially, only local area of damage affected, but process then extends out as more fibrous tissue forms in vessel walls
c. Lymph stasis and build-up of protein in the interstitium overwhelms the normal neutrophil and macrophage response, provoking diffuse scarring
d. Intensive neoangiogenesis associated with migration of endothelial cells causes further damage
e. Nonpitting edema results with increased density of skin
   1) Despite significant structural changes, up to 30% fluid overload in lymphatic system may occur before swelling is visible (Kelly, 2002)
   2) Some patients do not have symptoms at this stage until there is an increase in demand for lymphatic flow (exercise, lifting, air travel, increased temperature)
   3) Once symptoms develop, patient has permanent chronic fluid overload of impaired lymphatic drainage
   4) Swelling does not reduce with leg elevation

5. Stage III: elephantiasis
   a. Prolonged destruction of lymph vessels and obliteration of lymph nodes
   b. Often seen following repeated skin infections
   c. Skin has grotesque appearance: thick, bark-like, hard, and discolored, often with papillomas that leak spontaneously
   d. Limb more than doubled size of unaffected extremity; significant loss of function

C. Lymphangiosarcoma

1. Rare (<1%) sequela of longstanding peripheral lymphedema
   a. Initially thought to be exclusively related to treatment of breast cancer with radical mastectomy and radiation therapy (Stewart–Treves syndrome) (McHaffie et al., 2010; Robinson, Honda, & Bordeaux, 2011; Schirger & Gloviczki, 1996)
   b. Has been documented in other secondary lymphedemas as well as congenital or primary lymphedema (Witte & Witte, 2000)
2. Lymphedema thought to be the primary causative factor; neoplastic transformation of lymphatics (Gamble, Rooke, & Gloviczki, 2000)
3. Lesion: flat, bluish (looks like a bruise with no history of trauma); increases in size and develops satellite lesions with ulceration and crusting in center of initial lesion. Metastasis is usually rapid
4. Diagnosis requires immediate proximal amputation and radiation therapy; wide excision merely promotes blood-borne metastases; high fatality rate
5. Kaposi sarcoma (a vascular tumor similar to Stewart–Treves syndrome and usually associated with HIV disease) has origin from lymphatic endothelium (Witte & Witte, 2000)
6. Other malignancies reported in association with chronic lymphedema: non-Hodgkin and Hodgkin lymphoma, squamous cell carcinoma, and malignant melanoma (Gamble et al., 2000)

D. Chylous Reflux

1. Abnormal retrograde transport of intestinal lymph
2. Cholesterol and long-chain triglycerides are absorbed by lymphatic system; any disruption of mesenteric lacteals, cisterna chili, or thoracic duct leads to chylothorax, chylous ascites, or chyluria
3. If high-grade obstruction present, peripheral lymphatics dilate and lipid-rich lymph refluxes into soft tissues of pelvis, scrotum, and lower extremities: chylous vesicles and edema

E. Classification: several classifications used to describe severity (Mohler & Mondry, 2013), American Physical Therapy Association (APTA) and National Cancer Institute's Common Terminology Criteria for Adverse Events (CTCAE).

1. APTA: uses girth or circumferential measurements limb to limb
   a. Mild: maximum difference <3 cm
   b. Moderate: 3.5 cm
   c. Severe: >5 cm
2. CTCAE: based on examination and functional limitations
   a. Grade 1: trace thickening/faint discoloration
   b. Grade 2: marked discoloration, leathery skin, limiting activities of daily living
   c. Grade 3: severe symptoms limiting self-care

III. Etiology and Precipitating Factors

A. Primary Lymphedema: congenital or unknown cause; classified by age of onset

1. Congenital (Shinawi, 2007)
   a. Present at birth
   b. 10% to 15% of primary lymphedema cases
   c. Milroy disease
      1) Present at birth
      2) Familial sex-linked form of lymphatic aplasia (absence of vessels)
      3) Genetic abnormality of vascular endothelial growth factor receptor-3, which plays an important role in lymphatic development (Mohler, 2004)
      4) Associated with intestinal lymphangiectasia and cholestasis
   d. Turner syndrome: congenital lymphedema may also occur in patients with this disorder
      1) Dysmorphic features of webbed neck, nail dysplasia, high palate, short fourth metacarpal
2. Praecox
   a. Onset at or near puberty
   b. 70% to 80% of primary lymphedema cases (Rudkin & Miller, 1995)
   c. Meige disease: hereditary lymphedema praecox
      1) Autosomal dominant disorder usually affecting females 10:1 over males
      2) Bilateral mild edema of ankles and legs to knee level
      3) May be associated with other anomalies (e.g., extra eyelashes [distichiasis])

4) Associated with mutations in the FOXC2 gene
5) Impairment is result of agenesis (lack of growth) of valves that normally prevent lymphatic backflow
6) FOXC2 also expressed in venous valves; approximately 50% of patients with lymphedema-distichiasis also have venous insufficiency and valvular incompetence (Mohler, 2004)

3. Tarda: onset after age 35 (Rockson & Dean, 2011)
4. Primary lymphedema may also be classified by lymphangiographic findings
   a. Hypoplastic: 80%; lymphatics are narrowed and reduced in number; seen in Meige disease; slow progression of disease, which responds to conservative measures
   b. Hyperplastic: less than 10% of cases; lymphatics are dilated and increased in number because of obstruction or incompetent valves (Rudkin & Miller, 1995); usually affects males; bilateral involvement; megalymphatics with involvement of mesenteric system may occur with subsequent chylous reflux
   c. Proximal occlusion of aortoiliac or inguinal lymph nodes: 10%; unilateral involvement affecting entire limb; affects males and females; rapid progression which responds poorly to conservative measures

B. Secondary Lymphedema

1. Results from well-defined disease process that causes obstruction or injury to lymphatic system
2. Filariasis: most common secondary cause worldwide, affecting over 100 million people
   a. Caused by one of three lymphatic-dwelling parasites: *Wuchereria bancrofti, Brugia malayi,* or *Brugia timori;* endemic in tropical and subtropical regions
   b. Nematode worm larvae transmitted to humans by mosquitoes or black fly bites
   c. Adult filarial live, reproduce, and die in lymphatic vessels
   d. Death of parasite causes local inflammation, then chronic inflammation, damaged and blocked lymphatics
3. Surgery
   a. Surgical excision and irradiation of the axillary or inguinal lymph nodes as part of treatment for malignancy is the most common etiology in North America and Europe (Gloviczki & Wahner, 2000)
   b. Breast, cervical, and prostate cancer; soft tissue tumor; and malignant melanoma with nodal dissection (Apollo, 2007; Foeldi, 2012; Lockwood-Rayermann, 2007; Tada, Teramukai, Fukushima, & Sasaki, 2009)
   c. Well-documented correlation between degree of dissection and development of lymphedema, but patients may develop lymphedema even with newer tissue-sparing techniques (e.g., lumpectomy with sentinel node biopsy). Other factors, such as use of chemotherapy and radiation, contribute to scar tissue formation
4. Trauma
   a. Destruction of lymphatic nodules and vasculature by traumatic injury reduces transport capacity below level of normal lymphatic fluid load

b. Trauma can initiate infectious process, which further challenges lymphatics and can lead to more scarring
c. Pelvic fracture, liposuction, brachial plexus injury, burns and thermal injury, crush injury

5. Tumor (benign or malignant)
   a. Obstruct lymph nodes and vessels
   b. Metastasize to lymph nodes and through lymphatic channels
6. Iatrogenic damage during diagnostic or therapeutic procedures
   a. Radiation therapy
      1) Contributes to tissue fibrosis and decreased circulation of lymph in involved area
      2) Decreases availability of collateral channels
      3) Shrinks lymph nodes and hinders regeneration of lymph vessels; unable to respond to trauma or infection in the future
   b. Direct destruction during surgical procedures, groin punctures, use of tourniquet on limb
7. Infection
   a. Increased local blood flow and capillary permeability challenges lymphatic system
   b. Recurrent infections, especially cellulitis or lymphangitis, contribute to tissue destruction and fibrosis
   c. Defective immune response in patients with inadequate lymphatic flow or replacement of normal lymph tissue and nodes with fat and scar tissue from previous infections or injury felt to be responsible for increased susceptibility for recurrent infections
8. Chronic venous insufficiency: fluid overload from damaged venous system can initiate or worsen lymphedema (Foeldi, 2012; Piller, 2009)
9. Other causes: tuberculosis, contact dermatitis, rheumatoid arthritis, infection after snake or insect bite (Gloviczki & Wahner, 2000)

C. Precipitating Factors

1. Stimulus or trigger that causes initial onset of symptoms varies between at-risk individuals (e.g., postmastectomy patient). For people with normal lymphatic circulation, these events do not generally cause chronic swelling.
2. Local or systemic events that cause hyperemia of the involved limb: hot packs, hot tub, summer weather, handling hot food, aggressive massage, overuse of limb, infection, soft tissue sprains, or strain.
3. Alterations in barometric pressure
   a. Airplane travel: interstitial fluid pools while limb is dependent and lowered cabin pressure may exacerbate an incompetent lymphatic system
   b. Scuba diving: significant decrease in hydrostatic pressure as individual surfaces
   c. Application of external pressure that might affect limb hydrostatic pressure: use of tight clothing, aggressive massage, sleeping for long periods on at-risk limb, tight blood pressure cuff on at-risk limb
4. Breakdown of skin integrity: pet scratches, gardening, insect bites, contusions, injections, intravenous cannulation
5. Change in weight and body fluid volumes: pregnancy, weight gain, chronic venous insufficiency, chronic illness, such as heart failure or chronic obstructive pulmonary disease (COPD), medications such as calcium channel blockers

IV. Assessment

A. Risk Factor Assessment

1. Family history: any first or second degree relative with known lymphedema suggests primary etiology
2. Secondary causes or incidents as listed in precipitating factors, especially cancer and cancer interventions
3. Age
   a. Age decreases force of lymph pumps and circulation generally slows in all systems; fatigue and structural changes result with less efficient uptake of all fluids (Kelly, 2002).
   b. Studies vary regarding effect of aging on development of lymphedema in at-risk individuals, but aging seems to be linked to progression of lymphedema after onset (Kelly, 2002).
4. Obesity (Fife, Benavides, & Carter, 2008; Greene, Grant, & Slavin, 2012)
   a. Slower circulation leads to biosynthesis of fat.
   b. Obese patients and those who gain weight following a cancer diagnosis are at greater risk of developing lymphedema (Kelly, 2002).
5. Infection: onset or recurrence of infection, especially cellulitis, may be the initiating trigger or exacerbate lymphedema
   a. Protein-rich lymph fluid facilitates bacterial growth.
   b. Repeated infections can lead to scarring of existing lymphatics and nodes, resulting in onset or worsening of lymphedema.
   c. Erysipelas from beta-hemolytic streptococcal infection is the most common skin infection (Witte & Witte, 2000).

B. Patient History

1. Subjective findings
   a. Swelling in affected area: usually painless, gradual onset, although patient may not notice insidious changes early in course of disease
   b. Feeling of heaviness or fullness of one or more extremities
   c. Pain or paresthesia may be present: if severe, suspect infection or neuritic pain secondary to nerve compression or damage from surgical or radiation intervention
   d. Increased perspiration or watery discharge through uninjured skin: active lymphatic exudation in late or complicated cases
   e. Symptoms of skin infection may be first sign of lymphedema: warm, red, tender skin with or without lymphangitic streak, macular or maculopapular erythematous rash with well-defined borders of involvement, fever, flu-like symptoms
   f. Decreased mobility caused by limb heaviness: difficulty carrying out daily activities
   g. Diminished suppleness of skin; dry, taut skin; bark-like thickened fibrotic skin in advanced stages
2. History of etiologic or precipitating factors as previously listed
   a. History of presenting symptoms: triggers for swelling (e.g., lifting, infection, trauma.); onset; duration; pain or limitations; any previous treatments attempted
   b. Past medical history or comorbid conditions: venous disease; cardiac disease including hypertension; renal or hepatic disease; diabetes

TABLE 23-1 Differential Diagnosis of Chronic Leg Swelling

Systemic Causes	Local Causes
Cardiac failure	Chronic venous insufficiency
Hepatic failure	Lipedema (excess fat)
Renal failure	Congenital vascular malformation: Klippel–Trénaunay syndrome
Hypoproteinuria	Arteriovenous fistula
Hyperthyroidism or myxedema	Trauma
Allergic disorders	Snake or insect bite
Idiopathic cyclic edema	Infection, inflammation
Hereditary angioedema	Hematoma
Drugs	Dependency
Antihypertensives: methyldopa, nifedipine, hydralazine	Rheumatoid arthritis
Hormones: estrogen, progesterone	Postrevascularization edema
Monoamine oxidase inhibitors	Soft tissue tumor
	Reflex sympathetic dystrophy

Adapted from Gloviczki, P., & Wahner, H. W. (2000). Clinical diagnosis and evaluation of lymphedema. In R. B. Rutherford (Ed.), *Vascular surgery* (5th ed., pp. 2123–2142). Philadelphia, PA: W.B. Saunders.

mellitus; malignancy; rheumatologic or dermatologic disorders; nutritional deficits; past surgeries (especially abdominal or pelvic)

c. Medication history and all current therapeutic drugs
d. Social or functional history: tobacco and alcohol use, habits, physical fitness level or exercise capacity, occupation and possible exposure to carcinogens, self-care, and home management
e. Systems review to exclude other conditions contributing to extremity swelling: especially heart failure, chronic respiratory conditions, venous disease

3. Differential diagnosis (see Table 23-1)
   a. Extrinsic compression of circulatory system by mass or malignancy. For patients over 40 with new-onset lymphedema, malignancy should be excluded as 94% of upper extremity and 52% of lower extremity lymphedemas are secondary to cancer, with or without surgery or radiation therapy (Felty & Rooke, 2004).
4. Subjective findings (see Fig. 23-2)
   a. Primary and secondary lymphedema often is similar in appearance.
   b. Diagnosis is usually made on basis of history and physical examination without use of confirmatory tests, except as needed to exclude other conditions, such as venous thrombosis or heart failure.
      1) Special imaging techniques using magnetic resonance lymphangiography may have some benefit (refer also to section V, C2- noninvasive tests) (Lu, Xu, & Liu, 2010).
   c. Visible and measurable swelling of part or entire length of limb: pathognomonic shape of limb caused by distribution of edema.
      1) Bilateral limb measurements every 4 cm for entire length of extremity
      2) Typical changes include concentric edema with loss of normal contour (limb looks straight and pole-like), sparing at ankle or wrist joint, significant hindfoot edema compared to forefoot with "buffalo hump" appearance, toes are tense with sausage shape or "squared"

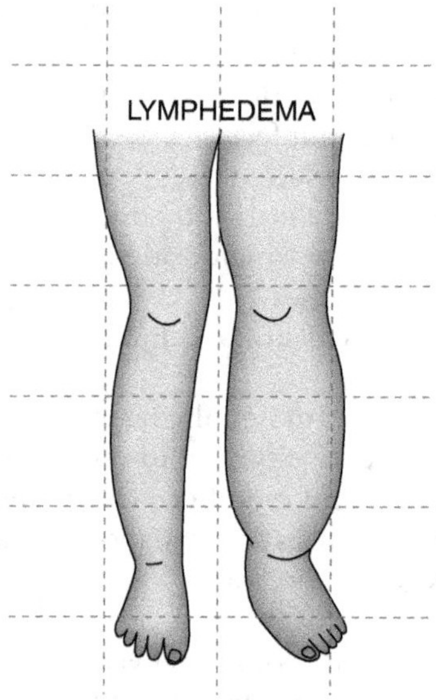

FIGURE 23-2. Lymphedema.

3) Stemmer sign: inability to pick up skin on toes
4) Fluid distribution in lymphedema differs from venous insufficiency or other causes of dependent edema, which have more fluid collection in foot and ankle with gradual decrease proximally

d. Pitting or nonpitting edema depending on stage of disease
e. Classification for edema (see Table 23-2)

C. Physical Examination

1. Inspection
   a. Skin: in early stage of lymphedema, skin is often slightly warm with pinkish-red color caused by increased vascularity; may be difficult to distinguish from early skin infection
      1) In later stages, skin thickens, has hyperkeratosis with lichenification, peau d'orange changes
      2) Verrucae or small vesicles that may drain clear lymph fluid (lymphorrhea) develop over time and indicate longstanding disease, usually with hyperplasia and lymphatic valvular incompetence
      3) If drainage is milky (chylorrhea), suspect lymphangiectasia and reflux of chyle
      4) Primary lymphedema patients often have yellow nails; may be associated with pleural effusion (yellow nail syndrome)

TABLE 23-2 Edema is Not Detectable Until Interstitial Volume Exceeds 30% Above Normal

1+	Edema barely detectable
2+	Slight indentation remains following skin depression
3+	Deeper fingerprint returns to normal in 5–30 sec
4+	Extremity may be 1.5–2 times normal size

Adapted from Kelly, D. G. (2002). *A primer on lymphedema*. Upper Saddle River, NJ: Prentice Hall/Pearson Education.

5) Severe clubbing, transverse ridging, friability of nails, and decreased rate of nail growth
6) Tinea pedis and tinea corporis often present and may be site of recurrent skin infections: assess for cracks, fissures between toes and on plantar surface of feet; look under skin folds for bright red skin with confluent rash and odor
7) Chronic dry eczematous dermatitis or excoriations common on lower extremities
8) Assess for evidence of cellulitis or lymphangitis (refer to Subjective Findings)
9) Ulcers rare until lymphedema is advanced; skin maintains higher degree of elasticity than in venous conditions

b. Joint integrity and mobility, posture and gait, use of supportive devices
c. Neurologic examination: balance, mentation, cognition, sensory and reflex integrity; pain scale

2. Palpation
   a. Pulses difficult to assess in affected limb because of degree of swelling: auscultate with hand-held Doppler to assess patency of arterial system
   b. Skin: assess turgor, texture, pitting versus nonpitting edema, warmth, papillomas, or bullae
      1) Stemmer skin fold test: thickened skin folds at base of second toe or second finger are resistant to lifting, a positive Stemmer sign. A negative skin fold test does not exclude lymphedema.
   c. Lymph nodes: cervical, axillary, inguinal
   d. Abdomen: masses or organomegaly
   e. Any areas suspicious for tumor involvement (e.g., neck or chest wall in patient with history of or suspicion for breast cancer)
   f. Musculoskeletal examination: joint swelling, crepitus with mobility
3. Percussion
   a. Chest: areas of dullness that may suggest pleural effusion or consolidation
   b. Abdomen: organomegaly
4. Auscultation
   a. Heart sounds for evidence of murmur, rub, gallop
   b. Chest: assess for adequate air exchange, presence of rales, or congestion
   c. Doppler evaluation of pulses in affected limb; may require ankle–brachial index to determine adequacy of arterial circulation

D. Considerations Across the Life Span

1. Pediatric and young adult patients
   a. Congenital primary lymphedema may be present at birth
      1) Rare, 11% of primary cases (Feins, 1997)
      2) Usually affects multiple extremities and has poorest prognosis because of decreased number of functioning lymphatics (Feins, 1997)
      3) Parents or caregivers provide daily compression therapy, encouraging children to participate as soon as possible around age 3 to 4 to prevent decreased activity level, social isolation, and poor self-esteem
   b. Lymphedema praecox
      1) Most common primary lymphedema

2) 85% present before age 35 with onset usually at or near puberty through early twenties; begins concurrently with growth spurt as decreased number of functioning lymphatics are overwhelmed by increased hydrostatic pressure
3) 15% present after age 35; lymphedema tarda
4) Since young patients are usually very active, assess for inciting incident (e.g., sports injury or trauma)

c. Psychosocial assessment: significant physical and psychosocial impact on patient's life because of impairment of mobility, heavy unsightly limbs, and need for daily compression therapy; assess for activities, history of depression, coping mechanisms
d. Surgery may be indicated if conservative measures fail (refer to Section VIII)

2. Women of childbearing age
   a. Pregnancy not contraindicated but will likely exacerbate condition because of increased systemic fluid volume and uterine extrinsic compression on lower extremity vessels
      1) Consistent compression therapy throughout pregnancy with increased periods of leg elevation
      2) Increased strength of waist-length compression garment; minimum of 30 to 40 mm Hg
      3) Low-salt diet
   b. Because of increased risk of thromboembolism (stasis, immobility in advanced lymphedema), caution advised regarding use of oral contraceptives
3. Elderly
   a. When lymphedema suddenly develops in patient over 60, accurate diagnosis should be obtained rapidly to evaluate for cardiac, liver, renal, metastatic disease, or mechanical obstruction.
   b. Management of lymphedema with traditional compression therapies may be hindered by other co-morbidities.
      1) Congestive heart failure: if uncompensated, distal compression is absolutely contraindicated; if compensated, diligent monitoring for signs of exacerbation warranted
      2) Osteoarthritis: limits range of motion and dexterity; patient may need assistance for home therapies, application of compression garments, and skin inspection
      3) Obesity: increases risk of skin infection because of increased flora (especially Candida) in skin folds and limitations in bathing and inspecting skin
      4) Diabetes mellitus: extra diligence regarding foot care and monitoring for skin infections, especially if patient is neuropathic
   c. Decreased responsiveness of immune system predisposes to increased frequency of skin infections and lack of usual signs (e.g., fever). May present with confusion or mental status change
   d. If lymphedema has been present for many years, skin will be extremely hypertrophic (woody), often with crevices, bullae; may require whirlpool or manual debridement
      1) Other skin conditions, such as psoriasis, pose additional challenges in the elderly (Kaya, Akbayrak, Bakar, & Topuz, 2010)
   e. Increased risk of lymphangiosarcoma after longstanding secondary lymphedema (Gloviczki & Wahner, 2000)

V. Pertinent Diagnostic Testing

A. Goals of Diagnostic Evaluation

1. Establish diagnosis
2. Assess lymphatic function
3. Document objectively the severity of the condition (Rockson, 2003)

B. Laboratory Tests: generally not required to establish diagnosis in moderate to severe lymphedema, which is based on characteristic appearance of limb and history. Reasonable tests to exclude other conditions, evaluate for signs of infection or impact of lymphedema management on other existing co-morbidities include:

1. Complete blood count
2. Renal and liver profile
3. Glucose
4. Thyroid studies: TSH, total T3 and T4
5. Electrocardiogram and chest x-ray
6. X-ray of affected limb may be warranted

C. Noninvasive Tests

1. Venous duplex ultrasound to rule out venous obstruction
2. Lymphoscintigraphy
   a. Technique: radioactive colloid (e.g., technetium Tc 99 m human serum albumin) injected into web space of foot or hand. Patient often experiences very intense stinging sensation lasting approximately 10 seconds. Patient instructed to exercise limb with either foot ergometer or squeeze ball for 5 minutes initially and then 1 minute out of every 5 minutes for 1 hour. Images of lymphatic system obtained with gamma camera and computer to assess rate of lymph flow and lymph node uptake speeds. Images obtained at intervals of 30 minutes, 1, 3, and 6 hours (Felty & Rooke, 2004)
   b. Interpretation
      1) Evidence of proper injection: if tracer present in liver prior to 1 hour, suspect intravenous (rather than subcutaneous) injection
      2) Appearance time of activity in regional lymph nodes after tracer injection: normal transit time is 15 to 60 minutes to groin or axilla from injection site
      3) Absence, presence, and pattern of lymph channels in limb; number, size, and symmetry of regional lymph nodes in groin or axilla
      4) Pattern of nodes and channels in pelvis and abdomen and liver activity
   c. Results
      1) Normal: visible ascending tracer, bilateral symmetry, tracer visible at regional nodes within 1 hour and in liver within 3 hours
      2) Abnormal: slow or no removal of tracer from injection site, presence of collaterals or dermal back-flow, reduced or absent uptake in regional nodes, or abnormal tracer accumulation suggesting extravasation, lymphocele, or lymphangiectasia
      3) Unable to distinguish between primary and secondary etiology with this test but can determine aplasia, hyperplasia, or hypoplasia in primary lymphedema states (Gloviczki & Wahner, 2000)

   d. No reported morbidity with this procedure; considered reliable and safe alternative to invasive testing (Kelly, 2002; Schirger & Gloviczki, 1996)
3. Computed tomography (CT scan): refer to Chapter 5, Vascular Diagnostic Studies, for test description and patient preparation
   a. Greatest value is to exclude obstructing mass in secondary lymphedema
   b. May also demonstrate honeycomb appearance of subcutaneous tissue, caused by either lymphatic channels or free fluid accumulating in tissue spaces, but test cannot determine cause of swelling
4. Magnetic resonance imaging (MRI) (Lohrmann, Foeldi, & Langer, 2011; Lu et al., 2010)
   a. Useful for identification of congenital vascular malformations and soft tissue tumors
   b. For patient with swollen limb, useful in differentiating insufficiency; lipedema (excess subcutaneous fat); and lymphedema (honeycomb appearance in subcutaneous layer)
   c. Complements findings on lymphoscintigram: delineates nodal anatomy, larger lymphatic trunks, soft tissue changes, and nodes or channels proximal to site of lymphatic obstruction
   d. Supermagnetic agents (iron oxide) show promise in improving imaging of lymphatic anatomy (Gloviczki & Wahner, 2000)
5. Abdominal or pelvic ultrasound: evaluate for extrinsic compression from mass or tumor

D. Invasive Tests: lymphangiography

1. Developed by Servelle in 1943; considered "gold standard" for imaging lymphatics
2. Technique: Area to be cannulated is locally anesthetized with 1% lidocaine; small incision made on dorsum of foot or hand after 1 mL of isosulfan blue dye has been injected subcutaneously to identify lymphatics; lymph vessel is dissected under magnification and 30-gauge needle inserted into vessel for constant infusion of lipid-soluble contrast material at rate of 1 mL in 8 minutes for maximum amount of 7 mL per limb; serial films are taken of limb, proximal regional nodes, pelvis, abdomen, chest, and lumbars. Additional films are taken several hours later. Contrast may remain in lymph channels for several months.
3. Interpretation
   a. Normal: dye fills superficial medial lymphatics and most of regional nodes (5 to 15 in thigh) with visualized valves every 5 to 10 mm; lateral and deep lymphatics not seen in normal patients; nodes have ground-glass appearance; proximal lymphatics (iliacs) fill within 30 to 45 minutes; thoracic duct fills several hours later
   b. Abnormal: visualization of deep lymphatics suggests obstruction of superficial channels (these are paired and follow main blood vessels); in primary lymphedema, distal obliteration more common than proximal or pelvic lymphatic obstruction; backflow of contrast into dilated skin lymphatics seen
   c. Longstanding lymphedema: fibrotic changes of dilated distal lymphatics seen in both primary and secondary lymphedema
   d. Lymphangiectasia: dilated, incompetent lymphatics require extra contrast to fill vessels; decreased number of pelvic nodes; contrast

may reflux into mesenteric lymphatics; thoracic duct may be absent, occluded, or dilated and tortuous (Gloviczki & Wahner, 2000)

4. Complications
   a. Lengthy and uncomfortable
   b. Obstructive lymphangitis and progression of lymphedema has been reported (Felty & Rooke, 2004; Gloviczki & Wahner, 2000)
   c. Pulmonary embolism from oily contrast via spontaneous lympho-venous anastomosis
   d. Use of ethiodized oil contraindicated if patient has iodine allergy
   e. Long-term staining of extremity
   f. Cellulitis or local infection at procedure site
5. Indications
   a. Rarely used for diagnosis of lymphedema
   b. Beneficial if patient is candidate for microvascular lymphatic reconstruction
   c. Preoperative evaluation of patient with lymphangiectasia and chylous reflux
   d. Best test to use for evaluation of thoracic duct and identification of pelvic, abdominal, and thoracic lymphatic fistulae

E. Special Procedures

1. Fluorescent microlymphography (Kelly, 2002)
   a. Subepidermal injection near medial malleolus of fluorescent tracer
   b. Fluorescent microscope and video camera record diffusion of fluorescent substance
   c. Superficial cutaneous lymph capillaries and lymph system functions can be imaged and observed
2. Volumetric or circumferential measurements of limb
   a. Circumferential measurements every 4 cm of both extremities for comparison
   b. Computerized programs available for calculation of limb volumes, or may use water displacement to assess volumetric differences between extremities (limb is submerged in water tank and volume of water displaced is measured)
   c. Tonometry: tension-measuring device that presses on the skin; the greater the tension, the less compliant the skin, suggesting fibrotic changes; helpful in assessing subclinical changes of skin prior to limb volume increase

VI. Medical and Nonoperative Management

A. No Known Cure or Ability to Restore Normal Lymphatic Flow

B. Therapeutic Goals

1. Reduce affected limbs to near-normal size
2. Maintain normal skin tone
3. Maintain normal limb function
4. Prevent complications, especially recurrent infection
5. Educate patient and family in self-care of this chronic condition

C. All nonoperative therapies use limb elevation, compression therapy or garments, and skin care (Foeldi, 2012).

1. Limb elevation and bed rest:
   a. 45 degrees or above level of heart using foam wedge or sling while recumbent; caution regarding lightheadedness upon arising
   b. Recommended: 20 minutes 2 to 3 times per day for outpatients
   c. Inpatient or home bedrest for exacerbations: limb volume significantly reduces with several days of bedrest and elevation except in advanced cases
2. Compression therapy: increases venous and lymphatic flow; prevents reaccumulation of fluid
   a. Nonelastic compression bandaging
      1) Multiple layers of nonstretch or short-stretch wraps applied to limb; only stretch 70% or less of length of bandage, providing more resistance to fluid accumulation and thus decreasing limb size
      2) Gradient compression wrap technique: highest pressure at distal portion with gradual taper
      3) Additional foam padding applied over bony prominences or areas of fibrosis to further soften tissue
   b. Elastic compression garments: selected according to stage of lymphedema; worn during day after limb is maximally reduced by other therapeutic interventions
      1) Stage I: class I, 20 mm Hg pressure for arm; class II, 30 to 40 mm Hg for leg
      2) Stage II: class II or class III, 40 to 50 mm Hg
      3) Stage III: custom-made class III
   c. Other nonelastic compression devices
      1) Useful for patients who cannot apply elastic garments or compression bandages, or as adjunctive therapy
      2) Circ-Aid (Shaw Therapeutics, NJ): series of Velcro interlocking straps applied sequentially up limb; may be used alone or in combination with elastic garment for additional support (Lawrence, 2008)
      3) Reid Sleeve: multiple air cell chambers in sleeve; secured to limb with wide Velcro straps; often used as replacement for bandages if patient unable to wrap limb independently
   d. Pneumatic compression pump: single or multi-chambered sleeve with intermittent inflation of compartments to mobilize fluid from distal to proximal portion of limb (see Fig. 23-3)
      1) Pump pressure adjusted to just above venous and below arterial mean pressures: 30–40 mm Hg
      2) Outpatient treatment time usually 1 hour twice or three times daily with limb elevated
      3) May be used intensively during in-patient care for 3 to 4 hours of treatment time with careful monitoring of skin, hemodynamics, and cardiac status
      4) Compression wraps or garments used between pump sessions
      5) Useful for patients who cannot participate in bandaging or massage therapy or travel to treatment center
      6) Recommended compression pump features: sequential gradient pressure (multiple chambers with highest pressure at end of limb);

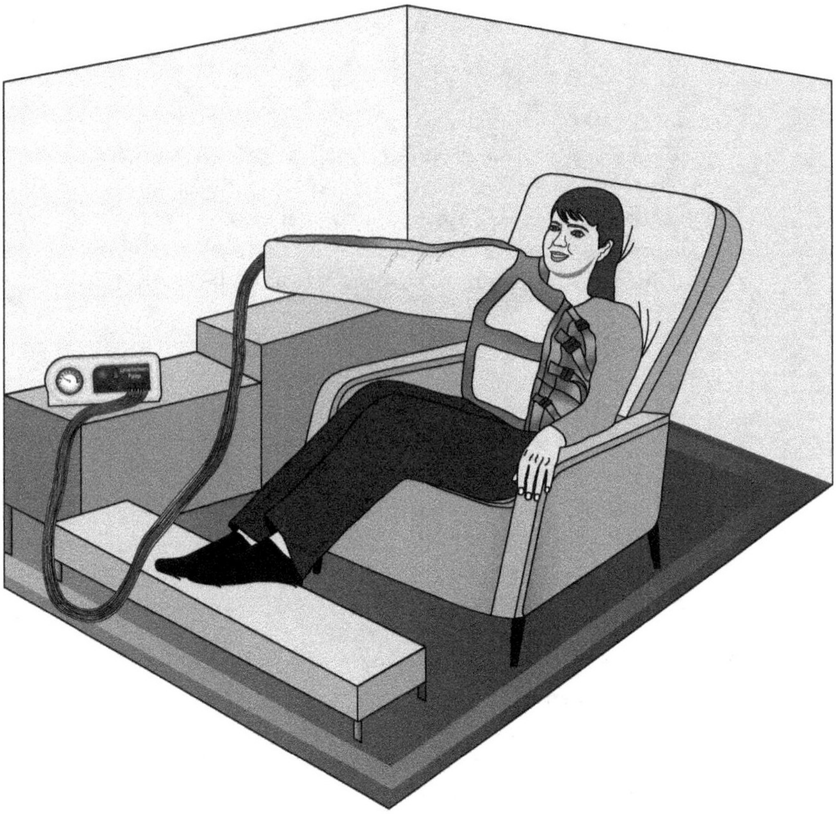

FIGURE 23-3. Lymphedema pump

adjustable pressure setting that allow for a rest cycle for vessel refilling; short rest and compression cycles (on for 30 seconds, rest for 5 seconds)

7) Pump cannot move fluid beyond root of limb: need to assess for fluid collection in trunk, pelvis, abdomen, chest, or neck
8) Precautions: initial training by experienced therapist required; immediately discontinue if patient experiences dyspnea, chest pain, or skin breakdown or neurologic changes of limb during session; skin changes at root of limb indicate formation of ring of fibrosis caused by inability of lymph fluid to exit limb
9) Contraindications: uncompensated heart failure, active skin infection, thrombophlebitis or DVT, pelvic surgery with swelling of groin or abdomen, arterial occlusive disease
10) A newly designed sequential pneumatic pump utilizing high pressure has been trialed on a small number of patients with mean reduction of 75% but this has not been replicated (Modaghegh & Soltani, 2010)

3. Skin care
   a. Daily cleansing with pH balanced, nondrying soap
   b. Careful inspection for evidence of infection or breakdown
   c. Liberal use of lanolin skin lubricants; should not contain alcohol or perfumes
   d. Podiatric care

e. Use of antifungal creams or powders to prevent and treat tinea pedis
f. Aggressive treatment of any wounds; immediate cleansing, topical antibiotic ointment, extra compression over site, close monitoring for signs of infection

D. Manual Lymph Drainage (MLD) (Foeldi, 2012)

1. Developed by Dr. Emil Vodder in 1930s as method of manually moving lymph fluid from one body part to another (Felty & Rooke, 2004).
2. Certified therapist uses light touch (as opposed to deep muscular massage) to move fluid gently through area of obstruction into other channels.
3. Body is divided into lymphatic regions, which are "cleared" or opened prior to limb massage in order to stimulate proximal flow and prepare central channels to receive distal flow. Flow is constantly directed toward main thoracic duct (terminus).
4. MLD causes lymphatic dilation and increasing contractility.
5. Special attention may be given to areas of fibrosis to soften tissue.
6. Minimum of 1 hour treatment daily for 2 to 4 weeks; some centers require twice daily treatments.
7. Limb is bandaged between massage sessions.
8. Patient or family is instructed in self-massage technique for lifetime home therapy.
9. Contraindications: treatment is postponed until these conditions are controlled or resolved.
   a. Neck treatment: cardiac arrhythmia, hyperthyroidism, hypothyroidism, hypersensitivity of carotid sinus
   b. Abdominal treatment: pregnancy, recent abdominal surgery, abdominal complication after radiation therapy, Crohn disease, diverticulitis, aortic aneurysm, undiagnosed abdominal pain
   c. Lower extremity: DVT or phlebitis, at discretion of medical provider; may begin therapy within weeks to months after episode

E. Complex Decongestive Therapy (CDT) (see Fig. 23-4)

1. Combination of MLD, compression bandaging of limb, exercises done while bandaged, and skin care
2. Two-phase program
   a. Intensive phase: 2 to 4 weeks of daily or twice daily lymphatic massage, compressive bandaging 24 hrs/day except during bathing or skin care, exercise in bandages, skin care with instruction in self-bandaging and limb elevation
   b. Maintenance phase: life-long self care with bandage application at night, compression garment during day, self-massage, exercise, and skin care
3. Exercises performed while bandaged to propel lymph flow toward central circulation with aid of muscle contraction
4. Swimming (aqua therapy) may be added as a low-resistance activity that promotes lymph flow through muscle contraction combined with water pressure in pool (Shimony & Tidhar, 2008)
5. Response to treatment
   a. Ideally, 40% to 70% limb size reduction toward normal

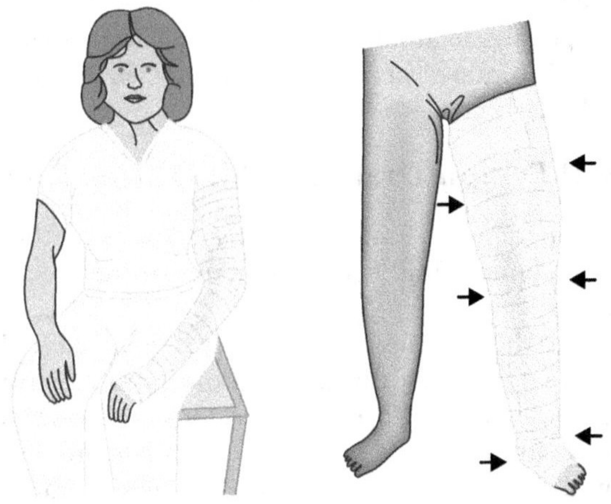

FIGURE 23-4. Upper extremity and lower extremity wrapping for decongestion of lymphedema.

b. Limb considered maximally reduced when there has been no change in limb volume or size with two consecutive measurements or treatments (Felty & Rooke, 2004)
c. Results highly variable. Observational studies show reduction in limb volumes ranging from 33% to 68% (Carmelli & Bartoletti, 2011; Mohler & Mondry, 2013)
d. Requires high level of motivation and commitment by patient and family
e. Periodic follow-up care by medical provider and lymphedema therapist required

F. Diet

1. Weight control
   a. Maintenance of ideal body weight improves lymphedema management.
      1) Excess adipose tissue promotes fluid retention.
      2) Obesity limits mobility, impairs venous return, and promotes bacterial or fungal skin infection.
   b. Maintenance of ideal body weight improves management of co-morbidities, especially diabetes mellitus, coronary artery disease, pulmonary conditions, arthritis, and congestive heart failure.
2. Low-fat, low-salt diet recommended with calorie intake appropriate for age and activity level.
3. No specific dietary supplements (e.g., grape seed extract or bioflavonoids) have been shown in clinical trials to be beneficial for lymphedema management; often marketed without benefit of government regulation for safety and purity.

G. Medications

1. No medications have been developed specifically for lymphatic fluid reduction.
2. Diuretics are not recommended for long-term therapy unless other medical conditions (e.g., hypertension, heart failure) warrant use.
   a. Do not remove excess protein in interstitial space; therefore, lymph fluid in subcutaneous tissue remains unaffected.

b. Hemoconcentration may be serious side-effect (Gamble et al., 2000)
c. May be useful in the following situations:
    1) Early lymphedema when edema is still pitting
    2) Women whose lymphedema worsens around time of menses
    3) Patients in terminal stages of malignancy

3. Benzopyrones: flavonoids and coumarin (not to be confused with Coumadin)
    a. Used for over 20 years in Europe and Australia as adjunctive therapy to compression; thought to promote protein breakdown.
    b. Patient needs to take drug for at least 6 months before benefit noted and remain on drug indefinitely.
    c. US clinical trials have shown no benefit over placebo; pulled off market by Food and Drug Administration (FDA) because of liver toxicity.
    d. Newer agent, purified, micronized flavonoids fraction (PMFF), does not have hepatotoxicity and shows promise in increasing lymphatic transport; further investigation is needed (Gamble et al., 2000).
4. Antibiotic therapy
    a. Essential for treatment of complications of cellulitis, lymphangitis.
    b. Agents needed to cover common skin organisms: group A streptococcus most common; staphylococcus, penicillin, 250 to 500 mg four times daily, or cephalexin, 500 mg three to four times daily, for minimum of 10 days.
    c. Patients with recurrent infections need to initiate antibiotic at first sign of illness; keep them at home.
    d. Suppressive antibiotic therapy regimens
        1) Used for more than 4 to 6 episodes per year
        2) Example: 1 week of antibiotic out of the month, or continuous low-dose daily therapy for refractory cases
        3) If patient still has break-through infection episode, switch to a different antibiotic; alternate between two or three agents to avoid development of antibiotic resistance
        4) Always look for source (cracks in skin, fungal infection of nails)
5. Antifungal agents: topical creams recommended for tinea pedis, tinea corporis; use in interdigital space and under skin folds to control fungal and yeast infections as these are common sites for secondary bacterial infections.
6. Filariasis infections
    a. Diethylcarbamazine (DEC) or ivermectin initiated at time infection discovered.
    b. Population-wide treatment using combination therapy of DEC plus ivermectin or albendazole (a newer antihelminthic agent) have been advocated (Gamble et al., 2000).
    c. Other public health measures also effective and important to control spread of disease: control of mosquito breeding, use of protective clothing, prophylactic antifilarial medications.

H. Other Treatment Considerations

1. Psychological impact (Finnane, Hayes, Obermair, & Janda, 2011; Kim, 2011)
    a. Primary: younger patients feel ugly, unaccepted, self-conscious, angry, afraid, unlucky, frustrated regarding lack of cure or cause

b. Secondary: if result of cancer therapy, often feel overwhelmed by prospects of lifetime of disfigurement after having undergone rigors of cancer treatment; serves as constant reminder of cancer; psychosocial maladjustment persists despite lymphedema intervention (Woods, Tobin, & Mortimer, 1995)
c. Increased sense of loss: self-esteem, friends, favorite activities, jobs or financial stability, sexual desire or image
d. Increased anxiety: infection and complications, ability to perform routine activities, budget or financial concerns, insurance reimbursement, recurrence of cancer
e. Assess and treat for situational depression or anxiety

2. Functional impact
   a. Limitations of mobility or sports participation because of increased heaviness, aching, or pain.
   b. Job opportunities limited: prolonged sitting or standing contraindicated; must be able to change positions, elevate limb when able, avoid heavy lifting and excess heat; may need to change occupations after diagnosis.
   c. Lost time from work because of complications, especially infection.
   d. Include physical and occupational therapists in assessment and intervention planning.

I. **Evidence** is beginning to support weight bearing/lifting exercise or resistance training as safe and beneficial, especially in regards to improvement of cardiovascular fitness and quality of life (Katz et al., 2010; Kunkel, 2010; Mohler & Mondry, 2013).

VII. Surgical Management

A. Fewer than 10% of Patients are Candidates for Surgical Interventions (Felty & Rooke, 2004).

1. Performed when traditional medical therapeutic measures fail and patient develops progressive disability.
2. Patients with recurrent lymphangitis (with or without sepsis) may also benefit.
3. No procedure offers a cure; results are palliative and may not be cosmetically appealing.

B. Goals of Surgery

1. Reduce extremity size
2. Improve limb function
3. Decrease frequency of infections

C. Types of Procedures

1. Reduction or excisional procedures: removal of excess tissue to decrease limb volume
2. Lymphatic reconstructions to improve flow, drainage

D. Reduction Procedures

1. Homans procedure: resection of portion of edematous skin and subcutaneous tissue
   a. Staged excision beneath skin flaps
   b. While some long-term studies show lasting improvement, other case studies show only modest improvement or even regression to preoperative limb size (Heffel & Miller, 2000; Mohler & Mondry, 2013).
   c. Poor postoperative results when used for arm lymphedema (Heffel & Miller, 2000).
2. Charles procedure: complete excision of skin, subcutaneous tissue, and fascia; remaining muscle layer covered with split-thickness skin graft taken from donor site
3. Thompson procedure: buried dermis flap
   a. Portion of lymphedematous subcutaneous tissue is resected beneath skin flaps; flap edge is de-epithelialized then buried in underlying muscle compartment.
   b. Buried dermis permits formation of lymphatic connections between subdermal lymphatics of the flap and deep lymphatics of the muscle compartment.
   c. Muscle contractions promote lymphatic flow.
   d. Buried flap acts as barrier to regeneration of deep fascia.
4. Techniques for various procedures are not standardized; results are surgeon dependent.

E. Lymphatic Reconstructions

1. Direct lymphatic reconstructions
   a. Lymphovenous anastomoses
      1) Direct end-to-end anastomosis of femoral lymph node to tributary of femoral vein using microsurgical technique
      2) Indicated for patients with early secondary lymphedema with no previous cellulitis or lymphangitis and no significant tissue fibrosis
      3) Preoperative lymphoscintigraphy required to confirm presence of proximal lymphatic obstruction and identify flow patterns
      4) High occlusion rate at 4 weeks
   b. Lymphatic grafting
      1) Lymphatic-to-lymphatic (lympholymphatic) anastomosis
      2) Patency rates documented beyond 3 years (lymph does not have platelets to promote clotting) (Gloviczki & Noel, 2000)
      3) Suitable for arm or leg
   c. Lymphatic microsurgery
      1) Limited experience with this technique
      2) Minimal limb size reduction of 5% at 2 months and 2% at 1 year (Mohler & Mondry, 2013)
2. Indirect lymphatic reconstructions: based on ability of lymphatic system to form spontaneous lymphatic anastomoses to improve collateral drainage to regions of normal flow
   a. Omental flap
      1) Omentum sewn over area of obstructed lymph tissue
      2) Poor long-term results; multiple complications including bowel obstruction, pulmonary embolism, wound infection

b. Mesenteric bridge
    1) Indications: patients with fibrotic occlusion or surgical excision of iliac nodes
    2) Technique: segment of ileum is opened, mucosa removed, bowel wall sewn over transected inguinal lymph nodes; end-to-end ileostomy restores continuity of small bowel
    3) Limited studies show long-term patency with limb size improvement lasting over 5 years (Gloviczki & Noel, 2000)
c. Autotransplantation of lymphatic tissue as a free flap
    1) Used in postmastectomy lymphedema
    2) Transplantation of free axillary lymph node flap from contralateral axillary fossa to affected arm; anastomoses created with subclavian artery and vein
    3) Limited series of patients showed 75% improvement both clinically and by lymphoscintigraphy; more experience needed to assess efficacy (Gloviczki & Noel, 2000)

3. No proof of long-term effectiveness for any of these procedures; use of these procedures remains controversial (Gloviczki & Noel, 2000)

F. **Liposuction:** removal of fatty tissue with mechanical suction technique; highly controversial because of unknown effects on lymphatic drainage and disturbance of microcirculation

G. Operations for Chylous Disorders

1. Surgical interventions for treatment of abnormal accumulation of chyle in various body parts: chylous ascites, chylothorax, or chylocutaneous fistula
    a. Secondary causes: malignant tumors (lymphoma), trauma to mesenteric lymphatic or thoracic duct (during vascular surgical procedures)
    b. Primary chylous disorders: congenital lymphangiectasia or megalymphatics with or without obstruction of thoracic duct
        1) Reflux of chyle into extremities, mesentery, perineum, or genitals
        2) May also have protein-losing enteropathy, chylopericardium, reflux of chyle into lungs and bronchi
        3) Medical treatment: medium-chain triglycerides diet, parenteral nutrition, replacement of lost proteins and calcium
2. Only surgical intervention offers long-term improvement
3. Procedure: ligation of incompetent retroperitoneal lymph vessels with oversewing of lymphatic leak

H. **Low Level Laser Therapy:** limited experience with low level laser therapy shows some promise for treatment of lymphedema praecox (Mahram & Rajabi, 2011)

I. Future Therapies

1. Mouse model research with VEGFR-3 mutation, similar to congenital hereditary primary lymphedema (Milroy disease)
2. Virus mediated therapy with gene for VEGF-C (activates VEGFR-3) led to generation of functional lymphatic vessels (Karkkainen et al., 2001)

VIII. Nursing Management

A. Fluid Volume Excess Related to Underlying Disease Process

1. Assess for defining characteristics as previously described
   a. Increased limb swelling with loss of bony anatomical landmarks as noted by circumferential measurements taken every 4 cm
   b. Skin changes: fibrosis; signs of infection
2. Expected patient outcomes: optimal decrease in edema
3. Interventions
   a. Elevate extremity above level of heart while supine
   b. Use of foam wedge at foot of bed
   c. Administer diuretics as prescribed for early onset lymphedema
   d. Instruct patient regarding correct application of compression wraps or garments (see Fig. 23-5)
   e. Collaborate with certified lymph therapist to instruct patient regarding correct use of intermittent pneumatic compression pump or MLD massage and potential complications (Langbecker, Hayes, Newman, & Janda, 2008)
   f. For patient undergoing corrective lymphedema surgery, maintain bedrest for 24 to 48 hours preoperatively and as directed by surgeon postoperatively (up to 10 to 14 days) with DVT prophylaxis instituted per protocol
4. Evaluation
   a. Edema is decreased
   b. Patient can apply compression wraps or stockings and demonstrates consistent use
   c. Patient uses compression pump therapy or MLD massage consistently and correctly

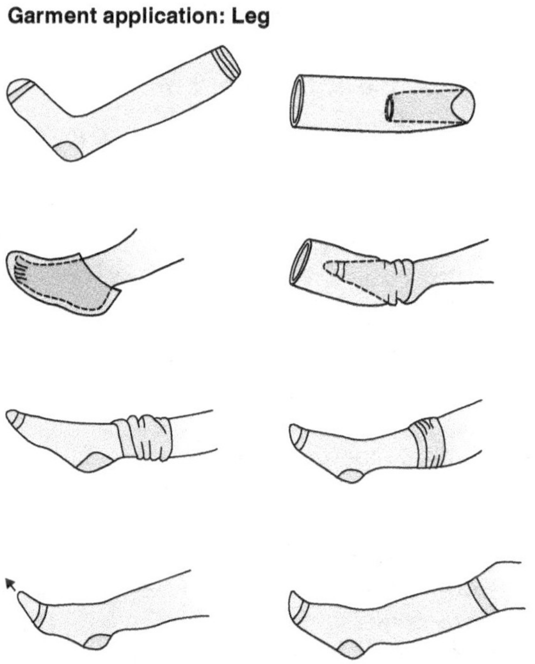

FIGURE 23-5. Application of a compression garment.

B. Potential for Infection Related to Increased Susceptibility Secondary to Interruption of Skin

1. Assessment for defining characteristics
   a. Break or lesion in skin
   b. Increased swelling or edema
   c. Red, erythematous, or inflamed skin, with or without rash or streaking
   d. Skin is tender with light touch
   e. History of prior cellulitis or lymphangitis
2. Expected outcome: absence of infection
3. Nursing interventions
   a. Assess skin per unit standard of care (suggest at least every shift for in-patient) or as condition indicates.
   b. Assess for redness, warmth, tenderness, and fever.
   c. Provide meticulous skin care with pH balanced soap and alcohol-free lubricants; provide special attention to interdigital areas on feet.
   d. Emphasize importance of properly fitting clothing and shoes to prevent trauma, excess tightness from bands.
   e. Avoid using nonprescribed or nonrecommended topical ointments or creams, especially homemade products.
   f. Administer antibiotics as ordered.
   g. Treat fungal infections promptly.
   h. For patient undergoing procedure, identify "at-risk" limb with patient identification bracelet, or sign above bed.
   i. For patient undergoing corrective lymphedema surgery, maintain meticulous skin and wound care pre- and postoperatively.
4. Evaluation of nursing care
   a. Skin infections and lesions are treated promptly.
   b. Secondary complications (i.e., sepsis) are avoided.
   c. Patient describes measures to prevent infection.
   d. Patient demonstrates care of skin.

C. Potential Body Image Disturbance Related to Changes in Body Appearance

1. Assessment
   a. Comments and feelings about appearance expressed
   b. Perception of effect on lifestyle
2. Expected outcome: communication of changes in body appearance and demonstration of coping skills
3. Nursing intervention
   a. Provide emotional support to patient.
   b. Encourage verbalization of feelings about appearance and perceptions.
   c. Validate perceptions as appropriate.
   d. Discuss and suggest means of coping with changes.
      1) Creative methods of adapting clothing to fit edematous limb
      2) Alter shoes to fit
      3) Promote active lifestyle within patient's capacity
      4) Encourage daily exercise, both of affected limb and aerobics
4. Evaluation of nursing care
   a. Open communication of feelings and perceptions
   b. Implementation of adaptive response to lymphedema

IX. Patient Teaching

A. Disease Prevention

1. Measures to reduce edema and prevent exacerbations
   a. Regular and correct use of compression therapy, lymphedema exercises in wraps, and MLD or pumps as previously described
   b. Use of elastic compression garments as prescribed, worn during waking hours and removed at night. Skin inspection and care before and after application; may apply nonelastic, short-stretch bandages or alternative wraps (e.g., Reid sleeve) for nighttime use
   c. Elevate limb above heart for 20 minutes two to three times daily
   d. Avoidance of heat: sun exposure or sunburn, hot showers, sauna or hot tubs; use oven mitts, protective clothing; sun screen, air conditioning, fans or cool towels in summer
   e. Avoidance of overuse of limb: heavy or repetitive lifting or work against resistance (e.g., shoveling snow, pushing vacuum over thick carpet, throwing hay bails or wood); avoid heavy handbags (carry on unaffected arm); balance heavy objects on unaffected side
   f. Avoidance of tight clothing or jewelry; no blood pressure cuff on affected limb
   g. Avoid sports injuries and treat sprains immediately with ice to affected site 15 minutes four times daily for 48 hours; elevate, notify medical provider; additional physical therapy may lessen swelling
   h. For postmastectomy care, patient should wear supportive bra with no underwire; shoulder strap padding may be necessary; avoid heavy prosthesis
   i. Report any new swelling immediately
   j. Avoid prolonged immobility, especially while traveling; move limb through exercises and stretches every 1 to 2 hours
   k. Wear a Lymphedema Alert bracelet
2. Measures to prevent infection
   a. Keep limb as clean as possible; wash hands frequently, applying lotion after each washing to avoid over-drying of skin; dry thoroughly but gently.
   b. Avoid needle sticks or invasive procedures in high-risk limb.
   c. Check skin folds for signs of infection, rash; keep dry and apply anti-fungal powder as needed.
   d. Podiatric and nail care: soak feet for 10 minutes prior to cutting nails; avoid trimming too close and cutting cuticles; avoid astringents; inform manicurist of condition; inspect feet and treat all fungal infections promptly; use anti-fungal powders to prevent recurrent tinea.
   e. Wear clean socks or stockings; change shoes mid-day.
   f. Avoid trauma, burns, cuts, pet scratches, insect bites (apply repellent as needed); treat every break in the skin seriously and seek medical care if needed.
   g. Wear cotton-lined household rubber gloves for cleaning chores, especially washing dishes and bathroom; avoid skin exposure to strong chemicals.
   h. Wear canvas or leather gloves for outdoor work or gardening; avoid thorn injuries.
   i. Shave with electric razor; change blades frequently.

j. Wound care: wash with warm water and soap; apply antibacterial ointment and sterile dressing; inspect closely for signs of infection, especially cat scratch; monitor temperature.
k. For diabetics, maintain normal blood glucose as much as possible; do not use affected limb for glucose testing or insulin injections; use caution with compression bandages or garments because of increased potential for circulatory compromise and neuropathy.
l. For patients with history of recurrent skin infection, keep prescribed antibiotic available at all times, especially when traveling.

B. Health Promotion

1. Diet: drink 2 to 3 quarts of water daily; avoid salt, fatty foods, and alcohol; eat six or more servings of fruits and vegetables daily; high fiber foods encouraged; do not eliminate protein from diet.
2. Weight: maintain ideal body weight (body mass index between 19 and 24).
3. Exercise: regular daily exercise for minimum of 30 to 40 minutes encouraged; walking, swimming, biking, water aerobics recommended; include stretches and deep breathing with appropriate warm-up and cool-down times; strenuous exercise may increase swelling, consult therapist. Certain activities (e.g., golf, bowling, tennis) may be pursued with close monitoring of affected limb.
4. Avoid smoking to prevent burn injury, decreased circulation, adverse medical outcomes.
   a. Rest and sleep position: avoid sleeping on affected side; affected limb straight rather than flexed or curled; rest during day as needed as a heavy limb is tiring; plan minimum of 8 hours rest at night
   b. Regular medical examinations: annually and as needed to detect complications, institute appropriate therapy; partner with lymphedema therapist to plan care

C. Home Care Considerations

1. Patient motivation essential to successful management
2. Partner may be needed to implement home care, especially compression wraps or garment application
3. Treatment of suspected infection
   a. Call medical provider immediately; if not available, seek emergency care
   b. Institute early antibiotic therapy; depending on severity of symptoms, may require oral or intravenous therapy
   c. Remove all wraps, bandages, garments
   d. Do not use pneumatic compression pump or massage therapy until infection resolved
   e. Keep affected part elevated as much as possible
   f. Check temperature twice daily; notify provider if >102°F, patient develops chills, or worsening symptoms (e.g., vomiting)
   g. Drink 3 quarts of fluids daily
   h. Contact medical provider if not improved after 5 days of home antibiotic therapy
   i. Following infection, limb will be more edematous; additional therapy may be required for reduction; do not attempt to wear compression garments if too tight until limb reduced to previous size

j. For recurrent infection, contact medical provider for prophylactic antibiotic regimen

4. Travel considerations
   a. Air travel is associated with increased swelling because of changes in cabin pressure.
   b. Exercise every 1 to 2 hours; change positions, walk, stretch, move limbs.
   c. Wear compression garment, even if at-risk limb is edema-free.
   d. Drink extra water; avoid caffeine and alcohol to prevent dehydration.
   e. Carry low-salt, low-fat, nutritious food; avoid fast food meals.
   f. Arrange for extra leg room if needed.
   g. Carry antibiotics as prescribed if prone to recurrent infection.
   h. If traveling to hot, wet climate, carry insect repellent; be aware if there is increased risk of filariasis in country of destination (India, Malaysia, New Guinea, Africa, China, Brazil); take DEC within 30 days of exposure if needed.
5. Emotional support
   a. List problems and losses that result from chronic lymphedema condition (e.g., clothing, job, fun activities, financial concerns, self-esteem, friendships, sexual desire).
   b. Provide for appropriate grieving regarding losses.
   c. Seek support from family, friends, counselor, medical provider, support groups.
   d. Identify strengths and build achievable goals based on positive attributes.
   e. Keep home records of lymphedema plan and response to therapy to foster sense of self-care and authority.
   f. Participate in advocacy for lymphedema research, insurance coverage, congressional bills.

CASE STUDY

S.R., a 54-year-old male, is referred to the vascular surgery clinic with chief complaint of new onset of painless swelling of the entire left leg. He is no longer able to wear his usual shoe or socks. The limb is slightly more swollen in the later part of the day after work but does not significantly reduce after sleeping through the night with the leg elevated. Walking is not limited but he complains of heaviness and aching in the limb, especially with standing at his job as a butcher. He denies recent injury, episodes of DVT, wounds, or skin infections. Review of systems is negative for fevers or chills, recent loss of weight or appetite, exertional dyspnea or cough, chest pain or pressure, or any gastrointestinal complaints. His past medical history is significant for surgical treatment of prostate cancer followed by radiation therapy 2 years prior to this visit. He has chronic urinary incontinence and erectile dysfunction postoperatively.

Immediate examination includes the following:

Wt: 81 kg. Ht: 74 inches. BMI: 22.3
Integumentary: pink, dry, free of bruises or rash; skin on left leg is taut, shiny, bright pink but without warmth or redness and is intact
Lymphatics: No cervical, axillary or groin nodes
Cardiovascular: BP: 126/74; P: 66, regular. Normal cardiac examination. Brisk carotid upstroke with no bruits. Distal pulses of upper and lower extremities are 4+ except for nonpalpable

pulses on left popliteal, dorsalis pedis, and posterior tibial due to degree of swelling. Doppler examination reveals brisk, triphasic signals at all levels on left leg. Nonpitting edema of entire left leg with blunting of bony landmarks at digits, ankle, and knee. Measurements of both legs obtained every 4 cm: maximum circumferential variance of 5 cm at mid-calf and 7 cm at mid-thigh level on left compared with right leg.

Respiratory: rate 12; clear, full effort

Gastrointestinal: soft, nontender, no organomegaly or palpable masses, normal bowel sounds in all quadrants

Genitourinary: rectal examination: no palpable masses; prostate absent. Negative fecal occult blood

Neurologic: no deficits; distal sensation to light touch, vibration, pinprick intact; walks with limp, favoring left leg; normal balance

Musculoskeletal: full range of motion of all extremities, with exception of difficulty with full flexion of left ankle and knee because of degree of limb swelling; no joint pain, warmth, erythema, or arthropathy

Social history: 60 pack year smoking history, currently smoking 1.5 packs per day. Drinks two beers each evening. Lives with wife and four teenage children. Likes to play golf but has not been able to enjoy playing for past 2 months because of leg swelling.

Family history: father deceased, age 67, ruptured AAA; mother, 78, hypertension and osteoarthritis. One brother, age 56, healthy. Children all healthy.

Laboratory values: normal chemistry panel and complete blood count. PSA nondetectable.

Diagnostic tests: venous duplex ultrasound is negative for deep vein thrombosis in the left leg.

Chest x-ray is normal with no cardiac enlargement or pulmonary congestion

Diagnosis: left leg lymphedema secondary to prostate cancer therapy

Review Questions

1. Lymphedema is usually diagnosed based on clinical evidence or appearance of affected body part rather than diagnostic tests.
   a. True
   b. False
2. Does Mr. R. have primary or secondary lymphedema?
3. Mr. R. most likely has what stage of lymphedema?
   a. Stage I
   b. Stage II
   c. Stage III
4. Which therapeutic interventions might be considered for management of Mr. R's lymphedema?
   a. Pneumatic compression pump and elastic compression garment
   b. MLD massage and short-stretch compression bandaging
   c. Leg elevation and diuretic therapy
   d. Low-salt diet and leg exercises with ankle weights
   e. a and b
   f. All of the above
5. In addition to therapeutic management, what other issues should be addressed in planning Mr. R's care?
   a. Evaluation of family history risk factors
   b. Smoking cessation
   c. Employment change
   d. Recreation activities
   e. All of the above

6. Which of the following are essential elements of patient education for patients with lymphedema?
   a. Limiting fluid intake to 1,500 mL/day
   b. Daily skin inspection for signs of infection and leg elevation when nonambulatory
   c. Limiting protein intake in his diet to prevent further protein accumulation in subcutaneous tissue
   d. Wearing elastic compression support stocking 24 hrs/day except for bathing and skin care

Answers/Rationales

1. a. True. Nonpitting edema, absence of normal contour, and blunting of bony anatomical landmarks are classic features of lymphedema. Diagnostic tests are generally not necessary to support the diagnosis, although may be used to rule out other medical problems, such as extrinsic compression from tumor or DVT.
2. Secondary, which is associated with a known cause for lymphatic obstruction or malfunction. The most common etiology of secondary lymphedema in industrialized nations is cancer and cancer therapy. Primary lymphedema is either congenital or has no known etiology. The most common type of primary lymphedema is lymphedema praecox, which develops around the time of puberty to the early 20s.
3. b. Stage II, nonpitting on pressure and does not reduce with elevation. Skin is still smooth, but fibrosis has likely begun to affect subcutaneous tissues. In Stage I lymphedema, skin will pit with light pressure and the limb size reduces with elevation. In Stage III lymphedema, edema is nonpitting and advanced fibrosis has changed the appearance of the skin, which becomes woody and hypertrophic.
4. a and b. Therapeutic interventions that have demonstrated positive benefit for management of lymphedema include compression therapies and MLD used in combination with skin care and compression bandaging using short-stretch wrap materials. Leg elevation is also beneficial but diuretics are seldom effective: unless used in the early stages of the disease and to manage other medical conditions, such as hypertension. Mr. R. does not have hypertension. Salt-restricted diets are recommended but leg exercise should not be performed against resistance, which could worsen leg swelling.
5. e. All of the above. Mr. R's father died of ruptured AAA. An evaluation for AAA is appropriate for this patient. Smoking cessation is strongly encouraged to minimize his risk of recurrent cancer and cardiovascular disease. His job requires long hours of standing, which contributes to increased swelling and associated discomfort. He enjoys golfing and should be encouraged to continue this activity, along with daily use of an elastic compression garment and monitoring for effects of activity on leg edema. Mr. R. will require significant counseling and assistance to make necessary changes to achieve optimal therapeutic outcomes.
6. b. Daily skin inspection for signs of infection and leg elevation when nonambulatory is crucial for prevention of complications of cellulitis and leg swelling. Fluid intake of 2 to 3 L/day is encouraged, but protein limitation is not beneficial to prevention of progression of lymphedema. Compression support garments are to be worn during waking hours only and removed at night. Short-stretch compression bandaging may be used 24 hrs/day during intensive phase of CDT, as well as at night for maintenance therapy.

REFERENCES

Apollo, K. (2007). Clinical challenges: Lower extremity lymphedema in a patient with gynecologic cancer. *Oncology Nursing Forum, 34*(5), 937–940.

Carmelli, E., & Bartoletti, R. (2011). Retrospective trial of complete decongestive physical therapy for lower extremity secondary lymphedema in melanoma patients. *Supportive Care in Cancer, 19*(1), 141–147.

Feins, N. R. (1997). The surgical management of 324 children and young adults with lymphedema. *Surgical Rounds,* 63–72.

Felty, C. L., & Rooke, T. W. (2004). Lymphedema. In V. Fahey (Ed.), *Vascular nursing* (4th ed., pp. 33–46). St. Louis, MO: W.B. Saunders.

Fife, C. E., Benavides, S., & Carter, M. J. (2008). A patient-centered approach to treatment of morbid obesity and lower extremity complications: An overview and case studies. *Ostomy Wound Management, 54*(1), 20–22, 24–32.

Finnane, A., Hayes, S. C., Obermair, A., & Janda, M. (2011). Quality of life of women with lower-limb lymphedema following gynecological cancer. *Expert Review of Pharmacoeconomics & Outcomes Research, 11*(3), 287–297.

Foeldi, M. (2012). *Foeldi's textbook of lymphology: For physicians and lymphedema therapists* (3rd ed.). Munich, Germany: Elsevier.

Gamble, G. L., Rooke, T. W., & Gloviczki, P. (2000). Non-operative management of chronic lymphedema. In R. B. Rutherford (Ed.), *Vascular surgery* (5th ed., pp. 2142–2152). Philadelphia, PA: W.B. Saunders.

Gloviczki, P. (2000). Lymphedema: An overview. In R. B. Rutherford (Ed.), *Vascular surgery* (5th ed., pp. 2105–2109). Philadelphia, PA: W.B. Saunders.

Gloviczki, P., & Noel, A. A. (2000). Lymphatic reconstructions. In R. B. Rutherford (Ed.), *Vascular surgery* (5th ed., pp. 2159–2174). Philadelphia, PA: W.B. Saunders.

Gloviczki, P., & Wahner, H. W. (2000). Clinical diagnosis and evaluation of lymphedema. In R. B. Rutherford (Ed.), *Vascular surgery* (5th ed., pp. 2123–2142). Philadelphia, PA: W.B. Saunders.

Greene, A. K., Grant, F. D., & Slavin, S. A. (2012). Lower extremity lymphedema and elevated body-mass index. *New England Journal of Medicine, 366*(22), 2136–2137.

Heffel, D. F., & Miller, T. A. (2000). Excisional operations for chronic lymphedema. In R. B. Rutherford (Ed.), *Vascular surgery* (5th ed., pp. 2153–2159). Philadelphia, PA: W.B. Saunders.

Karkkainen, M. J., Saaristo, A., Jussila, L., Karila, K. A., Lawrence, E. C., Pajusola, K., . . . Alitalo, K. (2001). A model for gene therapy of human hereditary lymphedema. *Proceedings of the National Academy of Sciences of the United States of America, 98*(22), 12677–12682.

Katz, E., Dugan, N. L., Cohn, J. C., Chu, C., Smith, R. G., & Schmitz, K. H. (2010). Weight lifting in patients with lower-extremity lymphedema secondary to cancer: A pilot and feasibility study. *Archives of Physical Medicine & Rehabilitation, 91*(7), 1070–1076.

Kaya, S., Akbayrak, T., Bakar, Y., & Topuz, S. (2010). Effects of complex decongestive physiotherapy on an older female patient with psoriasis-related primary lymphedema. *Topics in Geriatric Rehabilitation, 26*(2), 171–175.

Kelly, D. G. (2002). *A primer on lymphedema.* Upper Saddle River, NJ: Prentice Hall/Pearson Education.

Kerchner, K., Fleischer, A., & Yosipovitch, G. (2008). Lower extremity lymphedema update: Pathophysiology, diagnosis, and treatment guidelines. *Journal of the American Academy of Dermatology, 59*(2), 324–331. Retrieved from href="http://www.ncbi.nlm.nih.gov/pubmed?term=Kerchner%20K%5BAuthor%5D&cauthor=true&cauthor_uid=18513827">

Kim, S. J. (2011). The long-term effects of complex decongestive physical therapy on lower extremity secondary lymphedema and quality of life. *Journal of Physical Therapy Science, 23*(1), 155–159.

Kunkel, K. R. (2010). Identification and impact of standard treatment protocols on the impairments and activity limitations related to lower extremity lymphedema. *Open Access Dissertations.* Paper 403. Retrieved from http://scholarlyrepository.miami.edu/cgi/viewcontent.cgi?article = 1402&context = oa_dissertations, accessed August 10, 2013.

Langbecker, D., Hayes, S. C., Newman, B., & Janda, M. (2008). Treatment for upper-limb and lower-limb lymphedema by professionals specializing in lymphedema care. *European Journal of Cancer Care, 17*(6), 557–564.

Lawrence, S. (2008). Use of a VELCRO wrap system in the management of lower limb lymphoedema/chronic oedema. *Journal of Lymphoedema, 3*(2), 65.

Lockwood-Rayermann, S. (2007). Lymphedema in gynecologic cancer survivors: An area of exploration? *Cancer Nursing, 30*(4), E11–E18.

Lohrmann, C., Foeldi, E., & Langer, M. (2011). Diffuse lymphangiomatosis with genital involvement-evaluation with magnetic resonance lymphangiography. *Urologic Oncology, 29*(5), 515–522.

Lu, Q., Xu, J., & Liu, N. (2010). Chronic lower extremity lymphedema: A comparative study of high-resolution interstitial MR lymphangiography and heavily T2-weighted MRI. *European Journal of Radiology, 73*(2), 365–373.

Mahram, M., & Rajabi, M. (2011). Treatment of lymphedema praecox through Low Level Laser Therapy (LLLT). *Journal of Research in Medical Sciences, 16*(6), 848–851.

McHaffie, D. R., Kozak, K. R., Warner, T. F., Cho, C. S., Heiner, J. P., & Attia, S. (2010). Stewart-Treves syndrome of the lower extremity. *Journal of Clinical Oncology, 28*(21), e351–e352.

Modaghegh, M. D., & Soltani, E. (2010). A newly designed SIPC device for management of lymphoedema. *Indian Journal of Surgery, 72*(1), 36–40.

Mohler, E. R. (2004). Lymphedema. Retrieved from www.uptodate.com, accessed April 12, 2013.

Mohler, E. R., & Mondry, T. E. (2013). Clinical manifestations and diagnosis of lymphedema. Retrieved from www.uptodate.com, accessed April 12, 2013.

Newton, H. (2011). Chronic oedema of the lower limb: Pathophysiology and management. *British Journal of Community Nursing, 16,* S4–S12.

Piller, N. (2009). Phlebolymphoedema/chronic venous lymphatic insufficiency: An introduction to strategies for detection, differentiation and treatment. *Phlebology, 24*(2), 51–55.

Robinson, M. R., Honda, K. S., & Bordeaux, J. S. (2011). Angiosarcoma in an obese woman with worsening lymphedema after weight-loss and skin-reduction surgeries. *Journal of the American Academy of Dermatology, 65*(2), 448–449.

Rockson, S. (2003). Lymphatic disease. In M. A. Creager & E. Braunwald (Eds.), *Atlas of vascular disease* (2nd ed., pp. 241–253). Philadelphia, PA: Current Medicine.

Rockson, S., & Dean, S. M. (2011) Lymphedema. In *Manual of vascular diseases* (2nd ed.). Philadelphia, PA: Lippincott Williams & Wilkins.

Rudkin, G. H., & Miller, T. A. (1995). Lymphatic disease. In C. B. Ernst & J. C. Stanley (Eds.), *Current therapy in vascular surgery* (3rd ed., pp. 973–982). St. Louis, MO: Mosby.

Schirger, A., & Gloviczki, P. (1996). Lymphedema. In J. R. Young, J. W. Olin, & J. R. Bartholomew (Eds.), *Peripheral vascular diseases* (2nd ed., pp. 525–538). St. Louis, MO: Mosby.

Shimony, A., & Thidhar, D. (2008). Aqua lymphatic therapy for managing lower extremity lymphedema. *Journal of the American Academy of Dermatology, 59*(6), 1092.

Shinawi, M. (2007). Lymphedema of the lower extremity: Is it genetic or nongenetic? *Clinical Pediatrics, 46*(9), 835–841.

Tada, H., Teramukai, S., Fukushima, M., & Sasaki, H. (2009). Risk Factors for lower limb lymphedema after lymph node dissection in patients with ovarian and uterine carcinoma. *BMC Cancer, 9*, 47.

Weiss, R. (2007). How many lymphedema cases are there in the United States? Retrieved from www.lymphnotes.com/article.php/id/401/, accessed August 6, 2013.

Witte, C. L., & Witte, M. H. (2000). Lymphodynamics and pathophysiology of lymphedema. In R. B. Rutherford (Ed.), *Vascular surgery* (5th ed., pp. 2110–2122). Philadelphia, PA: W.B. Saunders.

Woods, M., Tobin, M., & Mortimer, P. (1995). The psychosocial morbidity of breast cancer patients with lymphoedema. *Cancer Nursing, 18*(6), 467–471.

RELEVANT WEBSITES

American Cancer Society: www.cancer.org
American Society of Lymphology: www.lymphology.com
Lymphatic Research Foundation: www.lymphaticresearch.org
Lymphoedema Association of Australia: www.lymphoedema.org.au
National Lymphedema Network: www.lymphnet.org

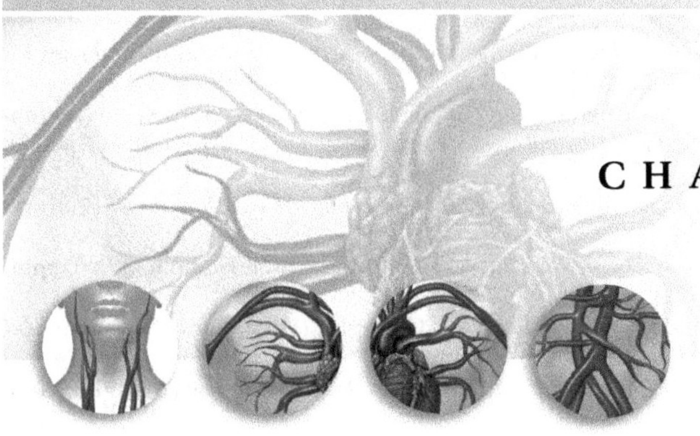

CHAPTER 24

Vascular Trauma

Michelle Tinkham

First Edition Author: *Isobel Green*

OBJECTIVES

1. Recognize the significance of vascular injuries in the community and identify the characteristic physical signs and symptoms of acute vascular trauma.
2. Demonstrate an understanding of the nursing management of patients with venous and arterial injuries.
3. Describe the mechanism of vascular injury and the indications for invasive and noninvasive vascular studies.
4. Demonstrate a confident approach to the assessment, evaluation, potential complications, and prevention of iatrogenic vascular trauma.
5. Discuss surgical and endovascular treatments.

Overview/Introduction

Trauma is the leading cause of death in persons under the age of 44. Trauma accounts for approximately 164,112 deaths yearly (Emergency Nurses Association, 2007). Recent increases in violent crimes, together with an increase in high-speed motor-vehicle accidents, have not only resulted in an increase in vascular trauma, but also a change in the types of injuries sustained. In marked contrast to the predominance of extremity vascular trauma documented during wartime, many neck and trunk vascular injuries are currently being observed (Gupta, Rao, & Sieunarine, 2001). In addition, there has been an increase in the number of vascular injuries due to self-injection of a variety of substances by intravenous drug users, and complications from endovascular procedures leading to dire consequences for the vascular system.

I. Mechanism of Injury

The mechanism and severity of vascular injuries are the determining factors in management.

A. Penetrating Trauma

1. Most common cause of injury to arterial and venous structures
   a. Gunshot wounds account for 55% of vascular injuries

b. Knife wounds account for 35% of vascular injuries
c. Iatrogenic injuries have increased in number because of more frequent interventional radiological procedures (Hallet, Brewster, & Clement Darling, 1995)

2. Causes localized damage to vessels in the case of knife wounds and low velocity missiles. High-velocity missiles (e.g., from a hunting rifle) can create a wide area of explosive cavitation damage around the missile path extending for an area 30 to 40 times the size of the missile (Hallet et al., 1995)

B. Blunt Trauma

1. Refers to an injury in which there is no communication with the outside environment
2. Most commonly caused by motor-vehicle accidents, falls, assaults, and contact sports
3. May cause damage by fracture fragments or fracture dislocations causing excessive and sudden stretch contusions of arteries (Hallet et al., 1995)
4. Prognosis usually more serious than for penetrating injuries because the mechanism of injury is more difficult to diagnose and treat
5. Can often be the cause of accidental death (Payne, 1994)

C. Blast Injuries

1. Refers to injuries from explosions
2. Often associated with military and terrorism but may also be industrial accidents
3. Most common blast injury in US is from fireworks

II. Risk Factors

A. Age

B. Gender

C. Race

D. Alcohol

E. Violence and Self-Inflicted Injury

F. Tobacco and Drug Use

III. Iatrogenic Vascular Damage

A. Frequently Involves Femoral and Brachial Vessels Serving as Access Sites for Arteriography and Endovascular Procedures (Caps, 1998)

B. Injuries

1. Hematoma
2. Hemorrhage
3. Arteriovenous fistula
4. Arterial occlusion
5. Acute limb ischemia
6. Distal embolization
7. Nerve compression

C. Risk Factors

1. Difficulty in maintaining accurate hemostatic pressure in the groin due to obesity (Caps, 2000)
2. Advanced age of patients
3. Severe atherosclerosis
4. Concurrent use of anticoagulant therapy
5. Previous procedures

IV. Assessment

Primary goal and first priority is patient survival.

A. Evaluate Ventilatory Status and Stabilize Airway

B. Identify Circulatory Compromise and Provide Fluid Resuscitation

C. Observe for Hemorrhage and Establish Control

D. Establish Mechanism of Injury (Hess, 1999)

V. Physical Examination

A. Purpose

1. Determine location and extent of injury
2. Identify location of entrance and exit wounds
3. Document presence of hematoma or hemorrhage

B. Signs of Trauma

1. Hard signs
   a. Observed pulsatile bleeding
   b. Palpable thrill
   c. Visible, expanding hematoma
   d. Continuous murmur
   e. Six P's: pain, pallor, pulselessness, paresthesia, paralysis, and poikilothermia (Nunnelee, Sander, Oetker, Auer, & Troop, 1994)
2. Soft signs
   a. Significant history of hemorrhage or shock
   b. Proximity of penetrating injury to major vascular structure

c. Small, nonpulsatile and nonexpanding hematoma
d. Bony injury or proximity penetrating wound
e. Neurological abnormality (Glasgow Coma Scale)
f. Decreased pulse compared to a contralateral extremity (Bjerke, Jakubs & Stuhlmiller, 2003; Perry & Bongard, 2002)
g. Revised Trauma Score (Emergency Nurses Association, 2007)

VI. Considerations Across the Life Span

A. Most are Young and Male

B. Most Injuries Occur Suddenly

C. Injuries Often a Result of Drug or Alcohol Abuse

D. Most Injuries are Iatrogenic Injuries in Older Age Group

E. Number of Comorbidities has Significant Effect on Outcomes

VII. Pertinent Diagnostic Testing

A. Laboratory Tests

1. Essential
   a. Full blood count
   b. Typing and crossmatching
   c. Electrolytes, urea, and creatinine
   d. Prothrombin time and activated partial thromboplastin time
   e. Blood glucose
   f. Arterial blood gas
2. Recommended
   a. Blood alcohol
   b. Toxicology
   c. Amylase
   d. Creatine kinase (Bjerke et al., 2003)

B. Noninvasive Tests

Advanced ultrasound technology for patients with soft signs of vascular injury
1. Chest x-ray
2. CT/MRI

C. Invasive Tests (CTA/MRA)

1. Arteriography considered in cases involving:
   a. Stable patients with multiple levels of injury
   b. Extensive bone or soft tissue injury
   c. Shotgun injuries

d. Potential injuries to the subclavian or axillary arteries
e. Pre-existence of peripheral artery disease
f. Penetrating chest and abdominal injuries
g. Injuries to extremities

2. Most patients with hard signs of vascular injury require immediate transfer to the operating room (Britt, Weireter, & Cole, 2001)

VIII. Medical Management (nonoperative management)

A. Options for Medical Management are Extremely Limited

1. Fluid resuscitation to maintain volume
2. Vasopressors to maintain blood pressure

B. Use Temporary Intraluminal Balloon Tamponade to Reduce Hemorrhage

C. Place Percutaneous Stent for Acute Traumatic Arterial Injury (Hood & Blair, 1998)

D. Nonsurgical Management of Vascular Trauma Remains Controversial (Brohi, 2002)

IX. Surgical Management (operative management)

A. Extremity Vascular Injuries

1. Injuries to subclavian, axillary, brachial, superficial femoral, profundus femoral, and popliteal arteries should always be repaired if possible
2. Injuries to the radial or ulnar arteries should be repaired if the other vessel is not functioning or is also injured (Cohen, 1998)
3. Lower-extremity injuries account for 30% to 50% of all vascular injuries (Payne, 1994)
4. Advanced ischemia is established within 6 to 8 hours after arterial disruption or occlusion (Hallet et al., 1995)

B. Intra-Abdominal Vascular Injuries

1. Frequently associated with injuries to other intra-abdominal organs
2. Mortality after surgical intervention for injuries to abdominal aorta can be as high as 50% to 70%
3. Mortality after surgical intervention for injuries to inferior vena cava can be as high as 30% to 53% (Hood & Blair, 1998)
4. Iliac arteries are often repaired by end-to-end anastomosis, depending on the amount of tissue loss
5. Injuries to renal, superior mesenteric, and coeliac axis arteries are usually repaired with the use of autogenous graft if necessary (Cohen, 1998)
6. Injuries to hepatic or splenic vessels may require intracaval shunting or splenectomy

C. Carotid Artery Injuries

1. Severe neurological deficit; ligation of artery recommended
2. Mild or no neurological deficit; repair usually safe and recommended (Cohen, 1998)
3. Surgical technique determined by nature of the injury and similar to those for carotid dissection
4. Majority of cases repaired by direct suture
5. Occasionally segmental resection with end-to-end anastomosis necessary
6. Other techniques include:
    a. Bypass with autogenous saphenous vein or synthetic material
    b. Patch angioplasty
    c. Transposition using external carotid artery (Payne, 1994)
    d. Covered stent or detachable balloon
7. May have additional trauma such as C-spine injury
8. Consider transcranial Doppler (TCD) monitoring

D. Vertebral Artery Injuries

1. Relatively rare
2. Often associated with other injuries to cervical structures
3. Direct surgical repair and exposure of vessel difficult because of intimate relationship with cervical vertebrae
4. If the patient has sustained both carotid and vertebral injuries, the carotid repair takes priority (Hood & Blair, 1998; Payne, 1994)

E. Thoracic Vascular Trauma

1. Most common causes of blunt injuries to intrathoracic structures are motor-vehicle accidents
2. May require immediate treatment for tension pneumothorax or cardiac tamponade
3. Knife stabbings followed by gunshot wounds are most common causes of penetrating thoracic vascular injuries
4. Underlying cause of tamponade often needs to be determined and controlled by thoracotomy (Hood & Blair, 1998; Payne, 1994).

F. Venous Injuries

1. Most commonly injured veins:
    a. Superficial femoral (42%)
    b. Popliteal (23%)
    c. Common femoral (14%)
2. End-to-end or lateral venorrhaphy usually performed unless the patient is hemodynamically unstable
3. More extensive venous injury may require repair with an interposition or panel graft (Brohi, 2002)

G. DVT/PE

1. 50% of trauma patients experience DVTs
2. Some DVTs occur after orthopedic or abdominal repairs
    a. 10% to 30% occurs proximal to injury

   b. 40% to 80% occurs in calf
   c. 1% fatal PE occurrence (Hallet, Mills, Earnshaw, & Reekers, 2004)
3. Consider prophylaxis use of retrievable inferior vena cava filters

H. Pseudoaneurysm (false aneurysm)

1. Most occur following catheterization of the femoral artery for cardiac or radiological procedures
2. Development can be insidious in trauma patients
3. Usually detected by ultrasound scanning or CT
4. Easily differentiated from hematoma by duplex ultrasound
5. Most require autogenous patch angioplasty or suture repair (Hood & Blair, 1998)

I. Arteriovenous Fistula

1. Often presents late
2. An audible thrill or palpable bruit may be detected
3. Can remain asymptomatic for some time in deeply placed veins
4. Surgical repair involves dividing the fistula, then repairing the venous and arterial injuries with lateral sutures
5. An autogenous patch angioplasty is sometimes required (Hood & Blair, 1998; Payne, 1994)

J. Thoracic Outlet Syndrome (Hallet et al., 2004)

1. 86% of these patients have a history of trauma
2. Clavicle injuries (auto accidents) can put subclavian vein at risk
3. Axillo-subclavian vein thrombosis

K. Nerve Injuries

1. Occur in approximately 50% of upper-extremity and 25% of lower-extremity vascular injuries
2. The nerve injury determines the long-term prognosis and ultimate functional status of the injured extremity
3. Immediate repair is rarely possible for most penetrating and blunt nerve injuries
4. Primary amputation, rather than reconstruction, is often considered in limbs with massive orthopedic, nerve, and soft tissue injuries (Weaver, Papanicolaou, & Yellin, 1996)

L. Compartment Syndrome and Fasciotomy

1. Most common site is anterior compartment of the lower leg
2. Acute arterial trauma can cause an abrupt increase in compartmental pressure (Payne, 1994)
3. More likely to represent a delayed response after a period of ischemia
4. Early recognition critical in avoiding limb loss
5. Surgical intervention via fasciotomy usually performed if pressures are greater than 30 mm Hg (Brohi, 2002; Caps, 2000)

M. Secondary Lymphadema

1. Tissue loss containing lymph nodes
2. Common after degloving injuries

X. Nursing Management

A. Diagnosis and Evaluation

1. Requires astute physical assessment and management skills
2. Initial resuscitation, assessment, and evaluation essential to a positive outcome
3. In multiple traumas, attention diverted from occult vascular injuries
4. Should proceed concurrently with management of other serious injuries (Hallet et al., 1995; Payne, 1994)
5. Teamwork is essential element of all trauma care
6. Clinical features suggesting great vessel involvement (Moore, 2006)
   a. Cardiac arrest
   b. Shock
   c. Cardiac tamponade
   d. Wide mediastinum
   e. Recurring hemothorax

B. Intervention

1. Depends on type and severity of injuries
2. ACLS primary/secondary ABCD
3. Airway establishment first priority
4. Complete neurovascular assessment
5. Restore, monitor, and maintain fluid and electrolyte balance
6. Always prepare for expeditious transfer of patient to operating room

C. Expected Patient Outcomes

Overall mortality rate currently in 5% range (Hallet et al., 1995). Principal factors include:

1. Initial identification and management
2. Extent and site of injury
3. Time from injury to repair
4. Age and preinjury health status of the patient
5. Postprocedure management
6. Complications
   a. Shock
   b. Sepsis
   c. Infection

XI. Patient Teaching and Home Care Considerations

A. Continue to Monitor Posthospitalization for Complications.

Pay special attention to possible graft infection and delayed healing of the wound

B. Provide Patients and Families with Specific Instructions Regarding:

1. Wound-care techniques and infection-control procedures
2. Principles of hygiene
3. Likely signs and symptoms indicating potential or actual vascular complications

4. Pain management
5. Ongoing rehabilitation
6. Appropriate access to vascular team and follow-up requirements, keeping in mind that patients may live some distance from where their injuries were sustained and treated
7. Long-term effects of the injury
8. Importance of possible continued radiological follow-up if endovascular procedure or need for possible reinterventions

XII. Ethical Issues

A. Family Presence During Resuscitation

B. Organ Donation

C. Nursing Care of Grieving Patients and Family Members

D. Care and Stress Management of Trauma Team Members

CASE STUDY

TRAUMA CALL

Trauma call 5 minutes. An 18-year-old male found by runner at 0500 with penetrating trauma to abdomen, extremities, and chest from multiple small caliber gunshot wounds. Victim unconscious for undetermined amount of time. Witness called 911.

CLINICAL PRESENTATION

Patient is unresponsive with a blood pressure of 90/50 mm Hg, pulse of 118 beats/min; labored shallow breathing, respirations 22 breaths/min. Pupils equal and reactive. Multiple abrasions on face and limbs, possible assault. Possible head trauma as well as thoracic and abdominal injuries. Possible vascular injury to extremities from gunshots.

INITIAL INVESTIGATION

Chest x-ray showed left pnuemothorax with foreign body

Cervical x-ray showed no C-spine injury

CT to abdomen showed free air to sigmoid colon area with multiple foreign bodies (probable bullet fragments)

X-ray to left shoulder showed no fractures. Probable soft tissue injury only.

MRA to right lower extremity shows disruption in flow from femoral artery. Probable dissection from bullet fragment.

CBC, CMP, UA, Type and Cross 4 units, Toxicology screen preformed. Blood chemistry within normal limits. Toxicology screen shows alcohol and marijuana.

Physical examination: Physical examination revealed a large hematoma of the right upper thigh. This hematoma appeared to be expanding. No pedal pulses in right foot. Intravenous lines were inserted, and the patient was resuscitated with 3 L of Normal Saline. His blood pressure was 120/80 following the infusion.

RELEVANT HEALTH HISTORY

Prior health history was unknown. Awaiting contact of next of kin.

SUMMARY OF SIGNIFICANT INJURIES

Bowel and Spleen injury: Trauma surgeon alerted and patient prepared for immediate transfer to Operating Room
Thoracic injury: Thoracic trauma surgeon consulted
Vascular injury: Right thigh—Vascular surgeon consulted

OPERATIVE FINDINGS AND REPAIR

Small laceration found to sigmoid bowel and splenic laceration. Sigmoid Colectomy with Splenectomy performed. 19 fr. JP drain placed
Chest tube placed to left chest to intermittent suction
Fem-Pop bypass with in situ vein to right leg. All performed by trauma surgeon

NURSING MANAGEMENT AND CLINICAL COURSE

Following surgery, the patient was transferred to the surgical intensive care unit. He was intubated and ventilated. Nursing documentation noted the following:

- His chest was clear, and he was saturating at 99%. Drainage to chest tube was minimal.
- Peripheral pulses were returned to right foot. Right leg felt warm and color normal.
- He was hemodynamically stable and in sinus bradycardia.
- His neurovascular observations were stable.
- Foley catheter was placed in the ER. His urinary output was satisfactory. Some hematuria was noted on arrival but resolved.
- His nasogastric tube was on free drainage.
- His abdomen was soft but bowel sounds had not yet returned. Minimal drainage to JP drains.
- His dressings were dry and intact.
- He was sedated and kept pain-free with intravenous morphine. Ventilator weaning protocols were started on postoperative day 1.
- His ongoing laboratory tests remained stable.

SECONDARY DIAGNOSIS AND EVALUATION

No additional injuries were noted. Gunshot wound to left shoulder was soft tissue and wound was cleaned and closed.

CLINICAL COURSE AND PROGRESS

Postoperative day 1: Patient was weaned off the ventilator the following postoperative day. He complained to pain to his right leg and abdomen. He was started on a morphine PCA.

Postoperative day 3: His bowel sounds returned and he was given clear liquids. He tolerated this diet and his NG tube was removed. His diet was advanced as tolerated. Physical therapy evaluated him and light ambulation was encouraged once a day. His chest tube was removed with no signs of distress.

Postoperative day 4: His diet was advanced to regular. His JP drain was removed. He was ambulating several times a day and his pain was controlled with PO meds.

Post-op day 5: He was discharged home with family.

REHABILITATION AND FOLLOW-UP

Follow-up with the trauma surgeon in 1 week.

SIGNIFICANT SOCIAL HISTORY

Patient agreed to alcohol/drug rehabilitation. He and his family were encouraged to seek counseling as well.

CONCLUSION

Patient was reportedly shot by rival gang over drug deal. He did attend counseling and drug rehabilitation and with the support of his family, was attempting to cut his gang ties and return to school. He was made a full recovery from his injuries.

Review Questions

1. The overall mortality rate for vascular trauma is in the range of:
   a. 5%
   b. 15%
   c. 20%
   d. 40%
2. Blunt trauma can often be the cause of accidental death because:
   a. there can be localized damage to vessels
   b. it can cause extensive bone and soft tissue injury
   c. it is more difficult to diagnose and treat
   d. it can lead to the development of an arteriovenous fistula
3. The primary goal and first priority in trauma assessment is:
   a. blood pressure control
   b. patient survival
   c. pain management
   d. management of vascular injuries
4. Following arterial disruption or occlusion, advanced ischemia becomes established within:
   a. 8 to 10 hours
   b. 4 to 6 hours
   c. 2 to 4 hours
   d. 6 to 8 hours
5. Trauma is the leading cause of death in patients who are:
   a. over age 34
   b. under age 24
   c. over age 64
   d. under age 44
6. An important risk factor for iatrogenic vascular injury is:
   a. alcohol abuse
   b. cigarette smoking
   c. obesity
   d. diabetes
7. Hematomas are easily differentiated from false aneurysms by:
   a. duplex ultrasound
   b. palpation
   c. plain radiograph
   d. arterial blood gas
8. Signs of vascular injury include all of the following except:
   a. expanding hematoma
   b. inflammation
   c. palpable thrill
   d. pallor

9. Most patients who sustain lower-extremity trauma require:
   a. an elective arterial bypass
   b. primary amputation
   c. urgent surgical intervention
   d. intraluminal balloon tamponade
10. Injuries resulting from direct vascular intervention include all of the following except:
   a. arterial occlusion
   b. venous occlusion
   c. hematoma
   d. nerve compression

Answers/Rationale

1. a. Rapid transport of trauma patients to major surgical centers has decreased the average time from injury to treatment for most vascular injuries (Hallet et al., 1995).
2. c. Because this mechanism of injury is more difficult to diagnose and treat, it is often more deadly than a penetrating injury (Payne, 1994).
3. b. Survival of the patient is the primary goal even if the extremity injury is limb-threatening. (Hess, 1999).
4. d. Advanced ischemia becomes established within 6 to 8 hours after arterial disruption or occlusion (Hallet et al., 1995).
5. d. Trauma is the leading cause of death in persons under the age of 44 (Caps, 2000).
6. c. Obesity is a risk factor due to the difficulty in maintaining accurate hemostatic pressure in the groin (Caps, 2000).
7. a. Hematomas are easily differentiated from false aneurysms by duplex ultrasound (Nehler, Taylor, & Porter, 1998).
8. b. See text: Signs of trauma (1a–e, 2a–f) (Bjerke et al., 2003; Perry & Bongard, 2002).
9. c. Most patients with lower-extremity trauma require urgent surgical intervention (Payne, 1994; Savage & Walker, 1995).
10. b. See text: III. Iatrogenic Vascular Damage, B. Injuries.

REFERENCES

Bjerke, H. S., Jakubs, E. J., & Stuhlmiller, F. E. (2003). Extremity vascular trauma. Retrieved from http://www.emedicine.com/med/topic2812.htm

Britt, L. D., Weireter, L. J., Jr., & Cole, F. J. (2001). Newer diagnostic modalities for vascular injuries. *Surgical Clinics of North America, 81*(6), 1263–1279.

Brohi, K. (2002). Peripheral vascular trauma. Vascular trauma basics. Retrieved from http://www.trauma.org/vascular/PVTintro.html, accessed February 29, 2012.

Caps, M. T. (1998). The epidemiology of vascular trauma. *Seminars in Vascular Surgery, 11*(4), 227–231.

Caps, M. T. (2000). The epidemiology of vascular trauma. In R. B. Rutherford (Ed.), *Vascular surgery* (5th ed., pp. 857–862). Philadelphia, PA: W.B. Saunders.

Cohen, J. R. (1998). Vascular trauma. In R. Faust & J. Cohen (Eds.), *Vascular surgery* (3rd ed., pp. 47–51). Baltimore, MD: Williams & Wilkins.

Emergency Nurses Association. (2007). *Trauma nurse core course* (6th ed.). Des Plaines, IL: ENA.

Gupta, R., Rao, S., & Sieunarine, K. (2001). An epidemiological view of vascular trauma in Western Australia. *Australian and New Zealand Journal of Surgery, 71*, 461–466.

Hallet, J. W., Brewster, D. C., & Clement Darling, R., Jr. (1995). Vascular trauma. In J. Hallet, D. Brewster, & R. Clement Darling, Jr (Eds.), *Handbook of patient care in vascular surgery* (3rd ed., pp. 290–297). Boston, MA: Little, Brown and Company.

Hallett, J. W., Mills, J. L., Earnshaw, J. J., & Reekers, J. A. (2004). *Comprehensive vascular and endovascular surgery.* London, UK: Mosby (Elselvier).

Hess, A. V. (1999). Treatment of vascular injuries from penetrating and nonpenetrating trauma. *Hand Clinics, 15*(2), 249–295.

Hood, J. M., & Blair, P. H. (1998). Vascular trauma. In J. Beard & P. Gaines (Eds.), *Vascular and endovascular surgery* (pp. 171–199). London, UK: W.B. Saunders.

Moore, W. (2006). *Vascular and endovascular surgery: A comprehensive review* (7th ed.). Philadelphia, PA: Saunders Elsevier.

Nehler, M. R., Taylor, L. M., & Porter, J. M. (1998). Iatrogenic vascular trauma. *Seminars in Vascular Surgery, 11*(4), 283–293.

Nunnelee, J., Sander, R., Oetker, D., Auer, A., & Troop, B. (1994). Emergency department nursing vascular assessment: A retrospective study. *Journal of Vascular Nursing, 12*(2), 35–37.

Payne, J. (1994). Vascular trauma. In V. Fahey (Ed.), *Vascular nursing* (2nd ed., pp. 536–557). Philadelphia, PA: W. B. Saunders.

Perry, M. O., & Bongard, F. S. (2002). Vascular trauma. In W. S. Moore (Ed.), *Vascular surgery* (6th ed., pp. 677–695). Philadelphia, PA: W. B. Saunders.

Savage, L. S., & Walker, E. (1995). Vascular trauma on the rise. *Journal of Vascular Nursing, 13*(4), 106–111.

Weaver, F. A., Papanicolaou, G., & Yellin, A. E. (1996). Difficult peripheral vascular injuries. *Surgical Clinics of North America, 76*(4), 843–859.

SUGGESTED READING

Spade, K., Aziz, F., & Sumpio, B. E. (2008). The use of retrievable inferior vena cava filters in the trauma population. *International Journal of Angiology, 17*(1), 23–26.

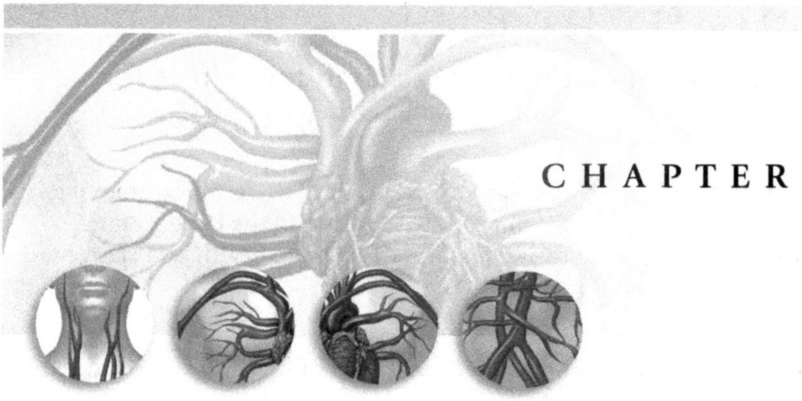

CHAPTER 25

Amputation

Cynthia Christensen

OBJECTIVES

1. Identify risk factors for amputation.
2. Identify early interventions to reduce the risk for amputation.
3. List postoperative interventions for decreasing secondary complications.
4. Describe the essential factors necessary for successful rehabilitation after amputation.
5. Describe the impact amputation has on a person's life.

There are approximately 2 million Americans with some form of limb loss, more than 185,000 new amputations each year in the United States and more than 250,000 amputees worldwide in the United Nations registry (Ketz, 2008; Wehmer & Jones, 2014). Amputations can be described as primary (performed as an initial procedure) and secondary (performed after revascularization) (MacVittie, 1998).

I. Introduction

A. Amputation should be performed at the level that allows for complete healing but will also permit the most efficient use of the limb.

1. Upper-extremity amputations account for 15% to 20% of all amputations (Krupski, 2000).
2. Lower-extremity amputations (LEA) comprise the majority of amputations and will be the focus of further discussion.
   a. Approximately two thirds are below the knee (Fitzgerald, 2000; Fletcher et al., 2002).
   b. Approximately 33% are above the knee (Fitzgerald, 2000).

B. About 30% to 60% of the LEA Occurs in Persons with Diabetes Mellitus (Amputation and Amputation Surgery, 2011; Complications of Diabetes in the US, 2011; Deery & Sangeorzan, 2001; Helt & Jacobsen, 1999; Munro, 2001; Wehmer & Jones, 2014).

C. **The Incidence of LEA is Twice as High for Men as for Women** (Carrington et al., 2001; Krapfl, Gohdes, & Burrows, 2003).

D. **In the United States,** African Americans have two to three times the risk for diabetes-related LEA compared with whites in the United States. This may be accounted for by inequalities in access to health care (Leggetter, Chaturvedi, Fuller, & Edmonds, 2002).

E. **Native American's** (Krapfl et al., 2003) rate of LEA is 3.5 times higher than for non-Hispanic whites.

F. **Eighty Percent of Americans Requiring LEA have Peripheral Artery Disease (PAD)** (Bryant, 2001) and may go through four stages of development:

1. Asymptomatic PAD
2. Claudication
3. Rest pain
4. Tissue necrosis
5. Most persons progress directly from stage 1 to stage 3 or 4 (Nehler, Hiatt, & Taylor, 2003)

G. **It is Estimated that 5% of Persons with Intermittent Claudication will Progress to Critical Limb Ischemia and Amputation** (Lawson, 2005).

H. **Vascular Patients** who have had one amputation have a 20% to 50% chance of a contralateral amputation in 1 to 3 years and a 39% to 68% mortality rate within 5 years (Datta, 2001; Deery & Sangeorzan, 2001; MacVittie, 1998). The survival rate is lower in persons with diabetes mellitus, especially with end-stage kidney disease or other comorbidities. The 1- and 5-year survival rates are 50% and 15%, respectively (Zgonis, Stapleton, Jeffries, Girard-Powell, & Foster, 2008).

I. **Approximately 33%** of persons with acute preoperative ischemia will require an amputation with mortality rates of 5% to 11% (Keshelava et al., 2009).

J. **Absent Sensation** on the sole of the foot has been related to a 10-fold risk of foot ulcer development and a 17-fold risk of amputation (Wehmer & Jones, 2014).

K. **Persons with Diabetes Who have Recurrent Ulcers have a 5% to 15% Risk of Amputation** (Amputation and Amputation Surgery, 2011).

II. Etiology/Precipitating Factors (see Table 25-1)

TABLE 25-1 Etiology and Precipitating Factors for LEA

Peripheral artery disease[a]
Diabetic foot ulceration[a]
Peripheral neuropathy[a]
Trauma
Infection
Impaired wound healing
Limited joint mobility
Malignancy
Thermal injury
Congenital malformations
Cutaneous fungal infections
High glycosylated hemoglobin level
Contributing medical conditions causing neuropathy:
1. Thyroid disease
2. Spinal stenosis
3. Amyloidosis
4. Alcoholism
5. Vasculitis
6. Diabetes mellitus
Contributing medical conditions causing peripheral edema:
1. Congestive heart failure
2. Venous insufficiency
3. Congenital lymphedema
4. Hypothyroidism
Contributing medical conditions causing decreased peripheral perfusion:
1. Peripheral artery disease
2. Congestive heart failure
3. Buerger disease
4. Scleroderma
Medications that cause neuropathy:
1. Chemotherapy
2. Antiretrovirals
Medications that decrease arterial flow:
1. Beta-blockers
2. Alpha-agonists

[a]Most common factors (Gibson, 2001).
Bryant (2001); Carrington et al. (2001); Deery & Sangeorzan (2001); Gibson (2001); Watts et al. (2001).

III. Assessment

A. Risk Factors and Primary Prevention

1. Risk factors for LEA include diabetes mellitus, hypertension, coronary artery disease, past and present tobacco use, end-stage renal disease requiring hemodialysis, dyslipidemia, foot ulcer, heel crack, or plantar callous (Abou-Zamzam, Teruya, Killeen, & Ballard, 2003; Calle-Pascual et al., 2001; Carrington et al., 2001; Deery & Sangeorzan, 2001).
   a. A severe diabetic foot infection has a 25% increased risk of major LE amputation (Zgonis, Stapleton, Girard-Powell, & Hagino, 2008).
   b. Smokers are twice as likely as nonsmokers to develop critical limb ischemia leading to amputation (Muir, 2009).

c. Persons with peripheral artery disease and diabetes are more likely to develop impaired wound healing and neuropathy making them a higher risk for gangrene resulting in a higher rate of amputation (Muir, 2009).

2. Primary prevention includes reduction in the incidence of disease by eliminating or controlling risk factors. This includes:
   a. Better control of dietary factors resulting in tighter control of hypertension, glycosylated hemoglobin levels and dyslipidemia; smoking cessation, exercise, and foot care (Lawson, 2005; Muir, 2009).
   b. Comprehensive foot care programs that include risk assessment, foot care education and prevention, treatment of foot problems, and referrals to specialists can reduce amputation rates by 45% to 85% (Complications of diabetes in the US, 2011).
   c. Ninety percent of diabetic foot ulcers will heal when treated with appropriate antibiotics, restoration of arterial perfusion, and aggressive wound care including off-loading of the ulcer (Deery & Sangeorzan, 2001).

B. Patient History

1. Subjective findings include:
   a. Numbness, burning, itching, tingling, crawling, prickling
   b. Pain burning or sharp; may be worse at night or with recumbent position. Persons with pain may sleep sitting in a chair for relief
   c. Staining of socks or foot odor
   d. Leg swelling with or without dependent position
   e. History of previous foot ulceration, infection, or surgery
   f. Claudication
   g. Footwear usage in and outside the house
   h. Report of tobacco usage (Deery & Sangeorzan, 2001; Gibson, 2001)
2. Objective findings include:
   a. Impaired monofilament sensation
   b. Impaired vibration perception
   c. Absent Achilles tendon reflex
   d. Callous foot deformities
   e. Inappropriate footwear
   f. Absent pedal pulses and/or decreased capillary refill
   g. Presence of edema, infection, necrosis or gangrene (Deery & Sangeorzan, 2001; Muller et al., 2002; Spollett, 2006; Zgonis et al., 2008)

C. Physical Examination

1. Inspection
   a. General inspection for loss of hair on the legs and feet; dry skin or venous stasis dermatitis; presence of foot deformities, such as small muscle wasting, hammer/claw toes, bony prominences, prominent metatarsal heads, Charcot arthropathy, and limited joint mobility
   b. Inspect feet, including all toe web spaces for ulceration, excessive moisture leading to maceration, dryness predisposing skin to cracking and tearing, focal erythema as a sign of pressure, friction fracture, or infection.

   c. Examine footwear for presence of foreign bodies, abnormal wear pattern, or internal staining suggesting an open wound. Bulging of shoes suggests poor fit while an irregular wear pattern can indicate biomechanical abnormalities (Carrington et al., 2001; Deery & Sangeorzan, 2001; Wehmer & Jones, 2014).
2. Palpation of legs and feet is done to assess for temperature changes, degree of pulses, and for capillary refill (Carrington et al., 2001; Deery & Sangeorzan, 2001; Muir, 2009; Wehmer & Jones, 2014)

D. Consideration Across the Life Span.

Lower-extremity amputations performed as a result of injury, trauma, malignancy, battlefield wounds, or congenital malformations may occur at any age. Nontraumatic indications for LEA occur around the sixth decade of life with a dramatic increase in the eighth decade (Bryant, 2001; Calle-Pascual et al., 2001; Marks & Michael, 2001; Wehmer & Jones, 2014)

IV. Pertinent Diagnostic Testing.

Testing is done not only to aid in wound healing, but to aid in the selection of the amputation site.

A. Noninvasive Tests Include:

1. Segmental Doppler systolic blood pressure measurements; toe pressure may be the most helpful, especially in the presence of arterial calcification
2. Laser Doppler velocimetry to evaluate blood flow
3. Skin perfusion pressure measured by:
   a. Laser Doppler measurement
   b. Photoelectric measurement
4. Thermographic measurement of skin temperature
5. Measurement of transcutaneous oxygen tension
6. Measurement of transcutaneous carbon dioxide tension
7. Common peroneal motor nerve conduction velocity
8. Vibration perception threshold
9. Traditional radiography
10. Pulse volume recordings (Bacharach, 2001; Carrington et al., 2001; Durham, 2000; Gibson, 2001; Muir, 2009; Nehler et al., 2003; Wehmer & Jones, 2014; Zgonis et al., 2008)

B. Invasive Test Include:

1. Fluorescein dye measurements
2. Isotope measurements of:
   a. Skin perfusion pressures
   b. Skin blood flow
3. Bone scan
4. 24-hour leukocyte scan
5. Angiography to determine possibility of limb salvage through revascularization
6. Computerized tomography (CT)
7. Magnetic resonance imaging (MRI)
8. MRI with angiography (Bacharach, 2001; Durham, 2000, MacVittie, 1998; Muir, 2009; Wehmer & Jones, 2014; Zgonis et al., 2008)

C. Laboratory Tests Include:

1. Complete blood count with differential
2. Metabolic panel
3. Sedimentation rate
4. C-reactive protein (Wehmer & Jones, 2014; Zgonis et al., 2008)

V. Medical/Surgical Management.

Revascularization for nontraumatic distal extremity disease is the first choice when applicable. Bypass to plantar arteries is not only feasible but may result in prolonged patency and limb salvage. Approximately 14% to 20% of persons with critical lower limb ischemia are not suited for reconstruction due to occluded crural and pedal arteries, which results in amputation (Keshelava et al., 2009; Roddy et al., 2001). Revascularization may be inappropriate in some cases such as in persons who are wheelchair bound, neurologically impaired, or have extremely limited life expectancy (Abou-Zamzam et al., 2003).

A. Medical Management Before Amputation

1. Smoking cessation as early before surgery as possible until healing is complete
2. Control of diabetes using sliding scale insulin as necessary
3. Control of hypertension
4. Control of pain
   a. Prolonged pain may result in poor nutrition.
   b. There is some evidence that preamputation pain increases the risk for phantom limb pain.
5. Treatment of infection
   a. It can be difficult to distinguish between colonization of exposed tissue and infection.
   b. A surface culture on an undebrided ulcer may demonstrate only skin bacteria.
   c. Culture of tissue should be done following sterile debridement with bone curetting if indicated.
   d. Empiric antibiotics should be initiated until culture and sensitivities are available (Attinger et al., 2002; Bacharach, 2001; Bloomquist, 2001; Datta, 2001; Deery & Sangeorzan, 2001; Gibson, 2001; Lawson, 2005; MacVittie, 1998; Zgonis et al., 2008).

B. Indications for Amputation

1. Severe, acute ischemia secondary to unreconstructable arterial disease or failed revascularization.
2. Irreversible tissue compromises secondary to acute and prolonged ischemia.
3. Chronic ischemia resulting in rest pain, gangrene, nonhealing skin lesions, and osteomyelitis or tissue infection unresponsive to aggressive wound care and antibiotics.
4. Massive muscle necrosis.
5. Phlegmasia cerulea dolens—rare.
6. Nonvascular intractable pain—rare (Durham, 2000; Helt & Jacobsen, 1999; Honkamp, Amendola, Hurwitz, & Saltzman, 2001).

C. Selection of Level of Amputation. Clinical judgment and diagnostic testing are used in the determination of the level of amputation. The goal of level selection is to identify the most distal site at which the amputation will reliably heal and also yield a stump that may be readily fitted with a prosthesis. Major amputation increases the energy of ambulation by 10% to 40% for below-knee amputations, 50% to 70% for above-knee amputation, and 60% if ambulating on crutches without a prosthesis (Attinger et al., 2002; Durham, 2000). Persons with a more proximal amputation seem to have more functional impairment than those with a more distal amputation (Amputation and Amputation Surgery, 2011; Peters et al., 2001; Wehmer & Jones, 2014).

D. Techniques

1. General principles of amputation include:
   a. Choosing a site after demarcation
   b. Debridement of nonviable tissue
   c. Appropriate use of antibiotics
   d. Gentle handling of tissues
   e. Preservation of all blood supply
   f. Avoidance of hematoma formation through hemostasis
   g. Approximation of skin edges and shaping of incision to promote a smooth stump to decrease prosthesis irritation
   h. Limitation of tension on sutures (Durham, 2000; Helt & Jacobsen, 1999)
2. Surgical approaches include:
   a. Open amputation, generally utilized for trauma or majorly infected tissue; the wound is packed and traction is applied to flaps to prevent skin and muscle retraction. A guillotine amputation also may be done in which all tissues are cut at the same level. Both techniques allow for drainage and observation of tissue but require a second surgical procedure for closure.
   b. Closed amputation is the most commonly used technique. The incision is made through healthy tissue and skin flaps are shaped for primary closure.
   c. Nonsurgical amputation or autoamputation. Usually reserved for small, well-demarcated areas, such as a toe. If the gangrenous limb does not become secondarily infected it is allowed to demarcate, mummify, and eventually fall off. The mummified limb will not separate until healing occurs at the line of demarcation.
   d. Above-knee amputation. A fish-mouth incision is used creating equal anterior and posterior flaps. The soft tissues are elevated from the femur and retracted allowing the bone to be divided and smoothed. Ligation and division of the nerves are performed with gentle traction on the nerve so that the nerve remnant will retract well into the thigh. Blood vessels are ligated carefully. The skin and deep fascia are drawn distally and the incision primarily closed. A drain may or may not be used. The sutures are placed loosely to allow for expansion of edema (see Fig. 25-1).
   e. Below-knee amputation. A long posterior myocutaneous flap is fashioned from the calf muscles. The tibia is divided in the upper third section and the front edge is beveled at a 45- to 60-degree angle. The fibula

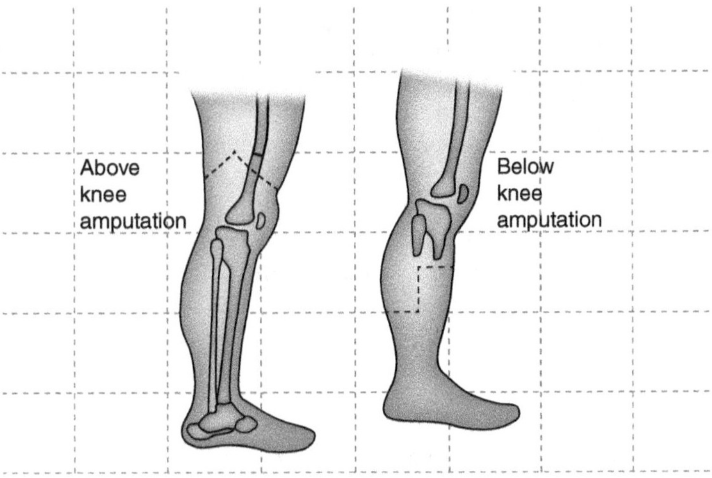

FIGURE 25-1. Levels of amputation.

is divided one half to 1 in shorter than the tibia. Both bones are filed smooth. The flap is brought anterior for closure creating a pad for the bone and a rich blood supply to the incision. The remaining tissues are handled in the same matter as for an above-knee amputation (see Fig. 25-1) (Durham, 2000; Helt & Jacobsen, 1999).

f. To achieve the best fit for a functional prosthesis the bone must extend 22 to 28 cm below the tip of the greater trochanter or 12 to 15 cm above the knee joint for above-knee amputation and extend 11 to 15 cm below the patella for a below-knee amputation (see Fig. 25-1) (Amputation and Amputation Surgery, 2011; Gibson, 2001).

g. Distal infections may heal with a more limited amputation such as:
   1) Symes amputation—through the ankle joint that retains the fatty heel pad for weight bearing
   2) Transmetatarsal amputation
   3) Toe or Ray amputation—resection of the toe(s) and part of the metatarsal (see Fig. 25-2) (Wehmer & Jones, 2014; Zgonis et al., 2008)

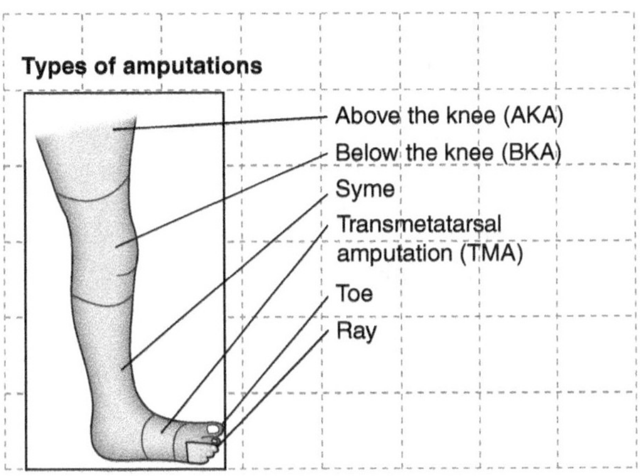

FIGURE 25-2. Types of amputations.

E. Complications

1. General complications of amputation include:
   a. Death
   b. Stump trauma
   c. Swelling
   d. Deep vein thrombosis
   e. Decubitus heel ulcers
   f. Decubitus sacral ulcers
   g. Bone erosion
   h. Chest infection
   i. Angina
   j. Myocardial infarction
   k. Stroke (Amputation and Amputation Surgery, 2011)
2. Early complications include:
   a. Excessive pain
   b. Infection
   c. Poor wound healing
   d. Flexion contractures
   e. Inadequate or insufficient muscle stabilization causing a stump with too much bone prominence, too flabby, or loss of control
3. Late complications include:
   a. Stump congestion secondary to a poor fitting prosthetic socket
   b. Bulbous stump may complicate prosthesis fitting causing pressure and skin breakdown
   c. Calluses and cysts
   d. Neuroma
   e. Bone spurs
   f. Osteoporosis
   g. Bone overgrowth
   h. Adherent scar

VI. Nursing Management

A. Preoperative. Nursing care should include maintaining fluid balance and nutrition, infection control, avoidance of trauma, preservation of mobility, and prevention of venous thrombosis. The nurse also should help the patient understand the need for amputation, the proposed surgery, pain control methods, rehabilitation plans, and individual goals. Pain control is essential to help the patient rest and be as comfortable as possible. The use of a bed cradle and foam pads may help relieve pain from pressure of blankets. There is a phenomenon called pain memory that suggests phantom sensations felt postoperatively may mimic the pain felt before surgery making preamputation pain control a priority. There is evidence that relief of pain for approximately 72 hours prior to amputation may reduce the frequency and intensity of postamputation phantom pains. Medications such as calcitonin and ketamine have some promise in preventing phantom pain (Bloomquist, 2001; Bryant, 2001; Datta, 2001; Gibson, 2001; Helt & Jacobsen, 1999; Wehmer & Jones, 2014)

B. Postoperative (see Table 25-2)

TABLE 25-2 Postamputation Nursing Interventions

Nursing Diagnosis	Expected Patient Outcome	Interventions	Evaluation
Potential for infection related to ischemia, preoperative infection, incision	Remain free of infection	Assess for signs and symptoms of infection Locally or systemically	No signs or symptoms of infection
Alteration in nutrition related to ischemia, pain, increased energy needs	Maintain weight	Control pain, offer favorite foods, drinks, and protein snacks when able	Weight is maintained. Prealbumin is in normal range
Potential for blood loss related to amputation	Remain free of excessive drainage from incision	Monitor dressing for drainage, outline any drainage noted, reinforce dressing as needed, avoid bumping limb, have a tourniquet near in the event of excessive bleeding	Hemoglobin will be within 1 g/dL of preoperative Hgb, no hematoma formation
Potential alteration in tissue perfusion related to ischemia	Maintain tissue perfusion	Monitor for cool skin, tingling, pallor, poor capillary refill, petechiae, cyanosis at incision line, mottling of limb	Incision remains intact, warm, appropriate in color with brisk capillary refill
Potential for muscle contraction related to amputation	Remain free of muscle contractures	Avoid using pillows under hips and limb stump or bending knee gatch. Have patient lie prone several times a day for 20 min. Position legs close together to avoid hip adduction	Hip and limb remain mobile without contractures
Potential alteration in skin integrity related to bedrest, loss of limb	Skin will remain intact	Compare postoperative risk assessment to preoperative assessment noting specific changes. Utilize trapeze for position change. Elevate nonoperative heel off bed. Utilize pressure-relieving mattress as indicated, reposition every 2 hrs	Skin is intact
Potential alteration in fluid balance related to trauma of amputation	Maintain fluid balance	Do not allow the patient to sit for more than 1 hr, change position every 2 hrs. Avoid a dependent stump position, utilize compression dressing per surgeon's order	Limb is free of edema

TABLE 25-2 Postamputation Nursing Interventions (continued)

Nursing Diagnosis	Expected Patient Outcome	Interventions	Evaluation
Alteration in comfort related to amputation, ischemia, and preoperative pain	Pain will be controlled or relieved	Ask patient to indicate the location and intensity of pain. Each type of pain may require a different therapy. Pain may be: 1. Incisional-controlled with methadone epidural infusion, patient-controlled analgesia pump, or intermittent opiate analgesia. 2. Coexisting musculoskeletal pain from performing activities without one limb and guarding the residual limb from injury-controlled with nonsteroidal anti-inflammatory drugs (NSAIDs), heat, cold, and the meds used for incisional pain. 3. Phantom pain—it is important to acknowledge that phantom pain is real. The incidence of phantom pain increases with age of amputee. Analgesics are seldom effective for pain relief. Medications for relief include NSAIDs, local anesthetics, steroid injections, beta-blockers, anticonvulsants, baclofen, antidepressants, and capsaicin cream. Alternative modalities include anxiety relief; early exercising; desensitizing the stump by massage, finger tapping, ultrasound, hot and cold contrasting baths; acupuncture, hypnosis, biofeedback, therapeutic touch, distraction, massage, meditation, transcutaneous electrical nerve stimulation; proper stump wrapping. Surgical alternatives may be considered but have little success and include sympathectomy, cordotomy, neuroma excision, deep brain, and spinal stimulation	Report of ≤3 on a 1–10 scale

Bloomquist (2001); Bryant (2001); Datta (2001); Gibson (2001); Helt & Jacobsen (1999); Ketz (2008); MacVittie (1998); Marshall et al. (2002); Mayo Clinic Phantom Pain (2011); Wehmer & Jones, 2014.

C. Nursing Management—Rehabilitation

1. The likelihood of achieving a successful prosthetic fitting in the geriatric population is poor, especially in persons greater than 85 years old. Preoperative mobility, age >70 years; comorbidities such as renal and cardiac diseases or dementia make it unlikely a person will walk after amputation. Extreme frailty, severe cardiorespiratory disease, severe dementia, fixed flexion contractures, and severe arthritis are absolute contraindications to prosthetic rehabilitation (Amputation and Amputation Surgery, 2011; Datta, 2001; Fletcher et al., 2002).
2. Rehabilitation is an action-oriented process involving an interdisciplinary team consisting of a surgeon, physiatrist, physical therapist, nurses, amputee volunteers, prosthetist, nutritionist, social worker, patient, and the patient's significant others. Rehabilitation begins preoperatively with the focus on maintaining mobility of unaffected limbs, preventative care for the unaffected limb, general conditioning exercises to improve strength along with cardiac and respiratory reserves, psychosocial assessment.
3. Postoperative rehabilitation begins in the acute care setting and continues through outpatient or at home therapies (Datta, 2001; Helt & Jacobsen, 1999) (see Table 25-3).

TABLE 25-3 Postamputation Rehabilitation

Nursing Diagnosis	Expected Patient Outcome	Inervention	Evaluation
Alteration in balance related to removal of limb, altered sense of gravity, phantom pain sensation	Maintain balance	Transfer and get up slowly to reduce risk for falls, especially at night. Provide proper lighting for transfers and walking	No falls noted
Alteration in fluid balance related to trauma of amputation	Maintain fluid balance	See Table 25-2. Use ace wraps over dressing for compression. When incision is healed, surgeon may switch to a stump shrinker sock with graduated pressure to help shrink and shape it for fitting in a prosthesis. Be sure there are no wrinkles in ace wrap or shrinker sock	Limb is free of edema
Potential alteration in skin integrity related to loss of limb	Skin will remain intact	See Table 25-2. Avoid use of lotion or oils on stump as they may cause folliculitis with prosthesis use. Assess for proper footwear to protect other limb from increased pressure and damage from wheelchair or crutch use. Massage skin of thigh toward incision line and after healed-over incision to prevent adherence of underlying tissue to the skin, which could tear when prosthesis is worn. Frequent assessment of skin is necessary especially when using an early walking aid and prosthesis	Skin and incision are intact Patient is able to demonstrate wound care and care of unaffected limb

TABLE 25-3 Postamputation Rehabilitation (continued)

Nursing Diagnosis	Expected Patient Outcome	Inervention	Evaluation
Alteration in body image related to amputation	Patient will have a positive body image	Be aware of the phases of grieving, reassure patient their reaction is normal. Be sensitive to patient's desire not to see stump initially. Be aware that body image affects a patient's expression of sexuality and he or she may want to discuss this. Assess for signs of prolonged depression and use antidepressants as ordered	Patient is motivated and participates in care and therapies
Alteration in comfort related to amputation	Pain will be controlled or relieved	See Table 25-2. Antidepressants are helpful for chronic pain. Utilizing massage, finger tapping helps decrease pain and psychologically accept stump. Optimizing prosthetics can minimize dysfunctional posture and secondary stress and improve psychological feelings	Report of ≤3 on a 1–10 scale
Alteration in mobility related to amputation	Patient will be as independent in mobility as they are able	Physical therapy begins postoperative day 1–2 with exercises for bed mobility, joint movements, and transferring. Between days 3 and 5 stump exercises, muscle strengthening and ROM, sitting balance and general cardiovascular exercises. As soon as there is surgical clearance the patient is fitted with an early walking aid, a type of temporary prostheses that allows for stump desensitization; improved standing and walking balance, reduces edema, and provides a morale boost. When the incision is healed, at 6 to 8 wks the stump can be measured for the first prosthesis. It is important to work with a prosthetist that the patient likes. There are many styles of prosthesis to fit the patient's mobility goals. Physical therapy continues until the patient is safely walking with the prosthesis. Before discharge equipment needs are identified and procured such as crutches, wheelchair, shower-tub bench, and hand-held shower, safety bars, and hand rails. Refer patient to DMV for handicapped parking permit and validation of license as indicated. Continue with outpatient physical therapy and home nursing care as needed	Patient is safely ambulating with prosthesis and assistive devices as needed

Bloomquist (2001); Bryant (2001); Datta (2001); Gibson (2001); Helt & Jacobsen (1999); Mayo Clinic Phantom Pain (2011); Wehmer & Jones, 2014.

VII. Patient Teaching

A. **Disease Prevention** should be encouraged through lifestyle changes, including smoking cessation, control of hyperlipidemia and hyperglycemia, and care of the unaffected limb. To encourage therapy at home, pictures of exercises and skin care procedures; high-protein, high-carbohydrate menus;

and a list of resources should be provided. Instruct patients to call their physicians if they notice cracks, blisters, sores, rashes, redness, increased stump pain, increased skin temperature, or odor (Bryant, 2001; Gibson, 2001). Refer to chapter 22 Diabetic Foot Management for foot care guidelines.

B. **Home Care Considerations** include wound care, maintenance of nutritional status with increased energy needs, and the ongoing process of being correctly fitted with a prosthesis. Patients should be aware of the psychological changes that may occur. Patients may experience a loss of control, self-esteem, potential income loss, and social and leisure losses. Patients also should know that although one chronic wound has been eliminated, there are many remaining issues, such as skin care and pain control that need their continued diligence to minimize effects. Evaluate home environment for safety issues such as rugs on floors that can lead to tripping, choice of shoes to avoid slipping, having a chair available when in the bathroom, shower, or dressing area to assist with balance and fatigue issues. Having personal items within easy reach can prevent falls from reaching. Do not rush persons learning to ambulate. Plan ahead to help achieve successful activities. The National Amputee Foundation has Tips for the New Amputee Their Families and Friends (http://www.nationalamputation.org) that provides helpful information for amputees from amputees. Amputee support groups can provide general reassurance and practical advice for prosthesis and stump care (Bloomquist, 2001; Fitzgerald, 2000; Gibson, 2001; Mayo Clinic Phantom pain, 2011; Wehmer & Jones, 2014).

CASE STUDY

A 67-year-old African-American man presents with an open wound on his right heal: he denies injury or history of edema. The wound has been present for approximately 3 weeks. He has been using an antibiotic ointment and adhesive bandage over it, but it continues to get larger. He also states he has had increased urination and thirst. His past medical history includes hypertension and smoking. He has not seen a physician for 5 years.

Review Questions

1. What interventions need to be done to heal this wound and prevent the need for amputation?
   a. Continue antibiotic ointment with wrapped bandage and limit walking
   b. Change to saline wet-to-dry dressing changes and encourage him to quit smoking
   c. Assess arterial perfusion and serum glucose, use antibiotics as appropriate, debride wound if necessary, and off-load ulcer
   d. Continue antibiotic ointment and bandage, control hypertension, and encourage smoking cessation
2. Which of the following would not be a common diagnosis related to this nonhealing wound?
   a. Peripheral artery disease
   b. Peripheral neuropathy
   c. Venous stasis ulcer
   d. Diabetic foot ulcer

3. Which of the following is not a possible indication for amputation?
   a. Osteomyelitis
   b. Recurrent venous ulcers with intolerance to compression therapy
   c. Acute ischemia secondary to unreconstructable arterial disease or failed revascularization
   d. Chronic ischemia resulting in rest pain

Answers/Rationales

1. c. Interventions used for arterial wound healing include assessing arterial perfusion with revascularization if indicated; use of appropriate antibiotics; control of hypertension, dyslipidemia, and hyperglycemia; and aggressive wound care, including off-loading of the ulcer (Calle-Pascual et al., 2001; Deery & Sangeorzan, 2001; Muir, 2009; Watts et al., 2001; Zgonis et al., 2008).
2. c. The three most common diagnosis related to nonhealing wounds are peripheral artery disease, diabetic foot ulceration, and peripheral neuropathy (Gibson, 2001).
3. b. Indications for amputation include: severe, acute ischemia secondary to unreconstructable arterial disease or failed revascularization; irreversible tissue compromise secondary to acute and prolonged ischemia; chronic ischemia resulting in rest pain, gangrene, nonhealing skin lesions; and osteomyelitis or tissue infection unresponsive to aggressive wound care and antibiotics (Durham, 2000; Helt & Jacobsen, 1999; Keshelava et al., 2009).

REFERENCES

Abou-Zamzam, A. M. Jr, Teruya, T. H., Killeen, J. D., & Ballard, J. L. (2003). Major lower extremity amputation in an academic vascular center. *Annals of Vascular Surgery, 17*, 86–90.

Amputation and Amputation Surgery. (2011). www.vascular.co.nz. Retrieved from http://www.vascular.co.nz/Amputation%20surgery.hym, accessed March 26, 2011.

Attinger, C. E., Ducic, I., Neville, R. F., Abbruzzese, M. R., Gomes, M., & Sidawy, A. N. (2002). The relative roles of aggressive wound care versus revascularization in salvage of the threatened lower extremity in the renal failure diabetic patient. *Plastic and Reconstructive Surgery, 109*, 1281–1289.

Bacharach, J. M. (2001). Severe occlusive peripheral arterial disease and critical limb ischemia. Part II amputation. In A. T. Hirsch (Ed.), *Primary care series: Peripheral arterial disease and intermittent claudication* (pp. 68–71). New York, MA: Excerpta Medica.

Bloomquist, T. (2001). Amputation and phantom limb pain: A pain-prevention model. *American Academy of Nurse Anesthetists Journal, 69*(3), 211–217.

Bryant, G. (2001). Stump care. *American Journal of Nursing, 101*, 67–71.

Calle-Pascual, A. L., Garcia-Torre, N., Moraga, I., Diaz, J. A., Duran, A., Monux, G., . . . Maranes, J. D. (2001). Epidemiology of Nontraumatic Lower-Extremity Amputation in Area 7, Madrid, Between 1989 and 1999: A population-based study. *Diabetes Care, 24*, 1686–1689.

Carrington, A. L., Abbott, C. A., Griffiths, J., Jackson, N., Johnson, S. R., Kulkarni, J., . . . Boulton, A. J. (2001). A foot care program for diabetic unilateral lower-limb amputees. *Diabetes Care, 24*, 216–221.

Complications of Diabetes in the United States. (2011). National diabetes fact sheet 2011. Center for disease control web site. Retrieved from http://www.cdc.gov/diabetes/pubs/pdf/ndfs-2011.pdf, accessed March 26, 2011.

Datta, D. (2001). Amputation, rehabilitation and prosthetic developments. In J. Beard & P. A. Gaines (Eds.), *Vascular and endovascular surgery* (pp. 89–102). London, UK: W. B. Saunders Company Limited.

Deery, H. G., & Sangeorzan, J. A. (2001). Saving the diabetic foot with special reference to the patient with chronic renal failure. *Infectious Disease Clinics of North America, 15*, 953–981.

Durham, J. R. (2000). Lower extremity amputation levels: Indications, determining the appropriate level, technique, and prognosis. In R. B. Rutherford (Ed.), *Vascular surgery* (pp. 2185–2213). Philadelphia, PA: W. B. Saunders Company.

Fitzgerald, D. M. (2000). Peer visitation for the preoperative amputee patient. *Journal of Vascular Nursing, 18*, 41–44.

Fletcher, D. D., Andrews, K. L., Hallett, J. W. Jr., Butters, M. A., Rowland, C. M., & Jacobsen, S. J. (2002). Trends in rehabilitation after amputation for geriatric patients with vascular disease: Implication for future health resource allocation. *Archives of Physical Medicine & Rehabilitation, 83*, 1389–1393.

Gibson, J. (2001). Lower limb amputation. *Nursing Standard, 15*, 47–52.

Helt, J., & Jacobsen, J. (1999). Amputation in the vascular patient. In V. A. Fahey (Ed.), *Vascular nursing* (3rd ed., pp. 416–444). Philadelphia, PA: W. B. Saunders Company.

Honkamp, N., Amendola, A., Hurwitz, S., & Saltzman, C. L. (2001). Retrospective review of eighteen patients who underwent transtibial amputation for intractable pain. *The Journal of Bone & Joint Surgery, 83-A*(10), 1479–1483.

Keshelava, G., Gigilashvili, K., Chkholaria, A., Pagava, G., Janashia, G., & Beselia, K. (2009). Foot venous system arterialization for salvage of non-reconstructable acute ischemic limb: A case report. *Journal of Vascular Nursing, 27*, 13–16.

Ketz, A. K. (2008). Pain management in the traumatic amputee. *Crtical Care Nursing Clinics of North America, 20*, 51–57.

Krapfl, H., Gohdes, D., & Burrows, N. R. (2003). Lower extremity amputation episodes among persons with diabetes New Mexico, 2000. *Journal of the American Medical Association, 289*, 1502–1503.

Krupski, W. C. (2000). Overview of extremity amputations. In R. B. Rutherford (Ed.), *Vascular surgery* (pp. 2175–2180). Philadelphia, PA: W. B. Saunders Company.

Lawson, G. (2005). The importance of obtaining ankle-brachial indexes in older adults: The other vital sign. *Journal of Vascular Nursing, 23*, 46–51.

Leggetter, S., Chaturvedi, N., Fuller, J. H., & Edmonds, M. E. (2002). Ethnicity and risk of diabetes-related lower extremity amputation. *Archives of Internal Medicine, 162*, 73–78.

MacVittie, B. A. (1998). *Vascular surgery*. St. Louis, MO: Mosby.

Marks, L. J., & Michael, J. W. (2001). Science, medicine, and the future: Artificial limbs. *British Medical Journal, 323*, 732–735.

Marshall, H. M., Jensen, M. P., Ehde, D. M., & Campbell, K. M. (2002). Pain site and impairment in individuals with amputation pain. *Archives of Physical Medicine & Rehabilitation, 83*, 1116–1119.

Mayo Clinic. Phantom pain. (2011). Mayo Clinic Web site. Retrieved from http://www.mayoclinic.org/diseases-conditions/phantom-pain/basics/lifestyle-home-remedies/con-20023268. Accessed 5-22-14.

Muir, R. L. (2009). Peripheral arterial disease: Pathophysiology, risk factors, diagnosis, treatment, and prevention. *Journal of Vascular Nursing, 27*, 26–30.

Munro, R. (2001). Time to limber up. *Nursing Times, 97*(26), 14–15.

Nehler, M. R., Hiatt, W. R., & Taylor, L. M., Jr. (2003). Is revascularization and limb salvage always the best treatment for critical limb ischemia? *Journal of Vascular Surgery, 37*, 704–708.

Peters, E. J., Childs, M. R., Wunderlich, R. P., Harkless, L. B., Armstrong, D. G., & Lavery, L. A. (2001). Functional status of persons with diabetes-related lower extremity amputations. *Diabetes Care, 24*(10), 1799–1804.

Roddy, S. P., Darling, R., III, Chang, B. B., Kreienberg, P. B., Paty, P. S., Lloyd, W. E., & Shah, D. M. (2001). Outcomes with plantar bypass for limb-threatening ischemia. *Annals of Vascular Surgery, 15*(1), 789–783.

Spollett, G. R. (2006). Diabetic neuropathies: Diagnosis and treatment. *Nursing Clinics of North America, 41*, 697–717.

Tips for the new amputee and their families and friends. (2011). National Amputation Foundation Web site. Retrieved from http://www.nationalamputation.org./, accessed March 26, 2011.

Watts, S. A., Daly, B., Anthony, M., McDonald, P., Khoury, A., & Dahar, W. (2001). The effect of age, gender, risk level and glycosylated hemoglobin in predicting foot amputation in HMO patients with diabetes. *Journal of the American Academy of Nurse Practitioners, 13*, 230–235.

Wehmer, M. A. & Jones, D.C. (2014). Amputation: Helping patients successfully recover from surgery. *Mosby Nursing Consult-Clinical Updates Web site*. Retrieved from http://www.nursingconsult.com, accessed May 23, 2014.

Zgonis, T., Stapleton, J. J., Girard-Powell, V. A., & Hagino, R. T. (2008). Sugical management of diabetic foot infections and amputations. *Association of Operating Room Nurses Journal, 87*(5), 935–946.

Zgonis, T., Stapleton, J. J., Jeffries, L. C., Girard-Powell, V. A., & Foster, L. J. (2008). Surgical treatment of charcot neuroarthropathy. *Association of Operating Room Nurses Journal, 87*(5), 971–986.

RELEVANT WEBSITES

www.nationalamputation.org
www.nlm.nih.gov/medlineplus/ency/article/000006.htm
www.mossresourcenet.org/amputa.htm
www.disabilityresources.org/AMPUTATION.html
http://ndep.nih.gov/materials/pubs/feet/feet.htm
http://www.amputee-coalition.org

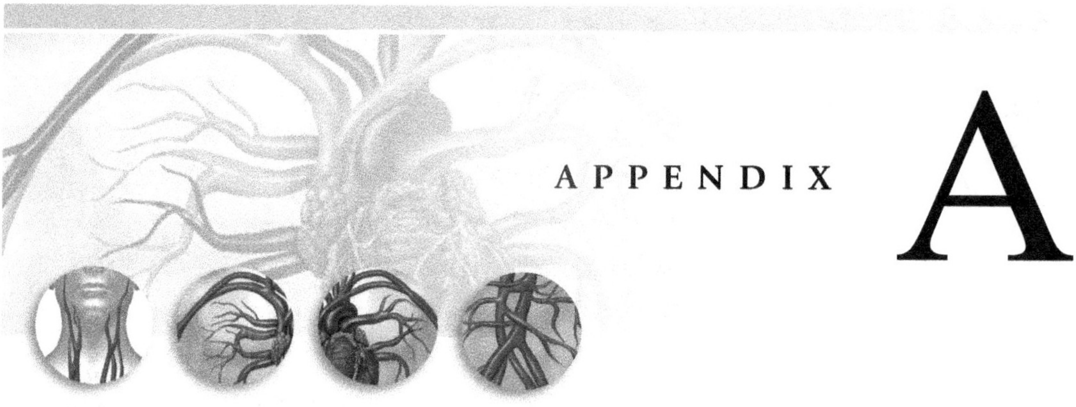

APPENDIX A

Overview of Topical Wound Treatments

Virginia Capasso
Christine M. Pontuso

Classification	Indication	Description	Advantages	Precautions
Debriding Agents				
Santyl (Healthpoint) (Alvarez et al., 2002; Shi & Carson, 2009; Smith, 2008)	Debridement of yellow fibrinous tissue	Ointment containing collagenase	Hastens removal of necrotic tissue; does not injure healthy tissue	– Requires cross-hatching to penetrate black eschar – Mupirocin can be mixed with Santyl
Medi-honey (DermaSciences) (C. Liscio, personal communication, August 3, 2013)	Debridement of black or yellow necrotic tissue	Gel of manuka honey which rehydrates and loosens necrotic tissue (autolytic debridement); osmotic effect replenishes *plasminogen* at wound surface, where it is converted to active plasmin which breaks the adhesion of necrotic tissue	Inexpensive	Osmotic effect can produce a large amount of exudate which requires absorbent secondary dressing to avoid periwound maceration
Antimicrobial Dressings				
Moisture-donating				
Example: Medi-honey (DermaSciences) (Biglari et al., 2012; Lusby, Coombes, & Wilkinson, 2005; Robson, Dodd, & Thomas, 2009)	Broad spectrum antimicrobial	Low water activity does not support growth of bacteria and fungi; glucose oxidase produces gluconic oxidase and H_2O_2; acidic pH, 3.9	Multiple modes of action may reduce bacterial resistance	As osmotic effect dilutes gel, may become bacterial food, malodorous and messy

(continued)

Classification	Indication	Description	Advantages	Precautions
Gel with ionic silver				
Examples: SilvaSorb (Medline) (Gago et al., 2008; Heggers et al., 2005; Tkachenko & Karas, 2012; Widgerow, 2011)	Partial- and full-thickness wounds, including pressure ulcers, leg ulcers, diabetic foot ulcers, graft wounds and donor sites, first- and second-degree burns, surgical wounds, skin tears, lacerations, and abrasions	Microlattice hydrogel matrix containing silver chloride	– Releases silver at a controlled level for broad spectrum antimicrobial action – Maintains moist environment; hydrogel matrix may hold significant amount of wound exudate	Allergy to metals, specifically silver
Absorbent cadexomer Iodine				
Examples: Iodoflex/ Iodosorb (Smith & Nephew) (Chow, Lemos, & Einarson, 2008; O'Meara, Al-Kurdi, Ologun, & Ovington, 2010; Ubbink, Westerbos, Evans, Land, & Vermeulen, 2008)	Wounds with moderate to heavy exudate and/or requiring antimicrobial dressings (e.g., venous stasis ulcers)	Iodinated (0.9%) paste absorbs 6 mL of exudate per gram of paste used. Bonded iodine is bactericidal for staphylococcus, including methicillin-resistant *Staphylococcus aureus* (MRSA), streptococcus, and pseudomonas	Reduces or eliminates odor	– Allergy to iodine, shellfish, contrast medium – Hyperthyroidism is relative contraindication
Alginate or fiber with ionic silver				
Examples: Silvercel (Systagenix), Acticoat Absorbent (Smith & Nephew) Aquacel Ag (Convatec) (Bell & Hart, 2007; Castellano et al., 2007)	Lightly to moderately exuding acute and chronic wounds which are at risk of infection	While fiber absorbs exudate and traps bacteria, silver ions are released from sodium carboxymethylcellulose (Aquacel) or sterilized brown seaweed (calcium alginate), exerting a sustained antimicrobial effect against a wide range of organisms thus preventing colonization of the dressing and providing an antimicrobial barrier to protect the wound	When compared to standard care, silver dressings may reduce wound size, odor, pain	Avoid concurrent use of petroleum-based products which bind silver and make it unavailable to the wound

Classification	Indication	Description	Advantages	Precautions
Moisture-donating Dressings				
Wet-to-wet gauze dressings (Hackl et al., 2013; Milne, Hagan, & Ciccarelli, 2007; Spear, 2008; Svensjo, Pomahac, Yao, Slama, & Eriksson, 2000)	Primary or secondary dressings for a dry wound bed with minimal exudate	Usually a loosely woven unfilled 100% cotton fabric, which is dampened with normal saline, then covered with a dry/or, wet gauze dressing depending on the amount of moisture in the wound bed. Gauze is packaged as both sterile and nonsterile	Option for inexpensive dressing supplies that protects and mechanically debrides the wound bed by lifting necrotic tissue and bacteria; promotes new tissue growth by increasing moisture in the wound; absorbs wound exudate; prevents early wound closure	Requires frequent dressing changes to prevent periwound maceration thus may be time-consuming, making compliance low If cut, loosely woven fabric may shed lint in wound
Nonadherent gauze dressings				
Examples: Oil of emulsion (Curad) Xeroform (Kendall) Adaptic/Adaptic Touch (Systagenix) (Case Study Series, 2013; Coviden Product Information, 2012; Malpass, Snelling, & Tron, 2003; Terrill & Varughese, 2000; Vogt, Uhlyarik, & Schroeder, 2007)	Used to protect delicate or fragile tissue with no exudate to moderate exudate	Petroleum-based gauze or mesh to protect delicate tissue	Improves dry periwound skin and helps provide a moist wound environment. Prevents skin tears when removing old dressings	Do not use with silver as petroleum will bind silver and make it unavailable. Important: Xeroform may contain povidone iodine contraindicated in patients allergic to iodine
Amorphous hydrogel				
Examples: Curasol (Healthpoint) (Capasso & Munro, 2003; Cohn et al., 2004; Dumville, O'Meara, Deshpande, & Speak, 2013)	– Dry, desiccated wound bed – Minimal to small amount of exudate	Clear, viscous wound gel	Provides moisture to a dry wound bed increasing availability of enzymes and growth factors that promote debridement and cell growth	Important to balance amount of hydrogel and dressing change frequency in order to promote healing and avoid periwound maceration May relieve or increase pain depending on type of wound and formulation of gel

(continued)

Classification	Indication	Description	Advantages	Precautions
Moisture-absorbing Dressings				
Wound fiber				
Example: Aquacel (Convatec) (Kunugiza, Tomita, Moritomo, & Yoshikawa, 2010; Williams, 1999)	For acute or chronic wounds that have minimal to moderate exudate	Sterile, nonwoven absorbent pad or ribbon dressing composed of sodium carboxymethylcellulose	Absorbs drainage and bacteria from wound bed to form a gel substance that conforms to the wound bed and promotes a moist environment to enhance cell growth	Important to evaluate amount of exudate and balance with dressing, change frequency to prevent periwound maceration
Example: Mesalt (Molnlycke) (Molnlycke Health Care Products, 2003; Upright, Salton, Roberts, & Murphy, 1994)	For acute or chronic wounds with heavy exudate and/or infection, beefy red wound bed, with or without softened yellow fibrinous tissue	Sterile, nonwoven absorbent pad or ribbon dressing containing 15% (hypertonic) sodium chloride	Absorbs and stimulates exudate production to promote desloughing. The hypertonic dressing may create a nonspecific bactericidal environment	May cause pain in superficial wounds due to the hypertonic NaCl Also, with prolonged use, may cause bleeding due to inflammatory response
Alginates				
Example: Curasorb (Kendall) (Dumville, O'Meara, Deshpande, & Speak, 2012; Hindhede & Meuleneire, 2012; Faucher, Safar, Baret, Philippe, & Farid, 2012; Sweeny, Miraftab, & Collver, 2012; Verall, Coulborn, & Bree-Aslan, 2010)	For moderate to heavy exudate, beefy red wound bed, with or without softened fibrinous tissue	Alginate is sterilized brown seaweed that has been formed into a fibrous nonwoven pad or ribbon to absorb wound exudate	Absorbs wound exudate to prevent periwound maceration. Once fluid is absorbed, fibrous dressing transforms to a gel that autolysis the necrotic tissue in the wound bed	Patients may complain of odor since it has no bactericidal properties, and additional odor controlling dressings (e.g., Carboflex) or odor controlling gel (e.g., metronidazole gel) may need to be added
Foam				
Example: Mepilex (Molnlycke) (Banks, Bale, Harding, & Harding, 1997; Tsao, Lo, Harmod, & Lee, 2013; Vanscheidt, Sibbald, & Eager, 2004)	For red, superficial wounds with moderate to heavy wound exudate, such as venous stasis ulcers	Polyurethane foam that protects and absorbs	Prevents skin tears and breakdown around wound margin, absorbs wound fluid in an absorbent pad in the center, maintains a moist environment. Comfortable for patients to wear and easy to use	Hypersensitivity to silicone

Classification	Indication	Description	Advantages	Precautions
Secondary Dressings				
Gauze (Cowan & Stechmiller, 2009; Rippon, Davies, & White, 2012)	Used as a primary or secondary dressing for wounds with minimal exudate	Sterile or nonsterile, 100% loosely woven cotton fabric pad	Wicks away fluid from wound bed and absorbs fluid into dressing	Requires frequent dressing changes to prevent periwound maceration. When cut, loosely woven fabric may shed lint
Transparent occlusive film/vapor-permeable dressing Example: Tegaderm (3M) (Cosker, Elsaved, Gupta, Mendonca, & Tayton, 2005; Ravenscoft, Harker, & Buch, 2006)	Used as a primary dressing for stage I pressure ulcers, IV sites, skin tears, and as a secondary dressing for wounds with no exudate to minimal exudate	Secondary, transparent occlusive dressing that helps protect wound/skin and prevent skin tears	Provides an impermeable barrier to outside contamination by fluid or bacteria; facilitates autolysis by providing a moist environment	Contraindicated in third-degree burns
Hydrocolloid dressings				
Examples: Duoderm (Convatec) (Cuschieri, Debos, Miller, & Celis, 2013; Lisle, 2002)	For wound beds with red, yellow fibrinous and necrotic tissue with minimal to moderate exudate	Hydrocolloid dressing coated with polyurethane film	Provides a barrier to bacteria and water. Reduces the risk of skin breakdown due to friction and shear	Allow margin of 2.5 cm around wound edges. Contraindicated with known anaerobic bacteria in wound
Hydrogel island wound dressings				
Example: Curagel (Covidien) (Leaper, Brennan, Simpson, & Foster, 2013)	For pressure ulcers, diabetic ulcers and venous stasis ulcers as well as partial/full thickness wounds to provide protection and maintain a moist wound environment	Clear gel wafer	Soothing, may reduce wound pain. Provides protection and helps maintain a moist wound environment	Contradicted in infected and/or heavily exudate in wounds

(continued)

Classification	Indication	Description	Advantages	Precautions
Foam with silicone adhesive				
Examples: Mepilex Border Lite or Sacrum (Molnlycke) (Sanatmaria et al., 2013; Waring, Biefeldt, Matzoid, Wilhem, & Butcher, 2011)	For acute and chronic wounds with minimal to moderate exudate	Adhesive, nonadherent, absorbent dressing with soft tacky silicone borders which help secure the dressing but prevent skin tears during removal	Prevents skin tears and breakdown around wound margin while absorbing wound fluid in an absorbent pad in the center and maintaining a moist environment. Comfortable for patients to wear and an easy dressing to use	Hypersensitivity to silicone
Wound-modulating Treatments				
Negative pressure wound therapy				

Example: VAC dressing (KCl), SNaP (Spiracur) (Acosta & Monsen, 2012; Lerman, Oldenbrook, Ryu, Fong, & Schubart, 2010; Vig et al., 2011)	Superficial to deep cavity with or without shallow undermined areas
	- Stage 3/ stage 4 pressure ulcers
	- Vascular wounds
	- Neuropathic ulcers
	- Dehisced wounds
	- Split-thickness mesh skin grafts
	- Muscle flaps
		Continuous or intermittent negative pressure (at 75–125 mm Hg) provides peak blood flow four times that of non–NPWT-treated wounds, promotes repetitive release of biochemical messengers that play role in wound healing, mechanical stretch of cells that increase rate of cellular proliferation. This stretch also encourages neoangiogenesis, uniform wound size reduction, and eventually epithelialization. Removes stagnant wound fluid, decreasing bacterial colonization. Transparent dressing that secures the NPWT to the wound protects from bacterial invasion	- Reduces frequency of dressing changes to two to three times per wk, if transparent occlusive film remains sealed
			- Canister contains wound exudate, decreasing risk of maceration and contamination
				Precautions:
				high risk for bleeding/ hemorrhage
				- anticoagulants, platelet aggregation inhibitors
				- friable vessels/ infected blood vessels
				- vascular anastomosis
				- infected wounds
				- osteomyelitis
				- exposed vessels, tendons, and ligaments
				- sharp edges in the wound (i.e., bone fragments)
				- spinal cord injury (stimulation of sympathetic nervous system)
				- enteric fistulas
				- patients requiring
				  - MRI
				  - hyperbaric oxygen
				  - defibrillation
				  - patient size and weight
				  - use near vagus nerve (bradycardia)
				  - circumferential dressing application

Classification	Indication	Description	Advantages	Precautions
				– mode of therapy: intermittent versus continuous negative pressure Contraindications: – untreated osteomyelitis – nonenteric and unexplored fistulas – malignancy in the wound – exposed vasculature – exposed nerves – exposed – anastomotic site – exposed organ – >30% nonviable tissue within the wound bed
Keratin products				
Examples: Keragel (Keraplast) Keramatrix Kerasorb (Pechter et al., 2012; Tang, Sierra, Kelly, Kirsner, & Li, 2012)	Dry, lightly or moderately exudating partial or full thickness wounds: – Stage 1–4 pressure ulcers – venous stasis ulcers – mixed etiology vascular wounds – diabetic ulcers – donor sites/grafts	Soft, hydrophilic keratin, derived from New Zealand sheep wool, which interacts with wound fluid to create a moist wound healing environment Keratin activates keratinocytes at the wound edge. The activated keratinocytes produce keratins 6, 16, and 17 that promote cell growth, migration, and differentiation and provide structural stability to epithelial cells and various tissues	Keragel is inexpensive ($17/20 g); Keramatrix ($90/4" × 4") and Kerasorb ($70/4" × 4") are more expensive. Dressings can be changed every 2–3 d	– Caution with history of wool allergy – Risk of periwound maceration in the setting of moderate to large amount of gel/exudate
Platelet-derived growth factor				
Example: Regranex (Systagenix) (Smiell et al., 1999; Steed, 1995; Ziyadeh, Fife, Walker, Wilkinson, & Seeger, 2011)	Diabetic/neuropathic foot ulcers containing small to moderately exudating beefy red tissue without devitalized tissue	Binding of the PDGF to its receptor sites initiates a range of molecular and cellular responses, such as chemotaxis, mitogenesis, and synthesis, necessary for wound healing	Diabetic foot ulcers treated with Regranex healed in one third less time than controls treated with gauze dressings moistened with NaCl	– In a retrospective review of patients treated with more than 3 tubes of Regranex, there was a five times higher likelihood of a cancer diagnosis than matched comparators who were not treated with

(continued)

Classification	Indication	Description	Advantages	Precautions
				Regranex. Results were not reproduced in a subsequent prospective study. However, the FDA maintains a black box warning about the potential risk for cancer – Regranex gel must be refrigerated – Pro-inflammatory effects of Regranex may produce bloody drainage in the wound – May not see any progress in wound closure for 1 mo after initiating – If wound is not completely closed in 20 wks, continued treatment with Regranex should be reassessed – Regranex may cost more than $1,500/15 g
Bioengineered Skin and Soft Tissue Substitutes				
Apligraf (Organogenesis) (Phillips et al., 2002; Veves, Falanga, Armstrong, & Sabolinski, 2001)	– Venous stasis ulcers of at least 1-mo duration that have not responded to standard ulcer therapy – Full thickness neuropathic diabetic foot ulcers of greater than 3 mos duration but without exposure of tendon, muscle, or capsule	Living bilayered skin substitute, which may be applied up to five times per wound at a frequency of every 1–5 wks	– Fibroblasts (dermal layer) stimulate production of collagen matrix – Keratinocytes (epidermal layer) multiply and differentiate to replicate architecture of human epidermis	– Contraindicated on infected wounds and in individuals with known hypersensitivity to bovine collagen or components of shipping medium – Expensive (over $1,500/30 cm^2)

Classification	Indication	Description	Advantages	Precautions
Epi-Fix (MiMedx) (Forbes & Fetterolf, 2012; Zelen, Serena, Denoziere, & Fetterolf, 2013)	Acute and chronic partial- and full-thickness wounds – diabetic foot ulcers – venous leg ulcers – arterial ulcers – pressure ulcers – inflammatory ulcers – burns – Mohs – scar revision	Dehydrated amniotic membrane allograft, delivers wound-healing growth factors (epidermal growth factor, transforming growth factors, fibroblast growth factor, platelet-derived growth factor A and B) that enhance – cellular proliferation – reduce inflammation – reduce scarring Available in 4 sizes	5-yr shelf life	– Areas with active or latent infection – A patient with a disorder that would create an unacceptable risk of postoperative complications – Allergies to aminoglycosides

REFERENCES

Acosta, S., & Monsen, C. (2012). Outcome after VAC therapy for infected bypass grafts in the lower limb. *European Journal of Vascular & Endovascular Surgery, 44*(3), 294–299.

Alvarez, O. M., Fernandez-Obregon, A. Rogers, R. S., Bergamo, L., Masso, J., & Black, M. (2002). A prospective, randomized, comparative study of collagenase and papain-urea for pressure ulcer debridement. *Wounds, 143*, 293–301.

Banks, V., Bale, S., Harding, K., & Harding, E. F. (1997). Evaluation of a new polyurethane foam dressing. *Journal of Wound Care, 6*, 266–269.

Bell, A., & Hart, J. (2007). Evaluation of two absorbent silver dressings in a porcine partial-thickness excisional wound model. *Journal of Wound Care, 16*(10), 445–448, 450–453.

Biglari, B., vd Linden, P. H., Simon, A., Aytac, S., Gerner, H. J., & Moghaddam, A. (2012). Use of Medihoney as a non-surgical therapy for chronic pressure ulcers in patients with spinal cord injury. *Spinal Cord, 50*(2), 165–169.

Capasso, V. A., & Munro, B. H. (2003). The cost and efficacy of two wound treatments. *AORN Journal, 77*(5), 984–992, 995–997, 1000–1004.

Case Study Series. (2013). *Using ADAPTIC TOUCH® non-adhering silicone dressing: Case studies.* London, UK: Wounds International.

Castellano, J. J., Shafii, S. M., Ko, F., Donate, G., Wright, T. E., Mannari, R. J., . . . Robson, M. C. (2007). Comparative evaluation of silver-containing antimicrobial dressings and drugs. *International Wound Journal, 4*(2), 114–122.

Chow, I., Lemos, E. V., & Einarson, T. R. (2008). Management and prevention of diabetic foot ulcers and infections: A health economic review. *Pharmacoeconomics, 26*(12), 1019–1035. doi:10.2165/0019053-200826120-00005

Cohn, S. M., Lopez, P. P., Brown, M., Namias, N., Jackowski, J., Li, P., ... Lopez, J. M. (2004). Open surgical wounds: How does Aquacel compare with wet-to-dry gauze? *Journal of Wound Care, 13*(1), 10–12.

Cosker, T., Elsaved, S., Gupta, S., Mendonca, A. D., & Tayton, K. J. (2005). Choice of dressing has a major impact on blistering and healing outcomes in orthopaedic patients. *Journal of Wound Care, 14*, 27–29.

Coviden Product Information. (2012). Xeroform occulsive petrolatum gauze [Data file]. Retrieved from http://www.kendallhq.com/kendallhealthcare/pageBuilder.aspx?contentID=79627&webPageID = 0&topicID = 79616&breadcrumbs = 0:121623,154339:0,155107:0# Features and Benefits, accessed August 20, 2013.

Cowan, L. J., & Stechmiller, J. (2009). Prevalence of wet-to-dry dressings in wound care. *Advances in Skin Wound Care, 22*, 567–573. doi:10.1097/01.ASW.0000363469.25740.74

Cuschieri, L., Debos, J., Miller, P., & Celis, M. (2013). Autolytic debridement of a large, necrotic, fully occluded foot ulcer using a hydrocolloid dressing in a diabetic patient. *Advance Skin Wound Care, 26*, 300–304. doi:10.1097/01.ASW.0000429779.48138.c0

Dumville, J. C., O'Meara, S., Deshpande, S., & Speak, K. (2012). Alginate dressings for healing diabetic foot ulcers. *Cochrane Database Systematic Review, 15*(2), CD009110. doi:10.1002/14651858.CD009110.pub2

Dumville, J. C., O'Meara, S., Deshpande, S., & Speak, K. (2013). Hydrogel dressings for healing diabetic foot ulcers. *Cochrane Database of Systematic Reviews, 12*(7), CD009101. doi:10.1002/14651858.CD009101.pub3

Faucher, N., Safar, H., Baret, M., Philippe, A., & Farid, R. (2012). Superabsorbent dressing for copious exuding wounds. *British Journal of Nursing, 21*(12), S22, S24, S26–S28.

Forbes, J., & Fetterolf, D. E. (2012). Dehydrated amniotic membrane allografts for the treatment of chronic wounds: A case series. *Journal of Wound Care, 21*(6), 290, 292, 294–296.

Gago, M., Garcia, F., Gaztelu, V., Verdu, J., Lopez, P., & Nolasco, A. (2008). A comparison of three silver-containing dressings in the treatment of infected, chronic wounds. *Wounds, 20*, 273–278.

Hackl, F., Kiwanuka, E., Philip, J., Gerner, P., Aflaki, P., Diaz-Siso, J. R., ... Eriksson, E. (2013). Moist dressing coverage supports proliferation and migration of transplanted skin micrografts in full-thickness porcine wounds. *Burns: The Journal of International Society for Burn Injuries*, pii: S0305-4179(13)00184-8. doi:10.1016/j.burns.2013.06.002

Heggers, J., Goodheart, R. E., Washington, J., McCoy, L., Carino, E., Dang, T., . . . Chinkes, D. (2005). Therapeutic efficacy of three silver dressings in an infected animal model. *Journal of Burn Care & Rehabilitation, 26*(1), 53–56.

Hindhede, A., & Meuleneire, F. (2012). A clinical case-series evaluation of a superabsorbent dressing on exuding wounds. *Journal of Wound Care, 21*, 574, 576–580.

Kunugiza, Y., Tomita, T., Moritomo, H., & Yoshikawa, H. (2010). A hydrocellular foam dressing versus gauze: effects on the healing of rat excisional wounds. *Journal of Wound Care, 19*, 10–14.

Leaper, D. J., Brennan, S. S., Simpson, R. A., & Foster, M. E. (2013). Experimental infection and hydrogel dressings. *Hospital Infection*, (Suppl. A), 69–73.

Lerman, B., Oldenbrook, L., Ryu, J., Fong, K. D., & Schubart, P. J. (2010). The SNaP Wound Care System: A case series using a novel ultraportable negative pressure wound therapy device for the treatment of diabetic lower extremity wounds. *Journal of Diabetes Science & Technology, 4*(4), 825–830.

Lisle, J. (2002). Debridement of necrotic tissue and eschar using a capillary dressing and semi-permeable film dressing. *British Journal of Community Nursing*, 29–30, 32, 34.

Lusby, P. E., Coombes, A. L., & Wilkinson, J. M. (2005). Bactericidal activity of different honeys against pathogenic bacteria. *Archives of Medical Research, 36*, 464–467.

Malpass, K. G., Snelling, C. F., & Tron, V. (2003). Comparison of donor-site healing under Xeroform and Jelonet dressings: Unexpected findings. *Plastic and Reconstruction Surgery, 112*, 430–439.

Milne, C., Hagan, J., & Ciccarelli, A. (2007). An examination of the antimicrobial effects of a 15% sodium chloride impregnated dressing on wounds: 1211. *Journal of Wound, Ostomy and Continence Nursing, 34*(3 Suppl.), S10.

Molnlycke Health Care Products. (2003). Wound care: Mesalt, mepliex border lite, mepitel [Data files]. Retrieved from http://www.molnlycke.com/us/Wound-Care-Products, accessed August 20, 2013.

O'Meara, S., Al-Kurdi, D., Ologun, Y., & Ovington, L. G. (2010). Antibiotics and antiseptics for venous leg ulcers. *Cochrane Database of Systematic Reviews, 20*(1), CD003557. doi:10.1002/14651858.CD003557.pub3

Pechter, P. M., Gil, J., Tomic-Canic, M., Paster, I., Stojadinovic, O., Kirsner, R., & Davis, S. C. (2012). Keratin dressings speed epithelialization of partial-thickness wounds. *Wound Repair and Regeneration, 20*(2), 236–242. doi:10.1111/j.1524-475X.2012.00768.x

Phillips, T. J., Manzoor, J., Rojas, A., Isaacs, C., Carson, P., Sabolinski, M., . . . Falanga, V. (2002). The longevity of a bilayered skin substitute after application to venous ulcers. *Archives of Dermatology, 138*(8), 1079–1081.

Ravenscroft, M. J., Harker, J., & Buch, K. A. (2006). A prospective, randomized, controlled trial comparing wound dressings used in hip and knee surgery: Aquacel and Tegaderm vs. Cutiplast. *Annals of the Royal College of Surgeons of England, 88*(1), 18–22.

Rippon, M., Davies, P., & White, R. (2012). Taking the trauma out of wound care: The importance of undisturbed healing. *Journal of Wound Care, 21*, 359–368.

Robson, V., Dodd, S., & Thomas, S. (2009). Standardized antibacterial honey (Medihoney) with standard therapy in wound care: Randomized clinical trial. *Journal of Advanced Nursing, 65*(3), 565–575.

Santamaria, N., Gerdtz, M., McCann, J., Freeman, A., Vassilou, T., DeVincentis, S., ... Knott, J. (2013). A randomized controlled trial of the effectiveness of soft silicone multi-layered foam dressings in the prevention of sacral and heel pressure ulcers in trauma and critically ill patients: The border trial. *International Wound Journal*, May 27. doi:10.1111/iwj.12101

Shi, L., & Carson, D. (2009). Collagenase Santyl ointment: A selective agent for wound debridement. *Journal of Wound, Ostomy, & Continence Nursing, 36*(6 Suppl.), S12–S16. doi:10.1097/WON.0b013e3181bfdd1a

Smiell, J. M., Wieman, T. J., Steed, D. L., Perry, B. H., Sampson, A. R., & Schwab, B. H. (1999). Efficacy and safety of becaplermin (recombinant human platelet-derived growth factor-BB) in patients with nonhealing, lower extremity diabetic ulcers: A combined analysis of four randomized studies. *Wound Repair & Regeneration, 7*(5), 335–346.

Smith, R. G. (2008). Enzymatic debriding agents: An evaluation of the medical literature. *Ostomy Wound Management, 54*, 16–34.

Spear, M. (2008). Wet-to-dry dressing-evaluating the evidence. *Plastic Surgery Nursing, 28*, 92–95. doi:10.1097/01.PSN.0000324782.18708.bd

Steed, D. L. (1995). Clinical evaluation of recombinant human platelet-derived growth factor for the treatment of lower extremity diabetic ulcers. Diabetic Ulcer Study Group. *Journal of Vascular Surgery, 21*(1), 71–78; discussion 79–81.

Svensjo, T., Pomahac, B., Yao, F., Slama, J., & Eriksson, E. (2000). Accelerated healing of full-thickness skin wounds in a wet environment. *Plastic and Reconstruction Surgery, 106*, 602–612.

Sweeney, I. R., Miraftab, M., & Collver, G. (2012). A critical review of modern and emerging absorbent dressings used to treat exuding wounds. *International Wound Journal, 9*, 601–612. doi:10.1111/j.1742-481X.2011.00923.x. Epub 2012 Jan 17.

Tang, L., Sierra, J. O., Kelly, R., Kirsner, R. S., & Lie, J. (2012). Wool-derived keratin stimulates human keratinocyte migration and types IV and VII collagen expression. *Experimental Dermatology, 21*(6), 458–460. doi:10.1111/j.1600-0625.2012.01505.x

Terrill, P. J., & Varughese, G. (2000). A comparison of three primary non-adherent dressings applied to hand surgery wounds. *Journal of Wound Care, 9*, 359–363.

Tkachenko, O., & Karas, J. A. (2012). Standardizing an in vitro procedure for the evaluation of the antimicrobial activity of wound dressings and the assessment of three wound dressings. *Journal of Antimicrobial Chemotherapy, 67*(7), 1697–1700.

Tsao, W. Y., Lo, S. F., Harmod, T., & Lee, R. P. (2013). [A comparison of the efficacy of different wound dressing management techniques in preventing pressure ulcers]. *Hu Li Za Zi, 60*, 65–75. doi:10.6224/JN.60.3.65

Ubbink, D. T., Westerbos, S. J., Evans, D., Land, L., & Vermeulen, H. (2008). Topical negative pressure for treating chronic wounds. *Cochrane Database of Systematic Reviews, 16*(3), CD001898. doi:10.1002/14651858.CD001898.pub2

Upright, C. A., Salton, C., Roberts, F., & Murphy, J. (1994). Evaluation of Mesalt dressings and continuous wet saline dressing in ulceration metastatic skin lesions. *Cancer Nursing, 17*, 149–155.

Vanscheidt, W., Sibbald, R. G., & Eager, C. A. (2004). Comparing a foam composite to a hydrocellular foam dressing in the management of venous leg ulcers: A controlled clinical study. *Ostomy Wound Management, 50*, 42–55.

Verall, D., Coulbom, A., & Bree-Aslan, C. (2010). Evaluating a super absorbent dressing in highly exuding wounds. *British Journal of Nursing, 19*, 449–453.

Veves, A., Falanga, V., Armstrong, D. G., & Sabolinski, M. L. (2001). Graftskin, a human skin equivalent, is effective in the management of noninfected neuropathic diabetic foot ulcers: A prospective randomized multicenter clinical trial. *Diabetes Care, 24*(2), 290–295.

Vig, S., Dowsett, C., Berg, L., Caravaggi, C., Rome, P., Birke-Sorensen, H., ... Runkel, N. (2011). Evidence-based recommendations for the use of negative pressure wound therapy in chronic wounds: Steps towards an international consensus. *Journal of Tissue Viability, 20*(Suppl. 1), S1–S18. doi:10.1016/j.jtv.2011.07.002

Vogt, K. C., Uhlyarik, M., & Schroeder, T. V. (2007). Moist wound healing compared with standard care of treatment of primary closed vascular surgical wounds: A prospective randomized controlled study. *Wound Repair & Regeneration, 15*(5), 624–627.

Waring, M., Biefeldt, S., Matzoid, K., Wilhem, K. P., & Butcher, M. (2011). An evaluation of the skin stripping of wound dressings adhesives. *Journal of Wound Care, 20*, 412, 414, 416–422.

Widgerow, A. D. (2011). Chronic wound fluid–thinking outside the box. *Wound Repair & Regeneration, 19*(3), 287–291.

Williams, C. (1999). An investigation of the benefits of Aquacel Hydrofibre wound dressing. *British Journal of Nursing, 8*(10), 676–677.

Zelen, C. M., Serena, T. E., Denoziere, G., & Fetterolf, D. E. (2013). A prospective randomised comparative parallel study of amniotic membrane wound graft in the management of diabetic foot ulcers. *International Wound Journal, 10*(5), 502–507. doi:10.1111/iwj.12097

Ziyadeh, N., Fife, D., Walker, A. M., Wilkinson, G. S., & Seeger, J. D. (2011). A matched cohort study of the risk of cancer in users of becaplermin. *Advances in Skin & Wound Care, 24*(1), 31–39.

SUGGESTED READINGS

Nguyen, C. V., Washington, C. V., & Soon, S. L. (2013). Hydrocolloid dressings promote granulation tissue on exposed bone. *Dermatology Surgery, 39*, 123–125. doi:10.1111/dsu.12021. Epub 2012 Dec 17.

Tachi, M., Hirabayashi, S., Yonehara, Y., Suzuki, Y., & Bowler, P. (2004). Comparison of bacteria-retaining ability of absorbent wound dressings. *International Wound Journal, 1*(3), 177–181.

Index

Page numbers followed by a "t" denote tables; Page numbers followed by a "f" denote figures.

B